Mental Health, Social Mirror

Mental Health, Social Mirror

Edited by

William R. Avison
Jane D. McLeod
Bernice A. Pescosolido

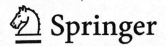 Springer

William R. Avison
Department of Sociology
The University of Western Ontario
London, ON, Canada

Jane D. McLeod
Department of Sociology
Indiana University

Bernice A. Pescosolido
Department of Sociology
Indiana University

Library of Congress Control Number: 2006929456

ISBN-10: 0-387-36319-X   e-ISBN-10: 0-387-36320-3
ISBN-13: 978-0-387-36319-6   e-ISBN-13: 978-0-387-36320-2

Preface

In 2004, the discipline of sociology celebrated the 100th anniversary of the founding of the American Sociological Association. In 2005, the Section on Medical Sociology celebrated 50 years since the formation of the Committee on Medical Sociology within the ASA. And, in 2003, the Section on the Sociology of Mental Health celebrated ten years since its founding within the American branch of the discipline. This brief accounting marks the American-based organizational landmarks central to concerns about how social factors shape the mental health problems individuals face as well as the individual and system responses that follow. This history also lays a trail of how the focus on mental health and illness has narrowed from a general concern of the discipline to a more intense, substantively-focused community of scholars targeting a common set of specific theoretical and empirical questions. While mental health and illness figured prominently in the writings of classical sociologists, contemporary sociologists often view research on mental health as peripheral to the "real work" of the discipline. The sentiment, real or perceived, is that the sociology of mental health, along with its sister, medical sociology, may be in danger of both losing its prominence in the discipline *and* losing its connection to the mainstream core of sociological knowledge (Pescosolido & Kronenfeld, 1995).

Perennial discussions about of the splintering of contemporary sociology into an increasing number of specialties with narrowly-focused concerns, and broader, national discussions about the place of the social sciences in an increasingly medicalized, "life sciences" research agenda (Collins, 1986; Mechanic, 2004; OBSSR, 2001; Pescosolido & Kronenfeld, 1995), make it opportune to consider where our field has been, where it stands now, and where it should move in the future. There are a number of fine volumes that catalogue our stock of knowledge in the sociology of mental health (e.g., Aneshensel & Phelan, 1999; Horwitz & Scheid, 1999). We saw no need to duplicate those efforts here. Instead, in this volume, we chart a new course for the sociology of mental health by reasserting the centrality of research on mental health to the broader discipline.

Our approach to this project was to issue a general call to mental health researchers to submit proposals for chapters that would address a variety of issues. This strategy has resulted in a volume that is somewhat selective rather than comprehensive in its coverage. Although the chapters in this collection are relevant to a number of specialties in sociology, they do not document the ways in which the sociology of mental health has contributed to all the areas of specialization in the discipline. We then asked our authors to consider the two-way process implied by our interests. First, we asked them, to draw from mainstream sociological theories and concepts to reconsider the potential of sociology to provide insights into critical problems in the etiology of mental illness, the use of services, and other key issues in the lives of persons affected by mental health problems as consumers, caretakers (formal and informal), and citizens. Second, we asked them to articulate the contributions that mental health research has made, and can make, to resolving key theoretical and empirical debates in important areas of sociological study. With this roadmap, our hope is that this volume builds bridges between the sociology of mental health, other subfields within the discipline, and the mainstream core of sociological theory.

We have divided the book into five sections that define the history, the issues, and reflections on the future of the sociology of mental health. In the first section, "Reflections through the Sociological Looking Glass," we analyze the theoretical and institutional trends that have produced the contemporary moment in the sociological study of mental health. Our opening chapter, "Through the Looking Glass: The Fortunes of the Sociology of Mental Health," traces the history of sociological research on mental health through the representation of mental health-related articles in our two flagship journals, the *American Journal of Sociology* and the *American Sociological Review*. Our review suggests that the sociological mainstream presents a very limited view of what researchers know about the social causes and consequences of mental health and illness, treatment processes and institutions, and community outcomes. "In "Sociology, Psychiatry and the Production of Knowledge about Mental Illness and Its Treatment," Pearlin, Avison, and Fazio consider the relative influence of biological and social factors, and the power of psychiatry versus sociology, in understanding the causes of mental health and illness. For more than 50 years, Leonard Pearlin has made important theoretical and empirical contributions to the sociology of mental health. His extensive experience with both the National Institute of Mental Health and university-based research affords him a unique perspective from which to examine the tensions between biological and sociological approaches to the study of mental health and illness. Pearlin and his colleagues identify reasons for the predominance of biological theories and assert the continued relevance of sociological insight in this new climate. Importantly, they conclude by suggesting how we could translate disciplinary difference and diversity into greater collaboration and scientific progress. Carmi Schooler closes the section with a chapter entitled, "The Changing Role(s) of Sociology (and Psychology) in the National Institute of Mental Health Intramural Research Program." Schooler's long-term association with the NIMH yields an insider's perspective on an organization that housed the sociologists who were critical in building a solid foundation for the sociology of mental health. Schooler details the shrinking attention and resources devoted to social science research, making a strong case for the costs to understanding mental health and illness.

The second section, "Sociological Theory and Mental Health" introduces major classical and contemporary debates in sociology as they have been, or could be, informed by research on mental health. Allan Horwitz begins in "Classical Sociological Theory, Evolutionary Psychology, and Mental Health" by reminding sociologists of the important disciplinary concepts that underlie research on mental health, asserting the complementarity of contemporary evolutionary psychological perspectives, and offering ways to integrate these perspectives into mental health research. Ann Branaman follows with a discussion of contemporary social thought, including theories of individualization, critical theories, and Foucauldian/postmodern perspectives, and their implications for research on mental health in "Contemporary Social Theory and the Sociological Study of Mental Health". These pieces locate the chapters that follow in a broad disciplinary context and demonstrate the interplay between sociological theory and the sociology of mental health.

The third section of the book, "The Social Origins of Mental Health and Mental Illness," takes on important sociological theories regarding the effects of macro-structural conditions and processes on individual mental health. Three chapters address the core of sociology by focusing on the effects of inequality and hierarchy. Muntaner, Borrell, and Chung take the widest view in "Class Relations, Economic Inequality and Mental Health: Why Social Class Matters to the Sociology of Mental Health." Rudy Fenwick and Mark Tausig focus more specifically on the macroeconomic environment, the labor market, and job conditions in "A Political Economy of Stress: Recontextualizing the Study of Mental Health/Illness in Sociology." They propose an innovative conceptual model for the study of stratification and mental health that draws on structural labor market theories. In a final chapter on stratification, "Race and Mental Health: Past Debates, New Opportunities," Teresa Evans-Campbell and her colleagues tackle the controversial issue of race. They draw on past conceptualizations of race to construct a compelling argument for giving greater attention to the unique experiences of specific racial and ethnic groups.

Two chapters on life course perspectives follow. In the most general of the two, "Life Course Perspectives on Social Factors and Mental Illness," Linda George reminds us of the importance of conceptualizing mental health and illness in dynamic terms, and introduces us to the basics of the life course perspective. In so doing, she presents a strong case for increased sociological attention to mental disorders whose temporal course can be charted precisely. Susan Gore and colleagues ("Transition to Adulthood, Mental Health, and Inequality") extend George's arguments by applying developmental theories to the study of inequality and mental health during the transition to adulthood, with special emphasis on pathways and turning points. Together, these two chapters illustrate the tremendous potential of life course perspectives on mental health and illness to enhance our understanding of the implications of social structure for individuals.

The final two chapters in this section emphasize the social psychological processes that link societies to their members. Robin Simon considers a relatively new area of research in sociology, the sociology of emotions. In "Contributions of the Sociology of Mental Health for Understanding the Social Antecedents, Social Regulation, and Social Distribution of Emotion", she considers how what we know from the sociology of mental health can be used to advance this new area of inquiry as well as the new insights from the sociology of emotions that can advance our understanding of mental health. Jane McLeod and Kathryn Lively present a comparable argument in "Social Psychology and the Stress Process," with special emphasis on the potential of symbolic interactionist principles to improve our understanding of how social structural conditions create distress.

In the fourth section, we turn to the topic of social responses: how social actors, organizations, and institutions respond to individuals with mental illness. We begin with a discussion of one of the central concepts in both the mainstream of sociology and the sociology of mental health, stigma. Drawing from Goffman's original definition that emphasizes the role of relationships, Bernice Pescosolido and Jack Martin rethink theories of stigma in "Stigma and the Sociological Enterprise". They urge sociologists of mental health to collaborate with other disciplines that have picked up on and developed concerns that sociologists have laid by the wayside. In "Social Integration: A Conceptual Overview and Two Case Studies," Stephanie Hartwell and Paul Benson present a similar review for another core concept in sociology, social integration. Cognizant of the many variants of the concept that appear in the literature, they organize them into a general conceptual model and illustrate the utility of their model in two of their ongoing studies. Moving into a more direct consideration of the treatment system, Donna McAlpine and Carol Boyer trace the history of research on mental health services utilization giving careful attention to shifts in theoretical frameworks and the resultant empirical research ("Sociological Traditions in the Study of Mental Health Services Utilization"). Teresa Scheid and Greg Greenberg follow with the importance of organizational structures for mental health care. In "An Organizational Analysis of Mental Health Care," they use historical periods and sectors of care provision to organize an exploration of how mental health care organizations offer a window to understand organizational process and effects. In turn, they provide insights and suggestions for the utility of organizational theory to guide our studies of the operation of changes in the mental health system. Finally, Philip Yanos and his co-authors delve into an important issue in mental health services research to address the recovery of persons with serious mental illness in "Recognizing a Role for Structure and Agency: Integrating Sociological Perspectives into the Study of the Recovery from Severe Mental Illness". They take as their starting point Fine's conceptualization of social structure, providing a comprehensive review of recent research which supports the utility of strongly suggests its utility.

The final section, "Mental Health, Social Mirror: Looking Forward, Reflecting Back" contains only one piece by Sheldon Stryker, the sociologist who developed identity theory, forged a generation of thought and empirical research, and trained at least two generations of sociologists, many of whom now produce the contemporary insights in the sociology of mental health. In "Mainstream Sociology and Sociological Specialties: Toward Understanding the Gap and Its Consequences,"

Stryker recounts the common history of the post World War II discipline, a time that shaped the work of a generation and which continues to form the give and take between the discipline and its subfields. The story of some of the examples are disheartening, others encouraging, but all speak to the critical interaction between the parent discipline, which sets a perspective, and its substantively-oriented subfields, which each offer a unique window into social life. The final chapter in this volume does so well what sociology tells us: It contextualizes the sociology of mental health in the broader landscape of the discipline. In that way, it offers a most fitting ending to the reflections in the looking glass.

References

Aneshensel, C. S., & Phelan, J. C. (1999). *Handbook of the sociology of mental health.* New York: Kluwer Academic/Plenum Publishers.

Collins, R. (1986). Is 1980s sociology in the doldrums? *American Journal of Sociology, 91*, 1336–1355.

Horwitz, A. V., & Scheid, T. L. (1999). *A handbook for the study of mental health.* Cambridge: Cambridge University Press.

Mechanic, D. (2004). The rise and fall of managed care. *Journal of Health & Social Behavior, 45*, 76–86.

Office of Behavioral and Social Sciences Research (2001). *Toward higher levels of analysis: Progress and promise in research on social and cultural dimensions of health: A research agenda.* Bethesda, MD: Office of Behavioral and Social Sciences Research.

Pescosolido, B. A., & Kronenfeld, J. (1995). Health, illness, and healing in an uncertain era: Challenges from and for medical sociology. *Journal of Health and Social Behavior, (Extra Issue)*, 5–33.

Acknowledgments

An edited book is often a labor of love, faith, and respect. So it is with this book. It grew out of our deep commitment to the power, accomplishments, and potential of the sociology of mental health to help unravel the complexities that mental health and mental illness bring to individuals, families, organizations, and societies. Our love for the field, stemming in part from the many existing contributions by sociologists, has instilled both a deep respect for our colleagues and an abiding faith that, together, we could show how closely tied the study of mental health and the study of sociology have been, are, and should continue to be. Not surprisingly, then, this book is the product of the combined efforts of many people. The journey from our solicitation of chapter proposals to the published volume was long and arduous but also exciting and inspiring due, in no small part, to our outstanding collaborators. Their work gave us a renewed appreciation for the intellectual caliber of mental health scholarship and for the continued relevance of mental health research to the discipline of sociology. On a more personal level, our work on this project deepened our ties to our colleagues, our ASA section and the larger discipline.

Our first thanks go to the scholars who contributed chapters. Their assigned task was neither simple nor easy: to consider the mutual relevance of mainstream sociology and research on mental health in their areas of expertise. Each set of authors brought a unique perspective to the task, building on their strengths as sociologists and as researchers committed to understanding the real-world implications of mental health and mental illness. The result is a volume that is rich with empirical information and theoretical insight.

Our thanks go also to the staff of the Indiana Consortium for Mental Health Services Research at Indiana University, who provided excellent technical support. In particular, Alex Capshew kept a watchful eye on the project from the beginning, Mary Hannah shepherded several chapters through the editing process, and Mala Subbaswamy worked magic on the figures. We could not have completed the book without their assistance.

Bill Avison wishes to acknowledge his wife, Julia McDonald, for her support and encouragement. The time devoted to this book has sometimes been at the expense of their time together. He is grateful for her understanding. He also wants to thank Jane McLeod and Bernice Pescosolido for their collaborative spirit, optimism, and energy. Bill would like to thank Carol Aneshensel, Len Pearlin, and Jay Turner for their support of this project in its formative stage. Finally, he wishes to acknowledge the continued support from the Department of Sociology at the University of Western Ontario and the Children's Health Research Institute.

Jane McLeod acknowledges the patience and support of her husband, Steve Krahnke, and her daughters, Sophie and Nell Krahnke. She is grateful for the time and space they gave her to write, read, and think while working on this book. She also wishes to thank Sheldon Stryker for encouraging her to pursue this project and the members of the Social Psychology, Health, and the Life Course workshop for giving her an intellectual home. Her weekly women's lunch group (Bernice, Eliza, and Pam) deserves special recognition for sustaining her with good humor throughout the year. Bill and Bernice made working on the book much more fun than she ever imagined it could be.

Bernice Pescosolido's thanks can be summed up, but never fully acknowledged in depth, in a series of acronyms: from JSF to JKM in the family, from the PPG to the SISR at IU, and from the NIMH to ASA in the larger scholarly community. Like Jane, she would like to thank the members of the Estrogen Summit for creating the kind of social safety net that all friends and colleagues should have to sustain their own mental health.

We wish to thank Teresa Krauss at Springer Publishing for her efforts in bringing this project to fruition. Springer's support for projects in the sociology of mental health is consistent with the theme of *Mental Health, Social Mirror*.

Finally, we acknowledge the sustained intellectual support of the American Sociological Association's Section on the Sociology of Mental Health. All three of us have served as Chair of the Section at one time or another, and we all value the stimulating and nurturing community it represents. Our contribution of the royalties from the sale of this volume to the Section cannot begin to match all we have received from its members.

Contents

Contributors

Robert H. Aseltine, Jr., Ph.D.
University of Connecticut Health Center
Division of Behavioral Sciences & Community Health, and
Institute for Public Health
Farmington, CT

William R. Avison, Ph.D.
The University of Western Ontario
Department of Sociology and
Children's Health Research Institute
London, ON, Canada

Paul R. Benson, Ph.D.
University of Massachusetts Boston
Department of Sociology
Boston, MA

Carme Borrell, M.D., Ph.D.
Agencia de Salut Publica de Barcelona
Barcelona, Spain

Carol Boyer, Ph.D.
Rutgers University
Institute for Health, Health Care Policy, and Aging Research
New Brunswick, NJ

Ann Branaman, Ph.D.
Florida Atlantic University
Department of Sociology
Boca Raton, FL

Haejoo Chung, M.Sc.
Johns Hopkins University
School of Public Health
Baltimore, MD

Teresa Evans-Campbell, Ph.D.
University of Washington
School of Social Work
Seattle, WA

Elena M. Fazio, M.A.
University of Maryland
Department of Sociology
College Park, MD

Rudy Fenwick, Ph.D.
The University of Akron
Department of Sociology
Akron, OH

Linda K. George, Ph.D.
Duke University
Department of Sociology
Durham, NC

Susan Gore, Ph.D.
University of Massachusetts Boston
Department of Sociology and Center for Survey Research
Boston, MA

Greg Greenberg, Ph.D.
VAMC
Northeast Program Evaluation Center
West Haven, CT

Stephanie W. Hartwell, Ph.D.
University of Massachusetts Boston
Department of Sociology
Boston, MA

Allan V. Horwitz, Ph.D.
Rutgers University
Department of Sociology and
Institute for Health, Health Care Policy, and Aging Research
New Brunswick, NJ

Edward L. Knight, Ph.D.
ValueOptions
Department of Recovery, Rehabilitation,
and Mutual Support
Colorado Springs, CO

Karen D. Lincoln, Ph.D.
University of Washington
School of Social Work
Seattle, WA

Kathryn J. Lively, Ph.D.
Dartmouth College
Department of Sociology
Hanover, NH

Jack K. Martin, Ph.D.
Indiana University
Karl F. Schuessler Institute for Social Research
Bloomington, IN

Donna D. McAlpine, Ph.D.
University of Minnesota
Department of Health Services
Minneapolis, MN

Jane D. McLeod, Ph.D.
Indiana University
Department of Sociology
Bloomington, IN

Carles Muntaner, M.D., Ph.D.
Centre for Addictions and Mental Health
Social Equity and Health Section, and
University of Toronto
Departments of Nursing, Public Health Sciences,
and Psychiatry
Toronto, ON, Canada

Leonard I. Pearlin, Ph.D.
University of Maryland
Department of Sociology
College Park, MD

Bernice A. Pescosolido, Ph.D.
Indiana University
Department of Sociology, and
Indiana Consortium for Mental Health Services Research
Bloomington, IN

David Roe, Ph.D.
University of Medicine and Dentistry of New Jersey
School of Health Related Professions
Department of Psychiatric Rehabilitation
Scotch Plains, NJ

Teresa L. Scheid, Ph.D.
University of North Carolina at Charlotte
Department of Sociology and Anthropology
Charlotte, NC

Elizabeth A. Schilling, Ph.D.
University of Connecticut Health Center
Division of Behavioral Sciences & Community Health, and
Institute for Public Health Research
Farmington, CT

Carmi Schooler, Ph.D.
Department of Health and Human Services
National Institutes of Health
National Institute of Mental Health
Intramural Rsearch Program
Section on Socioenvironmental Studies
Bethesda, MD

Robin W. Simon, Ph.D.
Florida State University
Department of Sociology
Tallahassee, FL

Sheldon Stryker, Ph.D.
Indiana University
Department of Sociology
Bloomington, IN

David T. Takeuchi, Ph.D.
University of Washington
School of Social Work and Department of Sociology
Seattle, WA

Mark Tausig, Ph.D.
The University of Akron
Department of Sociology
Akron, OH

Philip T. Yanos, Ph.D.
City University of New York
John Jay College of Criminal Justice
Department of Psychology
New York, NY

Part I
Reflections through the Sociological Looking Glass

1
Through the Looking Glass:
The Fortunes of the Sociology
of Mental Health

Bernice A. Pescosolido, Jane D. McLeod, and William R. Avison

From its very beginning, mental health has been central to the sociological understanding of society. Concerned about issues of life, death and well-being, the founders of sociology staked a claim for a new discipline concerned with how larger historical forces and new institutional structures shaped the fate of individuals. Marx (1964, p. 11) found alienation inherent in all modern institutions, but particularly when immersion in the workplace destroys a person's "inner life" (1964, p. 122). Durkheim (1951; 1954) wondered how the normlessness of modern life, anomie, would predispose individuals to suicide and he grappled with the loss of faith that he saw as endemic to the transition to modern society (see also Masaryk, 1970, on earlier, similar concerns). Simmel considered how the greater freedoms of modern society are accompanied by "psychological tensions or even a schizophrenic break" despite greater societal tolerance. He saw "external and internal conflicts [which] arise through the multiplicity of group-affiliations" that characterized the new social forms of the early 20th century (Simmel, 1955, p. 141). And following from this, Veblen linked social class (and particularly property ownership), social relationships and mental health. He believed that "(o)nly individuals with an aberrant temperament can in the long run retain their self-esteem in the face of the disesteem of their fellows" (Veblen, 1934, pp. 30–31).

These interests in no way imply that the founders of the discipline were fundamentally interested in mental health, illness or treatment, per se.[1] In fact, it is widely known that, for Durkheim, suicide was merely a strategic choice with which to make the case for the new discipline of sociology (Pescosolido, 1994). Others referred to mental illness only as a limiting case. For example, Weber, in his treatise on rationality, argued that only the behavior of "the insane" was truly unpredictable (Shils & Finch, 1949, p. 24). Robert E. Park's work with Ernest W. Burgess on concentric zone theory used mental illness as only one example to show how the dense urban centers of metropolitan areas produced the highest level of social problems, with corresponding decreases

---

[1] Nor could they have been. The restricted and vague conceptualization of mental illness that dominated the late nineteenth and early twentieth centuries precluded serious research interest in mental illness as the concept is understood today.

as distance from the core increased. Laying out issues of the self, status and roles in their *Introduction to the Science of Society* (Park & Burgess, 1921: 55), they suggested that "(t)he individual whose conception of himself does not conform to his status is an isolated individual. The completely isolated individual, whose conception of himself is in no sense an adequate reflection of his status, is probably insane" (p. 55).

Yet, neither does their dilettantish use of mental health and illness mean that the founders of the discipline have not influenced theory and empirical research in the sociology of mental health. Weber's basic ideas about the power of society to determine life chances, Marx's concern with the implications of economic exploitation for self-actualization, and Durkheim's analyses of social integration continue to shape influential research agendas in the Sociology of Mental Health (Weber, Gerth, & Mills, 1946). Rather, the relevant historical point is that early sociological interest in mental health, mental illness, and treatment reflected the major concerns that occupied the founders – the implications of the transition from agrarian to industrial society for individuals. Serious attention to mental health and illness, as topics in their own right, only began in the post-World War II boom that coincided both with the growth of the subfield of medical sociology and its link to the intramural program at the National Institute of Mental Health (see Bloom, 2002, for a general history of medical sociology; see Schooler in this volume).[2] Since that time, sociological research on mental health and mental illness has continued to evolve in tandem with its parent discipline and more general developments in mental health research (see Pearlin, Avison, & Fazio, in this volume).

In this introductory chapter, we consider the relationship of research in the Sociology of Mental Health to the sociological mainstream by reviewing historical trends in the quantity and substance of sociological research on mental health in the discipline's two major, generalist journals, the *American Journal of Sociology* and the *American Sociological Review*. In essence, we ask: What types of mental health research are represented in these journals? Or, to phrase it differently, if all we knew about mental health, mental illness, and its treatment was what we read in the *ASR* and the *AJS*, what would we know?[3] We observe substantial continuity in the topics that have been represented in the journals over the years along with the waxing and waning of specific substantive interests.

---

[2] The tie to medical sociology has continued even after the new ASA Section on the Sociology of Mental Health was formed in 1991. At the point of this writing, just over half of the members of the Section on the Sociology of Mental Health also belong to the Medical Sociology Section (54% of the 472 members) while almost one quarter of the Medical Sociology Section members also belong to the Mental Health Section (22% of the 1,164 members; Edwards, personal communication 2006). The overlap in membership between the two sections speaks to a close alliance in the interests of both subfields.

[3] We credit Susan Cotts Watkins and her Presidential Address in *Demography* (1993), in which she asked a similar question about the representation of gender issues in its flagship journal.

The Representation of Mental Health and Mental Illness in the Mainstream: An Historical View

Data

We reviewed articles in *AJS* from 1894 through part of 2005 (Volumes 1 to 110) and in *ASR* from 1936 through part of 2005 (Volumes 1 to 69) for mental health-related content. Our first task was to decide whether each article had sufficient content to be considered a "mental health" article. This task was not straightforward. In the early years of the journals, rates of mental illness or the numbers of psychiatrists were often included as one of many examples of a more general social phenomenon. We also struggled with how to deal with more generic topics such as "adjustment," "psycho-analysis," "Freud," "well-being," "mental," "suicide," and "disorganization" given changes in the cultural meaning and usage of such terms over time. In the end, we cast a wide net when identifying relevant articles. We decided that we would include arti-cles in our analysis if they targeted issues having to do with individual's health status or responses to illness and if they included some discussion of mental health or illness. This was true whether or not the articles were intended as specialty pieces. For exam-ple, much sociological research on suicide was considered "theory" rather than social psychiatry or social epidemiology. We included those articles, nonetheless, because they offer insight into how mental health-related issues are understood in the disci-pline. In contrast, we did not include early articles by Ogburn (1934; 1935) or others like it that presented many trends in social life, including rates of the "insane" (e.g., first admission to mental hospitals), but which gave no special attention to the latter.

With that decision made, we counted the numbers of such articles. We included research notes, reply and comment sets (as single units of analysis), and review symposia but not review essays or book reviews.[4] We followed the simple count with an in-depth analysis of each article to learn more about the texture of socio-logical attention to mental health and illness. What were the topics? What kinds of data did they use? How were articles framed, etc.? This approach yielded an informative and nuanced analysis of the mainstream sociological representation of mental health research during the 20th century, with a brief glance at the begin-ning of the 21st Century.

Historical Trends in the Representation of Mental Health and Illness

Of the roughly five thousand pieces (N = 4,977) that have appeared in the *AJS* since its founding, 144 or 2.9 percent included mental health content. On the other hand, the more recent *ASR* which also has over four thousand pieces (N = 4,434) presented 215, or 4.8 percent, articles on mental health topics.

---

[4] We counted articles of varying formats in order to accommodate the changes in formats that occurred in the journals, especially in the early era.

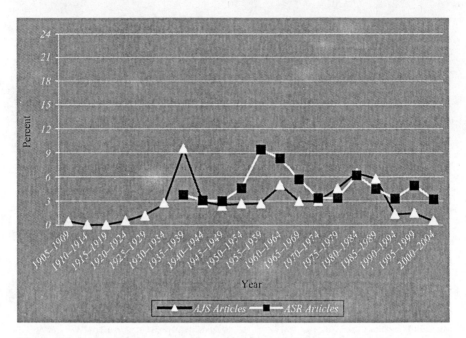

FIGURE 1.1. Representation of articles on mental health in sociology's mainstream journals.

Attention to mental health has not been constant over time: there have been peaks and valleys in mental-health related articles, as illustrated in Figure 1.1. Sociological interest in mental health began in earnest in the 1930s with very few articles appearing before that time. After that initial surge of activity, interest diminished until two later peaks in the post-World War II period and the 1980s. Most recently, there has been a troubling decrease, particularly in the *AJS*. These trends suggest that the fortunes of the sociology of mental health have waxed and waned throughout the published history of the discipline's mainstream.

What these figures cannot tell us, however, is what sociology has been learning from mental health research over these years. What images of mental health and illness have been represented? What topics have been covered? What major assertions have been made? To answer these questions, we review the content of mental health-related articles in six time periods that map the hills and valleys of mainstream sociological interest in mental health. Our review reveals a consistent interest in the social origins of mental illness, a broadening of the field to consider mental health as well as mental illness, and a movement of the field away from research on serious mental illness and its treatment.

The Earliest Years (1895–1930): Mental Illness and Morality

The first generation of articles in the *AJS* focused on the prevalence of mental illness. These articles adopted a decidedly moral tone that emphasized the social problems created by mental illness. The first article that focused exclusively on mental illness appeared in 1899 and addressed the "Prevention of Mental Diseases" (Morel & Henderson, 1899, *AJS*). In this article, the authors proposed diverse "social" measures to "prevent the increase of mental troubles in the degenerate and, at the same time, . . . diminish crime (p. 79)." These measures included special education services and the strategic selection of marriage partners. For example, neuropathic girls were advised to only marry men whose material situations would shield them from anxiety. With similar tone, Rentoul (1906 *AJS*) discussed how, under the claim that "insanity is on the increase," "we could prevent the present large total of mental degenerates from begetting degenerates" who are "the most dangerous citizens" (pp. 319–320). This moralistic tone appeared again in 1921 (*AJS*) when Laughlin included "the deranged" among the "socially inadequate" that needed to be "designated" and "sorted." Early sociological approaches to mental illness reflected the major social concerns *and* stereotypes of the time.

The First Peak of Interest (1925–1950): Social Determinants of Mental Illness

In the second quarter of the twentieth century, sociologists turned from their early moralistic prescriptions towards analyses of the social determinants of mental illness. This is the era in which many major themes in contemporary sociological research on mental illness were first introduced. Following on the heels of the discipline's founders, Ogburn and Winston (1928 *AJS*) presented data on the "startling fact" that lifetime mental hospital admissions rates were one in ten and related to "modern civilization" (p. 822). Jaffe and Shanas (1939, *AJS*) documented the inverse relationship between economic status and mental hospitalization, independent of sex, race and foreign-born status (see also Tietze et al. 1941 *AJS*; Dunham, 1944 *AJS*). Mowrer (1939 *ASR*) looked at the effect of the Depression on both suicide and "insanity." Tietze et al. (1942 *AJS*) examined residential mobility, and Dunham (1942 *AJS*) considered the impact of world conflict on American mental hospital admission rates (also Weinberg, 1946 *AJS*; Brookover, 1945 *ASR* on individual responses to world conflict).[5] In articles on suicide specifically, researchers began to see patterns by age, urban location, marriage/divorce, gender and occupation (Schmid, 1933 *AJS*; see Lunden, 1947 *AJS*; Porterfield, 1949 *ASR*). In this way, the discipline of sociology began to assert its relevance to understanding the distribution of mental illness in the population.[6]

---

[5] In another paper with close ties to the concerns of the day, Abel (1945 *ASR*) argued that Nazism was not attributable to mass mental illness.

[6] Additional themes included drug addiction as psychopathology (Lindesmith, 1940 *ASR*), marital difficulties (McLean, 1941 *ASR*), "poorly adjusted families" (Willoughby, 1942 *ASR*) and children (Mangus, 1948 *ASR*), and post-divorce adjustment (Goode, 1949 *ASR*).

In 1937, the classic piece by H. Warren Dunham (1937, p. 467 *ASR*) applied ecological methods from urban sociology to the study of schizophrenia in Chicago. He found that schizophrenia was concentrated in areas of "marked social disorganization," with no difference in ecological patterning for males and females, nor for local and sub-communities, nor across most types of schizophrenia (e.g., paranoid type). However, catatonic schizophrenia was most likely in "foreign-born and Negro communities" (p. 473). Overall, the rates were very skewed with "the bulk of communities having low rates and a few of the communities at the center of the city having high rates" (p. 473). In a similar vein, Faris (1938 *ASR*) found that socio-demographic characteristics, including race and foreign-born status, had more of an effect on mental hospitalization outside of the communities "in which that population is in the majority" (p. 204). Faris pointed to the role of social isolation and suggested that "(p)erhaps the real hope will never lie in the treatment of patients" but in the "stabilization" of communities (p. 209). Later, Demerath (1943 *ASR*) suggested social rejection of individuals as a cause of mental illness, a more individualistic interpretation of the social isolation argument (see also Clinard, 1949 *ASR*; Queen, 1949 *ASR*).

Yet, despite the assertion of a strong sociological perspective on mental illness, ambivalence regarding the relative importance of sociological and psychological factors in mental illness is also evident during these years. The first special issue on what we might consider "social psychiatry" appeared in *AJS* in 1936 with nine articles that addressed personal, individual or social disorganization. Countering the prevailing thinking of psychiatry, Blumer (1937, p.: 871 *AJS*) argued that individual disorder "gains its opportunity for expression where social disorganization prevails." Yet, only three years later, another issue of *AJS* was devoted to the integration of psychoanalytic theory into sociology, with Burgess (1939 *AJS*) asserting that "(a) final stage in the combination of psychoanalytic and sociological methods remains to be taken, that of cooperation of psychoanalysts and sociologists in joint research. The situation is becoming ripe for such a venture (p. 369)." Empirical research reflected this ambivalence, with suicide being related variously to insanity (Gargas 1932 *AJS*) and prosperity (Hurlburt, 1932 *AJS*), and rates of treated mental illness related to both birth order (Schuler, 1930 *AJS*), and "moral self-judgment" (Boisen, 1932 *AJS*).

Outside of research on the causes of mental illness, there were some stunning findings that addressed other issues still relevant today. Dunham (1939 *ASR*) concluded that there was only a negligible relationship between schizophrenia and criminal behavior. Treatment of mental illness was examined, including a consideration of methods to predict the length of hospitalization (Dunham & Meltzer, 1946 *AJS*) and numbers of treatment providers (Gregory, 1947 *AJS*). Winston (1938 *ASR*) documented "(m)arked inequalities in care of mental patients . . . from state to state" (p. 202) that reflected the inadequacy of expenditures for state hospitals.

As is evident from these examples, the research of this era concentrated primarily on ecological theory and ecological data, in keeping with more general trends in the discipline (see also, Queen, 1940 *ASR*; Schroeder, 1942 *AJS*; Clark,

1948, 1949 *ASR*). But by 1941, questions were being raised about the adequacy of hospital data to provide useful conclusions about the actual prevalence of mental illness (Owen at al., 1941 *AJS*).

The Post-World War II Peak (1950–1970): A Broadening of Interests

The end of World War II brought with it a general social interest in mental health (Mechanic, 1980) and new methods that allowed researchers to move beyond treatment statistics. In fact, measurement became a major issue with the development and introduction of new scales (e.g., the MMPI, Hathaway & Monachesi, 1952 *ASR*; also Manis et al., 1963, 1964 *ASR*; Dohrenwend, 1966 *ASR*) and the examination of both hospitalized and non-hospitalized cases (Kaplan et al., 1956 *ASR*). Clausen (1950:450 *ASR*) foreshadowed the important work in social epidemiology that was to come in his report on social sciences at the NIH: "Conceivably some sort of screening device may eventually be developed so as to be applicable in the community by someone other than an M.D. or Ph.D." (p. 450).

Research on the social predictors of mental illness extended earlier lines of research to individual-level data, with attention to social class (Hollingshead & Redlich, 1953, 1954 *ASR*; Dunham et al., 1966 *ASR*; Rushing, 1969 *ASR*), isolation and alienation (Jaco, 1954 *ASR*; Lowenthal, 1964 *ASR*; Summer & Hall, 1958 *ASR*), social mobility/migration (Hollingshead et al., 1954 *ASR*; Kleiner & Parker, 1959 *ASR*; Turner & Wagenfeld, 1967 *ASR*), as well as socio-demographics (e.g., Ikeda et al., 1962 *AJS*; Phillips & Segal, 1969 *ASR*; Bellin & Hardt, 1958 *ASR*). The range of mental health-related outcomes that were considered expanded beyond psychoses to other forms of mental illness (e.g., feral and autistic children; Bettleheim, 1959 *AJS*), paranoia (Bonner, 1950 *AJS*), and anxiety (Montague, 1961 *ASR*) and to general indicators of mental health. Personal adjustment (e.g., Stryker, 1955 *ASR*; Pan, 1951 *ASR*; Sewell & Haller, 1959 *ASR*), marital tension (Farber & Blackman, 1956 *ASR*), and stress (Jackson, 1962 *ASR*; Jackson & Burke, 1965 *ASR*) were the subject of nearly a dozen articles during this period.

The shift away from hospitalized rates of mental illness opened other new areas of inquiry outside of epidemiology. In particular, sociologists began to analyze individuals' use of mental health services. Raphael (1964 *AJS*) examined the role of the community acceptance of psychological and psychiatric explanations of mental illness; issues of "need" (e.g., stress) were considered (e.g., Mechanic & Volkart, 1961 *ASR*; Segal et al., 1965 *ASR*) and Kadushin pioneered the importance of social network ties (1966 *ASR*; see also Sampson et al., 1962 *AJS*). Research also went further into the mental hospital itself to look at resistance of staff to changes in treatment protocols (Pearlin, 1962 *AJS*), the social rhythms of patient behavior (Melbin, 1969 *AJS*; Perrucci, 1963 *ASR*) and social factors that predict the type and participation of patients in treatment options (Kandel, 1966 *AJS*; Myers & Schaffer, 1954 *ASR*). Research addressed the hospital as a total institution (Hillery, 1963 *ASR*), the climate of treatment settings and its impact on staff and patients (Street, 1965 *ASR*; Wallance & Raskis, 1959 *ASR*), the power of professional versus bureaucratic staff (Lefton et al., 1959 *ASR*), and the role and behavior of psychiatric nurses and attendants (Caudill 1961, *ASR*; Pearlin & Rosenberg, 1962 *AJS*; Simpson & Simpson, 1959 *ASR*; Melbin, 1961 *ASR*). Spotty but continued attention to lay providers appeared (e.g., the Puerto Rican spiritualist, Rogler & Hollingshead, 1961 *AJS*; clergy, Cummings & Harrington, 1961 *AJS*).

Finally, the effects of hospitalization on the community lives of individuals who had been treated were considered. Freeman and Simmons (1958 *ASR*), for example documented that the tolerance of former patients' significant others to "deviant behavior" was more important than their symptoms for predicting their ability to live successfully in the community. Lystad (1957 *ASR*) documented that treated schizophrenia affected the status mobility of upper SES individuals but not that of lower SES individuals, perhaps because of the limits already existing in the lower classes. Hardt and Feinhandler (1959 *ASR*) showed that lower SES was associated with a greater risk for continued, long-term hospitalization and Linn (1959 *AJS*) documented that the introduction of "tranquilizing drugs" into psychiatric treatment dampened, but did not eliminate, the magnitude of the effects of race, marital status, and sex on hospital release rates.

Extending the theme of community responses to persons with mental illness, an important set of articles revolving around issues of labeling theory, social reaction and stigma first appeared in this period. Becker (1962 *AJS*; see also Gibbs, 1962 *ASR*) argued that mental illness is a performance while Lefton et al. (1962 *AJS*) countered that behavior, not social class nor expectations, shaped the label of mental illness (see also Gove 1970, *ASR*). The first empirical reports of stigma among the public (Woodward, 1951, p. 464 *ASR*) documented a "gross failure to recognize serious mental symptoms" while Freeman (1961 *ASR*) examined attitudes among relatives of persons with mental illness. Rejection as a consequence of help-seeking (Phillips, 1963, 1964 *ASR*) rounded out discussions of stigma.

Finally, in keeping with long-standing disciplinary emphases, very important theoretical and empirical pieces on suicide appeared during this time (e.g., Powell, 1958 *ASR* on the role of occupation). Gibbs and Martin (1958, 1959, 1966 *ASR*, 1959 *AJS*) introduced the status integration theory of suicide and debated its utility with others (Chambliss & Steele, 1966 *ASR*). Questions about Durkheim's theory appeared (Dohrenwend, 1959 *ASR*; Selvin, 1958 *AJS*). For example, Johnson (1965 *AJS*) theorized that Durkheim's four-pointed typology could be folded into one cause, too little social integration. Methodological issues were also raised about the use of official rates and standard techniques (Simpson, 1950 *ASR*) in suicide research.

Throughout these years, sociologists continued their earlier discussion of the relevance of psychoanalytic theory by examining, integrating, and drawing lines between sociological perspectives and epidemiology (Hollingshead, 1961 *ASR*) and psychiatry (Bendix, 1952 *AJS*; Smith, 1957 *AJS*). For example, Simmons and Davis (1957 *AJS*) argued that the challenges to collaboration between clinical sciences and the social sciences were, ironically, not as much in perspective as in method, a point that continues to have relevance.

In many respects, then, the two decades following World War II represent the blossoming of sociological research on mental illness. Never before had sociologists pursued such a broad range of issues concerning mental illness.

Sociologists studied topics that integrated sociological ideas and methods from virtually all areas of the discipline to shed light on the causes and consequences of mental illness and on institutional responses.

The 1970s: A Stable Field

During this decade, the epidemiology of mental health and illness, societal reactions to mental illness, and suicide continued to dominate discourse and empirical research. The major debate in epidemiological research surrounded issues of gender. In a series of articles, Gove and colleagues (1973, 1974, 1976 *AJS*) postulated that the main role available to women, housewife, produced higher rates of mental illness, particularly neuroses and functional psychoses, because of its restrictive and unsatisfying character (1973, 1974, 1976 AJS). Dohrenwend and Dohrenwend (1976 *AJS*) countered with evidence that there was no gender difference in overall rates of mental illness, and argued, rather, that men and women experience different disorders. This debate continues today in mainstream sociological journals (Mirowsky & Ross, ASR 1995; Simon & Nath, 2004).

Research on psychological distress carried forward many earlier themes from research on mental illness. Webb and Collette (1977 *AJS*) found that rural areas appear to be more stressful, contrary to popular ideas about urban life. Likewise, economic strain (Pearlin & Radabaugh, 1976 *AJS*), unfavorable working conditions (Miller et al., 1979 *AJS*; Kohn & Schooler, 1973 *ASR*), unequal social status in marriages (Pearlin, 1975, 1977 *ASR*) and status inconsistency (Hornung, 1977 *ASR*) were all implicated in distress.[7]

The tradition of sociological research on suicide continued. Articles were published on the influence of changing technology and social integration on suicide rates (Miley & Micklin, 1971 *AJS*), as well as on the role of imitation (Phillips, 1974 *ASR*; 1979 *AJS*). Barnes (1975 *AJS*) investigated the influence of SES on suicide rates.

Beyond epidemiological research, labeling theory received substantial attention, particularly in the *ASR* (e.g., Dunham, 1971; Gove & Howell, 1974; Immershein & Simons, 1976; Scheff, 1974) with keen debate about its validity when applied to mental illness. Related empirical research began to move beyond the either-or character of the initial debate to present more nuanced understandings of societal reaction processes. For example, Rushing (1978 *ASR*) separated out voluntary from involuntary admissions to mental hospitals, and found that the effects of "status resources" such as SES on the type of admission were less pronounced for persons with severe disorders. With Ortega (1979 *AJS*), he went on to argue that the association of SES with mental illness held only for organic disorders and schizophrenia and proposed a sociomedical,

---

[7] The increasing emphasis on mental health rather than mental illness is also evident in a series of articles on the social correlates of self-esteem, especially in children and adolescents (Rosenberg and Pearlin 1978 *AJS*; Simmons et al. 1979, 1973 *ASR*).

rather than societal reaction, explanation for the association. Turner and Gartrell (1978 *ASR*) argued that socio-demographic differences in the length of psychiatric hospitalization reflected differences in social competence. Using very sophisticated methods, Wheaton (1978 *ASR*) took on the issue of social selection versus social causation with longitudinal data, finding the evidence favoring a modified social causation explanation.

Perhaps most striking during this period was the dramatic decline in attention to psychiatric treatment. Eaton (1974 *ASR*) studied long-term outcomes for persons with mental illness, and found support for theories of institutionalization. Light (1972 *AJS*) used psychiatrists as a case to investigate how professions manage failure (see also Light, 1975 *AJS*). With the exception of these two examples, there were no other articles on psychiatric treatment during the 1970s.

The 1980s: The Dominance of Distress

The 1980s saw another, but smaller, peak in attention to the Sociology of Mental Health along with a near complete retreat from the study of serious mental illness. Only three articles during this decade dealt with the epidemiology of mental illness rather than psychological distress. Eaton (1980 *AJS*) continued the earlier discussion about the role of social selection and social drift as explanations of the class differential in schizophrenia, finding that both processes are in operation. Link and colleagues (1986 *ASR*) presented evidence on schizophrenia consistent with the social causation hypothesis, finding "noisome" occupations to be critical for onset. Finally, Kadushin (1983 *ASR*) theorized and documented that different levels of context have different effects on paranoia among Vietnam era veterans: the larger social density of geographical areas shaped the appearance of PTSD in rural area while personal networks were important in urban areas.

What dominated the Sociology of Mental Health in mainstream journals was the etiology of distress. In particular, there was substantial interest in understanding gender differences in psychological distress. Drawing from Gove's gender theories of the 1970s, research addressed issues of marital power (Mirowsky, 1985 *AJS*), the role of women's labor force participation (Kessler & McRae, 1981 *ASR*), and women's education (Kessler, 1982 *ASR*). Overall, this body of research concluded that the effect of changing female roles on men's distress did not result from men's increased household responsibilities but rather from the clash of their changed circumstances with traditional gender roles (Kessler and McRae, 1982 *ASR*; Ross, Mirowsky, & Huber, 1983 *ASR*). Further, the connection between the traditional female role and distress was weaker in cultures that placed more emphasis on the family suggesting important contextual moderators (Ross, Mirowsky, & Ulbrich, 1983 *AJS*; see also Mirowsky & Ross, 1980 *AJS* on ethnicity more generally). The "cost of caring" hypothesis received empirical support (Kessler & McLeod, 1984 *ASR*; Lin & Ensel, 1989 *ASR*), suggesting that women's greater responsibility for the well-being of others carries a high psychological cost.

The research of this decade also reflects the emergence of the stress process paradigm (Pearlin, Menaghan, Lieberman, & Mullan, 1981) and its strong influence on sociological research on mental health. Studies of life events, both those that employed events checklists (Kessler & Cleary, 1980 *ASR*; Kessler & McLeod, 1984 *ASR*; Lin & Ensel, 1989 *ASR*; Thoits, 1981 *ASR*) and studies of single events (Furstenberg, Morgan, & Allison, 1987 *ASR*; Mutran & Reitzer, 1984 *ASR*; McCarthy & Hogge, 1984 *AJS*) became prominent. Research on multiple roles and mental health was also introduced, with studies finding that those who are more integrated gain more but also lose more in the face of change (Thoits, 1982 *ASR*).

The association of work and personality also received sustained attention in the research program of Kohn, Schooler, and their colleagues (Kohn & Schooler, 1982 *AJS*; Naoi & Schooler, 1985 *AJS*). Most notably, they introduced cross-cultural considerations. For example, Schooler and Naoi found that traditional jobs were less alienating in Japan than in the U.S. (Schooler & Naoi, 1988 *AJS*).

The one arena in which mental illness, rather than distress, continued to receive attention was with respect to issues of labeling and stigma. Thoits (1985 *AJS*) reconceptualized residual rule-breaking as violations of feeling or expression norms. In a series of papers, Link and colleagues documented that stigma only attached to those people who were labeled, even though their behaviors were similar to those of people who were not labeled (Link, 1982 *ASR*; 1987 *ASR*; Link & Cullen et al., 1987 *AJS*). In the end, modified labeling theory suggested that while labels may not create or produce mental illness, their application has dramatic effects on individuals across areas of employment, social relationships and mental health (Link, Cullen, Struening et al., 1989 *ASR*).

Finally, research on suicide continued to debate the importance of imitation with evidence that both supported (e.g., Bollen & Phillips, 1981 *AJS*, 1982 *AJS*; Phillips, 1982 *AJS*) and countered (Kessler, 1984 *AJS*) this idea. Further research suggested that it is only media coverage of celebrity suicides that has effects (Wasserman, 1984 *ASR*; Stack, 1987 *ASR*). The focus on the theory of status integration declined even as Gibbs (1982 *ASR*) documented that when the marital, parental and labor force integration were cross-classified, the theory was even more powerful. The focus on Durkheim's theory and, in particular, the role of religion continued to find support in its original thesis of the Protestant-Catholic difference (Breault, 1986 *AJS*) and in a reconsidered version which took into account American differences in denominationalism and social network ties created by religions (Pescosolido & Georgianna, 1989 *ASR*).

The Recent Face of Mental Health Research (The 1990s and the 21st Century)

The trend presented in Figure 1 suggests that mental health research is once again on the decline in mainstream sociological journals. Data from a recent American Sociological Association Task Force support the further assertion that this decline does not reflect changing interests of ASA members as mental health-related articles are currently underrepresented in proportion to membership in relevant ASA sections.[8]

Aneshensel, Rutter, and Lachenbruch (1991 *ASR*) contributed a paper at the beginning of the 1990s that clearly defined the distinction between sociological approaches to the study of mental health and biomedical or epidemiological perspectives. They argued that a sociological perspective documents the consequences of social structure and processes for mental health and illness. By contrast, biomedical or epidemiologic approaches attempt to identify the antecedents of specific illnesses. Over the past 15 years, the articles that have been included in *ASR* and *AJS* appear to have followed that sociological tradition. Research has pushed beyond a simple focus on socio-demographic predictors to consider the sociological processes that underlie observed associations. Focusing on gender, for example, Simon (2001 *AJS*) countered Gove's earlier contention that marriage benefits men more than women. Rather, she found that marriage is equally beneficial for men and women but that they respond differently to marital transitions. Umberson et al. (1996 *ASR*) concluded that the effects of social relationships on well-being do not differ for men and women. Mirowsky and Ross (1995 *ASR)* provided evidence that women experience all forms of distress more than men, countering claims regarding gender differences in emotional styles.

A more general interest in process is evident in research concerned with the associations of socio-demographic characteristics, religion, and stress with mental health (Burke, 1991 *ASR*; Idler & Kasl, 1992 *AJS*; Mirowsky & Ross, 1990 *AJS*; Turner, Wheaton, & Lloyd, 1995 *ASR*). The increasing influence of the life course perspective is evident, with research showing that experiences in childhood, adolescence, and early adulthood influence adult mental health

---

[8] In the summer of 2000, in the face of controversy about the *American Sociological Review*, then President Joe Feagin convened a task force to consider issues of topic and methods diversity in the discipline's flagship journals. Part of the report that was issued in 2003 examined data collected and analyzed by Mike Hout from the University of California, Berkeley and Erik Olin Wright from the University of Wisconsin, Madison. These data couple information on section membership in the ASA with the topics of articles in the *ASR* and the *AJS* during the 1990s. They can be used to determine which subfields of the discipline are over- and under-represented in the journals. The report included articles on mental health within the medical sociology category. As a result, the analysis overestimates the representation of mental health-related articles. Even with that bias, mental health-related articles as substantially underrepresented. Although 3.7 percent of ASA members belong to the Medical Sociology Section, only 0.3 percent of the articles in the 1990s addressed health, illness and healing. This mismatch represents the single largest gap between members' interests and articles in the flagship journal. In *AJS*, the 4 percent of articles on medical topics matches the 3.7 percent of the Medical Sociology Section membership. This apparent proportionate representation is due almost entirely to the presence of a special issue on Medical Sociology in 1992, edited by Donald W. Light. Importantly, of the nine articles in the "New Directions in the Sociology of Medicine" special issue, only one Idler & Kasl, 1992 *AJS*) is related to mental health issues.

(Cherlin et al., 1998 *ASR*; McLeod & Shanahan, 1993 *ASR*; Wheaton & Clarke, 2003 *ASR*). Research on contextual predictors of mental health, so visible in the early years of the discipline, has reappeared recently (Ross, Reynolds, & Geis, 2000 *ASR*), with evidence that neighborhood stability decreases distress in affluent neighborhoods but increases distress in disadvantaged neighborhoods.

The quantity of theoretically and methodologically sophisticated research on distress has not been matched by research on mental illness. Studies of the incidence of suicide are still represented in the mainstream journals but these studies are curiously divorced from "mental health" research. Pampel (1998 *ASR*) found that the sex difference in suicide in cross-national data narrowed initially as gender equality proceeded but then widened again over time. Further, birth cohorts with less integration and regulation have higher suicide rates, especially under situations of rapid social change (Stockard & O'Brien, 2002 *ASR*). And, in a spatial analysis, Baller and Richardson (2002 *ASR*) found that in both 19th century France and 20th century U.S., both integration and imitation processes seem to be in operation. What is new is the use of individual-level data in sociological studies of suicide. One such study questioned the Catholic-Protestant hypothesis in the Netherlands (van Poppel & Day, 1996 *ASR*). Another found that family integration and parental regulation were both implicated in youth suicidal ideation (Thorlindsdon & Bjarnason, 1998 *ASR*).

Mental illness also received attention in the continuing debate over the relative importance of social selection and social causation processes (with Miech and colleagues, 1999 *AJS*) reporting that the two processes are differentially relevant for different disorders) and in research on violence. With respect to the latter, Link and colleagues found a real but modest effect of mental illness on violent behavior among those with psychotic symptoms, more specifically those symptoms which represent an absence of "threat control overrides" (Link, Andrews, & Cullen, 1992 *ASR*; Link, Monahan, Stueve, & Cullen, 1999 *ASR*). Beyond these few exceptions, however, serious mental illness is not well-represented in mainstream sociological journals.

Similarly, treatment continues to receive little attention in *ASR* and *AJS*. Mental health providers were the subject of one cross-national investigation that found that individually-centered societies create more "professional psychology," even when social and economic resources are taken into account (Frank, Meyer, & Miyahara, 1995 *ASR*). Expanding the focus to systems, Liska and colleagues (1999 *AJS*) examined how the criminal justice and mental health systems are intertwined social control responses to deviant behavior. And, given the turn to comparative historical topics in the larger discipline, Sutton (1991 *ASR*) showed that organizational and political forces, rather than the perceive increase in "madness" resulted in the building of asylums at the turn of the 20th century. Finally, Pescosolido and Rubin (2000 *ASR*) questioned the utility of the postmodern critique by examining Simmel's conceptions of social forms and tracing the views and treatment of mental illness over historical periods to provide an answer.

Discussion and Conclusion: Mental Health Research in Mainstream Sociology

Our review suggests three main conclusions. First, throughout the history of the *AJS* and the *ASR*, social determinants of mental health and mental illness have received much more attention than social responses and consequences. Although there is continuing interest in stigma and labels, what little interest there was in help-seeking in early years has dwindled. Similarly, psychiatric providers, treatment organizations, and "the system" are virtually absent from mainstream sociological journals. Readers of these journals would learn much about the social conditions that foster despair, and about complexities in the association of social hierarchies with distress, but little about the organization or effectiveness of societal responses. Sociologists of mental health were integral to early research on the structure and functioning of mental hospitals, but that interest has not been followed through during the transition to community-based care.

Second, with respect to the social determinants of mental health and illness, what we know is constrained by a near-exclusive focus on distress to the neglect of serious mental illness. While comprehensive etiologies of serious mental illness may require consideration of both social and genetic factors (e.g., Caspi, Sugden, Moffitt, Taylor, Craig, Harrington, McClay, Mill, Martin, Braithwaite, & Poulton, 2003), it is nevertheless striking that very few studies in *ASR* and *AJS* include even research diagnoses as outcomes. Data from the National Comorbidity Survey (Kessler, Berglund, Demler, Jin, Merikangas, & Walters, 2005) confirm that mental disorders have important socio-demographic correlates which are unlikely to be explained by biological factors in isolation. Much as clinicians turned away from persons with serious mental illness to embrace the "worried well," sociologists have privileged analyses of distress over mental disorders in their mainstream publications (see George, this volume). The shift away from serious mental illness likely results from several factors—the dominance of the stress process paradigm, sociologists' continuing skepticism and mistrust of psychiatric definitions of mental illness, the relative ease of collecting data from community samples as compared to samples of people with serious mental illness, and the general privileging of epidemiological research over "services" research in the mental health research community. Regardless of its origins, however, the emphasis on distress in the sociological mainstream biases the discipline's knowledge of the social origins and consequences of mental illness.

Finally, we included suicide in our review but are struck by the isolated nature of research on this topic. While suicide is a fundamental concern of psychiatry, psychology, and the other "mental health" disciplines (e.g., social work), its examination within the mainstream sociological journals remains strangely distant from the sociology of mental health in two ways. First, the vast majority of pieces on suicide we reviewed were not written by sociologists who would identify themselves as sociologists of mental health, or even as medical sociologists (see Light, 1972 *AJS*; Pescosolido & Mendelsohn, 1986 *ASR*; Pescosolido & Georgiana, 1989

ASR, Timmermans, 2005, *ASR* as exceptions). Rather, most of these researchers see themselves as "suicidologists," "theorists," or "Durkheimians." Second, this research has focused almost exclusively on larger contextual effects; for example, ecological, cross-national, or longitudinal patterns.

Recently, suicide researchers have begun to argue that sociological research has been flawed because it did not focus on individuals (e.g., Thorlindson & B. Jamason, 1998, Van Poppel & Day, 1996), much as sociologists of mental health argued in the 1950s. Interestingly, though, sociologists of mental health have now moved on to embrace geographically-based, contextual-level variables, although now within multi-level analyses (e.g., Ross, 2000).

It is beyond the scope of this piece to suggest whether research on the sociology of mental health is proportionately representative of the research that has been done within the disciplinary journals, or across the entire spectrum of publication venues. That would be a much larger, and perhaps nearly impossible, task. However, even our brief look into the mainstream of the discipline suggests that what we would learn about the social causes and consequences of mental health and illness, treatment processes and institutions, and community outcomes is limited to a fraction of the issues that have concerned sociologists of mental health over the years and particularly, in the most recent decades. Our focus on the reflection back and forth in the looking glass of mental health and the mainstream presents a challenge, but one which this volume suggests sociologists of mental health are well-equipped to take on.

References

Bloom, S. W. (2002). *The word as scalpel: A history of medical sociology*. Oxford, New York: Oxford University Press.

Caspi, A., Sugden, K., Moffitt, T. E., Taylor, A., Craig, I. W., Harrington, H., McClay, J., Mill, J., Martin, J., Braithwaite, A. & Poulton, R. (2003). Influence of life stress on depression: Moderation by a polymorphism in the 5-htt gene. *Science, 301*, 386–389.

Durkheim, E. (1951). *Suicide*. New York: Free Press.

Durkheim, E. (1954). *The elementary forms of religious life*. New York: The Free Press.

Kessler, R. C., Berglund, P., Demler, O., Jin, R., Merikangas, K. R. & Walters, E. E. (2005). Lifetime prevalence and age-of-onset distributions of dsm-iv disorders in the national comorbidity survey replication. *Archives of General Psychiatry, 62*, 593–602.

Marx, K. (1964). *Selected writings in sociology and social philosophy*. London: McGraw-Hill.

Masaryk, T. G. (1970). *Suicide and the meaning of civilization*. Chicago, IL: University of Chicago Press.

Mechanic, D. (1980). *Mental health and social policy*. Englewood Cliffs, NJ: Prentice-Hall.

Ogburn, W. F. (1934). The background of the new deal. *American Journal of Sociology, 39*, 729–737.

Ogburn, W. F. (1935). Indexes of social trends and their fluctuations. *American Journal of Sociology, 40*, 822–828.

Park, R. L. & Burgess, E. W. (1921). *Introduction to the science of sociology*. Chicago: University of Chicago Press.

Pearlin, L. I., Menaghan, E. G., Lieberman, M. A. & Mullan, J. T. (1981). The stress process. *Journal of Health and Social Behavior, 22,* 337–356.

Pescosolido, B. A. (1994). Bringing Durkheim into the 21st century: A social network approach to unresolved issues in the study of suicide. In D. Lester (Eds.), *Emile Durkheim: Le suicide – 100 years later* (pp. 264–295). Philadelphia: The Charles Press.

Ross, C. E. (2000). Neighborhood disadvantage and adult depression. *Journal of Health and Social Behavior, 41,* 177–187.

Shils, E. & Finch, H. (1949). *Max Weber on the methodology of the social sciences.* New York: The Free Press.

Simmel, G. (1955). *Conflict and the web of group affiliations.* New York: Free Press.

Simon, R. W. & Nath, L. E. (2004). Gender and emotion in the United States: Do men and women differ in self-reports of feelings and expressive behavior? *American Journal of Sociology, 109,* 1137–1176.

Veblen, T. B. (1934). *The theory of the leisure class.* New York: The Modern Library.

Watkins, S. C. (1993). If all we knew about women was what we read in *Demography,* what would we know. *Demography, 30,* 551–577.

Weber, M., Gerth, H. & Mills, C. W. (1946). *From Max Weber: Essays in sociology.* Oxford University Press.

APPENDIX TABLE 1.1. Articles cited in *American Sociological Review.*

Author(s)	Year	Title
Faris, R.E.L.	1938	Demography of Urban Psychotics With Special Reference to Schizophrenia
Krout, Maurice H.	1938	A Note on Dunham's Contribution to the Ecology of Functional Psychoses
Winston, Ellen	1938	Indices of Adequacy of State Care of Mental Patients
Dunham, H. Warren	1939	The Schizophrene and Criminal Behavior
Mowrer, Ernest R.	1939	A Study of Personal Disorganization
Devereux, George	1939	Maladjustment and Social Neurosis
Queen, Stuart A.	1940	The Ecological Study of Mental Disorders
Lindesmith, A.R.	1940	The Drug Addict as a Psychopath
McLean, Helen V.	1941	The Emotional Background of Marital Difficulties
Hallowell, A.I.	1941	The Social Function of Anxiety in a Primitive Society
Willoughby, Raymond R.	1942	A Study of Some Poorly Adjusted Families
Demerath, N.J.	1943	Adolescent Status Demands and the Student Experiences of Twenty Schizophrenics
Fromm, Erich	1944	Individual and Social Origins of Neurosis
Abel, Theodore	1945	Is a Psychiatric Interpretation of the German Enigma Necessary?
Brookover, Wilbur B.	1945	The Adjustment of Veterans to Civilian Life
Green, Arnold W.	1946	The Middle Class Male Child and Neurosis
Dunham, H. Warren	1948	Social Psychiatry
Clark, Robert E.	1948	The Relationship of Schizophrenia to Occupational Income and Occupational Prestige
Mangus, A.R.	1948	Personality Adjustment of Rural and Urban Children
Clinard, Marshall B.	1949	The Group Approach to Social Reintegration
Queen, Stuart A.	1949	Social Participation in Relation to Social Disorganization
Goode, William J.	1949	Problems in Postdivorce Adjustment
Porterfield, Austin L.	1949	Indices of Suicide and Homicide by States and Cities: Some Southern-Non-Southern Contrasts with Implications for Research
Mowrer, Ernest R.	1950	Social Crises and Social Disorganization
Clausen, John A.	1950	Social Science Research in the National Mental Health Program
Weinberg, S. Kirson	1950	A Sociological Analysis of a Schizophrenic Type
Simpson, George	1950	Methodological Problems in Determining the Aetiology of Suicide
Alpert, Harry	1950	Suicides and Homicides
Pan, Ju-Shu	1951	Factors in the Personal Adjustment of Old People in Protestant Homes for the Aged
Stone, Carol Larson	1951	Sorority Status and Personality Adjustment
Woodward, Julian L.	1951	Changing Ideas on Mental Illness and Its Treatment
MacGreggor, Frances Cooke	1951	Some Psycho-Social Problems Associated with Facial Deformities
Dai, Bingham	1952	A Socio-Psychiatric Approach to Personality Organization
Reiss, Albert J. Jr.	1952	Social Correlates of Psychological Types of Delinquency
Hathaway, Starke R., and Elio D. Monachesi	1952	The Minnesota Multiphasic Personality Inventory in the Study of Juvenile Delinquents
Moberg, David O.	1953	The Christian Religion and Personal Adjustment in Old Age
Hollingshead, August B., and Frederick C. Redlich	1953	Social Stratification and Psychiatric Disorders

(*continued*)

APPENDIX TABLE 1.1. *Continued*

Author(s)	Year	Title
Hollingshead, August B., and Frederick C. Redlich	1954	Social Stratification and Schizophrenia
Myers, Jerome K., and Leslie Schaffer	1954	Social Stratification and Psychiatric Practice: A Study of an Out-Patient Clinic
Mowrer, Ernest R.	1954	Some Factors in the Affectional Adjustment of Twins
Hollingshead, A.B., R. Ellis, and E. Kirby	1954	Social Mobility and Mental Illness
Jaco, E. Gartly	1954	The Social Isolation Hypothesis and Schizophrenia
Hochbaum, Godfrey M.	1954	The Relation Between Group Members' Self-Confidence and Their Reactions to Group Pressures to Uniformity
Stryker, Sheldon	1955	The Adjustment of Married Offspring to their Parents
Kohn, Melvin L., and John A. Clausen	1955	Social Isolation and Schizophrenia
Schmid, Calvin F., and Maruice D. Van Arsdol, Jr.	1955	Completed and Attempted Suicides: A Comparative Analysis
Montague, Joel B. Jr.	1955	A Study of Anxiety Among English and American Boys
Adamson, LaMay, and H. Warren Dunham	1956	Clinical Treatment of Male Delinquents: A Case Study in Effort and Result
Rose, Arnold M.	1956	Neuropsychiatric Breakdown in the Garrison Army and in Combat
Kaplan, Bert, Robert B. Reed, and Wyman Richardson	1956	A Comparison of the Incidence of Hospitalized and Non-Hospitalized Cases of Psychosis in Two Communities
Farber, Bernard, and Leonard S. Blackman	1956	Marital Role Tensions and Number and Sex of Children
Lystad, Mary H.	1957	Social Mobility Among Selected Groups of Schizophrenic Patients
Powell, Elwin H.	1958	Occupation, Status, and Suicide: Toward a Redefinition of Anomie
Gibbs, Jack P., and Walter T. Martin	1958	A Theory of Status Integration and Its Relationship to Suicide
Freeman, Howard E., and Ozzie G. Simmons	1958	Mental Patients in the Community: Family Settings and Performance Levels
Bellin, Seymour S., and Robert H. Hardt	1958	Marital Status and Mental Disorders Among the Aged
Sommer, Robert, and Robert Hall	1958	Alienation and Mental Illness
Simpson, Richard L., and Ida Harper Simpson	1959	The Psychiatric Attendant: Development of an Occupational Self-Image in a Low-Status Occupation
Gibbs, Jack P., and Walter T. Martin	1959	On Status Integration and Suicide Rates in Tulsa
Sewell, William H., and A.O. Haller	1959	Factors in the Relationship Between Social Status and the Personality Adjustment of the Child
Dohrenwend, Bruce P.	1959	Egoism, Altruism, Anomie, and Fatalism: A Conceptual Analysis of Durkheim's Types
Kleiner, Robert, and Seymour Parker	1959	Migration and Mental Illness: A New Look

APPENDIX TABLE 1.1. *Continued*

Author(s)	Year	Title
Lefton, Mark, Simon Dinitz, Simon, and Benjamin Pasamanick	1959	Decision-Making in a Mental Hospital: Real, Perceived, and Ideal
Wallace, Anthony F.C., and Harold A. Rashkis	1959	The Relation of Staff Consensus to Patient Disturbance on Mental Hospital Wards
Hardt, Robert H., and Sherwin J. Feinhandler	1959	Social Class and Mental Hospitalization Prognosis
Brenner, Berthold	1960	On Suicide Rate Differentials in Tulsa
Sharp, Lawrence J.	1960	Employment Status of Mothers and Some Aspects of Mental Illness
Porterfield, Austin L.	1960	Traffic Fatalities, Suicide, and Homicide
Freeman, Howard E.	1961	Attitudes Toward Mental Illness Among Relatives of Former Patients
Mechanic, David, and Edmund H. Volkart	1961	Stress, Illness Behavior, and the Sick Role
Melbin, Murray	1961	Organization Practice and Individual Behavior: Absenteeism Among Psychiatric Aides
Hollingshead, August B.	1961	Some Issues in the Epidemiology of Schizophrenia
Caudill, William	1961	Around the Clock Patient Care in Japanese Psychiatric Hospitals: The Role of the Tsukisoi
Wood, Arthur L.	1961	A Socio-Structural Analysis of Murder, Suicide, and Economic Crime in Ceylon
Pearlin, Leonard I., and Morris Rosenberg	1962	Nurse-Patient Social Distance and the Structural Context of a Mental Hospital
Jackson, Elton F.	1962	Status Consistency and Symptoms of Stress
Gibbs, Jack P.	1962	Rates of Mental Hospitalization: A Study of Societal Reaction to Deviant Behavior
Manis, Jerome G., Milton Brawer, Chester Hunt, and Leonard Kercher	1963	Validating a Mental Health Scale
Breed, Warren	1963	Occupational Mobility and Suicide Among White Males
Kleiner, Robert, and Seymour Parker	1963	Goal-Striving, Social Status, and Mental Disorders: A Research Review
Mishler, Elliot G., and Nancy Waxler	1963	Decision Processes in Psychiatric Hospitalization: Patients Referred, Accepted, and Admitted to a Psychiatric Hospital
Hillery, George A. Jr.	1963	Villages, Cities, and Total Institutions
Perrucci, Robert	1963	Social Distance Strategies and Intra-Organizational Stratification: A Study of the Status System on a Psychiatric Ward
Phillips, Derek L.	1963	Rejection: A Possible Consequence of Seeking Help for Mental Disorders
Manis, Jerome G., Milton J. Brawer, Chester Hunt, and Leonard Kercher	1964	Estimating the Prevalence of Mental Illness
Lowenthal, Marjorie Fiske	1964	Social Isolation and Mental Illness in Old Age
Phillips, Derek L.	1964	Rejection of the Mentally Ill: The Influence of Behavior and Sex

(*continued*)

APPENDIX TABLE 1.1. *Continued*

Author(s)	Year	Title
Street, David	1965	The Inmate Group in Custodial and Treatment Settings
Segal, Bernard E., Robert Weiss, and Robert Sokol	1965	Emotional Adjustment, Social Organization and Psychiatric Treatment Rates
Jackson, Elton F., and Peter J. Burke	1965	Status and Symptoms of Stress: Additive and Interaction Effects
Johnson, Barclay D.	1965	Durkheim's One Cause of Suicide
Dohrenwend, Bruce P.	1966	Social Status and Psychological Disorder: An Issue of Substance and an Issue of Method
Dunham, H. Warren, Patricia Phillips, and Barbara Srinivasan	1966	A Research Note on Diagnosed Mental Illness and Social Class
Chambliss, William J., and Marion F. Steele	1966	Status Integration and Suicide: An Assessment
Gibbs, Jack P., and Walter T. Martin	1966	On Assessing the Theory of Status Integration and Suicide
Kadushin, Charles	1966	The Friends and Supporters of Psychotherapy: On Social Circles in Urban Life
Turner, R. Jay, and Morton O. Wagenfeld	1967	Occupational Mobility and Schizophrenia: An Assessment of the Social Causation and Social Selection Hypothesis
Wilkins, James	1967	Suicidal Behavior
Dohrenwend, Bruce P., and Edwin Chin-Shong	1967	Social Status and Attitudes Toward Psychological Disorder: The Problems of Tolerance and Deviance
Pierce, Albert	1967	The Economic Cycle and the Social Suicide Rate
Phillips, Derek L., and Bernard E. Segal	1969	Sexual Status and Psychiatric Symptoms
Rushing, William A.	1969	Two Patterns in the Relationship Between Social Class and Mental Hospitalization
Phillips, Derek L., and Kevin J. Clancy	1970	Response Biases in Field Studies of Mental Illness
Gove, Walter R.	1970	Societal Reaction as an Explanation of Mental Illness: An Evaluation
Dunham, H. Warren	1971	Comment on Gove's Evaluation of Societal Reaction Theory as an Explanation for Mental Illness
Mechanic, David	1971	Comment on "Mental Illness"
Gove, Walter R.	1971	Reply to Dunham and Mechanic
Harvey, Ted G.	1971	Comment on "Response Biases in Field Studies of Mental Illness"
Phillips, Derek L., and Kevin J. Clancy	1971	Reply to Harvey
Akers, Ronald	1972	Comment on Gove's Evaluation of Societal Reaction as an Explanation of Mental Illness
Gove, Walter R.	1972	Reply to Akers
Kohn, Melvin L., and Carmi Schooler	1973	Occupational Experience and Psychological Functioning: An Assessment of Reciprocal Effects
Simmons, Roberta G., Florence Rosenberg, and Morris Rosenberg	1973	Disturbance in the Self-Image at Adolescence
Gove, Walter R. and Patrick Howell	1974	Individual Resources and Mental Hospitalization: A Comparison and Evaluation of the Societal and Psychiatric Perspectives

APPENDIX TABLE 1.1. *Continued*

Author(s)	Year	Title
Eaton, William W. Jr.	1974	Mental Hospitalization as a Reinforcement Process
Phillips, David P.	1974	The Influence of Suggestion on Suicide: Substantive and Theoretical Implications of the Werther Effect
Scheff, T.J.	1974	The Labeling Theory of Mental Illness
Nettler, Gwynn	1974	On Telling Who's Crazy
Scheff, Thomas J.	1974	Reply to Nettler
Gove, Walter R.	1975	The Labeling Theory of Mental Illness: A Reply to Scheff
Chauncey, Robert L.	1975	Comment on "The Labeling Theory of Mental Illness"
Scheff, Thomas J.	1975	Reply to Chauncey and Gove
Pearlin, Leonard I.	1975	Status Inequality and Stress in Marriage
Townsend, J. Marshall	1975	Cultural Conceptions, Mental Disorders and Social Roles: A Comparison of Germany and America
Imershein, Allen W. and Ronald L. Simons	1976	Rules and Examples in Lay and Professional Psychiatry: An Ethnomethodological Comment on the Scheff-Gove Controversy
Scheff, Thomas J.	1976	Reply to Imershein and Simons
Gove, Walter R.	1976	Reply to Imershein and Simons (1976) and Scheff (1975)
Hornung, Carlton A.	1977	Social Status, Status Inconsistency and Psychological Stress
Pearlin, Leonard I., and Joyce S. Johnson	1977	Marital Status, Life-Strains and Depression
Turner, R. Jay, and John W. Gartrell	1978	Social Factors in Psychiatric Outcome: Toward the Resolution of Interpretive Controversies
Wheaton, Blair	1978	The Sociogenesis of Psychological Disorder: Reexamining the Causal Issues with Longitudinal Data
Rushing, William A.	1978	Status Resources, Societal Reactions, and Type of Mental Hospital Admission
Gove, Walter R., Michael Hughes, and Omer R. Galle	1979	Overcrowding in the Home: An Empirical Investigation of Its Possible Pathological Consequences
Simmons, Roberta G., Dale A. Blyth, Edward Van Cleave, and Diane Mitsch Bush	1979	Entry into Early Adolescence: The Impact of School Structure, Puberty, and Early Dating on Self-Esteem
Kessler, Ronald C., and Paul D. Cleary	1980	Social Class and Psychological Distress
Gove, Walter R., and Michael Hughes	1980	The Effects of Crowding Found in The Toronto Study: Some Methodological and Empirical Questions
Gove, Walter R., and Michael Hughes	1980	In Pursuit of Preconceptions: A Reply to the Claim of Booth and His Colleagues That Household Crowding in Not an Important Variable
Berk, Richard A., William P. Bridges, and Anthony Shih	1981	Does IQ Really Matter? A Study of the Use of IQ Scores for the Tracking of the Mentally Retarded
Thoits, Peggy A.	1981	Undesirable Life Events and Psychophysiological Distress: A Problem of Operational Confounding
Kessler, Ronald C., and James A. McRae, Jr.	1981	Trends in the Relationship Between Sex and Psychological Distress: 1957–1976
Vanfossen, Beth E., John Spitzer, and Dolores J. Jones	1981	Social Class and Emotional Distress

(*continued*)

APPENDIX TABLE 1.1. *Continued*

Author(s)	Year	Title
Boor, Myron	1981	Effects of United States Presidential Elections on Suicide and Other Cases of Death
Gibbs, Jack P.	1982	Testing the Theory of Status Integration and Suicide Rates
Kessler, Ronald C., and James A. McRae, Jr.	1982	The Effect of Wives' Employment on the Mental Health of Married Men and Women
Link, Bruce	1982	Mental Patient Status, Work, and Income: An Examination of the Effects of a Psychiatric Label
Bollen, Kenneth A., and David P. Phillips	1982	Imitative Suicides: A National Study of the Effects of Television News Stories
Kessler, Ronald C.	1982	A Disaggregation of the Relationship between Socioeconomic Status and Psychological Distress
Thoits, Peggy A.	1983	Multiple Identities and Psychological Well-Being: A Reformulation and Test of the Social Isolation Hypothesis
Kadushin, Charles	1983	Mental Health and the Interpersonal Environment: A Reexamination of Some Effects of Social Structures on Mental Health
Mirowsky, John, and Catherine E. Ross	1983	Paranoia and the Structure of Powerlessness
Wasserman, Ira M.	1983	Political Business Cycles, Presidential Elections, and Suicide and Morality Patterns
Ross, Catherine E., John Mirowsky, and Joan Huber	1983	Dividing Work, Sharing Work, and In-Between: Marriage Patterns and Depression
Mutran, Elizabeth, and Donald Reitzes	1984	Intergenerational Support Activities and Well-Being among the Elderly: A Convergence of Exchange and Symbolic Interaction Perspectives
Wasserman, Ira M.	1984	Imitation and Suicide: A Reexamination of the Werther Effect
Kessler, Ronald C., and Jane D. McLeod	1984	Sex Differences in Vulnerability to Undesirable Life Events
Wasserman, Ira M.	1984	Political Crisis, Social Integration and Suicide: A Reply to Boor and Fleming
Boor, Myron, and Jerome A. Fleming	1984	Presidential Election Effects on Suicide and Mortality Levels are Independent of Unemployment Rates
Thoits, Peggy A.	1986	Multiple Identities: Examining Gender and Marital Status Differences in Distress
Link, Bruce G., Bruce P. Dohdrenwend, and Andrew E. Skodol	1986	Socio-Economic Status and Schizophrenia: Noisome Occupational Characteristics as a Risk Factor
Miller, Karen A., Melvin L. Kohn, and Carmi Schooler	1986	Educational Self-Direction and Personality
Link, Bruce G.	1987	Understanding Labeling Effects in the Area of Mental Disorders: An Assessment of the Effects of Expectations of Rejection
Stack, Steven	1987	Celebrities and Suicide: A Taxonomy and Analysis, 1948–1983
Furstsenberg, Frank F. Jr.; S. Phillip Morgan, and Paul Allison	1987	Paternal Participation and Children's Well-being after Marital Dissolution

APPENDIX TABLE 1.1. *Continued*

Author(s)	Year	Title
Lin, Nan, and Walter M. Ensel	1989	Life Stress and Health: Stressors and Resources
Rosenberg, Morris, Carmi Schooler, and Carrie Schoenbach	1989	Self-Esteem and Adolescent Problems: Modeling Reciprocal Effects
White, Lynn, and John N. Edwards	1990	Emptying the Nest and Parental Well-Being: An Analysis of National Panel Data
Wheaton, Blair	1990	Life Transitions, Role Histories, and Mental Health
Aneshensel, Carol S., Carolyn M. Rutter, and Peter A. Lachenbruch	1991	Social Structure, Stress, and Mental Health: Competing Conceptual and Analytic Models
Sutton, John R.	1991	The Political Economy of Madness: The Expansion of the Asylum in Progressive America
Burke, Peter J.	1991	Identity Processes and Social Stress
Link, Bruce G., Howard Andrews, and Francis T. Cullen	1992	The Violent and Illegal Behavior of Mental Patients Reconsidered
McLeod, Jane D., and Michael J. Shanahan	1993	Poverty, Parenting, and Children's Mental Health
Girard, Chris	1993	Age, Gender, and Suicide: A Cross-National Analysis
Umberson, Debra, and Meichu D. Chen	1994	Effects of a Parent's Death on Adult Children: Relationship Salience and Reaction to Loss
Owens, Timothy J.	1994	Two Dimensions of Self-Esteem: Reciprocal Effects of Positive Self-Worth and Self-Deprecation on Adolescent Problems
Turner, R. Jay, Blair Wheaton, and Donald A. Lloyd	1995	The Epidemiology of Social Stress
Rosenberg, Morris, Carmi Schooler, Carrie Schoenbach, and Florence Rosenberg	1995	Global Self-Esteem and Specific Self-Esteem: Different Concepts, Different Outcomes
Mirowsky, John, and Catherine E. Ross	1995	Sex Differences in Distress: Real or Artifact?
Frank, David John, John W. Meyer, and David Miyahara	1995	The Individualist Polity and the Prevalence of Professionalized Psychology: A Cross-National Study
Van Poppel, Frans, and Lincoln H. Day	1996	A Test of Durkheim's Theory of Suicide–Without Committing the "Ecological Fallacy"
Umberson, Debra, Meichu D. Chen, James S. House, Kristine Hopkins, and Ellen Slaten	1996	The Effect of Social Relationships on Psychological Well-Being: Are Men and Women Really So Different?
Rosenfield, Sarah	1997	Labeling Mental Illness: The Effects of Received Services and Perceived Stigma on Life Satisfaction
Oates, Gary L.	1997	Self-Esteem Enhancement Through Fertility? Socioeconomic Prospects, Gender, and Mutual Influence

(*continued*)

APPENDIX TABLE 1.1. *Continued*

Author(s)	Year	Title
Thorlindsson, Thorolfur, and Thoroddur Bjarnason	1998	Modeling Durkheim on the Micro Level: A Study of Youth Suicidality
Cherlin, Andrew J., P. Lindsay Chase-Lansdale, and Christine McRae	1998	Effects of Parental Divorce on Mental Health Throughout the Life Course
Jang, Sung Joon, and Terence P. Thornberry	1998	Self-Esteem, Delinquent Peers, and Delinquency: A Test of the Self-Enhancement Thesis
Pampel, Fred C.	1998	National Context, Social Change, and Sex Differences in Suicide Rates
Simpson, Miles	1998	Suicide and Religion: Did Durkheim Commit the Ecological Fallacy, or Did Van Poppel and Day Combine Apples and Oranges?
Van Poppel, Frans, and Lincoln H. Day	1998	Reply to Simpson
Link, Bruce G., John Monahan, Ann Stueve, and Francis T. Cullen	1999	Real in Their Consequences: A Sociological Approach to Understanding the Association between Psychotic Symptoms and Violence
Amato, Paul R., and Juliana M. Sobolewski	2001	The Effects of Divorce and Marital Discord on Adult Children's Psychological Well-Being
Baller, Robert D. and Kelly K. Richardson	2002	Social Integration, Imitation, and the Geographic Patterning of Suicide
Stockard, Jean, and Robert O'Brien	2002	Cohort Effects on Suicide Rates: International Variations

APPENDIX 1. TABLE 1.2. Articles cited in *American Journal of Sociology*

Author(s)	Year	Title
Talbot, Marion	1896	Sanitation and Sociology
Tosti, Gustavo	1898	Suicide in the Light of Recent Studies
Millis, H.A.	1898	The Law Relating to the Relief and Care of Dependents. v. The Law Relating to the Care and Treatment of the Defective
Morel, Jules, and C.R. Henderson	1899	Prevention of Mental Diseases
Caldwell, W.	1899	Social and Ethical Interpretations of Mental Development
Macdonald, Arthur	1899	Alcoholic Hypnotism
Small, Albion W.	1900	The Scope of Sociology. I. The Development of Sociological Method
Small, Albion W.	1900	The Scope of Sociology. II. The Development of Sociological Method
Small, Albion W.	1900	The Scope of Sociology. III. The Problems of Sociology
Small, Albion W.	1900	The Scope of Sociology. IV. The Assumptions of Sociology
Small, Albion W.	1900	The Scope of Sociology. V. The Assumptions of Sociology
Small, Albion W.	1900	The Scope of Sociology. VI. Some Incidents of Association
Small, Albion W.	1901	The Scope of Sociology. VII. Classification of Associations
Ratzenhofer, Gustav	1904	The Problems of Sociology
Rentoul, Robert R.	1906	Proposed Sterilization of Certain Mental Degenerates
Laughlin, Harry H.	1921	The Socially Inadequate: How Shall We Designate and Sort Them?
Burrow, Trigant	1926	Insanity a Social Problem
Boisen, A.T.	1928	The Sense of Isolation in Mental Disorders: Its Religious Significance
Frank, Lawrence K.	1928	The Management of Tensions
Ogburn, William F., and Ellen Winston	1929	The Frequency and Probability of Insanity
Schuler, Edgar A.	1930	The Relationship of Birth Order and Fraternal Position to Incidence of Insanity
Lind, Andrew W.	1930	Some Ecological Patterns of Community Disorganization in Honolulu
Gargas, S.	1932	Suicide in the Netherlands
Hurlburt, Walter C.	1932	Prosperity, Depression, and the Suicide Rate
Boisen, A.T.	1932	The Problem of Values in the Light of Psychopathology
Schmid, Calvin F.	1933	Suicide in Minneapolis, Minnesota: 1923–32
Dollard, John	1934	The Psychotic Person Seen Culturally
Faris, Robert E.L.	1934	Cultural Isolation and the Schizophrenic Personality
Winston, Ellen	1935	The Assumed Increase of Mental Disease
Blumer, Herbert	1937	Social Disorganization and Individual Disorganization
Schilder, Paul	1937	The Relation Between Social and Personal Disorganization
Lawton, George	1938	The Study of Senescence: Psychiatric and Sociological Aspects
Jaffe, A.J., and Ethel Shanas	1939	Economic Differentials in the Probability of Insanity
French, Thomas M.	1939	Social Conflict and Psychic Conflict
Wittels, Fritz	1939	The Neo-Adlerians
Burgess, Ernest W.	1939	The Influence of Sigmund Freud Upon Sociology in the United States
Owen, Mary Bess, Robert E.L. Faris, and H. Warren Dunham	1941	Alternative Hypotheses for the Explanation of Some of Faris' and Dunham's Results

(continued)

APPENDIX 1. TABLE 1.2. *Continued*

Author(s)	Year	Title
Tietze, Christopher, Paul Lemkau, Marcia Cooper, and Ernest W. Burgess	1941	Schizophrenia, Manic-Depressive Psychosis and Social-Economic Status
Tietze, Christopher, Paul Lemkau, and Marcia Cooper	1942	Personality Disorder and Spatial Mobility
Schroeder, Clarence W.	1942	Mental Disorders in Cities
Dunham, H. Warren	1942	War and Personality Disorganizations
Dunham, H. Warren	1944	The Social Personality of the Catatonic-Schizophrene
Faris, Robert E.L.	1944	Reflections of Social Disorganization in the Behavior of a Schizophrenic Patient
Weinberg, S. Kirson	1946	The Combat Neuroses
Dunham, H. Warren, and Bernard N. Meltzer	1946	Predicting Length of Hospitalization of Mental Patients
Lunden, Walter A.	1947	Suicides in France, 1910–43
Gregory, W. Edgar	1947	The Chaplain and Mental Hygiene
Karpman, Ben	1947	A Psychiatrist Looks at the Social Scientists
Gough, Harrison G.	1948	A Sociological Theory of Psychopathy
Clark, Robert E.	1949	Psychoses, Income, and Occupational Prestige
Sutherland, Edwin H.	1950	The Diffusion of Sexual Psychopath Laws
McKeown, James Edward	1950	The Behavior of Parents of Schizophrenic, Neurotic, and Normal Children
Bonner, Hubert	1950	Sociological Aspects of Paranoia
Porterfield, Austin L.	1952	Suicide and Crime in Folk and in Secular Society
Bendix, Reinhard	1952	Compliant Behavior and Individual Personality
Straus, Jacqueline H., and Murray A. Straus	1953	Suicide, Homicide, and Social Structure in Ceylon
Clausen, John A., Melvin L. Kohn, and H. Warren Dunham	1954	The Ecological Approach in Social Psychiatry
Smith, Harvey L.	1957	Psychiatry in Medicine: Intra- Or Inter- Professional Relationships?
Simmons, Ozzie G., and James A. Davis	1957	Interdisciplinary Collaboration in Mental Illness Research
Gold, Martin	1958	Suicide, Homicide, and the Socialization of Aggression
Selvin, Hanan C.	1958	Durkheim's Suicide and Problems of Empirical Research
Bettelheim, Bruno	1959	Feral Children and Autistic Children
Gibbs, Jack P., and Walter T. Martin	1959	Status Integration and Suicide in Ceylon
Linn, Erwin L.	1959	Patients' Socioeconomic Characteristics and Release from a Mental Hospital
Porterfield, Austin L., and Jack P. Gibbs	1960	Occupational Prestige and Social Mobility of Suicides in New Zealand
Rosengren, William R.	1961	The Self in the Emotionally Disturbed
Rogler, Lloyd H., and August B. Hollingshead	1961	The Puerto Rican Spiritualist as a Psychiatrist
Wechsler, Henry	1961	Community Growth, Depressive Disorders, and Suicide
Becker, Ernest	1962	Socialization, Command of Performance, and Mental Illness

APPENDIX 1. TABLE 1.2. *Continued*

Author(s)	Year	Title
Sampson, Harold, Sheldon L. Messinger, and Robert D. Towne	1962	Family Processes and Becoming a Mental Patient
Lefton, Mark, Shirley Angrist, Simon Dinitz, and Benjamin Pasamanick	1962	Social Class, Expectations, and Performance of Mental Patients
Ikeda, Kiyoshi, Harry V. Ball, and Douglas S. Yamamura	1962	Ethnocultural Factors in Schizophrenia in the Japanese in Hawaii
Pearlin, Leonard I.	1962	Sources of Resistance to Change in a Mental Hospital
Cumming, Elaine, and Charles Harrington	1963	Clergyman as Counselor
Raphael, Edna E.	1964	Community Structure and Acceptance of Psychiatric Aid
Kandel, Denise Bystryn	1966	Status Homophily, Social Context, and Participation in Psychotherapy
Simon, Julian L.	1968	The Effect of Income on the Suicide Rate: A Paradox Resolved
Gibbs, Jack P.	1969	Marital Status and Suicide in the United States: A Special Test of the Status Integration Theory
Melbin, Murray	1969	Behavior Rhythms in Mental Hospitals
Gove, Walter R.	1970	Sleep Deprivation: A Cause of Psychotic Disorganization
Siegel, Bernard J.	1970	Defensive Structuring and Environmental Stress
Light, Jr., Donald W.	1972	Psychiatry and Suicide: The Management of a Mistake
Roman, Paul M.	1972	Sleep Deprivation, Drug Use, and Psychiatric Disorders
Miley, James D., and Michael Micklin	1972	Structural Change and the Durkheimian Legacy: A Macrosocial Analysis of Suicide Rates
Gove, Walter R., and Jeannette F. Tudor	1973	Adult Sex Roles and Mental Illness
Gove, Walter R.	1973	Sex, Marital Status, and Mortality
Clancy, Kevin, and Walter Gove	1973	Sex Differences in Mental Illness: An Analysis of Response Bias in Self-Reports
Light, Jr., Donald	1975	The Sociological Calendar: An Analytic Tool for Fieldwork Applied to Medical and Psychiatric Training
Barnes, Carl B.	1975	The Partial Effect of Income on Suicide is Always Negative
Simon, Julian L.	1975	Response to Barnes's Comment
Dinitz, Simon, Ann Davis, and Benjamin Pasamanick	1976	Comment on Braginsky's Review of Schizophrenics in the New Custodial Community
Dohrenwend, Bruce P., and Barbara Snell Dohrenwend	1976	Sex Differences and Psychiatric Disorders
Cooperstock, Ruth, and Penny Parnell	1976	Comment on Clancy and Gove
Seiler, Lauren H.	1976	Sex Differences in Mental Illness: Comment on Clancy and Gove's Interpretations
Gove, Walter R., and Kevin Clancy	1976	Response Bias, Sex Differences, and Mental Illness: A Reply
Pearlin, Leonard I., and Clarice W. Radabaugh	1976	Economic Strains and the Coping Function of Alcohol

(continued)

APPENDIX 1. TABLE 1.2. *Continued*

Author(s)	Year	Title
Gove, Walter R., and Michael R. Geerken	1977	Response Bias in Surveys of Mental Health: An Empirical Investigation
Gove, Walter R., and Jeanette Tudor	1977	Sex Differences in Mental Illness: A Comment on Dohrenwend and Dohrenwend
Dohrenwend, Bruce P., and Barbara Snell Dohrenwend	1977	Reply to Gove and Tudor's Comment on "Sex Differences and Psychiatric Disorders"
Webb, Stephen D., and John Collette	1977	Rural-Urban Differences in the Use of Stress-Alleviative Drugs
Roman, Paul M.	1978	Possible Effects of Using Alcohol to Control Distress: A Reanalysis of Pearlin and Radabaugh's Data
Pearlin, Leonard I., and Clarice W. Radabaugh	1978	The Sociological Study of a Social Problem: A Reply to Roman
Rosenberg, Morris, and Leonard I. Pearlin	1978	Social Class and Self-Esteem Among Children and Adults
Kett, Joseph F.	1978	Curing the Disease of Precocity
Rushing, William A., and Suzanne T. Ortega	1979	Socioeconomic Status and Mental Disorder: New Evidence and a Sociomedical Formulation
Phillips, David P.	1979	Suicide, Motor Vehicle Fatalities, and the Mass Media: Evidence Toward a Theory of Suggestion
Webb, Stephen D., and John Collette	1979	Rural-Urban Stress: New Data and New Conclusions
Miller, Joanne, Carmi Schooler, Melvin L. Kohn, and Karen A. Miller	1979	Women and Work: The Psychological Effects of Occupational Conditions
Eaton, William W.	1980	A Formal Theory of Selection for Schizophrenia
Mirowsky II, John, and Catherine E. Ross	1980	Minority Status, Ethnic Culture, and Distress: A Comparison of Blacks, Whites, Mexicans, and Mexican Americans
Hughes, Michael, and Walter R. Gove	1981	Living Alone, Social Integration, and Mental Health
Emerson, Robert M.	1981	On Last Resorts
Bollen, Kenneth A., and David P. Phillips	1981	Suicidal Motor Vehicle Fatalities in Detroit: A Replication
Phillips, David P.	1982	The Impact of Fictional Television Stories on U.S. Adult Fatalities: New Evidence on the Effect of Mass Media on Violence
Kohn, Melvin L., and Carmi Schooler	1982	Job Conditions and Personality: A Longitudinal Assessment of Their Reciprocal Effects
Demo, David H., and Ritch C. Savin-Williams	1983	Early Adolescent Self-Esteem as a Function of Social Class: Rosenberg and Pearlin Revisited
Carrier, James G.	1983	Masking the Social in Educational Knowledge: The Case of Learning Disability Theory
Ross, Catherine E., John Mirowsky, and Patricia Ulbrich	1983	Distress and the Traditional Female Role: A Comparison of Mexicans and Anglos
Johnson, David Richard, and Mary Holland Benin	1984	Ethnic Culture or Methodological Artifacts? A Comment on Mirowsky and Ross

APPENDIX 1. TABLE 1.2. *Continued*

Author(s)	Year	Title
Mirowsky, John, and Catherine E. Ross	1984	Meaningful Comparison Versus Statistical Manipulation: A Reply to Johnson and Benin
Kessler, Ronald C., and Horst Stipp	1984	The Impact of Fictional Television Suicide Stories on U.S. Fatalities: A Replication
McCarthy, John D., and Dean R. Hoge	1984	The Dynamics of Self-Esteem and Delinquency
Bachman, Jerald G., and Patrick M. O'Malley	1984	Black-White Differences in Self-Esteem: Are They Affected by Response Styles?
Naoi, Atsushi, and Carmi Schooler	1985	Occupational Conditions and Psychological Functioning in Japan
Thoits, Peggy A.	1985	Self-Labeling Processes in Mental Illness: The Role of Emotional Deviance
Mirowsky, John	1985	Depression and Marital Power: An Equity Model
Kaplan, Howard B., Steven S. Martin, and Robert J. Johnson	1986	Self-Rejection and the Explanation of Deviance: Specification of the Structure Among Latent Constructs
Breault, K.D.	1986	Suicide in America: A Test of Durkheim's Theory of Religious and Family Integration, 1933–1980
Link, Bruce G., Francis T. Cullen, James Frank, and John F. Wozniak	1987	The Social Rejection of Former Mental Patients: Understanding Why Labels Matter
Miller, Joanne, Kazimierz M. Slomczynski, and Melvin L. Kohn	1987	Authoritarianism as Worldview and Intellective Process: Reply to Ray
Gerard, Chris	1988	Church Membership and Suicide Reconsidered: Comment on Breault
Breault, K.D.	1988	Beyond the Quick and Dirty: Problems Associated with Analyses Based on Small Samples of Large Ecological Aggregates: Reply to Gerard
Schooler, Carmi	1988	The Psychological Effects of Traditional and of Economically Peripheral Job Settings in Japan
Faunce, William A.	1989	Occupational Status-Assignment Systems: The Effect of Status on Self Esteem
Kohn, Melvin L., Atsushi Naoi, Carrie Schoenbach, Carmi Schooler et al.	1990	Position in the Class Structure and Psychological Functioning in the United States, Japan, and Poland
Mirowsky, John, and Catherine E. Ross	1990	The Consolation-Prize Theory of Alienation
Hughes, Michael, and David H. Demo	1989	Self-Perceptions of Black Americans: Self-Esteem and Personal Efficacy
Idler, Ellen L., and Stanislav V. Kasl	1992	Religion, Disability, Depression, and the Timing of Death
Link, Bruce G., Mary Clare Lennon, and Bruce P. Dohrenwend	1993	Socioeconomic Status and Depression: The Role of Occupations Involving Direction, Control, and Planning
Parcel, Toby L., and Elizabeth G. Menaghan	1994	Early Parental Work, Family Social Capital, and Early Childhood Outcomes

(continued)

APPENDIX 1. TABLE 1.2. *Continued*

Author(s)	Year	Title
Miech, Richard A., Avshalom Caspi, Terrie E. Moffitt, Bradley R. Entner Wright, and Phil A. Silva	1999	Low Socioeconomic Status and Mental Disorders: A Longitudinal Study of Selection and Causation during Young Adulthood
Yabiku, Scott T., William G. Axinn, and Arland Thornton	1999	Family Integration and Children's Self-Esteem
Liska, Allen E., Fred E. Markowitz, Rachel Bridges Whaley, and Paul Bellair	1999	Modeling the Relationship Between the Criminal Justice and Mental Health Systems

2
Sociology, Psychiatry, and the Production of Knowledge about Mental Illness and Its Treatment

Leonard I. Pearlin, William R. Avison, and Elena M. Fazio

As in all areas of scientific activity, considerable change can be observed in what is known and what is assumed to be known about the causes and treatment of mental illness. Yet, while it can be asserted that our understanding of these matters is different now from what it was some decades ago, it is not a simple task to describe the changes or to identify the reasons for the directions they have taken. Part of the difficulty results from the fact that mental health and illness are large domains that draw the interests of multiple disciplines, each with it own shifting perspectives and agendas regarding causation and intervention. Among these disciplines, it is psychiatry and its allied bio-medical sciences whose causal conceptions and intervention stratagems have been most widely disseminated, accepted, and supported over the past 40 or 50 years. A major assumption that emerged within psychiatry over those years is that mental illness stems from the biological malfunctioning of individuals and, consequently, its amelioration is achieved by the biological modification of the organism through the use of drugs.

It might be asked why an examination of the changing contributions of the sociology of mental health should begin with a consideration of biological psychiatry. Partly it is because the paradigms that guide the work and thinking of biological psychiatry stand as useful points of comparison that help to define the sociology of mental health, its distinctive contributions to knowledge, and the conditions that influence its substantive directions. However, as we describe below, psychiatry and its reliance on biological explanations appear to be in the early stages of change. Indeed, we discuss later the possibility that the paradigmatic shifts that appear to be taking place in psychiatry will enlarge the niche within which the sociology of mental health does its work. This chapter, therefore, not only looks to the past and present in probing the production of knowledge and its underlying influences, but also speculates about the future.

An important caveat is in order at the outset. Beneath the generalities of some of our discussions is a great deal of diversity. Although these generalities might accurately describe major currents and themes within psychiatry or sociology, they are not always appropriate descriptions of individuals whose work lies within these disciplines. Biologically oriented psychiatrists, for example, may still see the utility of employing psychotherapeutic treatment, and those whose main calling is psychotherapy may not hesitate to place their faith in pharmaceutic interventions. It must be recognized, too, that many people engaged in psychiatric research are not psychiatrists but are, instead, geneticists, neuroscientists or other bio-medical personnel. No single statement can capture the range of substantive orientations and nuances encompassed by this diverse body of workers.

Although sociology does not have the disciplinary mix of psychiatry, it, too, is far from uniform in its interests. Thus, among sociologists whose work falls within the broad area of mental health, it is possible to identify social psychologists, social constructionists, epidemiologists, and scholars who champion either qualitative or quantitative methodologies. To note but a few of the interests spanning the field, there are such issues as stigma (Link, 1999), symbolic interaction (Rosenberg, 1992), exposure to stressors and hardships (Wheaton, 1994), and access to and utilization of health services (Aday, Fleming, & Andersen, 1984; Cook & Wright, 1995). Although our discussion focuses more on sociological research on the causes of mental health problems than on studies of the consequences of mental illness, this is not to suggest that the latter area of inquiry is unimportant. Indeed, other chapters in this volume document the contributions of sociological research on health services utilization (McAlpine & Boyer; Scheid & Greenberg) and the process of recovery from severe mental illness (Yanos, Knight & Roe). The extent of the differences *within* disciplines, however, should not obscure the profound differences that exist *between* them.

One of these differences, we submit, concerns the forces that have driven the changes that can be observed to have taken place in our knowledge and understanding of mental illness. A basic premise underlying our discussions, consistent with the sociology of knowledge (Merton, 1968), is that changes in scientific orientations come about not only through the thrust of discovery but also as a result of the changes in the social, economic, and institutional contexts in which fields of inquiry operate. Although the process of discovery within psychiatric research undoubtedly has contributed to changes in the understanding and knowledge of mental health, it is our view that in comparison to the sociology of mental health, changes in psychiatry have been driven at least as much by external forces as those that are internal to the field.

For its part, the sociology of mental health largely remains anchored to basic social theory. Over the decades, nevertheless, it has become cumulatively more sophisticated both in the basic knowledge it has produced and in the refinement of that knowledge. It is our contention, too, that the substance of this knowledge has been shaped more by forces internal to the discipline than by influences exerted by its external milieu - although sociology is certainly not insensitive to such influence. Beginning with a closer look at some of the fundamental contrasts in the perspectives of sociology and psychiatry, much of the remainder of this chapter presents arguments and evidence in support of these observations.

Sociology and Psychiatry: Some Paradigmatic Contrasts

Although the rather radical transformation through which psychiatry has gone in the past four or five decades resists simple descriptions, it is clear that there has been a movement from the couch to the laboratory. Correspondingly, etiological explanations that focused on psycho-social aspects of development in childhood have given way to those that are principally biological. This statement, it should be underscored, needs to be qualified by caveats noted above. First, it ignores the many individuals - practitioners and researchers alike – whose work embraces multiple perspectives or who otherwise are not part of the general historic trend toward biology. Second, it needs again to be reminded that not all psychiatric research is done by psychiatrists; the researchers whose work is devoted to the study of mental health and disorder are drawn from several fields, including genetics, the neurosciences, and biochemistry.

The professional diversity within the community of researchers and practitioners notwithstanding, a decided trend toward biological psychiatry can be detected. This is a marked departure from its major intellectual underpinning prior to and following World War II, an era in which psychoanalysis in its many modes was a prominent approach in the search for causal factors (Menninger, 1948). This search typically looks to painful experiences within important interpersonal relationships, especially those involving the family. Its major therapeutic tool, of course, is the uncovering of one's significant past and its connection to current psychological problems. This self knowledge, in turn, is presumed to ease the psychic pain and whatever disordered emotions and behavior might be associated with it.

Psychoanalytic orientations have largely been displaced by the causal assumptions underlying much of the thinking and practice of biological psychiatry. In contrast to scrutinizing the interpersonal history of the individual for the roots of disorder, biological psychiatry has tended in the past to begin and end its search for causation within the body. Correspondingly, its interventions are primarily aimed at pharmaceutically modifying the functioning of the biological substrata of the body, leaving individuals' external world out of the equation, both unexamined and, usually, unchanged. It can be recognized that these two types of mental health inquiry and practice contrast sharply not only with each other but also with the sociology of mental health, at least with regard to the search for the etiologies of disorder. Specifically, neither psychoanalysis nor biological psychiatry systematically considers large scale social arrangements and the conditions of life that result from them as particularly relevant to psychological disorder. In its effort to account for psychological disorder, sociologists are typically more interested in identifying social and economic conditions that help to account for the unequal distributions of disorders in community-based samples. The explanatory frameworks and intervention strategies of psychiatrists, whether at the couch or in the laboratory, are usually at a distance from such efforts.

As forewarned above, our sweeping description of psychiatry ignores the many nuances and pursuits that can be found within the profession, both as it once was and is currently becoming. Nevertheless, there can be no doubt that knowledge about disorder and treatment derived from cases on the couch has been joined, if not overtaken, by knowledge produced by the laboratory assay and clinical trials of biological and chemical materials (Kandel, 2005). In the course of the general transitions to biology and somatic interventions, the social environments of individuals and their experiences within these environments have faded from view. Without much exaggeration, it can be stated that biological psychiatry often separates mental disorder from its possible social and economic influences. As discussed later, changes in this regard appear to be underway; nevertheless, we believe that biological psychiatry has left and continues to leave a large gap in our understanding of the causes of disorder.

It is evident that the dramatic shifts that have occurred in psychiatry in the latter half of the last century place it at a pole that in critical respects is opposite that of the sociology of mental health. The contrast between the two disciplines can be clearly drawn by paraphrasing a position taken by C.W. Mills that has served for many years as an unspoken mantra of sociological investigators. Essentially, he asserted that the proper study of personal problems (i.e., mental disorder) is the study of social problems (Mills, 1959). To a substantial extent, sociological research into mental health implicitly echoes Mills in its effort to identify health-related hardships and stressors that are differentially found among people whose statuses in systems of inequality differ. The more this research can tell us about mental disorder and its distributions, the more we are able to learn about the larger society and the functions and dysfunctions of its social and economic arrangements. In this sense, mental disorder can truly serve as a social mirror, to borrow from the title of this book; it is a sensitive surface capable of reflecting social problems to which people are unequally exposed and the mental health consequences of these problems.

By contrast, the assumption that mental disorder originates in the brains or other malfunctioning organs of individuals effectively turns the Mills assertion on its head by implying that the proper study of social problems is the study of personal problems. That is, certain social problems – e.g., school failure, drug and alcohol abuse, premarital pregnancy and marital disruption, unemployment and occupational instability, domestic violence, homelessness, and criminality, to name a few – result from the aberrant dispositions or inadequacies of individuals. One might conclude from this sort of orientation that the treatment - or incarceration - of the deficient and troubled individuals is the way to rid the society of some of its noxious problems. Of course, it is reasonable to suppose that social problems may contribute to personal problems and, once established among large numbers of disadvantaged people, personal problems exacerbate those that are social.

There are many factors that potentially contribute to these polar positions in causal orientations, among them the evidence that there are, indeed, biological factors related to various disorders. The problem is that the evidence does not necessarily inform us as to the nature of the relationships or how they are formed. For example, biological factors may function as the mediating vehicle through which experiential circumstances impact mental health, or the same biological and experiential factors might interact with each other in a manner that undermines mental health or exacerbates mental disorder. Moreover, there may be instances in which both distress and biological functioning are each co-morbid consequences of socially rooted hardships. In any case, it is potentially misleading to jump to the assumption that biological factors that are correlated with disorder are the sole and exclusive cause of the disorder. Indeed, a growing body of studies indicate that it is unlikely that biological dispositions, genetic or otherwise, can qualify as the sole cause of any but few select disorders, such as Huntington's Chorea (Hayden, 2000). Indeed, studies indicate that many people possessing a gene or other bio-marker for a disorder do not, in fact, manifest the disorder (Roy-Byrne, 2005). Still other inquiries that are probing gene-environment interactions report that the expression of a biological condi-tion in mental disorder may require the presence of environmental and experi-ential conditions (Harris, 2005). Moreover, to support claims of sole causation it would be necessary to demonstrate that the distribution in the population of the genetic or other biological disposition is isomorphic with the epidemiologi-cal distribution of the disorder. Evidence for this kind of correspondence is understandably difficult to produce. In general, it appears that the fanfare with which the results of biological findings have often heralded is simply not warranted by the explanatory power of the findings (Merikangas & Risch, 2003). It may make for easy reading in the morning newspaper, but it can be misleading to the extent that it suggests that if X is present, Y must certainly follow. As sociological methodologists and researchers have repeatedly pointed out, X may be related to Y without being its primordial, direct, or unconditional cause (Aneshensel, 2002). As we discuss below, the questions and doubts currently being raised about the causal functions of biological factors point to directions for a line of inquiry that is likely to be undertaken by future sociological research into mental health.

We propose, then, that the weight of scientific discovery is insufficient by itself to account for the fascination with deterministic notions of the biological causes of mental disorder. As important as scientific discovery and developing technol-ogy have been in directing the trajectory of change in psychiatry, we believe it is necessary to look outside the profession itself in order to understand fully reasons for the changes that have taken place within it over the past several decades.

Social Change and the Production of Knowledge About Mental Disorder

It will be seen that some of the forces that have had a possible influential part in steering the course of psychiatry tend to be irrelevant to changes that can be discerned in the sociology of mental health. Specifically, it is our observation that the trajectories of psychiatry are more sensitive to influences external to the field than is the case for sociology. Though necessarily speculative, we submit that among the "outside" influences helping to illuminate the conditions behind the magnitude and direction of much of contemporary psychiatry are changes in the political and economic climate of the times. Keep in mind that if mental disorder is viewed as the consequence of faulty biological equipment of individuals, it logically follows that the prevention or amelioration of the disorder depends on the modification of the equipment. The responsibility for the correction falls to the professional worker and/or the faulty individual. This, of course, is sharply at odds with Mills' perspective, which would argue that since disorder is created by social problems, its prevention and amelioration depend on the correction of the social problems, a responsibility of the society and its institutions.

In the early years of the 21st century, Mills' perspectives and assumptions are likely to appear quite impractical and quixotic. However, there were circumstances in the not-too-distant past that made the assumption of these heavy responsibilities by the larger society more acceptable than is currently the case. Included among these circumstances, it seems, was the sense, not always spoken, that no problem was so great that it was beyond our national capabilities or resources to repair it, nor was any goal so remote that it was beyond our ability to reach it. This kind of collective understanding was probably nurtured both by the emergence of the Nation from the Great Depression and the determined national effort and enormous accomplishments that eventually led us to emerge from World War II as a victorious super power. It was further buttressed by the economic expansion that took place following the War. There was at the time of this era a spirit of collective empowerment and a highly optimistic view of the future that supported the widely accepted belief that as a nation we were able to achieve anything to which we seriously set our mind; no frontier was beyond our reach, including the moon. We do not want to idealize this era by creating the impression that it was a time of unblemished tranquility and optimism. In addition to hot and cold wars, there were many serious domestic problems that were dealt with inadequately or not at all, and it was a time, too, when people were demonized and persecuted for their political views. With it all, through much of the 1960s there were domestic programs and policies, however half-heartedly they might have been supported, that reflected a willingness to take on some responsibility for the correction of social problems and social injustices.

We have left this kind of ethos far behind us in the past 35 or 40 years. In more recent times the society has grown less certain of its ability to eliminate or ease institutionally rooted problems and, more important, it has substantially scaled back its sense of responsibility for the elimination or amelioration of these problems. Instead, it is argued that the causes and, therefore, the cures for what might ail individuals reside less in the problematic aspects of our social and economic arrangements than within the individuals themselves; troubled people are now more likely to be seen as needing to get their own acts together. As always, there are powerful interests that have a stake in keeping social and economic arrangements as they are and who are opposed to tinkering with what they believe is working in their behalf. Much of the research falling within biological psychiatry seems to be unreflectively congenial with—if not responsive to—these contemporary outlooks and values. At any rate, the heavy emphasis currently given to the biological underpinnings of mental disorder has certainly been consistent with current thinking about where personal problems begin and where responsibility for their amelioration lies. It's not the society and its institutions that bear some responsibility for psychologically troubled individuals; they are troubled either because their bodies have betrayed them or because they do not have the moral values or will to lift themselves from the ashes.

Of course, the correspondence between changes in prevailing values and ideologies and changes in the directions in which much of psychiatry seems to have moved is not meant to suggest that biology merely marched to the drumbeat of social and cultural changes over the past several decades. To the contrary, the discoveries of bio-markers and genes associated with disorder convince us that there may be biological concomitants of disorder and distress. As we argue above, what is questionable are the interpretations of these concomitants that place biological disorder as the primordial and sole cause of psychological disorder. The successful amelioration of disorders through pharmaceutical interventions, moreover, cannot by itself be taken as evidence of biological causation. Depression, for example, might be relieved by drugs that modify biological functioning, but this does not necessarily mean that the cause of the depression can be attributed to biological malfunctioning. The extent to which an exclusive causal role is imputed to biology represents a kind of explanatory imperialism that does not adequately bear the burden of close scrutiny. But it is an explanation whose support may in part stem from the fact that it does not go against the grain of contemporary values and political trends.

Although there is a correspondence between the shifts in the climate and values of the society and the faith that has been placed in biological psychiatry, it is unlikely that these shifts themselves have directly impacted the work or thinking of biological psychiatry. Whatever the association between macro changes in the society and those within the confines of psychiatry may be, it is likely that there was a confluence of other social, economic, and institutional circumstances that more directly and proximately influenced paradigmatic changes taken by the field. A circumstance that merits some consideration concerns the financial support for research into mental health, primarily as provided by the National Institute of Mental Health and its programs. One benchmark of change in this regard is provided by the support of social sciences in the intra-mural research program. Whereas these sciences once had a robust intellectual presence, they are now almost non-existent (see the chapter by Carmi Schooler). Moreover, it can be seen that the inclusion of social research in the extra-mural portfolio has decreased as the Institute's support for biological research increased (Kirk, 1999). Of course, the authorities at the National Institutes who establish programmatic directions do not and cannot make their decisions in isolation from surrounding institutions. In this regard, we are reminded that the Institutes are dependent on Congress and its committees, including those that regulate appropriations and budgets. One can understand that unlike the testimony they might have presented some decades earlier, Institute leaders who are seeking to justify their budget requests are reluctant to appear before Congressional bodies asking for money to pursue an agenda that focuses on social problems and their mental health consequences.

This does not mean that Institute authorities necessarily have serious reservations about biological psychiatry or that they are keeping their true feelings about the field expediently under wraps. To the contrary, there is reason to believe that the prevailing sentiment in that group has been one of strong and sincere commitment to biological psychiatry and its ability to explain mental disorder and treat mental illness. Indeed, this very commitment may unknowingly lead to a failure to accurately assess research findings and their implications. One example, documented by Horwitz (2005), concerns a public report issued by the NIMH about the results of a study of genetic contributions to the incidence of depression. Whereas the researchers in their published report were careful to emphasize that the expression of genes in depression depended on exposure to eventful stressors (Caspi, Sugden, Moffitt, Taylor, Craig, Harrington, McClay, Mill, Martin, Braithwaite, & Poulton, 2003), no mention of this was made in the announcement that was released. Instead, the announcement extolled the power of the genetic determination, while ignoring the experiential conditions regulating this power. We do not wish to imply that this kind of omission is deliberate, only that a scientific myopia is created by the uncritical devotion to the idea that the cause of depression lies entirely in the genes. Even where there is some acknowledgement that genetics alone is insufficient to account for mental illness, the attention given social factors is at most superficial. For example, Stephen Hyman, a former Director of NIMH, argues enthusiastically for psychiatric research that includes both genetic and environmental considerations (Hyman, 2000a) but his specification of what such a synthesis might look like is disappointingly sketchy (Hyman, 2000b; Kopnisky, Cowan, & Hyman, 2002). Thus, although Hyman (2000b) recognizes that advances in molecular biology and genomic science will require " ... greater attention to anatomy, physiology, pharmacology, and behavior" (p. 271), the value of attending to social structures and processes is noticeably missing.

Whatever the political and ideological influences may be, the elevation of biology and the diminished support for socially oriented research in the programs of NIMH to some extent stems from an effort to reestablish psychiatry as a strictly medical field. Like other medical specialties, it needed to establish diagnostic standards for the many disorders it recognizes; and also like other medical specialties, it looks to its various bio-medical allies to provide the "hard science" evidence for these disorders (Kirk, 1999). Planned or not, these trends have probably functioned to mark off a protected place for psychiatry that is separated from that occupied by other professions that are also engaged in the treatment of the persons with mentally illness. Clinical psychologists, psychiatric social workers, and people trained in counseling make up a large portion of the community of practitioners, especially those employing the talking therapies. A latent, if not intended, consequence of biologizing disorder is to distance psychiatry from fields that rely on psychotherapy as their modal treatment. When defined as a biological problem, mental disorder is understood as naturally demanding medical expertise and somatic intervention. Viewed from this perspective, no material reason can be found for psychiatric practitioners to take umbrage with their laboratory-based colleagues who have helped to create for them a protected niche in a competitive marketplace. Social and behavioral scientists, typically without a clientele to whom they provide professional services and on whom they must financially rely, are fortunately shielded from whatever marketplace influences befall psychiatry.

A related and crucial economic component in the nexus of conditions that have helped to redefine mental disorder and its causes concerns the conditions under which psychiatrists can be compensated for their work. One of these conditions concerns the length of time a patient may be treated for a disorder. Because a course of psychotherapy may require frequent sessions over an indefinite number of years, allowable compensation for this kind of treatment might be terminated before it is considered to be completed. From the vantage point of the patient/consumer, psychotherapy can eventually require individuals to rely more on their own deep pockets than on third-party payers. As a consequence, the practitioner who relies primarily on psychotherapy is more likely to be dependent on a clientele that is relatively affluent and, perhaps, fewer in number than that of a colleague relying mainly on somatic interventions. We do not wish to imply here that analytically oriented psychiatrists are exposed to economic hardships, for the compensation they receive from third-party payers is at a rate higher than that given non-psychiatrists who may be employing much the same treatment modality - other than having the right to prescribe medications. What we do suggest is that the emergence of biological psychiatry and its heavy reliance on somatic therapies can in part be interpreted as an adaptation to a system of compensation. Though not necessarily purposive or planned, modern psychiatry has taken a form congenial with economic constraints and imperatives that surround it.

The influence of insurers and managed care enterprises on the shaping of modern psychiatry can also be seen in their insistence that treatment and its compensation be for diagnostically specific ailments. Marital conflict, feelings of being an occupational failure, or a general ennui or dissatisfaction with life may motivate one to seek help, but unless a diagnostic tag can be attached to a complaint, it is unlikely that one's insurance—assuming one is fortunate enough to have insurance—will cover the cost. Psychiatry, in effect, was pressured to fall in line with other medical specialties by being more nosologically specific about the maladies it treats. The field seems to have responded to this pressure with a vengeance, producing in the Diagnostic and Statistical Manual a menu of hundreds of mental disorders (American Psychiatric Association, 2000). One consequence of tying compensation to diagnosis has been to edge psychiatry closer than it had been to main-stream medicine and its biological underpinnings. The advertisements sponsored by pharmaceutical companies exhorting people to ask their doctors if the pill they are marketing is good for what ails them is an additional force pushing psychiatry in this direction. And, of course, to those who ail, this marketing reinforces the understanding that their problem is one of biology and amenable to correction through biological interventions.

It is interesting that not only have consumers in general learned to accept biological psychiatry with a measure of uncritical faith, but persons with mental illness and their relatives may actively advocate in behalf of biological psychiatry. We refer in particular to relatives of persons with serious mental illness and others who have organized within the National Alliance on Mental Illness (1997) which tends to be in accord with the view of mental illness as a biologically rooted disease. It is understandable that family members who have reason to be sensitive to the stigma attached to mental illness would favor bio-medical explanations of mental illness. To the extent that stigma has a tone of moral condemnation and implies a notion of characterological degradation (Link, 1999; Scheff, 1966), the understanding of mental disorder as genetically driven may function to remove from the victim the onus of fault, willfulness, or moral shortcoming. Apparently, however, the branding of mental illness as a genetic anomaly, while associated with a greater understanding of the seriousness and persistence of the problem, also discourages close contact with siblings who are assumed to carry the same gene (Phelan, 2005).

The press and, to a lesser extent, other media, have also been partners in the definition and dissemination of psychological disorder as biologically determined (Conrad, 2001). Although they do not create the information, their uncritical acceptance of reports released by research groups and institutions about the genetic underpinnings of various disorders has helped to shape a public under-standing of mental illness as a product of flawed biology that can be corrected only by biological intervention. Such reports usually make easy-to-digest copy and the reader is not left to struggle with all of the uncertainties of heritability or the conditions that might regulate the influence of genetic factors. It is certainly less complicated, albeit more misleading, to assert baldly that researchers have found a gene that causes depression than to explain the complex interactions of genetic dispositions with disruptive events leading to depression. Again, the issue is not whether there are in fact biological concomitants of mental disorder but rather the exclusion from consideration of possible psycho-social influences and interventions.

Over recent decades, then, a kind of synergistic relationship seems to have developed among a number of forces external to psychiatry that have functioned to locate the causes and amelioration of mental disorder within the biological organism. As we have repeatedly emphasized, the purpose of these observations is not to deny or minimize the presence of biological factors in mental health and disorder, and certainly not to imply that somatic interventions systematically fail to relieve people of their inner miseries and dysfunctional behaviors. Instead, we have argued that there is a disconnect between the strength and persuasiveness of the evidence produced by biological psychiatry and the unquestioned acceptance and support it has received. If the directions taken by psychiatry over the past several decades cannot be explained solely by the impetus resulting from its discoveries, then it is reasonable to look at the possible role of external circum-stances, as we have done here, for explanations that help to account for its causal and treatment assumptions and their widespread acceptance. This is more than an irrelevant exercise. To the extent that the directions taken by psychiatry have led to the belief that the sources of people's mental health problems reside exclu-sively under the skin, they have had the consequence of diverting attention from social and economic problems and their deleterious impact on mental health.

This diversion is not consistent with what sociologists and others know about the etiology of disorder and it does not bode well for the creation of serious policies aimed at the prevention of disorder.

Continuities and Change in the Sociological Study of Mental Health

We now turn our focus from psychiatry to a more direct examination of the sociology of mental health, considering at a later point the possibility of strategic partnerships between the two fields. Our assessment of continuities and changes in the sociological study of mental health is not meant to be exhaustive. In the following discussion, we tend to focus somewhat more on issues concerning the social determinants of mental health than on developments related to the social consequences of mental illness. This should not be interpreted to imply that there is only limited sociological interest in research on the social sequelae of mental illness; recent reviews of the literature clearly attest to the contrary (Cook & Wright 1985; Mechanic, Schlesinger & McAlpine, 1995). Rather, our tendency to focus on research on the structural influences on mental health and illness admittedly reflects our own research interests and expertise.

At the outset, we can observe that there seems to be more continuity than change in sociology and the changes that have occurred appear to result more from the internal growth and sophistication of the field than from external social, cultural, political, and economic factors. However, the continuities that can be observed in the sociology of mental health should not be exaggerated, for considerable change can be observed in the substance and methods of the field. Probably one of the more dramatic changes took place in the latter part of the 1950s when the introduction of psychotropic drugs suddenly and completely brought to a halt studies of mental hospital organization and therapeutic communities. If Goffman had waited a few years, he would not have had the opportunity to write his piece on "the total institution" (Goffman, 1961). With a stroke on the prescription pad, the rather lively research into the complex relationships among hospital personnel and patients came to a halt. This remains a striking instance of how a technological innovation can impact an area of scientific inquiry.

It is certainly possible to track other changes that were once of great interest to sociologists but have largely disappeared from current literature. For example, organizational studies of the mental hospital (Stanton & Schwartz, 1954) have been casualties of the advent of psychotropic drugs and the ensuing transfer of persons with the mentally illness to the community (Brown, 1985). The identification of pathways to the mental hospital that was once an area of inquiry (Clausen & Yarrow, 1955) has largely disappeared, although there appears some revived interest in the links between community integration and social networks and service utilization (Pescosolido, Gardner, & Lubell, 1998). The earlier excitement about community mental health centers is virtually extinct, probably because their financial support has diminished and because treatment, where available, is more routinized, limited, and impersonal. It can further be observed that the very important community-and clinically-based studies, conducted as early as the 1930s (Faris & Dunham, 1939) and extending into the 1960s (Leighton, Harding, Macklin, Macmillan, & Leighton, 1963; Srole, Langner, Michael, Opler, & Rennie, 1962) seem to have given way to larger scale surveys. There are several possible reasons for these methodological shifts. One is that surveys, by casting a wide net, enable researchers to examine in some detail the multivariate worlds of people and the circumstances that connect their multiple statuses to their well-being. Another reason, difficult to exaggerate, concerns the availability of NIH financial support for the substantial costs of survey research.

Despite these and other notable alterations in the issues that have captured the attention of sociologists, there are current research concerns whose beginnings can be traced back to the earliest days of an emergent sociology of mental health. Some of these involve issues such as stigma and labeling (Link, 1999; Scheff, 1966), the legal system (Hiday, 1992), access to and utilization of care (Polgar & Morrissey, 1999), and the influence of social factors on diagnostic judgments (Brown, 1995; Loring & Powell, 1988). It is probably the search for etiologies of mental illness that has been most consistently a center of effort of sociological research. The starting point for much of the sociological studies of etiology has remained essentially as it was from the beginning: namely, the repeated observations that the incidence and prevalence of various mental and physical disorders are associated with people's status locations within social and economic systems (Eaton, 2000). It is the existence of such associations that provide much of the *raison d'etre* for a sociology of mental health. They signal that there is something about these hierarchically ordered statuses and their impact on the organization of experience that can result in mental disorder. If there were no associations between status placement and mental disorder, conversely, there would be far less to invite the scrutiny of sociologists.

Compared to psychiatry, then, the sociology of mental health has largely stayed the course, persistently engaged in the effort to explicate the status-disorder associations. There are several reasons for this continuity and why the sociology of mental health has not been influenced by the same external forces that have contributed to a changed psychiatry. First, sociologists are likely to be resistant to ideologies that point to individuals as significantly responsible for their own fates, either because of their willfulness or biological shortcomings. It is not simply because we are better or wiser than psychiatrists or others; rather, it is because such ideologies go against the fundamental theoretical and empirical grains of our discipline. To adopt an understanding of disorder as stemming from a game of biological roulette played by random individuals is simply inconsistent with what is known of the social patterns of a variety of disorders or with our theories of their social causation. Sociologists of mental health are not all of the same mind set in these regards, by any means, but some of the assumptions and implications underlying a biological psychiatry are fundamentally the antithesis of our disciplinary foundations.

A second and equally important reason for the basic continuities in the socio logy of mental health is that we are not exposed to the economic forces that act upon psychiatry (and other medical specialties). It is their good fortune that sociologists do not have a clientele nor do they depend for their sustenance on third-party payers. To the extent that academic scholars are able to follow their own intellectual noses without jeopardizing their livelihood, they are indeed in an enviable position. However, though different from practicing psychiatrists in this respect, the ability of sociologists to pursue their interests unfettered by extraneous forces may be somewhat constrained. For example, those of us largely dependent on NIH for the resources needed to pursue our interests may adapt our thinking and methods in ways that we believe will strengthen our chances for winning support in the competition for grants. Perhaps in some sub-tle and non-purposive ways our work does come to reflect these considerations, possibly in submitting proposals in response to program announcements in which we have but limited interest, or in including measures that seem to be in vogue with other disciplines and perspectives, or in avoiding ideas that may be innovative but carry considerable risk of failure.

Despite reliance on external funding, being comparatively shielded from extraneous marketplace demands means that many of the changes that can be noted in our specialty stem primarily from the refinement of knowledge and ideas and of methodological advances. With regard to the investigation of social factors contributing to disorder, a major development has been the heightened attention given to exposure to stressors and hardships as major harbingers of disorder. Research into life events during the 1960's and 1970's was an important spur to the emergence of this emphasis (Dohrenwend & Dohrenwend, 1974; Holmes & Rahe, 1967). Eventful experiences appeared at first blush to be amenable to easy and unambiguous measurement, and, moreover, there was some theoretical ratio-nale for their influence on well-being - namely, biological homeostasis (Selye, 1982). Most important, early investigations of life events turned up evidence that they mattered to psychological and physical health (Rahe, 1974). While still having a prominent place in stress research, the initial enthusiasm for research into life events and their effects on well-being leveled off as more was learned about the various methodological issues surrounding their measurement and as it became evident that many "events" more clearly reflect exposure to chronic or repeated stressors (Thoits, 1983).

Coextensive with the research into life events, the attentions of mental health researchers were branching out in a pair of related directions. One took into consideration not only disruptive life events as stressors but also the more chronic or repeated hardships, which, in fact, may occasionally be either consequences or forerunners of disruptive events. A second direction was toward what are referred to as moderating conditions, the resources that can protect people from the mental health impact of stressors. Coping and social support have had leading parts in this line of inquiry, joined in more recent years by certain self concepts and reli-gious beliefs and practices. A question that continues to guide much contempo-rary sociological research asks why people exposed to the same stressors do not necessarily manifest the same mental health consequences. Researchers often turn to differences in the possession of these protective resources to explain variations in mental health outcomes.

Paralleling some of these developments, finally, was the effort to bring some conceptual unity to the complex and changing interrelationships among people's socio-economic statuses, the various stressors to which they might be exposed, the social, personal, and material resources they are able to mobilize, and the mental health outcomes. The construction of an over-arching conceptual framework that includes these diverse components can be recognized as bearing the label of "the stress process" (Pearlin, Menaghan, Lieberman, & Mullan, 1981). The framework has been useful not only in providing a general view of the social and economic etiology of mental disorders, but also as it has been used in the study of particular status groups, institutions, and neighborhood contexts (Aneshensel & Sucoff, 1996; Schieman, 2005). Although the stress process framework has been widely adopted, it remains a work in progress with its components and their dynamic interrelationships undergoing continued elaboration and refinement.

It should be underscored that some conceptual and measurement issues stubbornly persist. One that deserves mention concerns the considerable uncertainty as to what represents reasonable indicators of mental health outcomes in sociological studies (Horwitz, 2002). First of all, although we are identified as sociologists of mental *health*, we deal immeasurably more with *illness* than health and, in fact, seem to know little about the latter. The one thing of which we can be fairly certain is that health is not merely the absence of illness. It also needs to be recognized that the constructs of mental illness, distress, or disorder are umbrellas for many different conditions. Indeed, in this paper we have been using the more generic terms, although they subsume a variety of mental dysfunctions that differ considerably in their nature and extent of the disabilities they entail. There is no doubt that we need to give greater consideration to the rationale for selecting the outcomes we choose to observe and, as others have urged, to expand the range of those that are employed in our inquiries (Aneshensel, Rutter, & Lachenbruch, 1991). This task goes beyond the debate as to whether we should use diagnostic criteria or symptom scales as dependent variables. It is more a matter of identifying measures that help to reveal whether different outcomes have different social and experiential precursors, whether the same precursors have multiple outcomes, and whether outcomes of the same precursors vary among people having different social and economic characteristics.

By no means should this be taken to suggest that we need to take into consideration all of the mental maladies found within the Diagnostic and Statistical Manual; many, if not most, have but limited incidence and/or are randomly distributed in the population, placing them outside sociological inquiry. If, as we believe, much of the business of sociologists of mental health is to understand the consequences of social arrangements for people's lives, we need to think more carefully about the range and specificity of consequences that best reveal what it is about these arrangements that is functional or dysfunctional and for whose well-being they are likely to matter.

There can be little doubt that our substantive knowledge about these complex issues has appreciably expanded over the past two or three decades. Much more is now known about mental health/illness and its many social influences and consequences. This expansion is the result of more conceptual specification, of greater methodological sophistication, and of the process whereby one question leads to others. Some of these questions to which the field has been led involve a more detailed examination of certain status groups. Thus, a perusal of the contents of the *Journal of Health and Social Behavior*, a major outlet for sociological research reports, reveals an increase in recent decades of investigations into gender and race/ethnicity and the health-related conditions that cluster around these statuses. What also stands as distinctly sociological areas of interest are studies that look for sources of stress and disorder within major institutional spheres such as family (Avison, 1999), occupation (Tausig, 1999), and economy (Kahn & Fazio, 2005). It is potentially useful to focus on the institutional domains in which exposure to stressors occurs because their impact on mental health may depend not only on the particular stressors they engender but also on the importance of the social institutions in which they arise.

Even as the scope of sociological investigations has expanded in recent decades, it appears that this has also been a period in which there has been considerable consolidation of knowledge. Specifically, there has been a steady accrual of new and refined information, but around issues and questions guided by theories and concepts that are largely unchanged. This observation is certainly open to challenge, but it does seem that despite knowing more, the way we think about the influences of social, economic, and experiential circumstances on mental health remains essentially unchanged over the past quarter century. We assume that research contributions of the sociology of mental health—or, for that matter, of any field of inquiry—can be described as being of two types. One expands our substantive knowledge of the field and the other changes the ways in which we think about the field. Even as our knowledge grows, we submit, the fundamental perspectives that guide our work remain essentially unchanged.

Anticipated Changes

What about the future of the sociology of mental health? At the outset, we disavow any special capacity to peer into the future; nevertheless, we offer some conjectures. First, it can be anticipated that the alliance between sociology and psychiatry will be expanded. There has always been some partnership between the two, largely formed by the expertise sociologists have brought and continue to bring to the epidemiological study of various disorders (Kessler, McGonagle, Zhao, Nelson, Hughes, Eshleman, Wittchen, & Kendler, 1994). This is an area of activity where psychiatry needs sociology; indeed, it is difficult to imagine that the training and experience of psychiatrists would enable them to construct and carry out by themselves large scale epidemiological inquiries involving representative samples.

There is another and equally important partnership that should grow in the future. Although, as we have argued, the deterministic role of biological factors in disorder is often exaggerated and not fully understood, we also have considerable faith in the self-correcting course of science. This faith is supported by the increasing indications that corrections are beginning to appear in bits and pieces, enough to arouse the sense that an uncritical embrace of mechanical biological causation is beginning to weaken. As in the case described by Horwitz (2005), evidence is likely to accumulate that expression of genetic and other biological dispositions in mental disorder, to the extent that they exist at all, depends on exposure to stressful life conditions. Indeed, there are interesting research reports that the very activation or inhibition of genetic influences may depend on exposure to stressful conditions; that is, the dispositional properties of genes may be closed down or stimulated by experiential factors (Kendler, Kessler, Walters, Maclean, Neale, Heath, & Eaves, 1995; Plomin & McGuffin, 2003). Even schizophrenia among adults may have intermingled biological and experiential roots. Thus, for example, there is some evidence that rates of schizophrenia are greater among those who in their earlier years faced conditions of famine (St. Clair, Xu, Wang, Yu, Fang, Zhang, Zheng, Gu, Feng, Sham, & He, 2005). Somewhat different but similarly interesting is research showing that a host of biological functions among members of different troops of the same species of primates, such as chimpanzees and baboons, vary with the stressful aspects of their social organization and the enforcement of authority hierarchies (Sapolsky, 2005). Whatever the inherent biological dispositions of the species may be, their activation and expression is shaped by their social and experiential milieu. The idea is certainly not new that social life and biological functioning are closely bound; there is a large literature documenting these bonds and the accumulated loads they impose on the organism (Seeman, McEwen, Rowe, & Singer, 2001). What is notable are the early signs that the recognition of these connections is beginning to penetrate and modify uncritical thinking about biology as the primordial and sole cause of mental illness.

The possibility of expanding our understanding of the convergence of experience structured by social arrangements and biological dispositions as they lead to mental disorder is quite exciting. But this possibility also places a burden on the sociologist of mental health. For example, the linkages between people's statuses in systems of inequality, and the health-related stressors and hardships that are associated with these statuses are quite complex and their influences on well-being may evolve over a considerable time span. It can be recognized that the chain of conditions that eventually come to be reflected in mental health and disorder can only be as strong as its weakest link. Our burden as sociologists is to specify in detail what is included in the global term "environment" within the gene/environment interaction. This is a task that can no more be left to the biologists than the exploration of the brain be left to sociologists. The complex human genome and its many thousands of biochemical components have been mapped and what awaits is a similar mapping of the equally complex macro and micro milieu that help to shape psychological development. In short, as social scientists it is up to us to conceptualize, identify, and measure appropriately the web of cultural, socio-economic, and experiential conditions that interact with or help to direct whatever biological dispositions to disorder there might be. It behooves us to insure that the links on the sociological side of the equation are at least equally robust as those on the biological and mental health sides. If we fail at this, we invite the erroneous conclusion that it is only the biology of people that matters to their mental health, not the nature of their socially and economically structured experiences.

The expansion of collaborative endeavors between sociologists and biologically oriented mental health researchers, then, has the potential to uncover the evolving interconnections between people's external social and economic circumstances and their internal biological circumstances as forerunners of mental disorder. Should such collaboration be successful, it is our guess is that it will be found that the social/experiential/biological interconnections are relevant not only to mental well-being and disorder, but to physical health and illness as well. Others appear to share this view. Thus, in their review of the effects of maternal behavior on defensive responses to threat and reproductive behavior among a variety of animal species, Cameron, Champagne, Parent, Fish, Ozaki-Kuroda, & Meaney (2005) find substantial evidence that challenged environments influence maternal-offspring behaviors. In turn, these interactions affect gene expression in the brain regions that control defensive and reproductive behaviors. They argue that the overwhelming weight of the evidence suggests that parental care influences gene expression and thus may affect health and well-being over the lifespan. In discussing the implications of this research for human health, they conclude that "ultimately, we will need to contend with the reality that neural development, function, and health are defined by social and economic influences, and that the success of interventions that ignore such forces will be seriously limited" (p. 860).

The separation of research into mental and physical health is to a substantial extent an artifact of the organization of the National Institutes of Health and does not reflect the intimate relationships between mental and physical well-being. It is likely, for example, that the very conditions that are inimical to mental health also have adverse consequences for physical health, though these effects might not become observable at the same time. Additionally, mental and physical health can exert mutual effects on one another. It is easily understood that a sustained threat to physical health, for example, will have mental health consequences, but it is also likely that sustained anxiety will take a toll on various biological sub-strata of the body, eventually undermining physical health. As far as sociology is concerned, an inclusive approach to well-being is reflective of the inseparability of mental and physical health. Sociological research into mental health will and should continue, but its process by which it comes to interface with physical health needs to come under closer scrutiny.

Still peering into the future, it is a good bet that sociologists engaged in research into health will place their work within a life-course context (George, 1999). Regardless of whether we are studying mental or physical health or both, there is now persuasive evidence that the health and mortality disparities that can observed among adults and elders are the consequence of conditions that evolve across the entirety of people's lives (Kahn & Fazio, 2005) and across family generations (McLeod, Nonnemaker, & Thiede Call, 2004). Indeed, some of the conditions that are eventually reflected in people's health may be in place prior to their births, including the household composition of the family of origin and parental educational and economic attainment. Sociologists, we believe, can make unique contributions to our understanding of health and health disparities by illuminating how the organization of the larger society and its institutional arrangements can structure the experiences of individuals at every stage of their lives and by demonstrating how these experiences, in turn, are related to health and its biological sub-strata.

Those of us who have been involved in research into mental health over the years have had the opportunity to be part of an exciting effort that has resulted in what is now a fairly mature specialty. While there may be periods where we seem to be carried along by the force of momentum, the future is no less challenging or exciting than the past.

Acknowledgment. This work is supported by NIA grant R01AG17461 (Leonard I. Pearlin, P.I.).

References

Aday, L. A., Fleming, G. F., & Andersen, R. (1984). *Access to medical care in the U.S.: Who has it, who doesn't.* Chicago: Pluribus Press.

American Psychiatric Association. (2000). *Diagnostic and statistical manual of mental disorders* (4th ed.). Washington, D. C.: American Psychological Association.

Aneshensel, C. S. (2002). *Theory-based data analysis for the social sciences.* Thousand Oaks, CA: Pine Forge.

Aneshensel, C. S., Rutter, C. M., & Lachenbruch, P. A. (1991). Social structure, stress, and mental health: Competing conceptual and analytic models. *American Sociological Review, 56,* 166–178.

Aneshensel, C. S., & Sucoff, C. A. (1996). The neighborhood context of adolescent mental health. *Journal of Health and Social Behavior, 37*(4), 293–310.

Avison, W. R. (1999). Impact of mental illness on the family. In C. S. Aneshensel, & J. C. Phelan (Eds.), *Handbook of the sociology of mental health* (p. 495). New York: Kluwer Academic/Plenum Publishers.

Brown, P. (1985). *Psychiatric deinstitutionalization and its aftermath.* London: Routledge and Kegan Paul.

Brown, P. (1995). Naming and framing: The social construction of diagnosis and illness. *Journal of Health and Social Behavior,* Extra Issue, 34–52.

Cameron, N. M., Champagne, F. A., Parent, C., Fish, E. W., Ozaki-Kuroda, K., & Meaney, M. J. (2005). The programming of individual differences in defensive responses and reproductive strategies in the rat through variations in maternal care. *Neuroscience and Biobehavioral Reviews, 29,* 843–865.

Caspi, A., Sugden, K., Moffitt, T. E., Taylor, A., Craig, I. W., Harrington, H., McClay, J., Mill, J., Martin, J., Braithwaite, A., & Poulton, R. (2003). Influence of life stress on depression: Moderation by a polymorphism in the 5-HTT gene. *Science, 301,* 386–389.

Clausen, J. A., & Yarrow, M. R. (1955). Paths to the mental hospital. *Journal of Social Issues, 11,* 25–32.

Conrad, P. (2001). Genetic optimism: Framing genes and mental illness in the news. *Culture, Medicine and Psychiatry, 25*, 225–247.

Cook, J. A., & Wright, E. R. (1995). Medical sociology and the study of severe mental illness: Reflections on past accomplishments and directions for future research. *Journal of Health and Social Behavior,* Extra Issue, 95–114.

Dohrenwend, B. S., & Dohrenwend, B. P. (1974). *Stressful life events—their nature and effects.* New York: John Wiley.

Eaton, W. W. (2000). *The sociology of mental disorders* (Third ed.). New York: Greenwood.

Faris, R. E. L., & Dunham, H. W. (1939). *Mental disorders in urban areas.* Chicago: University of Chicago Press.

George, L. K. (1999). Life course perspectives on mental health. In C. S. Aneshensel, & J. C. Phelan (Eds.), *Handbook of the sociology of mental health* (pp. 565–583). New York: Kluwer Academic/Plenum Publishers.

Goffman, E. (1961). *Asylums.* Garden City, NY: Anchor.

Harris, J. R. (2005). Introduction. *Journals of Gerontology: Series B Psychological Sciences and Social Sciences, 60B,* 5–6.

Hayden, M. R. (2000). Predictive testing for Huntington's disease: The calm after the storm. *The Lancet, 356,* 1944–1945.

Hiday, V. A. (1992). Civil commitment and arrests: an investigation of the criminalization thesis. *Journal of Nervous and Mental Disease, 180,* 184–191.

Holmes, T. H., & Rahe, R. H. (1967). The social readjustment rating scale. *Journal of Psychosomatic Research, 11,* 213–218.

Horwitz, A. H. (2002). Outcomes in the sociology of mental health and illness: Where have been and where are we going? *Journal of Health and Social Behaviour, 43,* 143–151.

Horwitz, A. V. (2005). Media portrayals and health inequalities: A case study of characterizations of gene x environment interactions. *Journals of Gerontology Series B: Psychological Sciences & Social Sciences, 60B,* 48–52.

Hyman, S. E. (2000a). The millennium of mind, brain, and behavior. *Archives of General Psychiatry, 57,* 88–89.

Hyman, S. E. (2000b). National Institute of Health goals for behavioral science. *Experimental and Clinical Pharmacology, 8,* 271–272.

Kahn, J. R., & Fazio, E. M. (2005). Economic status over the life course and racial disparities in health. *Journal of Gerontology: Series B: Psychological Sciences and Social Sciences, 60B,* 76–84.

Kandel, E. R. (2005). *Psychiatry, psychoanalysis, and the new biology of mind.* Washington, DC: American Psychiatric Publishing.

Kendler, K. S., Kessler R. C., Walters, E. E., Maclean, C., Neale, N. C., Heath, A. C., & Eaves, L. J. (1995). Stressful life events, genetic liability, and onset of an episode of major depression in women. *American Journal of Psychiatry, 152,* 833–842.

Kessler, R. C., McGonagle, K. A., Zhao, S., Nelson, C. B., Hughes, M., Eshleman, S., Wittchen, H.-U., & Kendler, K. S. (1994). Lifetime and 12-month prevalence of DSM-III-R psychiatric disorders in the United States. *Archives of General Psychiatry, 51,* 8–19.

Kirk, S. A. (1999). Instituting madness: The evolution of a federal agency. In C. S. Aneshensel, & J. C. Phelan (Eds.), *Handbook of the sociology of mental health.* New York: Kluwer Academic/Plenum Publishers.

Kopnisky, K. L., Cowan, W. M., & Hyman, S. E. (2002). Levels of analysis in psychiatric research. *Development and Psychopathology, 14,* 437–461.

Leighton, D. C., Harding, J. S., Macklin, D. B., Macmillan, A. M., & Leighton, A. H. (1963). *The character of danger: Psychiatric symptoms in selected communities*. New York: Basic Books.

Link, B. G. (1999). Labeling and stigma. In C. S. Aneshensel, & J. C. Phelan (Eds.), *Handbook of the sociology of mental health* (pp. 481–494). New York: Kluwer Academic/ Plenum Publishers.

Loring, M., & Powell, B. (1988). Gender, race, and DSM-III: A study of the objectivity of psychiatric diagnostic behavior. *Journal of Health and Social Behavior*, *29*, 1–22.

McLeod, J. D., Nonnemaker, J. M., & Thiede Call, K. (2004). Income inequality, race, and child well-being: An aggregate analysis in the 50 United States. *Journal of Health and Social Behavior*, *45*, 249–264.

Mechanic, D., Schlesinger, M., & McAlpine, D. D. (1995). Management of mental health and substance abuse services: State of the art and early results. *Milbank Quarterly*, *73*, 19–55.

Menninger, W. C. (1948). *Psychiatry in a troubled world: Yesterday's war and today's challenge*. New York: Macmillan.

Merikangas, K. R., & Risch, N. (2003). Will the genomics revolution revolutionize psychiatry? *American Journal of Psychiatry*, *160*, 625–635.

Merton, R. K. (1968). *Social theory and social structure*. New York: The Free Press.

Mills, C. W. (1959). *The sociological imagination*. New York: Oxford University Press.

National Alliance on Mental Illness. *About mental illness* (1997). (January 11, 2006); http://www.nami.org/Content/NavigationMenu/Inform_Yourself/About_Mental_Illness/ About_Mental_Illness.htm.

Pearlin, L. I., Menaghan, E. G., Lieberman, M. A., & Mullan, J. T. (1981). The stress process. *Journal of Health and Social Behavior*, *22*(4), 337–356.

Pescosolido, B. A., Gardner, C. B., & Lubell, K. M. (1998). How people get into mental health services: Stories of choice, coercion and "muddling through" from "first-timers." *Social Science and Medicine*, *46*, 275–286.

Phelan, J. C. (2005). Geneticization of deviant behavior and consequences for stigma: The case of mental illness. *Journal of Health and Social Behavior*, *46*, 307–322.

Plomin, R., & McGuffin, P. (2003). Psychopathology in the postgenomic era. *Annual Review of Psychology*, *54*, 205–228.

Polgar, M. F., & Morrissey, J. P. (1999). Mental health services and systems. In C. S. Aneshensel, & J. C. Phelan (Eds.), *Handbook of the Sociology of Mental Health* (pp. 461–479). New York: Kluwer Academic/Plenum Publishers.

Rahe, R. H. (1974). Life change and subsequent illness reports. In E. E. K. Gunderson, & R. H. Rahe (Eds.), *Life stress and illness* (pp. 58–78). Springfield, Illinois: Charles C. Thomas.

Rosenberg, M. (1992). *The unread mind: Unraveling the mystery of madness*. New York: Lexington Books.

Roy-Byrne, P. (2005). Epigenetic effects: A new way of explaining phenotypic differences in monozygotic twins. *Journal Watch Psychiatry*, *817*, 1.

Sapolsky, R. M. (2005). The influence of social hierarchy on primate health. *Science*, *30B*, 648–652.

Scheff, T. J. (1966). *Being mentally ill: A sociological theory*. Chicago: Aldine.

Schieman, S. (2005). Residential stability and the social impact of neighborhood disadvantage: a study of gender- and race-contingent effects. *Social Forces*, *83*, 1031–1064.

Seeman, T. E., McEwen, B. S., Rowe, J. W., & Singer, B. H. (2001). Allostatic load as a marker of cumulative biological risk: McArthur studies of successful aging. *Proceedings of the National Academy of Science*, *98*, 4770–4775.

Selye, H. (1982). History and present status of the stress concept. In L. Goldberger, & S. E. Breznitz (Eds.), *Handbook of stress* (pp. 7–17). New York: Free Press.

Srole, L., Langner, T. S., Michael, S. T., Opler, M. K., & Rennie, T. A. C. (1962). *Mental health in the metropolis: The midtown Manhattan study*. McGraw.

St Clair, D., Xu, M., Wang, P., Yu, Y., Fang, Y., Zhang, F., Zheng, X., Gu, N., Feng, G., Sham, P., & He, L. (2005). Rates of adult schizophrenia following prenatal exposure to the Chinese famine of 1959–1961. *The Journal of the American Medical Association*, *294*, 557–562.

Stanton, A., & Schwartz, M. (1954). *The mental hospital: A study of institutional participation in psychiatric illness and treatment*. New York: Basic Books.

Tausig, M. (1999). Work and mental health. In C. S. Aneshensel, & J. C. Phelan (Eds.), *Handbook of the sociology of mental health* (pp. 255–274). New York: Kluwer Academic/ Plenum Publishers.

Thoits, P. A. (1983). Dimensions of life events that influence psychological distress: An evaluation and synthesis of the literature. In H.B. Kaplan (Ed.), *Psychological stress: Trends in theory and research* (pp. 33–103). New York: Academic Press.

Wheaton, B. (1994). Sampling the stress universe. In W. R. Avison & I. H. Gotlib (Eds.), *Stress and mental health: Contemporary issues and prospects for the future* (pp. 77–114). New York: Plenum Publishing Corporation.

3
The Changing Role(s) of Sociology (and Psychology) in the National Institute of Mental Health Intramural Research Program

Carmi Schooler

This chapter details the history of the Laboratory of Socioenvironmental Studies (LSES) of the Intramural Research Program (IRP) of the National Institute of Mental Health (NIMH) – a topic that might at first glance seem of little interest to any but the relatively few who were part of that history. Nevertheless, for better or for worse, the history of the Laboratory is of very direct relevance to the field of sociology and of particular relevance to sociologists interested in mental health. The nature of the Laboratory's accomplishments illustrate what sociological researchers working within a government research setting, especially one focused on mental health issues, can add to our theoretical and practical knowledge of how environmental factors, especially those affected by a society's social structure, can affect normal and abnormal human functioning.

The history of the LSES's decline in size and resources provides an example of the problems that sociology faces in establishing and maintaining itself in present-day governmental and academic scientific settings, particularly biomedical ones. Furthermore, this example is not a trivial one, the intramural research programs of the National Institutes of Health (NIH), although not always well-known or under-stood outside of the NIH, are generally seen within the NIH as the most prestigious units within the various Institutes. Their relative successes and failures often appear to have a notable effect on the programmatic directions of the NIH programs that fund academic research. More generally, gaining some understanding of the chang-ing currents of scientific thought and medical values underlying the history and predicament of the LSES within the NIMH IRP tells us something of the nature of the losses that would occur, not only to sociology, but also to various of the 'sup-posedly' harder medical and biological sciences, should sociological research be substantially down-sized. As I hope I will make clear, such down-sizing would be especially harmful, if this means that sociology is squeezed out of relevant govern-ment and academic institutions where it can interact in a symbiotic and productive manner with other disciplines. An unfortunate bonus to my discussion of the LSES is that, as we shall see, the fates of other behavioral science researchers, as well as of the IRP units representing sub-disciplines of psychology that do not directly study brain function, closely parallel those of the sociologists of the LSES. Thus, the description of the LSES generalizes to other behavioral and social sciences.

The History of Socioenvironmental Studies at the NIMH

John Clausen, Melvin Kohn, Morris Rosenberg, Leonard Pearlin, Erwin Goffman; *Social Isolation and Schizophrenia* (Kohn & Clausen, 1955), *Social Class and Parental Values* (Kohn, 1959), *Asylums: Essays on the Social Situation of the Mental Patient* (Goffman, 1961), *Society and the Adolescent Self Image* (Rosenberg, 1965), Clas*s and Conformity* (Kohn, 1969), "The Structure of Coping" (Pearlin and Schooler, 1978), *Work and Personality* (Kohn & Schooler, 1983). All of these – I believe I can fairly say – illustrious sociologists and their seminally influential sociological works were part of the history of the LSES before the departure from the Laboratory in 1985 of Melvin Kohn, who in 1963 succeeded John Clausen to become the second chief of the LSES. After Kohn's departure—a departure that cannot reasonably be described as happy—the Laboratory was reduced to Section status (SSES), an organizationally significant reduction in status—but one that fortunately, because of other changes in the IRP bureaucratic structure, had essentially no practical consequences. What was essentially left is a one person fiefdom for a tenured intramural scientist. The Section now consists of me—the tenured scientist (half sociologist/half psychologist), a permanent colleague (officially designated as a Staff Scientist – a position that precludes being an independent investigator), a permanent research assistant, a program-assistant/secretary and two fellowship positions, one of which is generally used for a post-doctoral fellow and the other for a recent college graduate planning to go on to graduate school, who serves as a research assistant. There is a steady budget that comfortably covers the costs of data analysis and study planning and what can be seen as a hunting license to pursue sources of revenue that would pay the costs of data gathering (the possibility of extramural NIH funding, however, being legally excluded). In many ways this has been a pretty good sinecure—one that has allowed me to pursue a, I believe generally successful, research course of examining the determinants and effects of complex environments in different types of people in different social-structural and cultural settings. I have followed this course using research approaches ranging from experimental psychology, through sociology to comparative historical analysis. My sinecure does, however, have a couple of pretty big interrelated draw backs. One, is that the quadrennial review process that determines the resources, scope of research and, indeed, the continued existence of the Section is often carried out by people with limited knowledge of, and little interest in, basic sociological or social psychological scientific research (i.e., research whose direct aim is to come to an understanding of the phenomena being investigated by elucidating the rules governing them). A second is that my leaving, voluntary or otherwise, will almost certainly write finis to the role of sociology or of any kind of fairly basic social science research in the NIMH intramural program. It is worth noting that the LSES historically had several noted anthropologists in the program—William Caudill, Eliot Liebow, Melvin Ember—who left without being replaced, so that the presence of this social science in the NIMH intramural program has also been ended.

The NIMH Intramural Program Now

Briefly, both the past and probable future of psychology—at least of psychology that does not directly study brain function and does not pretty much fit under the rubric of cognitive neuroscience—generally parallels that of sociology. In the early days of the intramural research program – from mid 1950's to mid 1970's – the Laboratory of Psychology, which was dedicated to studying both normal and abnormal adult human psychology, was notably larger than the Laboratory of Socioenvironmental Studies and contained a similar proportion of quite notable researchers. Its remnants are also pretty much reduced to one researcher and supporting staff. The Laboratory of Developmental Psychology, which can be said to have played an equally illustrious role in the study of the psychological development of children, is gone, without leaving a trace.

Today the Intramural program can be fairly characterized as highly disease oriented, biologized, and reductionist—in the sense of seeing human behavior—both healthy and non-healthy—as essentially being determined by interrelated biological, biochemical and genetic processes. Among the researchers with this general orientation, there are some with a reasonably sophisticated knowledge of psychological processes—a primary example being Daniel Weinberger, head of the Genes, Cognition and Psychosis Program, whose important, and possibly even brilliant, theories on the origin and nature of schizophrenia take into account and deal with data and findings from neuromolecular to psychological, although not to sociological, levels of phenomena (e.g., Goldberg & Weinberger, 2004). It is also the case, that the IRP psychologists whose primary focus is on the basic neurobiological determinants of animal behavior include some who are acknowledged to be among the most influential and innovative in their fields. One example would Robert Desimone, who has recently left his position as head of the IRP, to take over directorship of the McGovern Institute for Brain Research at MIT. Among his accomplishments are highly influential studies of the pattern of firing of single neurons during different stages of monkeys' carrying out experimental cognitive tasks (for a review, see Desimone & Duncan, 1995).

Perhaps the best way to portray the present state of the Intramural Program is to show the listing of research units that is presented to the public on its website. Even a quick perusal of Table 3.1 provides a pretty accurate picture of the essentially biological and disease oriented research interests and priorities of the present NIMH IRP. The listing makes clear the IRP's lack of concern with normal healthy individual psychological functioning and its disinterest in how the functioning of both normal and mentally ill individuals may be affected by such socioenvironmental factors as: 1) the structure and functioning of the social systems of which they are a part, 2) individuals' positions in such structures or 3) the characteristics of the cultures in which the individuals and their social structures are embedded.

TABLE 3.1. NIMH intramural research programs.

Programs, laboratories, branches, independent sections and units
• Behavioral Endocrinology Branch
• Child Psychiatry Branch
• Genes, Cognition, and Psychosis Program
• Clinical Brain Disorders Branch
• Unit on Systems Neuroscience in Psychiatry
• Geriatric Psychiatry Branch
• Neuropsychiatry Branch
• Laboratory of Behavioral Neuroscience
• Laboratory of Brain and Cognition
• Laboratory of Cellular and Molecular Regulation
• Laboratory of Cerebral Metabolism
• Laboratory of Clinical Science
• Laboratory of Genetics
• Laboratory of Molecular Biology
• Laboratory of Neuropsychology
• Laboratory of Neurotoxicology
• Laboratory of System Neuroscience
• Biological Psychiatry Branch
• Clinical Neuroendocrinology Branch
• Experimental Therapeutics and Pathophysiology Branch
• Laboratory of Molecular Pathophysiology
• Molecular Imaging Branch
• Pediatric and Developmental Neuropsychiatry Branch
• Unit on Affective Cognitive Neuroscience
• Unit on Genetic Basis of Mood and Anxiety Disorders
• Unit on Genetics of Cognition and Behavior
• Unit on Neuroplasticity
• Section on Neuroendocrine Immunology and Behavior
• Section on Pharmacology
• Section on Socioenvironmental Studies
• Section on Clinical and Experimental Psychology
• Unit on Cognitive Neurophysiology and Imaging

The Decline of Sociology in the NIMH IRP

The Reality of the Decline

As is evident from my discussion of the past history of the NIMH IRP, the apparent disdain that characterizes the NIMH IRP's attitude towards sociology, as well as non-directly biologically oriented psychology, has not always been the case. In fact, while discussing the place of sociology and of Social Science during the early years of the IRP for an NIH sponsored history of NIMH's early years, Melvin Kohn described the attitudes of Robert Felix, the founding director of the NIMH and Seymour Kety—its first Scientific Director (i.e., head of the IRP and with the exception of Noble Prize winner Julius Axelrod, probably its most noted neurobiologically oriented scientist)—as follows:

It was certainly not happenstance that the director of the institute thought it necessary to include social science among its core disciplines, nor that the leaders of the intramural research program sustained that decision. On the contrary, it was breadth of imagination, a non-reductionist belief on the part of some very wise men that the social sciences might well have something important to contribute to our understanding of human behavior, and should therefore be included in the program (Kohn, 2004, p. 265).

Further proof of this early openness of the Intramural Program to social science is that a Social Psychologist – John C. Eberhart—was appointed as Scientific Director in 1961—a position he held for almost 20 years.

Why the Decline?

So why the decline of the place of sociology (and of non-directly-biological psychology) from an important position in the Intramural Program to a position where the time of their vanishing from the program is clearly foreseeable? Before discussing what I believe are contributing reasons for this decline, let me argue against two reasons that might seem plausible to some, but which I do not believe hold.

The first is that sociology (and non-directly-biological psychology) have not uncovered, and on principle cannot uncover, findings and develop theories that are relevant to our understanding of normal and abnormal human behavior. There is no need here to preach to the mostly converted, but I believe that in terms of relevant theories, methodologies and findings, basic sociology and basic non-biological psychology have much to contribute to our knowledge of abnormal, as well as normal human behavior. As I will briefly discuss at the end of at the end of this paper, what we are now finding out about the interaction of socioenvironmental and biological/genetic factors in determining human behavior strongly suggests that we should not put all of our resources into trying to gain a basic understanding of biology and genetics without paying substantial attention to trying to understand sociological and psychological level rules and processes. Sociological and psychological level rules and processes can no more be fully deduced from a knowledge of biochemistry than the rules and processes of biochemistry can be deduced from knowledge of Mendelev's Periodic Table of the Elements.

The second unlikely explanation is that the reduction of the place of sociology and psychology in the intramural program is the result of a politically and ideologically inspired government-wide effort intended to reduce the presumptive influence of the social sciences. Although there was evidence of such an intent in the early days of the Reagan administration—there is to my knowledge no evidence of a government wide interest in particularly reducing the influence of the social sciences compared to that of the other sciences. In fact, the NIH has been under a congressional mandate the last several years to increase its backing of the social sciences—a mandate which it, and the National Institute of General Medical Sciences in particular, have fairly steadfastly resisted.

So what are the explanations of the diminishing position of sociology in the NIMH intramural program? I use the plural "explanations" because I believe that the decline in the position of sociology (and the parallel decline of that of psychology) stem from a variety of causes and might even be described as over-determined. A major reason is the reductionist value system that seems to underlie the prestige hierarchy of the sciences. In the scientific community the more micro the level of phenomena that a particular science investigates the higher the level of esteem in which it is likely to be held. In this respect NIMH and NIH are definitely part of the scientific community. This tendency in the scientific community is paralleled in the medical community by a certain disdain by other medical special-ties for "incorporeal psychiatry" – a disdain to which the almost universal rejection of the psychoanalytic approach as a scientifically acceptable way of understanding human behavior has most probably contributed.

Undoubtedly also contributing to the high value placed in the National Institutes of Health on the study of relatively micro level phenomena is the commonly perceived high success rate of such approaches- a perception mostly based on reality. Paralleling, and in part underlying, this success rate is a variety of almost wondrous technical developments. Particularly relevant to the concerns of the NIMH are the real and exciting developments in the methodologies of brain imaging and the manipulation of animal genotypes. In addition, the field of psychiatry has been particularly influenced by the relative ease and success of psychopharmacological, as opposed to psychotherapeutic or psychosocial, treatments in ameliorating, if not curing, a wide range of mental disorders.

A different, but nevertheless related, cause for the decline of the position of sociology and non-biological psychology in both the intramural and extramural programs of NIMH is the very great and increasing influence of illness-based organizations and lobbying groups. Such groups play a central role in pressuring for and actually providing funding for mental health research. Almost every one of these groups is strongly focused on steering the maximal proportion of potentially available funds to studies that they see as directly relevant to finding a cure for their particular illness-of-concern. They tend to see the spending of money for studies that they do not believe to be directly relevant to curing their illness-of-concern as wasted money. In this context, basic sociological and psychological research on normal individuals is seen as such a waste of potential resources. In addition, since the basis of the recruitment to such organizations is very often the illness of a family member, such organizations, understandably, tend to be hostile to research that might suggest the importance of non-biological environmental factors in the development of their illness-of-concern—particularly those environ-mental conditions that might be seen as suggesting that behaviors of family members may contribute to the development of, or affect the course of, mental illness in general and their illness-of-concern in particular.

The Decline's Likely Continuation and Cost of the Loss

Given all of these facts, trends and pressures, how likely is there to be a rever-sal in the apparent path to extinction of sociology and non-directly biological psychology in the NIMH Intramural Program? My personal guess is that the

Dodo is as likely to make a comeback. If I am right in my prediction, a real price will be paid by both sociology and psychology. Going beyond disciplinary concerns and leaving aside the issue of whether gaining a basic understanding of the functioning of normal individuals is not in itself a worthy goal for the National Institute of Mental Health, abandoning the study of socioenvironmental and psychological level phenomena (and of their interaction) will lead to a net loss in our ability to understand and treat mental illness. This belief has been nothing if not reinforced by recent developments, and non-developments, in neuroscience and genetics.

One non-development is the paucity of testable hypotheses deriving from our experience with psychotherapeutic drugs. Although such drugs work and have been shown to work for almost half a century, and although there have been a plethora of hypotheses and dreams of Nobel Prizes, as of now there has been a notable lack of success in the development of strictly biological reductionist theories of the causes of any mental illness based on the known actions of any of the drugs.

On the other hand, evidence has been mounting of the existence of reciprocal relationships among neurobiological, psychological and socioenvironmental phenomena. For example, a series of studies have indicated that changes in chemical brain function brought about by behavioral interventions parallel those brought about by pharmaceutical interventions (an early example is Baxter, Schwartz, Bergman, Szuba, Guze, Mazziotta, Alazraki, Selin, Ferng, Munford, & Phelps, 1992). Experimental studies with animals have demonstrated that brain structures can be affected by exposure to complex environments in ways suggesting the development of more effective cognitive functioning (e.g., Kemperman, Kuhn, & Gage, 1997). Paralleling these findings, my own studies demonstrate that even in older people exposure to cognitively demanding environments can lead to increased levels of intellectual functioning as measured by standard psychometric tests (e.g., Schooler, Mulatu, & Oates, 2004). More generally, the last few years have seen mounting evidence of brain plasticity—indicating that environmental conditions can affect the nature and number of various types of brain cells and their interconnections well beyond what had generally believed to possible in the previous decades (for a review, see Mohammed, Zhu, Darmopil, Hjerling-Leffler, Enfors, Winblad, Diamond, Eriksson, & Bogdanovic, 2002).

Current trends and findings in the field of genetics also point to the importance of paying serious attention to the environment. Recent years have witnessed an increased interest among genetic researchers in understanding the processes through which genes affect development—processes that essentially represent gene X environment interactions (Cadoret, Winokur, Langbehn, Troughton, Yates, & Stewart, 1996; Caspi, McClay, Moffitt, Mill, Craig, Taylor, & Poulton, 2002; CDC Gene Interaction Fact Sheet, 2000). Furthermore, although the existence of a genetic contribution to various mental illnesses has been firmly established, the extent of the direct genetic contribution seems limited. Even using the somewhat questionable standard heritability index, the heritability for schizophrenia in industrial societies is about 50%. Serious doubts about the heritability index revolve around the likelihood that it seriously underestimates the effects of gene X environment interactions

(Dickens & Flynn, 2001). Taken together, genetic studies of mental illness strongly suggest that such illnesses have no simple genetic determinants. The best bet is that the genetic contributions to most of types of diagnosed mental illnesses depend on a variety of combinations of genes, and that most mental illnesses are the result of multiple and alternate interactions between genetic and environmental factors (with no particular gene being a sufficient or even a necessary cause). (For a biologically oriented version of such a view as it applies to schizophrenia, see Andreasen, 1999; for a psychologically oriented, biologically knowledgeable, somewhat tendentious, version that covers most psychoses, see Bentall, 2004). Given these recent trends in genetics and psychoneurobiology, it becomes even more problematic if the study of socioenvironmental processes is undervalued and the development of relevant and reliable socioenvironmental measures neglected. Such neglect becomes particularly troublesome in light of the mathematical fact that error in the measurement of an independent variable tends to underestimate its effects. Consequently when one is comparing the effects of, or examining the interactions between, supposedly well measured biological and genetic variables and poorly measured environmental ones, the effects of the biological and genetic variables will be overestimated in comparison to the effects the socioenvironmental ones and our knowledge of their interactions distorted. Good measurement requires good understanding of the processes being measured and good understanding of such processes depends on good basic research. Similar arguments could be made about gaining an understanding the nature of the relationship between psychological level processes and both socioenvironmental and biological genetic ones.

All the above would seem to make a strong and reasonable case for the meaningful presence of socioenvironmental, as well for non-biological psychological, studies in multidisciplinary, mental health oriented programs such as the NIMH IRP. Nevertheless, given the strengths of the trends and views arrayed against such a presence, the case is unlikely to be a winning one.

Acknowledgments. The views expressed in this paper are those of the author and not those of NIMH, NIH, DHHS or any other US government agency. I would like the thank Leslie Caplan and Nina Schooler for their careful readings of earlier versions of this paper. An oral version of the paper was presented August 16, 2005 at the Annual Meeting of the American Sociological Association.

References

Andreasen, N. C. (1999). A unitary model of Schizophrenia. *Archives of General Psychiatry, 56,* 781–787.

Baxter, L. J, Baxter, L. R., Schwartz, J. m., Bergman, K. S., Szuba, M. P., Guze, B. H., Mazziotta, J. C., Alazraki, A., Selin, C. E., Ferng, H. K., Munford, P., & Phelps, M. E. (1992). Caudate glucose metabolic rate changes with both drug and behavior therapy for obsessive-compulsive disorder. *Archives of General Psychiatry, 49,* 681–689.

Bentall, R. (2004). *Madness explained: Psychosis and human nature.* Penguin Global.

Cadoret, R., Winokur, G., Langbehn, D., Troughton, E., Yates, W., & Stewart, M. (1996). Depression spectrum disease, I: The role of gene-environment interaction. *American Journal of Psychiatry, 153*, 892–899.

Caspi, A., McClay, J., Moffitt, T., Mill, J., Martin, J., Craig, I. W., Taylor, A., & Poulton, R. (2002). Role of genotype in the cycle of violence in maltreated children. *Science, 297*, 851–854.

CDC. (2000). *Gene-Environment Interaction Fact Sheet*. Retrieved June 28, 2005, from http://www.cdc.gov/genomics/info/factshts/geneenviro.htm

Desimone, R., & Duncan, J. (1995). Neural mechanisms of selective visual attention. *Annual Review of Neuroscience, 18*, 193–222.

Dickens, W. T., & Flynn, J. R. (2001). Heritability estimates versus large environmental effects: the IQ paradox resolved. *Psychological Review, 108*, 346–369.

Goffman, E. (1961). *Asylums. Essays on the social situation of mental patients and other inmates*. New York: Doubleday Anchor.

Goldberg, T. E., & Weinberger, D. R. (2004). Genes and the parsing of cognitive processes. *TRENDS in Cognitive Sciences, 8*, 325–335.

Kempermann, G., Kuhn, H. G., & Gage, F. H. (1997). More hippocampal neurons in adult mice living in an enriched environment. *Nature, 386*, 493–495.

Kohn, M. L. (1959). Social class and parental values. *American Journal of Sociology, 64*, 337–351.

Kohn, M. L. (1969). *Class and conformity: A study in values*. Homewood, Ill.: Dorsey.

Kohn, M. (2004). *Reflections on the Intramural Research Program of the NIMH in the 1950s* (Vol. 62). Fairfax, VA: IOS Press.

Kohn, M. L., & Clausen, J. A. (1955). Social isolation and schizophrenia. *American Sociological Review, 20*, 265–273.

Kohn, M. L., & Schooler, C. (1983). *Work and personality: An inquiry into the impact of social stratification*. Norwood, NJ: Ablex Publishing Co.

Mohammed, A. H., Zhu, S. W., Darmopil, S., Hjerling-Leffler, J., Enfors, P., Winblad, B., Diamond, M. C., Eriksson, P. S., & Bogdanovic, N. (2002). Environmental enrichment and the brain. *Progress in Brain Research, 138*, 109–133.

Pearlin, L.I., & Schooler, C. (1978). The structure of coping. *Journal of Health and Social Behavior, 19*, 2–21.

Rosenberg, M. (1965). *Society and the adolescent self-image*. Princeton, NJ: Princeton University Press.

Schooler, C., Mulatu, M. S., & Oates, G. (2004). Effects of occupational self-direction on the intellectual functioning and self-directed orientations of older workers: Findings and implications for individuals and societies. *American Journal of Sociology, 110*, 161–197.

Part II
Sociological Theory and Mental Health

4
Classical Sociological Theory, Evolutionary Psychology, and Mental Health

Allan V. Horwitz

Introduction

Stressful life events and chronic stressors are typically the proximate sources of psychological distress (Avison & Turner, 1988; Brown, 2002; Dohrenwend, 2000; Turner, 2003). Yet, these stressors, as well as the coping resources that people use to deal with them, are themselves often the consequences of social locations that reflect broader patterns of social organization. One central goal of the sociology of mental health is to show how psychological well-being and distress result from such basic social arrangements and large-scale structural processes (Pearlin, 1989; Aneshensel, 1992). Few studies, however, illustrate how more proximate causes of distress and the demographic characteristics that produce variation in them are instances of more general dimensions of social life (Link & Phelan, 1995).

Revisiting the writings of the major classical sociological theorists—Durkheim, Marx, and Weber—can enrich studies in the sociology of mental health. The founders of the sociological discipline showed how seemingly individual traits reflected external and collective social forces. Their works suggest that stressors and consequent emotional distress stem from larger social processes of social integration, inequality, and cultural values as well as from the historical transformations in these processes. Tying mental health research to classical theory thus unites the field with the central themes in the broader sociological discipline. In this way, the sociology of mental health can become more integrated with a variety of fields in sociology, such as social stratification, economic and political sociology, and cultural sociology, which are more explicitly grounded in the classical tradition. In turn, the sociology of mental health can illuminate the mechanisms through which broader social processes influence individual states of mind. Together, classical theory and the sociology of mental health help explain a basic question about human existence: what accounts for psychological well-being and distress?

Several aspects of the classical tradition are salutary for the sociology of mental health. First, each classical theorist emphasized the fundamentally *social* aspects of the subject matter of the discipline. For Durkheim, social causes have an existence of their own that is independent of individuals because they retain the same intensity in the same environment as particular individuals change. Likewise, the Marxian emphasis on stratification is inherently social because it characterizes relationships, not individuals: dominance and dependence can only exist within interdependent relationships. Weber, as well, stressed how social action reflected values that are not idiosyncratic but depend on culture and social location.

Because the classical sociologists used a few basic themes—social integration, inequality, and cultural symbols—to interpret social life, a classical framework also realizes the basic aims of good scientific theory to develop parsimonious explanations of phenomena. Moreover, each classical theorist developed formulations of maximal generality that apply across all levels of social phenomena including macro-level differences across societies, meso level differences across units within societies, and micro differences across interpersonal relationships. Likewise, their interests cut across all social institutions, whether religious, political, occupational, or familial. Finally, each classical theorist developed propositions of maximal scope across time and space. All emphasized the importance of using comparative methods to produce general laws that are applicable to a wide range of social types.

Both the sociology of mental health and classical sociological theory explore the social conditions that facilitate or detract from psychological well-being. Evolutionary psychology provides a complementary perspective that shows how humans are genetically programmed to respond to the same social stimuli that classical social theory emphasize. Other biologically grounded theories, most notably behavioral genetics, focus on genetic reasons for behavioral differences among individuals (Plomin, DeFries, McClearn, & McGuffin, 2001). They tend to be reductionistic, viewing human behavior as a product of neurons, synapses, and biochemical processes inside the brain (Kandel, 1998). While these processes can help explain the causes of various mental disorders, they are usually not relevant to sociologists of mental health, who are typically concerned with the *normal* psychic consequences of stressful social arrangements.

In contrast to genetic accounts of individual differences, evolutionary psychology explains shared human traits that result from adaptations to social environments (Tooby & Cosmides, 1992; Freese, 2002). Its major tenet is that natural selection, operating over thousands of generations, has designed psychological mechanisms to respond to specific environmental challenges (Fodor, 1983; Pinker, 2002). *Contextuality* is an inherent aspect of these mechanisms; they are designed to activate in particular contexts and not to activate in others. Evolutionary psychology thus examines how shared genetic tendencies are differentially expressed in different environments (Buss, 1995). One of these tendencies is that people are hard-wired to pay attention to social roles, interactional needs, and cultural symbols (Turner, 2000). This focus on psychological similarity and environmental diversity is fundamentally compatible with a sociological perspective (Freese, Li, & Wade 2003).

Evolutionary psychology tries to specify the contexts in which depression, anxiety, and other emotionally painful states might have adaptive functions in analogous ways to the useful, albeit uncomfortable, defenses that pain, vomiting, or nausea provide against disease. The particular contexts that humans are naturally designed to respond to map remarkably well onto the major themes of the classical sociologists. One school of evolutionary thought regards depression as a naturally selected response to losses of valued attachments involving intimacy, love, and friendship. In this view, depression developed as a way of mobilizing social support from the group or of avoiding premature severing of important interpersonal ties (Hagen, 1999; Bowlby, 1980). Another school emphasizes how distress can be adaptive for subordinates in hierarchical relationships that feature unequal distributions of power, status, resources, respect, or prestige. The submissive qualities of distress responses presumably have greater survival values for persons in inferior positions than alternative responses would have in these circumstances (Price, Sloman, Gardner, Gilbert, & Rhode, 1994). A third perspective stresses how low moods can be adaptive after failures to achieve valued, but unreachable, social goals that provide coherence and purpose to life. Depression, in this view, can decrease investment in unsatisfying enterprises and prevent the premature pursuit of risky alternatives (Klinger, 1985; Nesse, 2000). These contexts, which reflect losses of valued attachments, resources, and goals, correspond to the major themes that Durkheim, Marx, and Weber, respectively, emphasized.

However, psychological mechanisms developed to adapt to problems stemming from social integration, stratification, and cultural coherence in ancient social environments, not in modern societies. Current manifestations of ancestral cues activate these mechanisms. Psychological traits that solved problems in ancestral environments must be executed in present environments where they may no longer be adaptive. This mismatch between contemporary social conditions and inherited mental mechanisms is a potent source of normal distress (Freese, 2002).

This chapter examines current research in the sociology of mental health in the complementary contexts of classical sociological theory, on the one hand, and evolutionary psychology, on the other. This broad purpose creates a number of limitations. First, no chapter can do justice to the range of classical theorists who are relevant to the study of mental health. This chapter ignores the major contributions of such seminal figures as Georg Simmel, W.E.B. DuBois, George Herbert Mead and many others. Moreover, the chapter only scratches the surface of the writings of the three theorists, Durkheim, Marx, and Weber, that it does cover. Third, it limits its survey of the sociology of mental health to studies that examine the impact of social factors on psychological well-being. This emphasis ignores other important branches of the field such as studies of how social factors define what conditions are labeled as signs of mental health or illness, how people define and seek help for mental problems, or how social factors shape the symptoms of various conditions (Horwitz, 1999; Pescosolido & Rubin, 2000). Finally, the chapter deals with the sorts of general psychological states of distress and well-being that naturally result from social arrangements. It has little to say about how social conditions affect the development of mental disorders that are dysfunctions of psychological systems.

I proceed by discussing the major themes found in the work of Durkheim, Marx, and Weber. For each theorist, I then show how their focus ties together a body of work in the sociology of mental health. Finally, in each section, I ground the themes of social integration, stratification, and values in genetically-based traits of the human species.

Social Integration

The Classical Tradition

Emile Durkheim sought the causes of human behavior in social structures of society that are not reducible to the characteristics of individuals who comprise them. Social facts are neither features of individuals nor universal properties of human nature but are certain ways of feeling, thinking and acting that individuals would not have if they lived in other human groups. Social groups are thus more than the sum total of their individual elements but comprise a different level of analysis that is *sui generis*.

Durkheim was intensely interested in the psychic consequences of social life. The basis of mental health and distress reside in variation in the degree to which individuals partake in collective social life. Durkheim focused on studying suicide rates, although his approach has far more general relevance. The proper objects of sociological study are the factors affecting the suicide rate in any social group, not idiosyncratic factors that lead one individual rather than another to commit suicide. "Indeed," Durkheim emphasized, "we must not forget that what we are studying is the social suicide-rate. The only types of interest to us, accordingly, are those contributing to its formation and influencing its variation" (1897/1951, p. 147). Although suicide is impossible if individual characteristics are opposed to it, most people have a "general, vague aptitude" for it that becomes manifest according to social circumstances (1897/1951, pp. 102–103). These characteristics can not, though, explain what causes a definite number of people to kill themselves in a particular group at a particular point in time. Mental health varies among different social categories of individuals because of their relationship to social forces, regardless of their particular biological or psychological characteristics. As long as social conditions remain relatively unchanged, rates of suicide should be constant over time.

Durkheim's *Suicide* is generally credited to be the first explicitly sociological empirical study of mental health and disorder. His great achievement was to link fundamental social processes with empirical indicators of rates of suicide across a wide variety of social contexts. Durkheim's central theme was that the nature of the connections that people have with each other and with social institutions affects the likelihood that they will commit suicide (Pescosolido & Levy, 2002). "Suicide," Durkheim (1897/1951) summarized, "varies inversely with the degree of integration of the social groups of which the individual forms a part" (p. 223).

Social integration affects mental health in two major ways. First, it satisfies affiliative needs through connecting people to socially given purposes and ideals, which are the major sources of human gratification. For Durkheim (1897/1951), "Social man is the essence of civilized man; he is the masterpiece of existence" (p. 213). Individuals are fundamentally social beings and their thought, values, morality, aspirations and the like all derive from society. The content of these beliefs is irrelevant: only how strongly they bond individuals to the collective conscience is important. "The more numerous and strong these collective states of mind are," Durkheim (1897/1951) explained, "the stronger the integration of the religious community, and also the greater its preservative value. The details of dogmas and rites are secondary. The essential thing is that they be capable of supporting a sufficiently intense collective life" (p. 170).

What Durkheim called *egoistic* suicides result from deficiencies in collective activity and meaning. Egoism arises when "the individual is isolated because the bonds uniting him to other beings are slackened or broken, because society is not sufficiently integrated at the points at which he is in contact with it" (1897/1951, p. 317). Specifically, egoistic suicides vary inversely with the degree of religious, familial, and political integration. Religion benefits mental health because it integrates individuals in caring social circles and provides ritual practices that reinforce coherent belief systems. Different religions, however, vary in the strength of their grip over their members. Catholics, for example, are less likely than Protestants to commit suicide because they share more common beliefs and practices while the latter religion permits more free inquiry among individuals. Integration is also a fundamental property of other groups including families and communities. Married persons commit fewer suicides than unmarried ones, although this is due less to the impact of the marital relationship than to the protective effect of family life (1897/1951, p. 189). The lower rate of suicide among married people results from parental, not spousal, roles: married people with children are especially unlikely to commit suicide. Likewise, rural areas have fewer suicides than urban ones because of their presumably more integrated nature. Times of war and revolution, as well, feature few suicides because of the growing intensity of collective life during their occurrence.

Social integration, however, has a curvilinear relationship with mental health. All social bonds create emotional dependence. Just as too little integration leads to isolation and despair, too much integration can create a situation where social demands overwhelm individuals to the extent that they take their own lives in what Durkheim called *altruistic* suicide. Examples are women who commit suicide after their husbands' deaths, cult members who kill themselves when their leader orders them to do so, soldiers who prefer death to humiliating defeat, or men who can no longer perform their occupational functions (1897/1951, p. 219). Altruistic suicides stem from social demands that are so oppressive that people kill themselves because they feel it is their duty.

Social integration affects mental health in a second way through regulating inherent human needs and desires. Durkheim believed that human nature leads people to have insatiable desires. Yet, happiness requires that needs be proportionate to means. Only strong collective rules can create limits on needs: "It is not human nature which can assign the variable limits necessary to our needs. They are thus unlimited so far as they depend on the individual alone. Irrespective of any external regulatory force, our capacity for feeling is in itself an insatiable and bottomless abyss" (1897/1951, p. 247). Note that Durkheim explicitly did not associate poverty with greater suicide rates, going so far as to say that: "Poverty may even be considered a protection" (1897/1951, p. 245). Poor people are unlikely to commit suicide because they are accustomed to limited aspirations so are not disappointed when their expectations are unfulfilled. Wealth, in contrast, stimulates needs, so that "the more one has, the more one wants" (1897/1951, p. 248).

Socially integrated social settings contain just and equitable norms that regulate human instincts and lead to states of contentment. Conversely, sudden changes in social life often lead to breakdowns in values and norms and, consequently, to distress. Modern, industrial societies are marked by constant crises that lead to the loosening of social regulations over natural desires. While egoistic suicides arise because people find no justification for life, *anomic* suicides occur because their activities lack regulation so their needs cannot be satisfied. Anomic suicides stem from periods of economic prosperity or depression that loosen social ties and deregulate controls over inherently unquenchable needs. Periods of both economic prosperity and economic disaster loosen moral regulation with consequent increases in suicide rates. Likewise, recently divorced men are deregulated from control over their aspirations and "he aspires to everything and is satisfied with nothing" (1897/1951, p. 271). In contrast, women's desires are naturally limited so do not suffer comparable deregulation after divorce; if men need restraint, women require liberty (1897/1951, p. 274).

For Durkheim, social bonds that are neither too weak nor too oppressive and socially promoted goals that are neither too vague nor too demanding optimize individual mental health. Good social institutions bring individuals into unity with society so that individuals do not perceive themselves as isolated but as part of a collective. In the modern world, neither the state nor religious groups are powerful enough to serve this purpose. Instead, Durkheim proposed that economic life be organized around occupational groups that would provide sources of attachment and regulation. Such groups would be especially well-positioned to exercise moral control because work is not distant and impersonal, is important to people, and involves the greater part of their lives (1897/1951, p. 379). As well, Durkheim believed that leveling gender differences in marriage could help reduce differences in unhappiness (1897/1951, p. 386). Social institutions that are sources of rational and just norms that check self-interested motives and desires can establish the conditions for happiness in modern life.

Sociology of Mental Health

A large literature in the sociology of mental health confirms the importance Durkheim placed on social integration as a fundamental cause of well-being. At the same time, it specifies the various ways in which integration leads to negative or positive psychological impacts. Studies of social relationships, social institutions, neighborhoods, and social support all indicate the fundamental power of Durkheim's insights.

One of the most consistent findings in the sociology of mental health is that attachments to other people are associated with positive mental health while their absence is related to distress. Generally speaking, social involvements of all sorts are associated with positive mental health. A huge literature, for example, indicates that married people have less distress than unmarried people (Mirowsky & Ross, 2003). The greater social integration married people gain through more supportive relationships and ties to community institutions largely account for this relationship (Umberson & Williams, 1999). In addition, marriage serves regulative functions that promote conformity to social norms, more conventional lifestyles, and lower levels of deviance of all sorts (Umberson, 1987; Horwitz & White, 1998). Moreover, because cohabitation has some, but not all, of the characteristics of marriage, it also has some, but not all, of the mental health benefits (Ross, 1995). Overall, people with more frequent contacts with family, friends, and neighbors report less distress (Lin, Ye, & Ensel, 1999). Likewise, people who are involved with voluntary organizations including churches, civic organizations, clubs, or recreational groups, have higher levels of well-being than those who are not (Rietschlin, 1998; Thoits & Hewitt, 2001). Participation in religious communities, as well, promotes mental health and protects against self-destructive behaviors (Pescosolido & Georgianna, 1989). In addition, *gains* in attachments result in mental health improvement: for example, single people who get married are better off than those who remain unmarried (Williams, 2003; Simon & Marcussen, 1999). One important qualification to Durkheim's emphasis, however, is that not social ties in themselves but only valued attachments are associated with positive mental health (e.g. Wheaton, 1990; Brown, 2002).

Much research in the sociology of mental health also links the loss of valued attachments to growing distress. Indeed, the three most stressful types of life events – the death of a spouse, divorce, and marital separation – all involve attachment losses (Holmes & Rahe, 1967). A large literature links the death of intimates to the development of grief (e.g. Archer, 1999). Transitions from marriage to separated, divorced, or widowhood statuses are also associated with growing distress (Williams, 2003; Simon & Marcussen, 1999). Likewise, breakups of romantic relationships are strong predictors of poor mental health among adolescents (Joyner & Udry, 2001; Keller & Nesse, 2004).

Considerable research in the sociology of mental health also reinforces Durkheim's emphasis on how the strength of social roles that tie individuals to collectivities is associated with psychological well-being. For example, people in mid-life have less distress than younger or older people because of their greater integration into valued social roles (Mirowsky & Ross, 2003). In contrast, young people, who are just entering careers or old people, who are just leaving them, have more distress. Durkheim's emphasis on the importance of clear and consistent social obligations also resonates with a large body of research that shows how poor mental health arises from conflict in meeting simultaneous, but conflicting, demands from work and family roles. Mothers who work outside the home, for example, face incompatible demands from their parental and occupational obligations (Lennon & Rosenfield, 1992; Menaghan, 1991). The claims of one role can make performance of other roles more difficult with consequent negative impact on mental health.

Recent research also shows how, as Durkheim predicted, too enveloping or too many social obligations can lead to distress (Thoits, 1986; Schwartz, 1991). Participation in all-encompassing religious cults, for example, often heightens self-destructive behavior (Pescosolido & Georgianna, 1989). Or, role overload creates burdens that can overwhelm individual abilities to meet demands. Family caregivers, for example, find it difficult to simultaneous meet their obligations as providers of support and as workers (Pearlin, Aneshensel, & LeBlanc, 1997). Working women with small children and husbands who do not share childcare responsibilities also have more distress than those either without children or with cooperative husbands (Mirowsky & Ross, 2003). This overload in part explains why Durkheim incorrectly expected that the presence of children would have a uniformly positive impact on mental health. Problems in fulfilling conflicting social roles stem less from individual characteristics than from the demands of social institutions that make parenting, caregiving, and homemaking difficult.

Studies of community characteristics were central in the early development of the sociology of mental health (Faris & Dunham 1939; Leighton, Harding, Macklin, Macmillan, & Leighton, 1963). After a long period of neglect, mental health research is starting to re-examine the impact of community level indicators of social integration on mental health using powerful new statistical models that separate community and individual level influences. The findings of this research indicate that residents of communities marked by high social integration and cohesion, strong ties among residents, orderly neighborhoods, and two-parent families have positive mental health, net of their own individual psychological characteristics (e.g. Aneshensel & Sucoff, 1996). Ross, for example, finds that neighborhoods that are clean and safe, feature well maintained buildings, and have respectful relationships are more conducive to positive mental health than disorderly neighborhoods (Ross, 2000). Conversely, neighborhoods without access to transportation, medical facilities, shopping, and organized leisure activities are more distressing for their elderly residents (Pearlin & Skaff, 1995). Low levels of community cohesion and connectedness give rise to distinctive stressors and have psychologically noxious effects, net of individual characteristics.

Considerable research also indicates that social integration not only directly predicts individual well-being but also helps people cope with the stressors that they experience (e.g. House, Landis, & Umberson 1988; Turner, 1999). One of the strongest relationships in the sociology of mental health is between the presence of social support and positive mental health. This relationship stems less from the direct impact of support on well-being than from the way that people with much support are better able to cope with the impact of stressful life events (Kessler & McLeod, 1985). As Durkheim realized, however, social support brings costs along with its strong benefits. People involved in supportive relationships reap emotional and instrumental gains but also accrue obligations to provide support to others. Social obligations can produce stressful demands such as caregiving responsibilities, role captivity, and worry over the well-being of others that strain mental health (Pearlin et al., 1997; Rook, 1992). For example, part of the reason women report more distress than men stems from their greater sensitivity to stressful life events that occur to others (Kessler & McLeod, 1984).

In general, then, the sociology of mental health strongly reinforces the Durkheimian emphasis on the importance of social integration in promoting well-being and its absence in leading to distress. This does not mean that the empirical derivations Durkheim drew from his theory were always correct. For example, his expectations that suicide rates would be higher in urban than in rural areas have not been confirmed (Goldsmith, Pellmar, Kleinman, & Bunney, 2002). Or, his belief that poverty is associated with well-being was clearly wrong. However, his incorrect predictions do not refute his general theory. One reason could be that Durkheim incorrectly operationized his general predictions: rural areas might not be more integrated than urban ones so that the general theory is still correct. Another reason is that the relationship of social integration with particular social processes changes in different contexts. For example, poor people in the 19th century might have had diminished expectations for realizing social goals with consequent better mental health. Conversely, the poor in current Western societies share in the desire to realize social expectations and so their impoverishment is no longer protective (Merton, 1938/1968). Durkheim's general theory that social integration is associated with mental health is almost certainly correct (Pescosolido & Georgianna, 1989; Lester, 1994; Stockard & O'Brien, 2002). Findings from attachment theory show how humans are hard wired to derive satisfaction from valued intimate relationships and to suffer when they are deprived of these relationships.

Evolutionary Perspectives

Durkheim believed that human instincts inherently conflicted with social institutions so that strong social ties were necessary to control insatiable human desires. Attachment theory, however, shows that needs for strong social attachments are innate aspects of human nature. Conversely, the absence of these ties is the source of misery. The many studies of the British psychiatrist John Bowlby and the large school of his followers indicate that humans are genetically programmed to acquire stable and secure attachments with parental figures during the first years of life (e.g. Bowlby, 1969/1982). Bowlby emphasized that infants are designed to need strong attachment bonds; when they are separated from their primary caregivers they develop intense sadness responses. He observed that healthy infants who were separated from their mothers initially reacted through crying and other expressions of despair. They protested the separation and searched for the lost attachment object. Their protests seemed to represent cries for help that were adaptive attempts to reengage the mother. These responses usually evoked sympathetic reactions from the mothers, who responded by attending to their infants' needs. When such efforts failed and separations were prolonged, however, infants reacted to the disruption in attachment by undergoing a period of despair ultimately marked by withdrawal and inactivity. Finally, the infants became remote and apathetic, similar to the symptoms of intense adult loss responses. Bowlby's work indicates that loss response mechanisms are naturally activated in infants after the loss of close attachments.

Infants who develop strong attachments with adults are not only more psychologically adjusted but are also protected against developing mental disorders as adults. Conversely, the failure to develop attachments or losing attachments in early life is associated with both psychological disturbance among children and with vulnerability to mental disorders in adulthood (Brown, Harris, & Bifulco, 1986). Brief separations from caregivers after birth are not harmful nor are those where substitute caregivers replace absent parents (Rutter, 1981). Prolonged separations, however, result in a state of profound detachment where young children cease to respond to parental figures when they are restored to their lives.

Research about the consequences of attachment breakdowns among primates shows how attachment needs predate the human species and so are inherited aspects of the human genome. As humans do, primates respond to separations from parental caregivers with a variety of pathological consequences (Harlow &Suomi, 1974; Suomi, 1991). These separations are associated with enhanced production of stress hormones, facial and behavioral expressions of sadness, and the same stages of protest, despair, and detachment noted among human infants that are removed from their caregivers (Bowlby, 1969). Adult primates that are separated from sexual partners or peers also show depressive reactions that are comparable to young primates separated from parents (Mineka & Suomi, 1978).

What adaptive function could explain the natural development of depressive responses after attachment losses? Bowlby (1980) believed that the pain of depressive feelings following attachment loss motivated people to vigorously seek reunion with the lost loved one and not to give up the lost tie. Grief at thoughts of loss was adaptive in ancient environments because it allowed social bonds to persist during the frequent temporary absences of one party and thus promoted the maintenance of social relationships. Another common explanation is that depressive feelings are adaptive because they function as a "cry for help" that calls attention to needy states and elicits social support. For example, some recent evidence indicates that postpartum depression arises under circumstances, such as poor infant health and a lack of social support, where it can lead others to provide more help to new mothers (Hagen, 1999).

The importance of attachments that Durkheim postulated is not unique to humans and stems from earlier periods of evolution. Although attachment theory has only been developed to explain particular bonds between intimates, loyalties to social groups should also be an evolutionarily selected trait (Buss, 1995). Humans seem to be programmed to thrive when they are deeply embedded in the social world but to naturally become distressed when they lose ties with valued intimates. Durkheim appropriately emphasized the mental health benefits of social enmeshment: he did not realize, however, that innate human needs and strong social bonds are complementary rather than contradictory.

Social Stratification

The Classical Tradition

Like Durkheim, Karl Marx was deeply concerned with understanding the social conditions that either realized or thwarted human potential. And, as Durkheim did, Marx believed that individuals are fundamentally social beings who could only be fulfilled through having satisfying social relationships. "The human essence," Marx stated, "is no abstraction inherent in each single individual. In its reality it is the ensemble of the social relations" (1845/1977, p. 157). Marx, however, focused on a different dimension of social life than Durkheim: the degree to which social institutions fostered dominance and subordination through the unequal distribution of rewards. Capitalist societies, in particular, fostered hierarchical relationships, inequitable distributions of power, and consequent widespread alienation among their members.

For Marx, human relationships reflected the forces and relationships of production in any given society (1932/1977). The forces of production are resources, labor, tools, and techniques that create material goods. Relations of production are forms of cooperation or domination and subjection that are closely related to the forces of production. The forces and relations of production together are the material base of society on which arise political, religious, familial, and cultural superstructures.

Marx's key premise is that the forces and relations of production, the state of society, and individual consciousness are always in contradiction as long as private property exists. Modern societies are based on private property and capital that give a small group of people power and control over most of the population. These economic forces gave rise to social classes so that: "The history of all hitherto existing society is the history of class struggles" (1847/1977, p. 222). The essence of modern, bourgeois societies is the relation of exploitation that underlies all forms of social relations. Laborers do not own what they produce, which belongs to owners. "No sooner is the exploitation of the labourour by the manufacturer, so far, at an end," Marx explains, "and he receives his wages in cash, than he is set upon by the other portions of the bourgeoisie, the landlord, the shopkeeper, the pawnbroker, etc." (1847/1977, p. 227). While Marx focused on unequal economic relationships, these relationships shape all other types of social interaction.

The major psychological consequence of inequality is the widespread alienation of humans not only from the products they produce but also from the natural world, other people, and their own human nature:

All these consequences follow from the fact that the worker relates to the product of his labour as to an alien object. For it is evident from this presupposition that the more the worker externalizes himself in his work, the more powerful becomes the alien, objective world that he creates opposite himself, the poorer he becomes himself in his inner life and the less he can call his own (1844/1977, pp. 78–79).

Alienated labor perverts human nature, creates misery, and makes people feel strangers to themselves.

For Marx (1932/1977), human liberation would only come after the abolition of the division of labor, private property, and social classes:

... in communist society, where nobody has one exclusive sphere of activity but each can become accomplished in any branch he wishes, society regulates the general production and thus makes it possible for me to do one thing today and another tomorrow, to hunt in the morning, fish in the afternoon, rear cattle in the evening, criticize after dinner, just as I have a mind, without ever becoming hunter, fisherman, cowherd, or critic (p. 169).

Communism supersedes private property and therefore emancipates human essence; it is the solution of the antagonism between man and nature and man and man. The end of alienation will come when workers change the world, realize their essential human nature, and regain their selves after they abolish the division of labor. For Marx, no change in consciousness can lead to human emancipation without a fundamental transformation in the actual conditions of social institutions.

Sociology of Mental Health

A large body of research confirms Marx's observations about the importance of both the conditions of work and the more general relationship of dominance and subordination to mental health. The characteristics of jobs are robustly associated with mental health in ways that Marx would have predicted. In particular, jobs that are autonomous, creative, complex, have much decision latitude, and involve control over others enhance well-being (Kohn, 1976; Link, Lennon, & Dohrenwend, 1993; Lennon & Rosenfield, 1992). These characteristics are most associated with non-alienating conditions of labor. Conversely, tedious, routine, and oppressive jobs where workers have little control or autonomy yet face high demands are associated with poor mental health (Lennon, 1994; Karasek & Theorell, 1990). Job characteristics also help explain gender differences in distress: women are more likely than men to hold jobs that are less flexible, complex, autonomous, and prestigious (Rosenfield, 1989; Lennon & Rosenfield, 1992).

A few studies indicate how job characteristics are associated with general structural features of economic formations and how changes in these formations result in changes in the nature of work and consequent mental health effects. Periods of unemployment, in particular, are associated with growing rates of other stressful life events and of distress (Catalano & Dooley, 1977; Reynolds, 1997). Economic downturns also affect the characteristics of jobs through increasing demands and job insecurity and decreasing decision latitude (Fenwick & Tausig, 1994). Broad economic transitions also lead to changes in the characteristics in employment such as temporary employment contracts, labor displacement, and deskilling technologies. Virtually no knowledge exists, however, about how macro-level economic changes such as the globalization of the economy, displacement of jobs to countries with cheap labor, and technological innovations lead to psychological consequences at the individual level.

Marx emphasized not just work conditions but how inequitable social relationships were products of economic organization. A core interest in the sociology of mental health has been how inequalities in income, power, and prestige affect mental health. The results are clear: low socio-economic status increases distress while high status enhances well-being (e.g. Link, Lennon, & Dohrenwend, 1990; Eaton & Mutaner, 1999; Dohrenwend, 2000; Mirowsky & Ross, 2003). Many reasons account for the strong association between socio-economic status and mental health in addition to alienating conditions of labor including the degree of economic hardship, inability to reach desirable societal goals, and senses of inequity. The impact of poverty extends far beyond economic deprivation to encompass unstable and undesirable employment, physically hazardous environments, marital instability, and unhealthy lifestyles (McLeod & Nonnemaker, 1999). Economic inequality, and resulting social relationships, are a fundamental cause of health disparities, including mental health disparities (Link & Phelan, 1995). A continuing, unresolved, debate exists on how much poverty, in itself, or inequality compared to relevant reference groups contributes to distress (Marmot & Wilkinson, 1999).

Marx's own work examined stratification within a limited economic context but hierarchy is a property of all social institutions and relationships. Recent work in the sociology of mental health has especially focused on the stratification of gender roles. Social positions characterized by lower power are accompanied by poor mental health and women are more likely than men to occupy such positions (Rosenfield, 1999). Many of the findings from research about the mental health of men and women can be deduced from their structural positions in dominance hierarchies.

Married women who are subordinate to their husbands report considerably higher rates of distress than those who are not (e.g. Gove & Tudor, 1973; Mirowsky & Ross, 2003). When, however, men and women are in relatively egalitarian relationships, rates of distress tend to equalize. Marriages marked by equity, sharing, and reciprocity feature comparable levels of mental health among partners (Rosenfield, 1980; 1989; Ross, Mirowsky, & Huber, 1983). When neither spouse dominates in a marriage and both share housework, both are less depressed (Mirowsky, 1985). As the conditions of actual life between men and women converge, differences in distress disappear as well. Thus, young, single men and women have relatively equivalent levels of distress because they have comparable roles (Mirowsky, 1996). At the other extreme, when men are subordinate to women, rates of distress among men actually exceed those of women (Rosenfield, 1992). Gender differences, in other words, can be deduced from power relationships, as Marx might have predicted.

Research regarding ethnic differences in mental health has been less successful than research on work, social class, and gender in showing how dominance and subordination relates to mental health. There seem to be no general patterns related to hierarchy that explain ethnic differences in mental health (Williams & Harris-Reid, 1999) possibly because of a number of mitigating factors including the ethnocentric frameworks people use to evaluate mental health, social support resources that ethnic groups provide their members, and the many cross-cutting identities that people hold.

Nevertheless, in general, subordinate social positions are clearly associated with poor mental health; conversely, dominance is related to psychological well-being. The reasons for these relationships could be related to the human genome.

Evolutionary Perspectives

A large evolutionary literature focuses on stratification systems and mental health, especially within primate societies (e.g. Gilbert, 1992; McGuire & Troisi, 1998; Stevens & Price, 2000). Primates share with humans social hierarchies with high and low status positions and situations of chronic social subordination. In both species, positions in these hierarchies are associated with similar psychological responses. Under most circumstances, dependent monkeys have far more depression-like behaviors than dominant ones as indicated by higher levels of stress hormones and lower levels of blood serotonin (Saplosky, 1989; McGuire & Troisi, 1998). Chronic social subordination is also associated with high stress hormones associated with depressive symptoms (Shively, 1998). Finally, when rank in status hierarchies changes, these physiological profiles change as well: the loss of rank in primate social hierarchies triggers the production of the neuro-chemical correlates of depression (Price et al., 1994).

For example, the research of psychiatrist Michael McGuire and colleagues indicates that induced changes in status positions among vervet monkeys are associated with markers related to depression. These primates feature strong and enduring hierarchical status relationships with one dominant male in each group (McGuire, Raleigh, & Johnson, 1983). The highest-ranking males have serotonin levels that are twice as high as those of other males in the group (Raleigh & McGuire, 1984). When experimenters withdrew the dominant males from the group, their serotonin levels fell, they refused food, showed diminished activity, and appeared to human observers to be depressed. Conversely, the serotonin levels of previously dependent monkeys who gained high status after the removal of the previously dominant male changed to values that characterized dominant males. Similar results have been obtained with female monkeys (Shively, 1998).

The nature of dominance hierarchies also shapes depressive responses: the behavioral and neurochemical advantages of high rank are only found in stable dominance hierarchies whereas in unstable hierarchies where the position of the dominant is precarious, high rank is not associated with fewer stress hormones (Sapolsky, 2005). As well, groups that feature much affiliative support show few differences in stress reactions among dominants and subordinates. "Consistently," Sapolky summarizes, "animals who are more socially stressed by the dominance hierarchy show indices of hyperactivity of the (glucocorticoid) system" (2005, p. 651).

Ethological studies indicate that depressive responses might have arisen as signals of acceptance of defeat in status contests that are ubiquitous in the animal world. The British psychiatrist John Price and his colleagues have developed the most convincing explanation of the adaptive functions of depressive reactions after losses in status contests (Price et al., 1994; Stephens and Price, 2000). Price connects the inhibited action, withdrawal, lack of self-assertion, nervousness, and anxiety of distressed states to primeval brain algorithms that assess relative strengths, weaknesses, power, and rank of organisms and adjust actions accordingly to produce responses of flight, fight, or submission in confrontations with other animals. Animals develop distress responses when they assess that they are weaker than their potential competitors. They cease competing with the dominant animal, accept their defeated status, and signal their submission to the winning party. The inhibited aspects of depressive reactions are adaptive responses to subordinate positions from which there is no possibility of escape.

The defeated party who has failed to defend territory or lost a status contest could respond with renewed anger and aggression rather than concede to the winner. However, the open expression of aggressive emotions and behaviors can lead to the serious injury or death. Many of the symptoms of distress involve behaviors that communicate that the loser will not confront the winner, will not attempt to gain dominance, and will give up the struggle. Submissive responses protect the loser from further aggression by showing the dominant animal it is safe from additional challenges and need not feel threatened. Subordinates that make submissive responses are more likely to survive and reproduce than those who respond more aggressively.

Human responses to changing social status should be more complex than those among non-human primates because of the importance of reference groups and justifying ideologies in shaping the degree of well-being (Festinger, 1954; Lennon & Rosenfield, 1994). Nevertheless, the general relationship between dominance and well-being and between dependence and depression seems to be an inherited aspect of the human genome. Evolutionary studies indicate that distress responses should be situation-specific; they are adaptive only when facing potential defeat at the hands of stronger adversaries. Thus, the inhibition that is at the core of depression would be naturally selected to occur in those contexts. These studies also explain the widespread findings that distress is more common among people at the bottom of status hierarchies, those who are in enduring states of subordination, and those who suffer loss events that involve the lowering of social status. Finally, the findings from primate studies that indicate depressive responses are most likely when subordinates cannot escape threatening conditions are congruent with studies showing a strong association between humiliation and entrapment and the development of depression among humans (Brown, 2002). Mental health, however, might not be a zero-sum game: it is perhaps optimized among all parties in situations that foster equal social relationships (Mirowsky, 1985).

Studies of inequality have become a core area of interest in the sociology of mental health. Recent studies, following Marx, now link social class and social stratification to broader social arrangements (Link & Phelan, 1995). Moreover, they show how chronic and persistent social stressors linked to inequitable social arrangements are more strongly linked to mental health than the acute life stressors the field has traditionally emphasized (Turner, Wheaton, & Lloyd, 1995). Understanding mental health disparities as consequences of systems of social inequality resonates with the core tenets of both classical theory and evolutionary perspectives.

Meaningfulness

Classical Theory

Unlike Durkheim, who viewed social life as a level unto itself that was external to particular individuals, and Marx, who reduced consciousness to material underpinnings, Max Weber strove to understand human action at the level of its meaning for subjects. Weber emphasized the key role of culture and, in particular, social values for understanding social action. Sociology, for Weber, is the science of social action that seeks to understand subjective meanings and motivations. "Subjective understanding," he wrote, "is the specific characteristic of sociological knowledge" (Weber, 1925/1968, p. 15). *Subjective* does not equate to individual but is fundamentally social because groups provide the values that motivate individuals and give meaning to existence. Sociology is the study of how the goals of human actions, together with the means people use to realize these goals, lead to meaningful conduct.

Weber's focus was to explain social action in its historical context. The most salient characteristic of meaning in the modern world stems from the rise of bureaucratic organizations, which are part of a broader trend toward the greater rationalization of life (Weber, 1925/1968). Rationalization is the systematic organization of people, resources, and ideas in the interests of instrumental efficiency and effectiveness. Bureaucracy is marked by a type of means-end relationship, which Weber called *instrumental rationality*, where the sole value is to maximize the achievement of practical goals.

Weber was centrally concerned with the spiritual impact of the spread of technocratic ideas and bureaucratic organization in the modern world: "The fate of our times is characterized by rationalization and intellectualization and, above all, by the 'disenchantment of the world' " (Weber, 1919/1958, p. 155). He famously used the metaphor of the "iron cage" to describe the human condition in a bureaucratized world where people were not only confined to narrow restricted roles but also had no satisfactory alternatives to these roles. Technique and efficiency become ultimate values but can never answer the most urgent questions about what people should believe in, how they should conduct their lives, and what the meaning of human existence is. In a previous age the "Puritan wanted to work in a calling; we are forced to do so" (Weber, 1920/1957, p. 181). While Weber viewed the rationalization of the modern world as inevitable, he did not believe it could provide satisfying answers to these fundamental questions. Worse, rationalization was spreading from depersonalized occupational roles found in business and professional life to more specialized, instrumental, and formally organized roles in all spheres of social life including families, schools, and voluntary organizations. The growth of rationalization, combined with the trend toward the individualization of meaning, led Weber to despair about prospects for attaining psychological well-being in the modern world.

While Weber wrote little on specifically mental health issues, he did create a powerful framework for showing the influence of values on psychological well-being. He directs attention to systems of cultural symbols that provide coherent patterns for the conduct of life. Human behavior must be understood through the subjective meanings it has for actors, which are oriented to different types of social goals (1925/1968). Realizing these goals is central for individual mental health. Achievements are always relative to people's expectations, which are socially generated and vary widely across societies. The higher expectations are, the more difficult they will be to realize. Historically, means and ends were congruent so that expectations and accomplishments were generally in line with each other. Widespread disjunction between ends and means only develops in modern, capitalist societies, which make the achievement of valued social goals more difficult. Conversely, mental health should be better in social formations that provide satisfying values as well as the means to realize these values.

Sociology of Mental Health

Possessing social values that provide meaning and purpose to life should be conducive to mental health. Relatively little work in the sociology of mental health, however, focuses on the relationships of social values to psychological well-being. Studies that do consider values usually view them as psychological characteristics of individuals rather than as socially generated properties of groups (Lazarus & Folkman, 1984). A few studies, however, take social values seriously (Pearlin, 1989).

One line of work studies how differences in the meaningfulness of social statuses are associated with variations in mental health (Burton, 1998). For example, widowhood is more detrimental to the mental health of recent cohorts of retired men than women because the value men place on occupational achievement leads widowhood to symbolize loneliness and the inability to manage daily affairs to them (Umberson, Wortman, & Kessler, 1992). Conversely, widowhood provides new opportunities for self-sufficiency for recent cohorts of older women. Men and women also have different value commitments about what constitutes "good" husbands and fathers and "good" mothers and wives, respectively, and these commitments have different mental health consequences (Simon, 1995). Similarly, the positive mental health effects of getting married are greater for people who believe in the desirability and importance of marriage than those who don't; conversely, the negative effects of marital loss are worse among people who hold these values (Simon & Marcussen, 1999). Values and goals must be contextualized in frameworks of historical time and relevant reference groups (Elder, 1974; Jackson, 2004). For example, marriage is especially beneficial and marital loss especially harmful for mental health during historical periods when beliefs about the permanence, desirability, and importance of marriage are culturally strong and pervasive and among social groups that hold these values (Simon & Marcussen, 1999).

An emphasis on values also points to the important of *nonevents*, life events that people want to happen, but do not take place (Wheaton, 1999). Childless people who desire to have children, single people who want to get married, or workers who expect to get promotions but do not all hold goals that are not realized. McLaughlin (2004) finds that women, but not men, who do not marry are more depressed than those who marry at normative ages. Likewise, not having children leads to more depression among women, but not men, although there are important subgroup differences in the impact of normative events and non-events on mental health. The study of unfulfilled goals is an important, but understudied, area in the sociology of mental health.

Another line of research follows from Merton's classic article "Social Structure and Anomie" (1938/1968), which showed how distress can result from the failure to realize valued social goals. All societies define legitimate and desirable goals, purposes, and values and the appropriate ways to realize these objectives. However, they vary considerably in the opportunities they provide members to attain these goals. By the 20th century, the achievement of economic success was decoupled from its religious roots in Calvinism and had become a value held out to all members of society. Only a small portion of people, however, actually have the means to become successful. Merton's analysis shows not only how distress is a natural outgrowth of the value system of society but also how variations in rates of distress across societies is a function of the degree to which they provide their members opportunities to reach social goals.

The achievement of economic success is a particularly important value in modern American society, although its importance varies across different social groups. Carr (1997) shows how value expectations in earlier periods of the life cycle affect the degree of psychological satisfaction in later periods. She finds that women in their mid 50's who have not met the occupational aspirations they held in their mid 30's have more distress and less purpose in life than women who achieve the goals they set earlier in life. Interestingly, surpassing one's earlier goals does not further enhance mental health. These processes are tied to historical contexts (Carr, 2002). Women who are members of cohorts that did not value achievement outside the home are more content with their statuses as homemakers; conversely, younger cohorts are more likely to put higher value pursuing careers and so have more room for disappointment when they do not realize their expectations.

In addition to studies of the value of economic success, another literature links religious values to mental health. The Weberian tradition shows how the importance of religion goes beyond the Durkheimian emphasis on involvement with religious groups to provide access to a unique system of symbols, a consistent body of knowledge, and a coherent world view. For example, Idler (1987) finds that men with strong senses of religiosity report less depression and disability than those who are less religious. Holding strong religious beliefs, especially among people with disabling conditions, is conducive to positive mental health (Idler, 1995).

Little work in the sociology of mental health goes beyond the study of religion to examine the importance of political loyalties, ethical commitments, moral and aesthetic standards, and other social values on psychological well-being. Likewise, few studies address how value transformations at the societal level affect mental health. For example, one reason for the extraordinarily high rates of distress among Native Americans could be the marginalization of their core belief systems in the modern world. Or, vanquished societies after wartime defeats undergo transformations in values with resulting collective deteriorations in mental health (Schivelbusch, 2004). A Weberian perspective suggests that changing cultural values at the social level are strongly related to variations in well-being and distress.

Evolutionary Perspectives

Evolutionary forces cannot account for particular cultural values, which are uniquely human. More generally, however, these forces show how distress naturally arises when organisms are blocked in their pursuit of incentives (Klinger, 1975). Because values provide key incentives for human behavior, people become distressed when they can neither achieve nor disengage from goals to which they are committed (Nesse, 2000). People who are blocked in pursuit of valued incentives naturally become depressed, which, paradoxically, helps them disengage from the original unproductive incentive and reengage in potentially more fulfilling goals. Klinger (1975, pp. 14–15) explains the adaptive value of depressed affect:

An organism would totally exhaust itself pursuing its first blocked goal if it did not incorporate a mechanism for annulling its commitment to an inaccessible incentive, thus ending that particular current concern. If, however, rest or the end of hard striving carries positive incentive value, it would be important that the disengagement process be affectively aversive in order to prevent failure from taking on a net positive incentive value, which would surely be a dangerous state of affairs. Depression, of course, embodies the properties of such a mechanism.

Distress can be adaptive when it makes people more likely to give up old goals and acquire new ones. Distress responses are especially likely to emerge after life crises when people are forced to reevaluate their futures, and in this context may be adaptive in helping individuals to avoid rash decisions, take all possible dangers into account, and not overestimate the chances of success in new activities. "In this situation," according to Nesse, "pessimism, lack of energy, and fearfulness can prevent calamity even when they perpetuate misery" (2000, p. 17). Distress decreases investments in unsatisfying life projects and also prevents the premature pursuit of alternative projects. To the extent that depressed affect was adaptive, people who become depressed after failures in major life projects should be instinctively reproducing responses that had certain advantages in early evolutionary environments (Keller & Nesse, 2005). Examining the mental health of people undergoing midlife corrections and crises, and turning points in the life course should be especially informative for the sociology of mental health (George, 1999; Stewart & Vandewater, 1999; Wethington, Kessler, & Pixley, 2004).

Rates of distress should vary to the degree that societies both provide fulfilling value systems and strong collective belief systems that help extricate people from the depression that follows from unfulfilled expectations. Early societies were unlikely to have provided their members with unachievable goals and they also featured strong belief systems and community rituals to help individuals disengage from depressed states (Nesse, 2000). Conversely, modern societies not only lack such collective ceremonies but also promote unrealizable goals without providing adequate means to reach these goals (Merton, 1938/1968). Social factors such as media exposure to unreachable goals promote distress, particularly among people who lack the resources to accomplish socially-valued ends. Social variation in psychological well-being and distress is a product of the human need for fulfilling values and goals, the degree that social arrangements provide these values and manage those people who fail to realize them, and the extent to which goals are replaceable.

The impact of systems of cultural meaning on mental health has not received commensurate attention with social integration or social inequality, perhaps because of the difficulties of integrating measures of meaningfulness into traditional survey research instruments. The important work of George Brown (2002), building on Weber's emphasis on *verstehen*, shows how sociologists of mental health can assess subjective meanings through objective methods. Tying such methods to the study of broader cultural systems would allow the field to fully realize the Weberian focus on the fundamental importance of meaningfulness for the study of mental health.

Conclusion

Classical sociological theory focuses on the major dimensions of social life that influence mental health—integration, stratification, and cultural systems of meaning. Rooting empirical studies in the sociology of mental health within these general processes has a number of advantages. The field of psychiatry emphasizes how abnormal individual experiences produce negative mental health consequences. In contrast, the classical tradition emphasizes how social stressors emerge from basic aspects of social organization. Even suicide is not the irrational result of abnormal individuals but the consequence of the way people are attached to social institutions. Normal, rather than abnormal, features of social life explain the roots of distress (Aneshensel, 1992).

Integrating the sociology of mental health with evolutionary theory also enhances its power to explain states of psychological well-being. Human emotions are programmed to respond to the dimensions of social life that classical theory emphasized. Because humans are naturally responsive to losses of valued attachments, status, and meaning, social conditions have profound impacts on mental health. George Brown, for example, finds a ten-fold divergence in rates of depression across different societies that directly maps onto the number of loss events found in these societies (Brown, 2002). Evolutionary studies also show how modern social arrangements pose particular problems to achieving psychological well-being. "The orienting insight that our minds were built for environments very different from today's," Freese notes, "suggests a potentially powerful route toward understanding the internal conflicts, frailties of will, susceptibilities to manipulation and other irrationalities so common in social life" (2002, p. 49).

Individuals now confront novel environments that inherited psychological responses were not designed to deal with. Contemporary social structures feature many changing relationships that are constantly being lost, mobility away from close kin, and few common rituals of solidarity. The number of situations where individuals are unable to achieve social goals and must try to disengage from unreachable expectations is much larger now than in the ancient environments in which the human genome was formed. The media allows status comparisons not just within well-defined local groups but also with innumerable others, many of whom will always seem to be of higher status than one's self. Few people in the contemporary world have the means to achieve the ideals of beauty, wealth, fame, and success that are held out to the public on a daily basis. The gap between objective reality and cultural ideals can lead to much distress.

Classical social theory and the sociology of mental health also point to different policy directions for promoting mental health and alleviating distress than the current societal emphases on individualized therapies. Durkheim, Marx, and Weber all emphasized that psychological well-being requires well-functioning social institutions. In particular, it is difficult to make lasting positive changes in individual well-being in the absence of changes in social institutions. For example, new institutional structures that provide effective help with childcare could do far more to promote mental health than providing a pill to an overwhelmed parent. Yet, modern medication and psychological therapies promote intra-individual solutions that might make problems stemming from individualism even worse (Horwitz, 1982). Although these therapies might help people cope with distress, the largest positive mental health effects should stem from macro-level changes that promote social integration, egalitarian structures, and meaningful, achievable values. Such institutional changes can be the most effective way for individuals to attain supportive relationships, fulfilling jobs, decent livings, and meaningful values that optimize well-being (Mirowsky & Ross, 2003).

Classical theory also points the sociology of mental health in new directions. All the classical theorists took comparative and historical approaches. The sociology of mental health, in contrast, focuses on studies in one context, usually contemporary U.S. society. Likewise, the classical sociologists always rooted individual consciousness within broader social institutions. They emphasized the importance for sociologists of using social-level variables to explain individual level dependent variables. In contrast, much research in the sociology of mental health uses psychological variables such as a sense of control, self-esteem, mastery, or perceived discrimination as independent or mediating variables. As Link and Phelan (1995, p. 84) emphasize:

To the extent that interest in mechanisms increases at the expense of more fundamental social conditions, medical sociologists may unwittingly contribute to the emphasis on individual factors and play into the hands of those who argue that social factors have only a modest role in disease causation.

Attention to the macro-level processes stressed in classical sociological theory can help direct sociologists away from focusing on individual-level explanatory mechanisms. In the classical tradition, psychological states would be the consequences of social forces rather than variables that explain other psychological states.

Finally, this chapter has tried to show how certain types of biological explanations are compatible with basic sociological principles. Although sociologists generally view biological explanations as competing with social ones, in fact, social processes and biological design are not antithetical; when it comes to psychological emotions, they are complementary (Massey, 2002). Although they had little knowledge of biology, Durkheim, Marx, and Weber all realized that basic human needs existed that social arrangements either fulfilled or frustrated. Human emotions are programmed to react to the degree of integration and isolation, equality and stratification, and meaningfulness and disenchantment in social arrangements.

The benefits of linking the sociology of mental health to classical theory run in both directions. The sociology of mental health can link classical theory to a large body of literature that specifies the mediating mechanisms that link broader social processes to distress and well-being. In addition, the sociology of mental health provides basic information about how well social institutions are working. "The maps of emotional high and low zones," Mirowsky and Ross stress, "tell us a great deal about the nature and quality of life in different social positions" (2003, p. 30). Moreover, sociology itself is enriched because mental health is the ultimate dependent variable of all sociological subfields (Wheaton, 2001). The sociology of mental health stands between the macro-processes classical theory emphasizes and the universal needs stressed in evolutionary psychology. As such it is poised to answer perhaps the most basic sociological question: what sorts of social arrangements optimize happiness and minimize distress?

Acknowledgments. I am grateful to Deborah Carr, Ira Cohen, Jeremy Freese, and Ellen Idler for their suggestions on an earlier draft of this chapter.

References

Aneshensel, C. S. (1992). Social stress: Theory and research. *Annual Review of Sociology, 18*, 15–38.

Aneshensel, C. S., & Sucoff, C. A. (1996). The neighborhood context of adolescent mental health. *Journal of Health and Social Behavior, 37*, 293–310.

Archer, J. (1999). *The nature of grief: The evolution and psychology of reactions to loss.* New York: Routledge.

Avison, W. R., & Turner, R. J. (1988). Stressful life events and depressive symptoms: Disaggregating the effects of acute stressors and chronic strains. *Journal of Health and Social Behavior, 29*, 253–264.

Bowlby, J. (1969/1982). *Attachment and loss, Vol 1: Attachment.* New York: Basic Books.

Bowlby, J. (1980). *Attachment and loss, Vol. 3. Loss: Sadness and depression.* London: Hogarth Press.

Brown, G. W. (2002). Social roles, context and evolution in the origins of depression. *Journal of Health and Social Behavior, 43*, 255–276.

Brown, G. W., Harris, T. O., & Bifulco, A. (1986). Long-term effect of early loss of parent. In M. Rutter, C. Izard, & P. Read (Eds.) *Depression in childhood: Developmental perspectives* (pp. 251–296). New York: Guilford.

Burton, R. P. (1998). Global integrative meaning as a mediating factor in the relationship between social roles and psychological distress. *Journal of Health and Social Behavior, 39*, 201–215.

Buss, D. M. (1995). Evolutionary psychology: A new paradigm for psychological science. *Psychological Inquiry, 6*, 1–30.

Carr, D. (1997). The fulfillment of career dreams at midlife: Does it matter for women's mental health? *Journal of Health and Social Behavior, 38*, 331–344.

Carr, D. (2002). The psychological consequences of work-family tradeoffs across three cohorts of men and women. *Social Psychology Quarterly, 65*, 103–24.

Catalano, R. A., & Dooley, D. (1977). Economic predictors of depressed mood and stressful life events. *Journal of Health and Social Behavior, 18*, 292–307.

Dohrenwend, B. P. (2000). The role of adversity and stress in psychopathology: Some evidence and its implications for theory and research. *Journal of Health and Social Behavior, 41*, 1–19.

Durkheim, E. (1897/1951). *Suicide: A study in sociology*. New York: Free Press.

Eaton, W. W., & Muntaner, C. (1999). Socioeconomic stratification and mental disorder. In A. V. Horwitz & T. L. Scheid (Eds.), *A handbook of the sociology of mental health and illness: Social contexts, theories, and systems* (pp. 259–283). New York: Cambridge.

Elder, G. H. (1974). *Children of the Great Depression*. Chicago: University of Chicago Press.

Faris, R. E., & Dunham, H. W. (1939). *Mental disorders in urban areas*. Chicago: University of Chicago Press.

Fenwick, R., & Tausig, M. (1994). The macroeconomic context of job stress. *Journal of Health and Social Behavior, 35*, 266–282.

Festinger, L. (1954). A theory of social comparison processes. *Human Relations, 7*, 117–40.

Fodor, J. A. (1983) *The modularity of mind*. Cambridge: MIT Press.

Freese, J. (2002). Evolutionary psychology: New science or the same old storytelling? *Contexts, 1*, 44–49.

Freese, J., Li, J.C., & Wade, L. D. (2003). The potential relevances of biology to social inquiry. *Annual Review of Sociology, 29*, 233–256.

George, L. K. (1999). Life course perspectives on mental health." In C.S. Aneshensel & J.C. Phelan (Eds.), *Handbook of the sociology of mental health* (pp. 565–584). New York: Kluwer/Plenum.

Gilbert, P. (1992). *Depression: The evolution of powerlessness*. New York: Guilford.

Goldsmith, S. K., Pellmar, T. C., Kleinman, A. M., & Bunney, W. E. (Eds.). (2002). *Reducing suicide: A national imperative*. Washington D.C.: The National Academies Press.

Gove, W. R., & Tudor, J. F. (1973). Adult sex roles and mental illness. *American Journal of Sociology, 78*, 812–835.

Hagen, E. H. (1999). The functions of postpartum depression. *Evolution and Human Behavior, 20*, 325–359.

Harlow, H. F., & Suomi, S. J. (1974). Induced depression in monkeys. *Behavioral Biology, 12*, 173–296.

Holmes, T. H., & Rahe, R. H. (1967). The Social Readjustment Rating Scale. *Journal of Psychosomatic Research, 11*, 213–18.

Horwitz, A. V. (1982). *The social control of mental illllness*. New York: Academic Press.

Horwitz, A. V. (1999). The sociological study of mental iIllness: A critique and synthesis of four serspectives. In C.S. Aneshensel & J. Phelan (Eds.), *Handbook of the sociology of mental health* (pp. 57–80). New York: Kluwer/Plenum.

Horwitz, A. V., & White, H. R. (1998). The relationship of cohabitation and mental health: A study of a young adult cohort. *Journal of Marriage and the Family, 60*, 505–514.

House, J. S., Landis, K. R., & Umberson, D. (1988). Social relationships and health. *Science, 241*, 540–545.

Idler, E. L. (1987). Religious involvement and the health of the elderly: Some hypotheses and an initial test. *Social Forces, 66*, 226–238.

Idler, E. L. (1995). Religion, health, and nonphysical senses of self. *Social Forces, 74*, 683–704.

Jackson, P. B. (2004). Role sequencing: Does order matter for mental health? *Journal of Health and Social Behavior, 45*, 132–154.

Joyner, K., & Udry, J. R. (2000). You don't bring me anything but down: Adolescent romance and depression. *Journal of Health and Social Behavior, 41*, 369–391.

Kandel, E. R. (1998). A new intellectual framework for psychiatry. *American Journal of Psychiatry, 155*, 457–469.

Karasek, R., & Theorell, T. (1990) *Healthy work: Stress, productivity and the reconstruction of working life*. New York: Basic Books.

Keller, M. C., & Nesse, R. M. (2005). Is low Mood an adaptation? Evidence for subtypes with symptoms that match precipitants. *Journal of Affective Disorders, 86*, 27–35.

Kessler, R. C., & McLeod, J. D. (1984). Sex differences in vulnerability to undesirable life events. *American Sociological Review, 49*, 620–631.

Kessler, R. C., & McLeod, J. D. (1985). Social support and mental health in community samples. In S. Cohen & S.L. Syme (Eds.), *Social support and health* (pp. 219–240). New York: Academic.

Klinger, E. (1975). Consequences of commitment to and disengagement from incentives. *Psychological Review, 82*, 1–25.

Kohn, M. L. (1976). Occupational structure and alienation. *American Journal of Sociology, 82*, 111–30.

Lazarus, R. S., & Folkman, S. (1984). *Stress, appraisal, and coping*. New York: Springer.

Leighton, D. C., Harding, J. S., Macklin, D. B., Macmillan, A. M., & Leighton, A. H. (1963). *The character of danger: Psychiatric symptoms in selected communities*. New York: Basic Books.

Lennon, M. C. (1994). *Women, work, and well-being: The importance of work conditions*. *Journal of Health and Social Behavior, 35*, 235–247.

Lennon, M. C., & Rosenfield, S. (1992). Women and mental health: The interaction of job and family conditions. *Journal of Health and Social Behavior, 33*, 316–327.

Lennon, M. C., & Rosenfield, S. (1994). Relative fairness and the division of housework: The importance of options. *American Journal of Sociology, 100*, 506–531.

Lester, D. (Ed.). (1994). *Emile Durkheim: Le Suicide one hundred years later*. Philadelphia: The Charles Press.

Lin, N., Ye, X., & Ensel, W. M. (1999). Social support and depressed mood: A structural analysis. *Journal of Health and Social Behavior, 40*, 344–59.

Link, B. G., Lennon, M. C., & Dohrenwend, B. P. (1993). Socioeconomic status and depression. *American Journal of Sociology, 98*, 1351–87.

Link, B. G., & Phelan, J. C. (1995). Social conditions as fundamental causes of distress. *Journal of Health and Social Behavior (extra issue)*, 80–94.

Marmot, M., & Wilkinson, R. G. (Eds.). (1999). *Social determinants of health*. New York: Oxford University Press.

Marx, K. (1844/1977). Economic and philosophical manuscripts. In D. McLellan (Ed.), *Karl Marx: Selected writings* (pp. 75–112). Oxford: Oxford University Press.

Marx, K. (1845/1977). Theses on Feuerbach. In D. McLellan (Ed.), *Karl Marx: Selected writings* (pp. 156–158). Oxford: Oxford University Press.

Marx, K. (1847/1977). The Communist Manifesto. In D. McLellan (Ed.), *Karl Marx: Selected writings* (pp. 221–247). Oxford: Oxford University Press.

Marx, K. (1932/1977). The German ideology. In D. McLellan (Ed.), *Karl Marx: Selected writings* (pp. 159–191). Oxford: Oxford University Press.

Massey, D. S. (2002). Emotion and the history of human society. *American Sociological Review, 67*, 1–29.

McLaughlin, J. (2004). *It's in the timing: The relationship between the temporal composition of family transitions and psychological well-Being*. Unpublished doctoral dissertation, Rutgers University, New Brunswick.

McGuire, M. T., Raleigh, M. J., & Johnson, C. (1983). Social dominance in adult male *Vervet* monkeys: General considerations. *Social Science Information, 22*, 89–123.

McGuire, M. &, Troisi, A. (1998). *Darwinian psychiatry*. New York: Oxford University Press.

McLeod, J. D,. & Nonnemaker, J. M. (1999). Social stratification and inequality." In C. S. Aneshensel & J. C. Phelan (Eds.), *Handbook of the sociology of mental health* (pp. 321–344). New York: Kluwer/Plenum.

Menaghan, E. G. (1991). Work experiences and family interaction processes: The long reach of the job? *Annual Review of Sociology, 17*, 419–444.

Merton, R. K. (1938/1968). Social structure and anomie. In R. K. Merton (Ed.), *Social theory and social structure* (pp. 185–214). New York: Free Press.

Mineka, S., & Suomi, S. J. (1978). Social separation in monkeys. *Psychological Bulletin, 85*, 1374–1400.

Mirowsky, J. (1985). Depression and marital power: An equity model. *American Journal of Sociology, 91*, 557–592.

Mirowsky, J. (1996). Age and the gender gap in depression. *Journal of Health and Social Behavior, 37*, 362–380.

Mirowsky, J., & Ross, C. E. (2003). *Social causes of psychological distress (2nd ed.)*. New York: Aldine de Gruyter.

Nesse, R. M. (2000). Is depression an adaptation? *Archives of General Psychiatry, 57*, 14–20.

Pearlin, L. I. (1989). The sociological study of stress. *Journal of Health and Social Behavior, 30*, 241–256.

Pearlin, L. I., Aneshensel, C. S., & LeBlanc, A. J. (1997). The forms and mechanisms of stress proliferation: The case of AIDS caregivers. *Journal of Health and Social Behavior, 38*, 223–236.

Pearlin, L. I., & Skaff, M. M. (1995). Stressors and adaptation in late life. In M. Gatz (Ed.), *Emerging issues in mental health and aging* (pp. 97–123). Washington DC: American Psychiatric Association Press.

Pescosolido, B. A., & Georgianna, S. (1989). Durkheim, suicide, and religion. *American Sociological Review, 54*, 33–48.

Pescosolido, B. A., & Levy, J. A. (2002). The role of social networks in health, illness, disease and healing: The accepting present, the forgotten past, and the dangerous potential for a complacent future. In J.A. Levy & B.A. Pescosolido (Eds.), *Social Networks and Health* (pp. 3–25). New York: JAI.

Pescosolido, B. A., & Rubin, B. A. (2000). The web of group affiliations revisited: Social life, postmodernism, and sociology. *American Sociological Review, 65*, 62–77.

Pinker, S. (2002). *The blank slate: The modern denial of human nature*. New York: Viking.

Plomin, R., DeFries, J. C., McClearn, G. E., & McGuffin, P. (2001). *Behavioral genetics, 4th ed.* New York: Worth Publishers and W.H. Freeman.

Price, J. L., Slomin, L., Gardner, R., Gilbert, P., & Rhode, P. (1994). The social competition hypothesis of depression. *British Journal of Psychiatry, 164*, 309–315.

Raleigh, M. J., & McGuire, M. T. (1984). Social and environmental influences on blood serotonin concentrations in monkeys. *Archives of General Psychiatry, 41*, 405–410.

Reynolds, J. R. (1997). The effects of industrial employment conditions on job-related distress. *Journal of Health and Social Behavior, 38*, 105–116.

Rietschlin, J. (1998). Voluntary association membership and psychological distress. *Journal of Health and Social Behavior, 39*, 348–55.

Rook, K. S. (1984). The negative side of social interaction: Impact on psychological well-being. *Journal of Personality and Social Psychology, 46*, 1097–1108.

Rosenfield, S. (1980). Sex differences in depression: Do women always have higher rates? *Journal of Health and Social Behavior, 21*, 33–42.

Rosenfield, S. (1989). The health effects of women's employment: Personal control and sex differences in mental health. *Journal of Health and Social Behavior, 30*, 77–91.

Rosenfield, S. (1992). The costs of sharing: Wives' employment and husbands' mental health. *Journal of Health and Social Behavior, 33*, 213–225.

Rosenfield, S. (1999). Gender and mental health: Do women have more psychopathology, men more, or both the same (and why)? In A. V. Horwitz & T. S. Scheid (Eds.), *A handbook for the study of mental health: Social contexts, theories and systems* (pp. 348–360). New York: Cambridge.

Ross, C. E. (1995). Reconceptualizing marital status as a continuum of social attachment. *Journal of Marriage and the Family, 57*, 129–140.

Ross, C. E. (2000). Neighborhood disadvantage and adult mental depression. *Journal of Health and Social Behavior, 41*, 177–187.

Ross, C. E., Mirowsky, J., & Huber, J. (1983). Dividing work, sharing work, and in-between: Marriage patterns and depression. *American Sociological Review, 48*, 809–823.

Rutter, M. (1981). *Maternal deprivation reassessed, 2nd ed.* London: Penguin.

Sapolsky, R. M. (1989). Hypercortisolism among socially subordinate wild baboons originates at the CNS level. *Archives of General Psychiatry, 46*, 1047–1051.

Sapolsky, R. M. (2005). The influence of social hierarchy on primate health. *Science, 308*, 648–652.

Schwartz, S. (1991). Women and depression: A Durkheimian perspective. *Social Science and Medicine, 32*, 127–140.

Schivelbusch, W. (2004). *The culture of defeat: On national trauma, mourning, and recovery.* New York: Picador.

Shively, C. A. (1998). Social subordination stress, behavior, and central monoaminergic function in female cynomolgus monkeys. *Biological Psychiatry, 44*, 882–891.

Simon, R.W. (1995). Gender, multiple roles, role meaning, and mental health. *Journal of Health and Social Behavior, 36*, 182–94.

Simon, R. W., & Marcussen, K. (1999). Marital transitions, marital beliefs, and mental Health. *Journal of Health and Social Behavior, 40*, 111–125.

Stevens, A., & Price, J. (2000). *Evolutionary psychiatry: A new beginning.* London: Routledge.

Stewart, A. J., & Vandewater, E. A. (1999). "If I had it to do over again": Midlife review, midcourse corrections, and women's well-being in midlife. *Journal of Personality and Social Psychology, 76*, 270–81.

Stockard, J., & O'Brien, R. M. (2002). Cohort effects on suicide rates: International variations. *American Sociological Review, 67*, 854–873.

Suomi, S. J. (1991) Adolescent depression and depressive symptoms: Insights from longitudinal studies with rhesus monkeys. *Journal of Youth and Adolescence, 20*, 273–287.

Thoits, P. A. (1986). Multiple identities: examining gender and marital status differences in distress. *American Sociological Review, 51*, 259–72.

Thoits, P. A., & Hewitt, L. N. (2001). Volunteer work and well-being. *Journal of Health and Social Behavior, 42*, 115–131.

Tooby, J., & Cosmides, L. (1992). On the universality of human nature and the uniqueness of the individual: the role of genetics and adaptation. *Journal of Personality, 58*, 17–68.

Turner, J. H. (2000). *On the origins of human emotions: A sociological inquiry into the evolution of human affect.* Stanford: Stanford University Press.

Turner, R. J. (1999). Social support and coping. In A. V. Horwitz & T. L. Scheid (Eds.), *A handbook for the study of mental health: Social contexts, theories, and systems* (pp. 198–210). New York: Cambridge University Press.

Turner, R. J. (2003). The pursuit of socially modifiable contingencies in mental health. *Journal of Health and Social Behavior, 44*, 1–17.

Turner, R. J., Wheaton, B., & Lloyd, D. A. (1995). The epidemiology of stress. *American Sociological Review, 60*, 104–25.

Umberson, D. (1987). Family status and health behaviors: Social control as a dimension of social integration. *Journal of Health and Social Behavior, 28*, 306–19.

Umberson, D., & Williams, K. (1999). Family status and mental health. In C.S. Aneshensel & J.C. Phelan (Eds.), *Handbook of the sociology of mental health* (pp. 225–253). New York: Kluwer/Plenum.

Umberson, D., Wortman, C. B., & Kessler, R.C. (1992). Widowhood and depression: explaining long-term gender differences in vulnerability. *Journal of Health and Social Behavior, 33*, 10–24.

Weber, M. (1919/1958). Science as a vocation. In H.H. Gerth & C.W. Mills (Eds.), *From Max Weber* (pp. 129–156). New York: Oxford University Press.

Weber, M. (1920/1958). *The Protestant ethic and the spirit of capitalism.* New York: Charles Scribner's Sons.

Weber, M. (1925/1968). *Economy and society, Vol. 1.* New York: Bedminster Press.

Wethington, E., Kessler, R. C., & Pixley, J. E. (2004). Turning points in adulthood. In O. G. Brim, C. D. Ryff, & R. C. Kessler (Eds.), *How healthy are we? A national study of well-being at midlife* (pp. 586–613). Chicago: University of Chicago Press.

Wheaton, B. (1990). Life transitions, role histories, and mental health. *American Sociological Review, 55*, 209–23.

Wheaton, B. (1999). The nature of stressors. In A. V. Horwitz & T. L. Scheid (Eds.), *A handbook for the study of Mental health: Social contexts, theories, and systems* (pp. 176–197). New York: Cambridge University Press.

Wheaton, B. (2001). The role of sociology in the study of mental health . . . and the role of mental health in the study of sociology. *Journal of Health and Social Behavior, 42*, 221–234.

Williams, D. R., & Harris-Reid, M. (1999). Race and Mental health: Emerging patterns and promising approaches. In A. V. Horwitz & T. L. Scheid (Eds.), *A handbook for the study of mental health: Social contexts, theories, and systems* (pp. 295–314). New York: Cambridge University Press.

Williams, K. (2003). Has the future of marriage arrived? A contemporary examination of gender, marriage, and psychological well-being. *Journal of Health and Social Behavior, 44*, 470–487.

5
Contemporary Social Theory and the Sociological Study of Mental Health

Ann Branaman

The analysis of the impact of modern life on subjective experience is common to both classical and contemporary social theory. While classical sociologists were concerned with the impact of the rapid social changes and emergent social conditions of the early modern era, contemporary social theorists focus on the conditions of life a century or so after classical social theory. Beginning with the Frankfurt School in the 1930s but picking up tremendously since the late 1960s, the linking of psychological tribulations to contemporary social conditions, the analysis of subjectivity as a site of social control, and a consideration of the psychological underpinnings and effects of domination and liberation have become prominent themes in social theory (Elliot, 2001). Within contemporary social theory, some of the classic themes re-emerge. Do contemporary social conditions enhance or restrict individuality, freedom, and psychic well-being? Is anomie the most significant threat to psychic well-being, or should mental distress be understood in terms of alienating societal systems of control and domination? These issues remain central.

My focus in this chapter is on the insights of contemporary social theory as they pertain to mental health issues. Contemporary social theory is, however, short on empirical knowledge of the actual experiences and proximate determinants of mental health of individuals. While theorizing about psychological matters with apparent insight, most social theorists know very little about mental health and illness. Thus, research in the sociology of mental health is essential for grounding, refining, challenging, or modifying the conceptions of social theorists. In this chapter, I not only identify contributions of contemporary social theory for thinking about mental health but also suggest ways in which research in the sociology of mental health provides relevant insight for contemporary social theorists.

Three widely recognized foci within the sociology of mental health are: the social origins of distress, the nature of mental health and illness, and mental health services. Contemporary social theory contributes to thinking about each of these areas of concern. In this chapter, I have chosen to focus on three broadly-defined schools of contemporary social thought: theories of individualization, critical theories, and Foucauldian/postmodern perspectives. These three perspectives highlight distinct ways of thinking about mental health, each of which are related to the three major foci of the sociology of mental health identified above. First, theories of individualization are most relevant for thinking about the social origins of mental distress, as they see contemporary life as producing psychic challenges and, often, distress in the lives of individuals. Second, critical theoretical perspectives contribute most to thinking about the nature of mental health and distress. In focusing on the ways in which structures of power and domination in the broader society produce distorting effects on the human psyche at the very same time that they mute discontent and promote "pseudo-happiness," they challenge conventional definitions of mental health and distress. And, third, Foucauldian/postmodern perspectives, because they view psychotherapeutic practices as an important site of power and social control, are most relevant for thinking about the social and personal implications of psychotherapeutic practices and discourse.

The Social Origins of Distress

A key insight of the sociology of mental health is that many people who experience mental distress may be responding normally to stressful life circumstances. Accordingly, research in the sociology of mental health has focused attention on the relationship between life conditions and mental health, demonstrating the negative impact of stressful life events as well as ongoing stressful life conditions. Sociologists have also shown that social roles, such as roles involving subordination to others, may be psychologically stressful and that absence of strong interpersonal ties makes individuals more vulnerable to distress (see Horwitz, 2002, for a brief review of these literatures). Mostly, however, this research has considered the impact of proximate social stressors that differentially affect individuals (e.g., divorce, poverty, unemployment) within particular societies at particular times. In contrast, contemporary social theorists present sweeping statements of the impact of current social conditions in advanced contemporary societies with little concern for individual or group differences. At least in part, this difference can be explained by the different aims of contemporary social theory and the sociology of mental health. Social theorists are more concerned with identifying pervasive conditions of social life, and, often, their reflections on their potential psychological impact are secondary. Sociologists of mental health, conversely, are *primarily* interested in mental health and the social factors that affect the mental health of individuals. While not so useful in understanding individual differences in mental health, contemporary social theory does highlight the question of whether contemporary life is more conducive to mental health or to distress.

Whether contemporary social life *is* in fact a psychologically taxing climate is debated. Maryanski and Turner (1992), for example, argue that the individualizing conditions of advanced industrial societies represent an increasingly *hospitable* climate, favoring the realization of the naturally individualistic tendencies of human beings. This position is not shared widely among social theorists, but does represent a debate echoing one implicit in the contrast between Durkheim ([1897] 1951) and Simmel ([1903] 1971; [1907] 1978), the former emphasizing the anomic and

distressful aspects of individualization and the latter placing relatively more emphasis on the possibilities for freedom and psychic individualization.

Whether or not the contemporary context is a climate more conducive to mental
health or to mental distress is, ultimately, an empirical question. Within the field of
psychology, research showing increasing anxiety, insecurity, and depression over the
second half of the 20th century has caused some to dub the contemporary period as
the "age of anxiety" (Spielberger & Rickman, 1990) and the "age of melancholy"
(Hagnell, Lanke, Rorsman, & Ojesjo, 1982; Klerman, 1978). Twenge (2000, 2002)
finds increasing levels of anxiety, dysphoria, and neuroticism among more recent
cohorts of young adults and children, providing empirical support for the view that
the contemporary period may be exceptionally conducive to mental distress. Other
research similarly documents cohort differences (used as a proxy for socio-cultural
environment) on various measures of psychological well-being (e.g., Dyer, 1987;
Klerman & Weissman, 1989; Lewinsohn, Rohde, Seeley, & Fischer, 1993; Twenge &
Campbell, 2001), also providing evidence useful for assessing the psychological
impact of the contemporary age.

In defining contemporary life in relation to problems of self-identity, the theorists of individualization – Zygmunt Bauman, Ulrich Beck and Elizabeth Beck-
Gernsheim, and Anthony Giddens – portray current social conditions as personally
challenging and, often, psychically distressing. Consistent with Durkheim's view
of anomie as a source of mental distress, they characterize contemporary life as
promoting anxiety and anomie; they also imply, however, that individualization
may enhance mental health by expanding opportunities for self-mastery.

Bauman portrays contemporary individuals as tormented by the problem of
identity. Although the achievement of identity has been an individual responsibility throughout the modern age, Bauman argues, the task is different and more
problematic in the contemporary age. Modernity de-traditionalized identity and
made the achievement of identity a personal task. The difference from the contemporary age, however, is that the "slots" to which individuals could aspire in
the earlier modern age were clearly defined. The individual *achieved* identity, and
could feel a solidity of identity, by living up to the expectations of occupation,
class, and gender. "The 'self-identification' task put before men and women once
the stiff frame of estates had been broken in the early modern era boiled down to
the challenge of living 'true to kind' ('keeping up with the Joneses'): of actively
conforming to the established social types and models of conduct, of imitating,
following the pattern, 'acculturating', not falling out of step, not deviating from
the norm" (Bauman, 2001, p. 145).

In the contemporary age of "liquid modernity," however, it is "not just the individual *placements* in society, but the *places* to which individuals may gain access
and in which they may wish to settle are melting fast and can hardly serve as
targets for 'life projects'" (Bauman, 2001, p. 146). Individuals are faced with
uncertainty about their prospects for sustaining the "marketability" of any chosen
identity and find it difficult to "hold onto" identity. Contemporary life conspires
"against distant goals, life-long projects, lasting commitments, eternal alliances,
immutable identities" (Bauman 1996, p. 51). Those who do best are those who

are able to "travel lightly," maintaining looseness of attachment (e.g., to others, to goals and values, to institutions, communities, or nations, and to self-identities) and staying ever 'on the move' (Bauman 2005, pp. 4–5). Here, Bauman is talking more about global capitalists maintaining loose commitments to workers, communities, and nations, but the same principle applies for thinking about the relationship between individuals and their identities. For loosely attached individuals, typically located at the top of the global power hierarchy, there may be pleasure as they perform the task of constructing and reconstructing their individualized identities with successful outcome. Even for them, however, anxiety cannot be put to rest. Since identities are constructed to a significant extent by means of consumption, to succeed in the individualized society costs lots of money; the key to staying in the game is the ability to maintain one's own "use-value," and this requires continual self-scrutiny and self-transformation. These more favorably positioned individuals, he argues, are haunted by "fears of being caught napping, of failing to catch up with fast-moving events, of being left behind, . . . of missing the moment that calls for a change of tack before crossing the point of no return" (Bauman 2005, p. 2).

For those less well-positioned, the enforced individualization of the contemporary age is anxiety-provoking in a different way and, likely, more depressing. There is a growing gap between "individuality as fate and individuality as a practical capacity for self-assertion" (Bauman 2001, p. 47). For the "global underclass," Bauman argues, individualization must seem a cruel joke; the only meaning that "individuality" could have for them is the experience of being cut adrift and left to their own devices in a hostile world (Bauman 2005, p. 23). Individuality is, Bauman emphasizes, a privilege. Many, including the masses in the middle, remain "stuck" and "fixed" in their "no-choice, no-questions-asked, assigned or imposed but in any case 'overdetermined' identities" (Bauman 2005, p. 26). Lacking the resources, capacities, and access to consumer markets necessary for the continual re-fashioning of identity, such individuals are likely to find painful the assault on their stable identities that the new individualization represents. They may resist individualization and hold tightly to their existing identities, yet cannot help but feel the devaluation of their "outdated models" of identity.

In sum, the explanation Bauman offers for the increasing levels of anxiety in the contemporary age is the precariousness of identity and the difficulty of sustaining goals and life-projects. For those at the top or near the top of global power hierarchies, the anxiety is driven by the need for hyper-vigilance in constructing, revising, and revamping identities in an effort to maintain "use-value" in the rapidly changing global marketplace. For those at the bottom or near the bottom, the fear is the realistic possibility (or, worse, realization) of being consigned to the waste heap of society, deprived and devalued. For those in the middle, the anxieties are a mixture of both (Bauman, 2005). Bauman suggests that Generation X, in particular, faces both sorts of anxieties intensely, feeling anxiety in the face of the threat of "redundancy" and depression in its realization (Bauman, 2004).

Beck and Beck-Gernsheim (1996, 2002) similarly focus on the stress, anxiety, and uncertainty experienced by individuals in the context of institutionalized individualization. Individualization, as they define it, involves the disintegration of previously existing social categories and forms of social integration such as class, social status, gender roles, family, and neighborhood (Beck & Beck, 1996, p. 24). "Individualization is a compulsion, albeit a paradoxical one, to create, to stage-manage, not only one's own biography but the bonds and networks surrounding it, and to do this amid changing preferences and at successive stages of life, while constantly adapting to the conditions of the labour market, the education system, the welfare state, etc. (Beck & Beck, 1996, p. 27). Similarly to Bauman, Beck and Beck-Gernsheim view individualization as a "precarious freedom." They characterize the contemporary individualized person as stressed and overtaxed, attributing this to uncertainty and the destruction of routine. They cite an extensive psychological literature that emphasizes the psychological relief afforded by internalized, preconscious or semi-conscious routines and argue that such routines support individuals in living their lives and discovering their identities (Beck & Beck, 1996, p. 29). As they see it, however, it is much less possible to take anything for granted these days, with the previously taken for granted "breaking down into a cloud of possibilities to be thought about and negotiated" (p. 30). "Think, calculate, plan, adjust, negotiate, define, revoke (with everything constantly starting again from the beginning): these are the imperatives of the 'precarious freedoms' that are taking hold of life as modernity advances" (p. 30).

Of the theorists of individualization, Giddens focuses most directly on the potential *positive* mental consequences of contemporary social conditions, although he is just as attuned as the others to darker possibilities. Giddens (2000) argues that individuals are forced to live more openly and reflectively as both public institutions and everyday life become released from the hold of traditions. The self becomes a "reflexive project," as contemporary individuals must make identity-shaping lifestyle choices in the absence of traditional guidelines. The project is ongoing; selves are constantly in revision as new lifestyle choices emerge and former ones become less viable in an ever-changing world (Giddens, 1991, p. 5). The positive side of reflexivity is the possibility it offers for a sense of mastery and self-authorship; the threat of personal meaninglessness, however, looms behind the reflexive project of the self, as individuals lack guidance and validation for the lives they lead and the selves they fashion (p. 32). While increased freedom to choose may enhance individuals' sense of life mastery, Giddens argues that "the dark side of decision making is the rise of addictions and compulsions" (Giddens, 2000, p. 64). All activities of life can become addictions and compulsions, precisely because they are not as structured by tradition and custom as they once were. "Addiction comes into play when choice, which should be driven by autonomy, is subverted by anxiety" (Giddens, 2000, pp. 64–65).

In sum, the theorists of individualization, considered collectively, link the anxiety and psychic distress experienced by contemporary individuals to various facets of the "individualized society." The most basic argument is that contemporary life and, with it, self-identity, has been de-traditionalized and individualized. This increases the anxiety of individuals, although it might also, under favorable circumstances, enhance an individual's sense of freedom and self-mastery. A second related argument is that an individual's life routines and life projects are not only more open to choice but also less sustainable, contributing to psychological distress and/or the development of addictions and compulsions. Third, because of de-traditionalization, individualization, and the instability and diversity of the contemporary world, contemporary individuals face "identity troubles" of various sorts. A final argument, emphasized most by Bauman, is that the pleasures, anxieties, and pains associated with identity construction in the contemporary age are socially stratified.

These arguments imply a number of empirical questions. The most basic one concerns the impact of de-traditionalization and individualization on mental health. Life course theorists have provided evidence of a "de-standardization of the life course" in the latter part of the 20th century in both Europe and the United States (Bruckner & Mayer, 2005; Buchmann, 1989; Heinz, 1991; Held, 1986; Mayer, 2004; O'Rand & Henretta, 1999; Shanahan, 2000). Although there is little direct evidence concerning the psychological effects of such de-standardization, the research does suggest an increased "turbulence" in life in comparison to the 30-year "Golden-Age" following World War II (Mayer, 2001; Myles, 2003). Twenge (2000, 2002) does not identify de-traditionalization or individualization as causes of increased rates on anxiety and depression among cohorts born after 1970, instead pointing to weakening of social bonds and non-economic environmental dangers; however, the increases in anxiety and depression she documents do occur conterminously with increased de-standardization. An interactive effect between de-traditionalization and mental health, further, is suggested by research indicating the increased importance of self-regulation to the successful navigation through crucial life course transitions. Heinz (2002) indicates the increased importance of "self-socialization" in the contemporary age, a process that could reasonably be thought to be affected by an individual's mental health. Further, Twenge, Zhang, & Charles (2004) show that the average college student in 2002 has a more external locus of control than 80% of college students in 1960; this might be seen as indirect evidence that detraditionalization and individualization do not, on the whole, contribute to an increased sense of freedom in determining one's own life fate.

A second issue concerns the relationship between routine, expansion of lifestyle choices, and mental health. The psychological evidence cited by Beck and Beck-Gernsheim indicating the psychological need for routine in daily life is straightforward. Further, research that emphasizes the importance of goals for positive mental well-being (Austin & Vancouver, 1996; Emmons, 2002; Karoly, 1999;) might be seen to support the idea that de-traditionalization could be psychologically taxing, at least if we accept Bauman's and Beck and Beck-Gernsheim's interpretation of it as interfering with sustaining goals, routine, and life projects. Not all agree, however, that de-traditionalization necessarily implies de-routinization. Campbell (1996) challenges this view, while Giddens (1991) suggests that routine only becomes destabilized at critical junctures. In any case, this psychological evidence is insufficient to fully address the crucial issues.

If routine is psychologically comforting, and if, as Beck and Beck-Gernsheim suggest, the experience of life as "a cloud of possibilities to be thought about and negotiated" interferes with sustaining routine in everyday life, then should we conclude that responsibility for making lifestyle choices adversely affects mental health? Research on locus of control casts doubt that individuals who experience life as a "cloud of possibilities" should be more distressed than those who experience little choice, as research shows that individuals with a more external locus of control are typically more depressed and anxious than individuals with an internal locus of control (Benassi, Sweeney, & Dufour, 1988; Seligman, 1975; Twenge et al., 2004). Yet, it would be a misreading of the theories of individualization to interpret the increased responsibility for making of life-shaping decisions as necessarily correlated with an increased sense of control over one's own life. Recall Bauman's contention of an increasing "gap between individuality as fate and individuality as practical capacity for self-assertion." And note that Beck and Beck-Gernsheim refer to a *cloud* of possibilities, not a *menu* with clearly demarcated selections and predictable outcomes. Even if individuals have choices, they may feel not only constrained but also experience lack of control over and an inability to predict the implications of their choices for their life trajectories. Thus, the documented increase in external locus of control among more recent cohorts may be fully compatible with increased responsibility for lifestyle choices. Giddens' contention that addictions are born of autonomy and freedom and represent "frozen autonomy" may seem insightful and appropriate for understanding *some* addictions and compulsions; however, if we consider the rising external locus of control among younger cohorts, it might seem just as reasonable to link addictions and compulsions to fatalism, thwarted opportunities, or derailed trajectories. As Bauman's work shows, however, anomie and fatalism need not be viewed as opposite, since anomie is more painful when opportunities and perceived control are absent.

A third major issue concerns the relationship between the "identity troubles" defined by the theorists of individualization and mental health. A key difficulty is the lack of guidelines for constructing identity and the uncertainty individuals face as they construct their identities within diverse and rapidly changing contexts. Kenneth Gergen (1991) has suggested that individuals may be overwhelmed by the multiplication of (actual and possible) identities and relationships in contemporary life, with the competing value orientations and demands that each of these entail. Although the theorists of individualization do not view the multiplicity of identities as an inherent source of distress, they do suggest that the diversity of contexts encountered by individuals and the multiple *possibilities* for identification pose a challenge for individuals as they attempt to construct a unified sense of self-identity and maintain a sense of value and viability in their chosen identity commitments. According to Giddens (1991), many make use of diversity in constructing a distinctive sense of identity and, thus, find multiple identities no barrier to achieving a unified sense of self-identity; yet, he notes that some individuals may react (pathologically) to such diversity either by clinging to a rigidly fixed identity or by losing all sense of self through chameleon-like conformity. Research on the impact of "multiple identities" on mental health contributes to thinking about this set of issues.

Research by Thoits (1983) and Linville (1987) shows that psychological well-being is enhanced by multiple identities. In contrast to Goode's (1960) classic theory of role strain and role conflict, Thoits' (1983) research shows the more identities individuals possess, the less likely they will experience psychological distress. Linville (1987) argues that greater self-complexity, defined as multiple and *weakly related* identities, serves as a buffer against stressful events that threaten a person in one of her self-aspects. Persons with greater self-complexity are less likely to experience depression, stress, physical symptoms, and other illnesses. Even if multiple, non-integrated identities pose no psychological threat, however, there remains the potential problem, suggested by nearly all of the theorists of individualization, of the lack of authoritative guidelines for constructing identity and the difficulty in "holding on" to identity in the face of rapid social change and changing standards. An explanation that Thoits (1983) provides for the psychologically beneficial effect of multiple identities is the guidance that these provide. "... *if one knows who one is (in a social sense), then one knows how to behave*. Role requirements give purpose, meaning, direction, and guidance to ones life. The greater the number of identities held, the stronger one's sense of meaningful, guided existence" (p. 175). The theorists of individualization, however, suggest that contemporary identities are less durable, no longer come with clear role requirements, and are less effective in providing purpose, meaning, direction, and guidance.

Indirectly, the research by Linville and Thoits lends support to Bauman's contention that those who do the best in the contemporary context are those who "travel lightly" and maintain "loose attachments." Linville's study shows that individuals who maintain multiple and *disconnected* identities, hence reducing investment in any particular identity, enjoy the greatest mental health. Their emotional reactivity to stressors *and* to positive events within any realm of their lives tended to be less extreme than the emotional reactivity of individuals who had fewer identities or who maintained an integrated set of identities. Thoits' (1983) research shows, further, that while multiple identities enhance psychological well-being, the psychological cost of loss of an identity is greater for those whose identities are more overlapping and integrated than for those whose identities are less connected. While maintenance of multiple *integrated* identities is most psychologically advantageous, then, this holds only so long as the identities are maintained. *If* the contemporary context is one in which it is difficult to sustain any identity, the implication is that more loosely connected identities would be, if not psychologically optimal, the safest bet.

Finally, Bauman's suggestions about the socially stratified distribution of the pleasures, fears, and anxieties associated with life's uncertainties offer a potentially helpful way of thinking about socioeconomic variations in mental health and distress. Research in the sociology of mental health, in general, demonstrates an inverse relationship between socioeconomic status and mental health (Eaton & Muntaner, 1999). With the exception of schizophrenia, for which social selection plays a significant role in explaining the greater rates among lower classes, research evidence generally supports the view that social stratification and other related structural factors have a causal influence on mental health (Dohrenwend, Levav, Shrout, Schwartz, Naveh, Link, Skodol, & Stueve, 1992; Eaton, 1986; Liem & Liem, 1978; Wheaton, 1978). A large body of research in the sociology of mental health focuses on the impact of stressful life experiences on mental health (e.g., Dohrenwend & Dohrenwend, 1974; Pearlin, 1989; Wheaton, 1994), and, in general, shows both a greater amount of chronic and systemic life stressors as well as greater vulnerability to stressors in lower social classes (Aneshensel, 1992; McLeod & Kessler, 1990; Turner, Wheaton, & Lloyd, 1995). Further, Wheaton (1980) finds a greater degree of "fatalism"— or external attribution—among lower class individuals and demonstrates the link between fatalism and increased vulnerability to psychological disorder. Broadly speaking, the literature on social stress, social status, and mental health is fully compatible with Bauman's interpretation of the anxiety-provoking and depressing nature of contemporary life for individuals less well positioned in socioeconomic hierarchies. Whether or not individualization and its associated ills, however, contribute to understanding the relationship between socioeconomic status and mental health, however, is difficult to determine. Further, Bauman makes no clear statement about the levels of psychic distress one would expect to see among the more privileged classes relative to the less privileged; even if the privileged do not experience as much fatalism and do experience more competence in navigating their way through contemporary life, Bauman believes that there are quite a number of reasons for them to feel anxiety. To adequately assess the extent to which Bauman's interpretations are helpful in making sense of the psychic distress of contemporary individuals and of their socioeconomic variations, we need to consider how these interpretations relate to existing definitions of social stressors used by sociologists of mental health and if they might contribute to defining additional sorts of stressors. Within the sociology of mental health, the definition of social stressors is an ongoing problem (Aneshensel, 1992; Turner et al., 1995); we might want to consider how the conceptions of Bauman and others might help to expand current definitions of systemic social stressors.

The Nature of Mental Health and Distress

A second core focus of the sociology of mental health is with the issue of defining mental health and mental illness (Mechanic, 1999; Wakefield, 1999). A distinct emphasis of the sociological perspective on mental health is that determinations of mental health and illness inevitably involve value-laden judgments of behavior that are shaped by culture and the wider social and historical context. The social constructionist tradition within the sociology of mental health has placed the greatest emphasis on the socially constructed nature of definitions of mental health and illness (e.g., Benedict, 1934; Conrad & Schneider, 1992;

Kirk & Kutchins, 1992; Scheff, 1966); the view that definitions of mental health and illness are shaped by the culture and socio-historical context is, however, broadly shared among sociologists of mental health, even as some are also concerned to develop more universally valid conceptions of mental health and illness (e.g., Horwitz, 2002; Wakefield, 1992a; 1992b). While also offering an analysis of the impact of contemporary social conditions on human subjectivity, critical social theories contribute a perspective on the nature of mental health and distress that is not only distinctive from the more predominant social constructionist perspective in sociology but also challenges conventional definitions of mental health and illness/distress.

While the main issue for social constructionists is the value judgments and cultural beliefs implicit in the definitions of mental health and illness that predominate in particular societies at particular historical times, critical theories are concerned instead with the meaning and implications of psychic distress for individuals and for the broader social order. Interestingly, the Frankfurt School theorists found the *absence* of manifest expressions of anxiety and misery in contemporary capitalist societies to be more disturbing than their presence. They argued that contemporary capitalist societies produced the "end of the individual," as individuals came to be enraptured with mass-mediated entertainment, consumer goods, and the conformist private life. In *Eclipse of Reason*, Horkheimer stated: "The substance of individuality itself, to which the idea of autonomy was bound, did not survive the process of industrialization" (Arato & Gebhardt, 1982). The "totally administered society", in Horkheimer's view, organized nearly all human activities and left little place for individual reflection or even for the formation of relationships or enjoyment of leisure experiences that were not subject to societal rationalization (Kellner, 1989). Horkheimer and Adorno (1972) held that the modern capitalist domination of nature inherently entailed domination of the nature of human beings, producing distortions in personality development and reducing human capacities for genuine pleasure, imagination, and autonomous thought (Horkheimer, 1974, p. vi).

Adorno (1991)focused on the culture industries as a core component of the "totally administered society," arguing that the culture industries promoted conformity and contributed to the decline of individuality. In place of genuine individuality, the culture industries promoted "pseudo-individuality," as individuals increasingly sought identity and personal expression through consumption of mass-produced goods and commodified leisure experiences. According to Herbert Marcuse, the culture industries and other aspects of the totally administered society obliterated intra-psychic conflict, creating the "one-dimensional man," or, in other words, an emergent society of people who were identified thoroughly with the existing society and did not seem to have any depth in their psychological make-up (Marcuse, 1955, 1964). Marcuse distinguished between "true needs" and "false needs," the former referring to "vital needs" which "have an unqualified claim for satisfaction" and the latter defined as desires for commodities that cannot fulfill advertisers' promises of happiness and fulfillment (Marcuse, 1964). He viewed liberation as involving a psychic transformation in which individuals realize their true needs and the limitations of the pseudo-satisfactions they have gained as they have pursued false needs. Marcuse was, however, pessimistic about the prospects of many people in advanced capitalist societies achieving such a transformation, given his belief that the existing society had effectively suffocated the needs which demand liberation (Marcuse, 1964, p. 7).

In general, the Frankfurt School theorists valorized misery, anxiety, and psychic suffering as indicating a realistic awareness of the violence that the existing world does to humanity. They viewed apparent happiness as "pseudo-happiness," as they did not see the world as it currently existed as conducive to real happiness. Mental distress, in their view, reflects a realistic awareness of the pathologies of social life and psychic resistance to structures of domination. Fromm (1941), in particular, explicitly argued that individuals who struggled against societal domination were psychologically healthier than those who conformed.

A similar sort of conception can be found in psychoanalytic-feminist social theory and post-colonial theory. Both focus on the psychic consequences of hierarchical relationships, problematizing the identity of both the dominant and subordinate parties, insofar as each has been formed in conformity to prevailing patterns of gendered and racialized hierarchy. According to psychoanalytic-feminist theory, gender hierarchy in the broader society as well as in the family and personal relationships leads, through a somewhat complicated psychodynamic process, to significant distortions in the personality development of both men and women (Benjamin, 1988, 1995; Chodorow, 1978, 1989; Dinnerstein, 1976). Briefly, women fail to establish an adequate level of autonomy and separate identity, making them vulnerable not only to interpersonal domination and devaluation but also to a suffocating over-identification with others; men, whose identities are constructed on the precarious basis of denigration of femininity and denial of dependence, are, at least on a deeper level, perpetually insecure. Thus, those who develop "normal" gender identity are, at least in some sense, psychologically crippled; the experience of psychological misery, by contrast, reflects a failure of identity within patriarchal terms (Mitchell, 1974; J. Rose, 1983, 1989). Similarly, the work of the post-colonial theorist Frantz Fanon (1986) identifies psychopathologies linked to colonialism and decolonization. In his view, both the colonizer and the colonized suffer neurotic patterns generated by colonial domination: the colonized suffers inferiorization, while the colonizer experiences phobias and anxieties. A component of Fanon's strategy to build a democratic and egalitarian postcolonial culture, thus, involves addressing these psychological effects.

In sum, the Frankfurt School, psychoanalytic feminist theory, and the post-colonial theory of Fanon, share the perspective that subjectivity is fundamentally distorted or damaged by societal patterns of domination, and share the critical vision of promoting alternative forms of subjectivity. Research in the sociology of mental health has explored the impact of relations of domination and subordination on mental health, showing that the experience of subordination in social relationships is a significant basis of psychological distress (Horwitz, 1982a). Gender differences in power, accordingly, have been offered as a primary explanation for gender differences in rates of mental distress (Mirowsky, 1985;

Rosenfield, 1999). In general, powerless positions are associated with greater mental distress, while dominant positions are associated with less distress. What distinguishes the analysis of the psychic effects of domination and subordination offered by psychoanalytic-feminist and post-colonial perspectives, however, is that they suggest ill effects of *both* dominant and subordinate positions. Brown (2003), in an article in which he applies critical race theory to the sociology of mental health, presents a similar argument when he proposes examining the potential pathological psychological effects of racial stratification on *both* whites and blacks.

The major implication of these critical perspectives for defining mental health and illness/distress is that mental distress, regardless of its intensity or duration, cannot necessarily be viewed as poor mental health. On the one hand, this point is consistent with the sociological emphasis on the importance of distinguishing normal responses to stressful life experiences from mental disorders, a point also articulated in the introductory pages of the DSM manuals, if not fully considered by practicing psychiatrists (Horwitz, 2002). On the other hand, however, the critical theorists suggest that the psychic damage inflicted in advanced capitalist societies is so thorough and insidious that distinctive "stressful life circumstances" need not be apparent, and that even those individuals who suffer intense psychic distress in the *absence* of readily identifiable stressors should not be pathologized. For the critical theorists, as we have seen, mental distress is an appropriate response to the psychologically damaging tendencies of contemporary societies, indicating *failure* to achieve comfortable identification with the inauthentic and problematic modes of identification on offer in contemporary society, and a positive sign that the individual's authentic human needs have *not* been entirely suffocated. Moreover, mental distress indicates a *higher* level of mental health compared to the absence of mental distress in the lives of individuals who more passively find identification with and "pseudo-happiness" on the terms of the societal status quo.

To use these critical theoretical perspectives as a basis for empirical research on mental health would pose methodological challenges. Many of the concepts used in these critical theoretical perspectives – i.e., "true" and "false" needs, "real" versus "pseudo-happiness", authentic versus inauthentic modes of being, distorted identities or "false" selves, etc. – are not ones that most scientifically-minded researchers would take seriously. Even within social theory, in which one finds a far greater comfort with abstraction, the kinds of distinctions made by the Frankfurt School theorists have been widely criticized and viewed as untenable (since they depend on value judgments that themselves will be rooted in particular cultural frameworks). Even if unacceptable to academics, however, distinctions such as these are employed not only by individuals in daily life but widely within psychotherapeutic discourse and by mental health professionals. In everyday life, people commonly judge others as superficial, fake, self-deceived, genuine, authentic, or real. Within psychotherapeutic contexts, judgments of unconscious motivations, repressed emotions, and defense mechanisms are quite routine, such that some patterns of motivation and behavior are thought to be authentic while others are seen as compensatory, defensive, or manifestations of a "false self." So, if such concepts are so widely used, might they not indicate something important that we should not categorically rule out of bounds when studying mental health? Nonetheless, they do pose problems, both of conceptualization and measurement.

These limitations notwithstanding, a distinction that mental health researchers have made between positive and negative mental health may be helpful in thinking about mental health and distress from the vantage point of critical theories. A number of mental health researchers have emphasized the point that mental health is not merely the absence of mental illness (Keyes, 2002a; Ryff & Singer, 1998). About one half of the adult population in the United States will not experience serious mental illness throughout life, while about 90% of the population will not experience major depression in any particular year. But this does not mean that the people who remain free of mental illness are mentally healthy. Keyes distinguishes between "flourishing" and "languishing." Flourishing indicates a "state in which an individual feels positive emotion toward life and is functioning well psychologically and socially" (Keyes, 2002b, p. 294). Languishing, by contrast, is a "state in which an individual is devoid of positive emotion toward life, is not functioning well psychologically or socially, and has not been depressed during the past year" (p. 294). A significant proportion of those who remain free of mental illness, he suggests, are languishers rather than flourishers.

The concept of languishing might be useful in making sense of the critical theorists' characterization of the lives of the many who experience "pseudohappiness" and "substitute gratifications." Although positive psychology researchers do not share the critical theorists' orientation and do not see contemporary advanced societies as inimical to human flourishing, it might be possible, nonetheless, to draw upon their research to assess the extent to which some of the characteristics of advanced industrial society identified by the critical theorists as psychically damaging —e.g., television and other forms of mass entertainment, consumerism, (pseudo-) individualism, status-seeking—are associated with languishing. If we studied the lives of "flourishers" and compared them to the lives of "languishers," would we find that flourishers are less likely, for example, to watch television, to be enraptured by consumer goods, to be as individualistic or competitive in the pursuit of power or status, or to relate to others in a hierarchical manner? A caveat, however, is that the critical theorists might consider the concept of languishing to be an inadequate indicator, as languishers are "devoid of positive emotion toward life" while the critical theorists indicate that pseudohappiness and substitute gratifications might mask the absence of genuine happiness and fulfillment.

An additional way in which critical theoretical perspectives might be applied towards thinking about mental health issues would be to use them as a basis for critical evaluation of concepts of mental health, both within research literatures as well as, perhaps more importantly, within psychotherapeutic settings. Given the emphasis that the critical theoretical perspectives place on the psychopathological effects of psychic conformity to the societal structures of domination, their perspectives call for evaluating the value judgments implicit in definitions of mental health and illness in a more politicized manner than has been typical within the constructionist tradition. In particular, the basic issue for the critical perspectives is the question of the extent to which any given standard of mental health promotes conformity to (or challenges) problematic structures of domination within the broader society. Relatedly, the critical theoretical perspectives suggest a need to critically evaluate psychotherapeutic practices, in which standards of mental health and illness are applied, in terms of their complicity with or opposition to societal structures of domination.

Throughout U.S. history, psychotherapeutic practices have been understood in both ways. From the early days of dynamic psychiatry through the early 1960s, psychotherapy was embraced by radical social critics and seen as critical of repressive social institutions and normative standards. By the 1960s, however, an "anti-psychiatry" movement (Chesler, 1972; Laing, 1960; Szasz, 1961) had emerged, indicting the entire "psychological establishment" for promoting individual adjustment to a repressive and unequal status quo (Horwitz, 2002). Later, in the 1970s, psychoanalytic-feminist social theory emerged, partially in opposition to the wholesale dismissal of psychoanalysis by feminists, and made the case for psychoanalysis as a tool for uncovering the psychic discontents of patriarchy. Overall, however, where do contemporary psychotherapeutic practices, and the standards of mental health and illness that they purvey, stand in relationship to the inequalities and problematic societal tendencies identified by critical theories?

While explicitly feminist, anti-racist, and other sorts of radical therapies are marginal within the mental health care field (Prilleltensky, 1994), the problematizing of hierarchical constructions of identity and the critique of dominant societal patterns and cultural values may be more common than rare within more "mainstream" therapeutic approaches. Research on positive psychology, for example, shows that individuals for whom "power strivings" are central goals tend to experience lower subjective well-being than individuals for whom power does not figure as a primary motivation (Emmons, 1991). Further, the experience of subordination is widely recognized as adversely affecting mental health. It is likely that many psychotherapists *do* recognize the mental stress associated not only with subordinate social roles but also with excessive "power striving," even if they limit their critiques of domination and subordination to psychological, interpersonal, and familial realms. Further, psychological values may often be presented in therapeutic contexts as *alternatives* to dominant cultural values. In *The Poverty of Affluence*, for example, psychologist Paul Wachtel (1983) suggests that "psychological values" may represent an alternative to the dominant consumerist values of contemporary society; he also, however, acknowledges the possibility that the emphasis on psychological growth within the mental health industries might be seen as just one more facet of the endless and problematic pursuit of "growth" in modern economies.

Critical theorists specialize in sniffing out domination and have emphasized the tendency of contemporary societies to mask domination with enticing offers of "liberation"; thus, they would not take overt critiques of hierarchy and challenges to dominant cultural values within psychotherapeutic practices at face value.

Nonetheless, if critical perspectives are going to be useful for evaluating contemporary psychotherapeutic practices and standards of mental health and illness, we need to get beyond the blanket critiques common among social critics and work on determining *if* and *how* therapeutic standards and practices are complicit with or critical of the power relations and societal dynamics problematized by critical theories. To address these issues in a relevant manner, we need not only develop theoretically-grounded criteria, but also attain deep knowledge of clinical perspectives on mental health and mental health care.

Conceptualizing the Therapeutic Process

A third major focus of the sociology of mental health is mental health care services. While the range of issues with which sociologists who study mental health care services are concerned are more numerous and diverse than what will be considered here, one major issue to which contemporary social theorists may provide insight is with the question of the sociocultural functions, meanings, and implications of mental health care. This issue is closely related to the discussion of the values implicit in definitions of mental health and illness in the last section. Psychotherapists themselves have called for recognition of the social, cultural, and ideological meanings implicit in various forms of mental health care (Fancher, 1995; Frank & Frank, 1991). In *Cultures of Healing*, for example, psychotherapist Robert Fancher (1995) evaluates the implicit cultural and political assumptions of four major "cultures of healing": psychoanalysis, behaviorism, cognitive therapy, and biological psychiatry. Reporting findings that type of therapeutic treatment makes little difference in the alleviation of the distress of patients, he argues that the type of therapy a patient receives is nonetheless important because each culture of healing promotes different beliefs, values, and ideals of living.

Concern with the political-ideological implications of mental health care, psychological discourse, and the emergence of what some have called the "psychological society" as well as, more particularly, with the basic question of the extent to which psychotherapeutic practices foster liberation from societal patterns of domination and social control or promote conformity to the status quo, as discussed in the previous section, has been pervasive in critical discourses on psychotherapy since the 1960s (see Prilleltensky, 1994, for a review of these critiques). A central theme is the indictment of psychotherapeutic practices and discourse for elevating individualistic understandings of personal problems and deflecting attention away from social structural bases of distress. Within the field of sociology, an early statement of this critique can be found in C. Wright Mills' (1959) classic *The Sociological Imagination* in which he argued that social and personal problems were increasingly being (inappropriately) understood in terms of the "psychiatric." Conrad and Schneider (1982) offer a similar sort of critique of the individualizing and depoliticizing impact of the "medicalization" of many sorts of deviant behaviors and personal problems.

Broadly, the central issue in these critiques and debates concerns the relationship between the psychotherapeutic process and social control. How is mental health care linked to societal systems of social control? Each of the three social theoretical perspectives I consider in this chapter speak to this issue in some fashion. For Foucault, however, the view of mental health professions as instruments of modern social control is most central, and so his work will receive the most attention in this section. The implications of critical theoretical perspectives for thinking about therapeutic practices were discussed in the previous section and will not be further discussed here. The theorists of individualization, however, interpret therapeutic practices differently than Foucault and question the applicability of Foucault's perspective in the contemporary period. Thus, I frame this difference of perspective as an important theoretical question for making sense of contemporary therapeutic practices.

Foucault's critical perspective on the emergence of psychiatry, psychology, and the human sciences is well-known among social theorists and sociologists of mental health, and has had a significant influence on historically-based analyses of mental health care (e.g., Caplan, 1998; Cushman, 1995; Herman, 1995; Lunbeck, 1994; N. Rose, 1989) as well as mental heath research within the constructionist tradition (e.g., Bayer, 1987; Figert, 1996; Scott, 1990). Foucault views the emergence of psychiatry and psychology as part of a larger modern transformation in the nature of discipline and social control. In *Madness and Civilization* (Foucault, 1965), he characterizes psychiatry as a "monologue of reason about madness" (p. xi). While psychiatry justifies itself as a humane and scientific endeavor, Foucault sees it as a method of social control aimed to induce the insane to judge themselves according to (social) standards of reason. Foucault views the insane as being subjected, via psychiatry, to a "gigantic moral imprisonment" (Foucault, 1965).

In *Discipline and Punish*, Foucault (1977) focuses on the emergence of modern disciplinary technologies after 1757, when moral control comes to be the primary means of social control. He identifies "hierarchical observation" and "normalizing judgment" as central mechanisms of modern discipline. Hierarchical observation involves intensive unilateral scrutiny of a subordinate (e.g., patient) by a superior (e.g., psychiatrist) and provides the basis for "normalizing judgment." Normalizing judgment entails evaluation of an individual's performance, behavior, characteristics, psychological makeup, etc. according to detailed standards of normality. Normalizing judgment aims not only at "offenses" or "infractions," as in prior disciplinary modes, but at any failure to perform optimally. Foucault saw these modern disciplinary processes as central to psychiatric social control. The psychiatric patient, for example, is judged and learns to self-monitor not only for "inappropriate" behavior but also for failure to realize optimal standards of mental health. Psychotherapeutic practices, thus, play a key role in constructing a self-monitoring and self-controlling modern subjectivity.

Foucault's (1976) critique of the "repressive hypothesis" in *History of Sexuality, Vol. 1* has crucial implications for understanding his view of the psychotherapeutic process. Focusing his attention explicitly on Victorian-era understandings of sexual repression, Foucault criticized the idea that frank discussion about sexuality and, more generally, the probing of the depths of the human psyche, entailed a release of psychically-damaging repression and thereby enhanced personal freedom. Instead, he viewed the idea of repressed impulses as a fiction constructed with the aim of intensifying self-monitoring and self-judgment according to prevailing standards of psychological normality. Although modern persons may view themselves as self-liberating as they probe their psyches, this self-conception reflects a misunderstanding of the nature of power. A central theme for Foucault is that power is not simply repressive (saying "no") but also productive. As individuals come to be fascinated with sexual matters and take great interest in monitoring and confessing their own desires, fantasies, and responses, they are, in fundamental ways, subject to *greater* social control. The modern emphasis on "knowing" the psyche, in Foucault's view, intensifies self-monitoring and constructs subjectivity according to modern normative standards. Some (more often those of higher social classes) actively seek out such control, in the name of self-knowledge, self-expression, and personal authenticity. For others who find themselves subjected to it following the commission of socially unacceptable behavior, the social control may be more explicit and direct. But, for Foucault, the social control is more *thorough* to the extent to which the psychotherapeutic subject actively participates and does *not* experience it as an alienating and external judgment. Foucault's perspective is, on this point, consistent with Horwitz's (1982b) theory of "therapeutic social control." Such control, Horwitz argues, is persuasive rather than coercive, emphasizing control of personality rather than control of behavior.

If we examine psychotherapeutic practices and discourse through a Foucauldian lens, the question of their political implications comes to the forefront, although in a different way than it does for the critical theorists. Instead of understanding individuals as having authentic selves or distinctive human desires and capacities that may be either liberated or dominated, Foucault views subjectivity as socially constructed and psychotherapeutic practices and discourse as playing a fundamental role in its construction. The idea of the "authentic self" to be discovered, known, and acted upon is an ideological ruse that serves to motivate individuals' self-discipline and facilitates social control. Implicitly, however, some sort of conception of authenticity lurks behind his critique of modern disciplinary techniques, especially the normalization promoted by the psychiatry, psychology, and the human sciences. Otherwise, why see this normalization as a form of violence to the self, as Foucault does? In later work, Foucault contrasts the practices or "technologies of the self" of the "politically active subject," to the "passive" subject which had been the center of critique in his earlier works (Foucault, 1982; 1988; Rabinow, 1984); he came to view the relationship of "self to self" as a useful point of resistance to domination, and envisioned the construction of an alternative type of subjectivity to the "normalized" form he saw as linked to the institutions of modernity and as promoted by modern psychotherapeutic practices (Foucault, 1988). What, precisely, this alternative form of subjectivity might look like, and how we might distinguish its characteristics from the passive and normalized subjectivity that Foucault problematizes, however, is not clear.

Arguably, a limitation of Foucault's work for thinking about mental health issues is the failure to pay attention to the actual experiences of mental distress that individuals may suffer. If there is any implicit notion of mental distress in Foucault's work, however, it would be the misery of the person who has been coercively constructed as "abnormal," "sick," and worthy of psychiatric intervention by modern discourses of normality. Particularly important, in Foucault's view, is that the "psy" disciplines create a fundamental transformation in the relationship of individuals to their behavior. Modern psychological discourse accords behavior, thoughts, and desires a fundamental status in determining a person's identity and, hence, makes intensive self-scrutiny and normalizing judgment necessary. This normalization, and, in particular, the tying of the individual's identity to her every thought, behavior, and desire, might be seen to cause misery much more than it would help to alleviate psychological pain. Foucault himself says nothing about this, unconcerned as he is with mental distress. However, we might nonetheless consider the possibility that some portion of psychological distress is a *product* of cultural standards of psychological normality. As sociologists of emotion have shown (e.g., Hochschild, 1983), powerful social norms dictating the propriety or "healthiness" of particular emotions in various contexts cause individuals to "have feelings about their feelings." When individuals feel bad about themselves for feeling an "unacceptable," "inappropriate," or "immature" emotion, particularly insofar as such emotions have, as Foucault argues, come to be seen as fundamental to self-identity, an additional layer of distress is added to what might or might not be on its own a stressful emotional experience. Applying the insights of the sociology of emotions to mental health, Thoits (1985) has argued that the experience of "emotional deviance" is a common basis of individuals' self-attributions of mental illness and professional help-seeking. Thus, it may be useful to follow Foucault and sociologists of emotion in carefully examining the role of emotion norms and standards of normal psychological development or normal "identity," as purveyed by therapeutic practices and discourses, in *producing* distress in individuals. This view represents, at a basic level, a contrast to the view of the theorists of individualization that much contemporary distress could best be understood in terms of an *absence* of standards.

Foucault's ideas have significantly influenced the development of postmodern thought in general, but, in particular, his thought has significantly influenced postmodern approaches to understanding psychotherapeutic practices. Burr and Butt (2000) provide a concise analysis of the implications of the postmodern perspective for thinking about psychotherapeutic practices. The postmodern perspective questions the presumed expertise of therapists, challenging the idea that therapists know what is best for clients. Accordingly, the postmodern perspective problematizes the asymmetric power relation often characteristic of therapy. The more appropriate type of therapeutic relation, from a postmodern perspective, is one that follows a "research supervisor/research student model" (Bannister, 1983; Burr & Butt, 2000). According to this model, the "researcher" (client) is presumed to know most about her project (her own self and life), and the role of the "supervisor" is to provide guidance on different ways the project might be approached. Drawing on the insights of Foucault, the postmodern perspective calls for scrutiny of the ways in which psychological constructions of normality and pathology affect the self-constructions of clients. It also calls for recognition of human diversity both between and within people. Instead of seeking a "deep, real self to be mined," a postmodern therapeutic approach emphasizes the relational nature of human experience and seeks to help individuals live meaningfully with fragmentation. It calls attention to our "vocabularies of self" and urges the exploration of alternative vocabularies. Postmodern psychology, finally, emphasizes the social and relational sources of individuals' psychological problems and so focuses on helping individuals to resituate themselves or to resist debilitating constructions of themselves that they may have adopted through problematic relationships. In short, postmodern psychology may be seen as an effort to avoid the very forms of therapeutic social control criticized by Foucault. So, one might reasonably ask how "postmodern" contemporary psychotherapeutic practices may have become and whether or not Foucault's view of the mental health professions as an instrument of normalizing social control continues to be a useful way to understand mental health care in the contemporary age.

In contrast to Foucault's perspective, the theorists of individualization do not conceptualize psychotherapeutic practices in terms of social control. Instead, they see individuals with very real psychological distress turning to psychotherapy to find guidance no longer provided by society. The responsibility that individuals hold for the reflexive making of self-identity under conditions of late modernity is, in essence, Giddens' explanation for the proliferation of psychotherapies and counseling in contemporary Western societies. As he puts it quite simply: "Self-identity has to be created and recreated on a more active basis than before. This explains why therapy and counseling of all kinds have become so popular in Western countries" (Giddens, 2000, p. 65). In Bauman's view, individuals seek out experts to provide authoritative advice on how to escape from the uncertainty characteristic of contemporary social life (Bauman, 1995, p. 80). While the individualization of the contemporary age involves increased individual responsibility for self-formation, the paradox is that individuals increasingly turn over this responsibility to professionals who "recommend" identities and ways of acquiring and holding them (Bauman, 1995, p. 82). Beck and Beck-Gernsheim (1996), see the destruction of routine as a primary source of psychological distress and understand the proliferation of psychotherapies as a product of individuals looking to authorities to answer the question "Who am I and what do I want?" (p. 31). In the late modern age, decisions about lifestyles come to have great ethical, and anxiety-provoking, significance. "Everyday life is being post-religiously deified" (p. 32), and seemingly we need therapeutic experts to help us find our salvation.

Whereas Foucault views psychotherapeutic practices as part of a larger system of modern discipline, Bauman argues that Foucault's conception of social control is not appropriate to the contemporary context. In Bauman's view, such control is no longer necessary; there is no longer a need to control people's wants and desires, to keep them commensurate with objective possibilities. Ambivalence is no longer a public enemy, he states, because the proliferation of wants and desires in the broader population in advanced societies fuels consumerism and is therefore entirely non-threatening to powerful global interests. Further, Bauman suggests that there is less need for the imposition of moral discipline on such populations as criminals, homeless, and the unemployed, as they are no longer a reserve army of labor but instead are inessential "waste" to be kept out of sight as much as possible. Ambivalence, however, remains a powerful private enemy – a source of confusion and distress for individuals; people turn to therapeutic experts in hopes of receiving guidance and support. Therapeutic experts, he says, are only too happy to provide systems of meaning and guidance to their clients and help them to "settle" the vexing questions that plague them. Both Bauman and Beck and Beck-Gernsheim view therapeutic intervention as an unsatisfactory attempt to provide private solutions to systemic contradictions, but neither would find the concept "normalization" to be an appropriate way to characterize the help that therapeutic experts provide.

Instead of seeing therapeutic practices as promoting normalization, Giddens sees psychotherapy as promoting a greater degree of reflexivity in the individual's relationships, construction of self, and making of important life decisions. Giddens and Beck and Beck-Gernsheim, as we have seen, focus on the stress that individuals may experience in the face of responsibility for a seemingly infinite array of self-constructing lifestyle choices and note the possibility for anxiety to subvert autonomy. Accordingly, the therapeutic process may be understood as working to expand individuals' freedom in living their lives in accordance with conscious and free choices. Giddens also suggests that therapeutic conceptions may promote more democratic orientations towards life, greater questioning of prevailing societal standards, thawing of "frozen" patterns in life and in relationships, and greater expectations for equality (Giddens, 1992).

The key theoretical question that emerges from these contrasting perspectives is the question of the appropriateness of viewing contemporary therapeutic practices as normalizing and disciplinary. Have contemporary therapeutic practices instead become more "postmodern," and/or do the interpretations of the theorists of individualization make more sense? Two relatively recent studies that draw heavily on Foucault's ideas are helpful for thinking about this question. In *Constructing the Self, Constructing America*, Cushman (1995) provides a cultural history of psychotherapy in the U. S. that indicates that therapeutic practices in American society were *never* particularly focused on social control, at least not in the way we typically think of social control. The view of therapeutic practices as social control through self-discipline, he suggests, *was* appropriate through the early part of the 20th century in *Europe*. Freud's dictum, "where id was, there ego shall be," was indicative of the modern European drive for self-mastery through rational self-control. The ultimate purpose of exploration of the unconscious mind, characteristic of Freudian psychoanalysis, was, in the European context, to *tame* the unconscious. Transported into the American context, however, Freud's ideas were transmuted; instead of taming unruly impulses, Americans were more interested in *liberating* them. Cushman characterizes the focus of therapeutic practices in the first half of the 20th century in the U.S. as focused on self-liberation, not self-domination. Corresponding to the sense of promise and optimism that Americans enjoyed in the late 19th century, Americans conceived of the human interior as "inherently good, saturated in spirituality, and capable of controlling the external world" (Cushman, 1995, p. 118); the key to well-being and prosperity was liberation of this enchanted human interior. In the second half of the 20th century, Cushman identifies another shift in focus of therapeutic practices. Increasingly individuals, particularly middle-class ones, come to experience what Cushman calls "the empty self," an experience of "interior lack, absence, emptiness and despair, the desperate yearning to be loved, soothed, and made whole by filling up the emptiness" (Cushman, 1995, p. 245); this he links to 20th century social changes, particularly the growth of consumerism. As individuals turn to psychotherapists (and to consumer goods) to soothe and fill up the emptiness, psychotherapeutic practices come to be understood accordingly. The emergence and influence of self psychology and object relations theory in the post-war period, in particular, is indicative of the view of the self as empty and of therapeutic practices as filling the void. Insofar as Cushman's interpretations of the cultural meanings of American psychotherapy are correct, then the view of therapeutic practices as agents of disciplinary social control does not fit so well in the American context and perhaps, also, not so well in the contemporary European context.

If we broaden our understanding of social control to fully grasp the meaning of Foucault's analysis, however, it would be misleading to argue that contemporary therapeutic practices, even if they do take the forms that Cushman suggests, do not function as instruments of social control. Cushman himself draws upon Foucault's thinking as one of the key theoretical foundations of his work; Foucault's key insight is, for him, that "each era produces a particular configuration of self and corresponding kinds of psychopathology" (Cushman, 1990, p. 600). The "empty self" is constructed by and contributes to the maintenance of a consumer-driven post World War II economy, thus illustrating rather than contradicting Foucault's perspective. While psychotherapists may see themselves as *responding* to and working to heal the individual's psychic emptiness, Cushman argues that psychotherapies (like advertising) also contribute mightily to reinforcing the conception and experience of the self as empty.

Hazleden (2003) similarly finds Foucault's perspective useful for understanding contemporary psychotherapeutic discourses, even when self-control is not a prominent theme. Despite the apparent tendency to emphasize self-love over self-control, Hazleden nonetheless believes that Foucault's concept "normalization" aptly describes psychotherapeutic discourse in contemporary advanced societies. Reviewing popular self-help books, she shows that these texts, while presenting themselves as guidebooks for discovering and properly nurturing the "true self" within, convey a set of specific messages about the *proper* relationship the individual should develop with oneself. They teach the individual to regard the self as of paramount importance, to consider love and nurturance of self a serious responsibility (not self-indulgence, but rather "hard work"), and to maintain self-sufficiency.

While these are not the sorts of messages we might associate with disciplinary social control, Hazleden argues (in a manner quite consistent with Foucault's perspective) that such messages *do* represent social control in that they define a *right* and a *wrong* way of relating to the self.

Drawing on Foucault, the key question is the extent to which contemporary mental health care functions as a system of social control, subjecting individuals to normalizing judgment. In actual therapeutic practice, *is* it common for therapeutic professionals to impose standards of psychological normality? If so, what is the nature of these standards? Do they involve ideals of living that reflect the therapists' own personal and cultural background? Do they, as the critical theories would lead us to ask, promote conformity or resistance to structures of inequality and domination in the broader society? Are they, as Foucault suggests, standards designed to maximize the individual's self-discipline and fitness for life within modern institutions? Or, might the standards of normality, at least in some therapeutic contexts, involve merely a therapeutic judgment that the degree of psychological pain and/or dysfunction experienced by the individual is not "normal"? It is not clear how appropriate it would be, in the face of debilitating mental illness, to understand a therapeutic judgment that a person's psychological functioning is impaired, to involve imposition of a problematic form of normalizing judgment. Waitzkin's (1989) work on ideology in medical practice, however, suggests that even such seemingly innocuous judgments may carry ideological freight. When doctors focus on symptoms and treatment, but ignore the troubled social reality at the root of a person's illness, the symptoms and treatment attain the aura of scientific fact while the problematic social relations become reified (Waitzkin, 1989, p. 224).

Drawing upon the theorists of individualization, the key issue is to assess their contention that confused individuals turn to psychotherapeutic experts for help in sorting out questions of identity, existential meaning, and life priorities. Even if *some* clients of psychotherapeutic services seek guidance from experts on such matters, to what extent are such questions a *pervasive* focus of therapeutic practices? Are some schools of therapeutic practice and or some practitioners more likely than others to emphasize such questions? Is confusion over identity, meaning, and life-purpose more relevant for understanding some types of mental distress more than others? Are those who seek therapy voluntarily more likely to focus on such questions than are those for whom treatment is involuntary? Further, are such questions more likely to figure into treatment with functional persons who seek therapy for help with ordinary problems of everyday living than they are in the treatment of individuals who suffer serious and debilitating mental illness? In short, are the anxieties and worries identified by the theorists of individualization simply those of the "worried well," or are they also useful in understanding serious mental illness? Further, if existential questions figure prominently in therapeutic treatment, what is the nature of the guidance that therapeutic experts provide? Is the mental health industry really an "answer factory," or are therapists more likely, in postmodern style, to eschew authoritative answers?

A tendency in social theory is to analyze psychotherapeutic practices, discourse, and ideology as a relatively monolithic entity serving a single function – e.g., challenging or supporting societal systems of domination, subjecting individuals to "normalizing" social control, providing individuals guidance as they make difficult life decisions – regardless of the type of therapy, the nature of the psychological problem, or the type of patient population. Within mental health professions, however, there is tremendous internal diversity that social theorists might take more seriously. As Fancher (1995) points out, there are somewhere between 50 and 500 different forms of psychotherapy, depending on how one counts; while there are likely common themes and orientations among many, surely also there are some differences in ideological implications or socio-cultural functions. Differences in the political/ideological orientations of individual psychotherapists, many of whom are "eclectic" in theoretical and practical orientations, are also important to consider (Fancher, 1995).

Severity of mental illness is another consideration, as well as whether or not treatment is voluntary or involuntary. Horwitz and Mullis (1992) argue that the rise of individualism has weakened the social control *and* social support for the seriously mentally ill, as the seriously mentally ill are less likely to receive long-term involuntary care in isolated mental health care facilities and are more likely to leave or be expelled from their families. Thus, Bauman's arguments about the impact of individualization in the lives of the socially marginal—the cutting adrift, the leaving to one's own devices, the lifting of moral control, the consigning to waste—are particularly apt for understanding the experiences of the seriously mentally ill in the contemporary period.

Conclusion

In this chapter, I have examined the contributions of contemporary social theorists to thinking about three broad concerns in the sociology of mental health: 1) the social origins of mental distress; 2) the nature of mental health and distress; and 3) conceptualizing therapeutic practices. I have drawn on three loosely defined theoretical perspectives: theorists of individualization, critical theoretical perspectives, and Foucauldian/postmodern theories. Each of these perspectives offers a distinct way of thinking about mental distress *and* therapeutic practices. The theorists of individualization portray contemporary individuals as suffering distress in the face of social conditions they see as promoting anxiety and anomie and view therapeutic practices as assisting individuals with the difficult task of sorting out the many life questions no longer answered by tradition and custom. The critical theories focus on psychic distortions that they attribute to structures of domination in contemporary societies and view therapeutic practices in terms of their role in promoting or challenging the individual's psychic complicity with such structures. The Foucauldian/postmodern perspective, focused less on mental distress, views therapeutic practices and discourse as promoting "normalization" and as constructing problematic forms of subjectivity linked to Western values of individualism, rationalism, instrumentality, denial and denigration of otherness, etc. (Rosenau, 1992).

Some of the questions and issues posed by contemporary social theorists cannot be fully or directly addressed with existing research on mental health and would, in any case, pose methodological difficulties. However, development of strategies to more fully utilize the theoretical perspectives I have considered here in empirical research on mental health could be useful not only for deepening our understanding of the impact of macro-structural social dynamics on mental health but also would contribute to greater precision and refinement in theoretical conception. As we have seen, existing research in the sociology of mental health contributes relevant knowledge and deserves to be given greater consideration by social theorists who include matters of self, psychology, mental health, and psychotherapies among their theoretical concerns. A thorough mining of research in the sociology of mental health and relevant psychological literature, in relation to the issues posed by contemporary social theorists, would, in itself, represent an important contribution, or at least a crucial first step, towards achieving a mutually-informative integration of contemporary social theory and the sociology of mental health.

References

Adorno, T. W. (1991). *The culture industry*. London and New York: Routledge.

Aneshensel, C. S. (1992). Social stress: Theory and research. *Annual Review of Sociology 18*, 15–38.

Arato, A., & Gebhardt, E. (Eds.) (1982). *The essential Frankfurt School reader*. New York: Continuum.

Austin, J. T., & Vancouver, J. B. (1996). Goal constructs in psychology: Structure, process, and content. *Psychological Bulletin, 120*, 338–375.

Bannister, D. (1983). The internal politics of psychotherapy. In D. Pilgrim (Ed.), *Psychology and psychotherapy* (pp. 139–150). New York: Routledge.

Bauman, Z. (1995). *Life in fragments: Essays in postmodern morality*. Cambridge, MA: Blackwell.

Bauman, Z. (1996). Morality in the age of contingency. In P. Heelas, S. Lash, & P. Morris (Eds.), *Detraditionalization: Critical reflections on authority and identity* (pp. 49–58). Cambridge, MA: Blackwell Publishers.

Bauman, Z. (2001). *The individualized society*. Malden, MA: Polity Press.

Bauman, Z. (2004). *Wasted lives: Modernity and its outcasts*. Malden, MA: Polity Press.

Bauman, Z. (2005). *Liquid life*. Malden, MA: Polity Press.

Bayer, R. (1987). *Homosexuality and American psychiatry: The politics of diagnosis*. Princeton, NJ: Princeton University Press.

Beck, U., & Beck-Gernsheim, E. (1996). Individualization and 'precarious freedoms': Perspectives and controversies of a subject-orientated sociology. In P. Heelas, S. Lash, & P. Morris (Eds.), *Detraditionalization: Critical reflections on authority and identity* (pp. 23–48). Cambridge, MA: Blackwell Publishers.

Beck, U., & Beck-Gernsheim, E. (2002). *Individualization: Institutionalized individualism and its social and political consequences*. London: Sage Publications.

Benassi, V. A., Sweeney, P. D., & Dufour, C. L. (1988). Is there a relation between locus of control orientation and depression? *Journal of Abnormal Psychology, 97*, 357–367.

Benedict, R. (1934). Anthropology and the abnormal. *Journal of General Psychology*, 10, 59–80.

Benjamin, J. (1988). *The bonds of love*. New York: Pantheon.

Benjamin, J. (1995). *Like subjects, love objects*. New Haven: Yale University Press.

Brown, T. N. (2003). Critical race theory speaks to the sociology of mental health: Mental health problems produced by racial stratification. *Journal of Health and Social Behavior*, 44, 292–301.

Bruckner, H., & Mayer, K. U. (2005). De-Standardization of the life course: What it might mean? And if it means anything, whether it actually took place? *Advances in Life Course Research 9*, 27–53.

Buchmann, M. (1989). *The script of life in modern society*. Chicago: University of Chicago Press.

Burr, V., & Butt, T. (2000). "Psychological distress and postmodern thought." In D. Fee (Ed.), *Pathology and the postmodern: Mental illness as discourse and experience* (pp. 186–206). London: Sage Publications.

Campbell, C. (1996). Detraditionalization, character, and the limits to agency. In P. Heelas, S. Lash, & P. Morris (Eds.), *Detraditionalization: Critical reflections on authority and identity* (pp. 149–170). Cambridge, MA: Blackwell Publishers.

Caplan, E. (1998). *Mind games: American culture and the birth of psychotherapy*. Berkeley: University of California Press.

Chesler, P. (1972). *Women and madness*. New York: Doubleday.

Chodorow, N. (1978). *The reproduction of mothering: Psychoanalysis and the sociology of gender*. Berkeley: University of California Press.

Chodorow, N. (1989). *Feminism and psychoanalytic theory*. New Haven: Yale University Press.

Conrad, P., & Schneider, J. (1992). *Deviance and medicalization*, 2nd ed.. Philadelphia: Temple University Press.

Cushman, P. (1990). Why the self is empty: Toward a historically situated psychology. *American Psychologist, 45*, 599–611.

Cushman, P. (1995). *Constructing the self, constructing America: A cultural history of psychotherapy*. Reading, MA: Addison-Wesley.

Dinnerstein, D. (1976). *The mermaid and the minotaur: Sexual arrangements and the human malaise*. New York: Harper & Row.

Dohrenwend, B. P. & Dohrenwend, B. S. (1974). *Stressful life events: Their nature and effects*. New York: Wiley.

Dohrenwend, B. P., Levav, I., Shrout, P. E., Schwartz, S. Naveh, G., Link, B. G., Skodol, A. E., & Stueve, A. (1992). Socioeconomic status and psychiatric disorders: The causation-selection issue. *Science, 255*, 946–952.

Durkheim, E. ([1897] 1951). *Suicide*. New York: Free Press.

Dyer, E. D. (1987). Ten-year differences in level of entering students' profile on the California psychological inventory. *Psychological Reports, 60*, 822.

Eaton, W. W. (1986). *The sociology of mental disorders*, 2nd ed. New York: Praeger.

Eaton, W. W., & Muntaner, C. (1999). Socioeconomic stratification and mental disorder. In A. V. Horwitz and T. L. Scheid (Eds.), *A handbook for the study of mental health* (pp. 259–283). New York: Cambridge University Press.

Elliott, A. (2001). *Concepts of the self*. Malden, MA: Blackwell Publishers.

Emmons, R. A. (1991). Personal strivings, daily life events, and psychological and physical well-being. *Journal of Personality, 59*, 453–472.

Emmons, R. A. (2002). Personal goals, life meanings, and virtue: Wellsprings of a positive life. In C. L. M. Keyes & J. Haidt (Eds.), *Flourishing: Positive psychology and the life well-lived* (pp. 105–128). Washington, D. C.: American Psychological Association.

Fancher, R. T. (1995). *Cultures of healing: Correcting the image of American mental health care*. New York: W. H. Freeman and Company.

Fanon, F. (1967). *Black skin, white masks*. New York: Grove Press.

Figert, A. E. (1996). *Women and the ownership of PMS: The structuring of a psychiatric disorder*. New York: Walter de Gruyter.

Foucault, M. (1965). *Madness and civilization: A History of insanity in the age of reason*. New York: Vintage.

Foucault, M. (1976). *The history of sexuality, vol. 1*. Harmondsworth: Penguin.

Foucault, M. (1977). *Discipline and punish: The birth of the prison*. London: Allen Lane.

Foucault, M. (1982). The subject and power. In H. Dreyfus & P. Rabinow, *Michel Foucault: Beyond structuralism and hermeneutics* (pp. 208–226). Brighton: Harvestor.

Foucault, M. (1988). The ethic of care for the self as a practice of freedom. In J. Bernauer & D. Rasmussen (Eds.), *The final Foucault* (pp. 1–20). Cambridge, MA: MIT Press.

Frank, J. D., & Frank, J. B. (1991). *Persuasion and healing*, 3rd ed. Baltimore: John Hopkins.

Fromm, E. (1941). *Escape from freedom*. New York: Rinehart.

Gergen, K. J. (1991). *The saturated self: Dilemmas of identity in contemporary life*. New York: Basic Books.

Giddens, A. (1991). *Modernity and self-identity: Self and society in the late modern age*. Stanford, CA: Stanford University Press.

Giddens, A. (1992). *The transformation of intimacy: Sexuality, love, and eroticism in modern societies*. Stanford, CA: Stanford University Press.

Giddens, A. (2000). *Runaway world: How globalization is reshaping our lives*. New York: Routledge.

Goode, W. J. (1960). A theory of role strain. American Sociological Review, 25, 483–496.

Hagnell, O., Lanke, J., Rorsman, B., & Ojesjo, L. (1982). Are we entering an age of melancholy? Depressive illnesses in a prospective epidemiological study over 25 years: The Lundby Study, Sweden. *Psychological Medicine, 12*, 279–289.

Hazelden, R. (2003). Love yourself: The relationship of the self with itself in popular self-help texts. *Journal of Sociology, 39*, 413–428.

Heinz, W. R. (1991). Status passages, social risks, and the life course: A conceptual framework. In W. R. Heinz (Ed.), *Theoretical advances in life course research, Vol. 1.* (pp. 9–22). Weinheim: Deutscher Studien Verlag.

Heinz, W. R. (2002). Self-socialization and post-traditional society. *Advances in Life Course Research 7*, 41–64.

Held, T. (1986). Institutionalization and deinstitutionalization of the life course. *Human Development, 29*, 157–162.

Herman, E. (1995). *The romance of American psychology: Political culture in the age of experts*. Berkeley: University of California Press.

Hochschild, A. R. (1983). *The managed heart: Commercialization of human feeling*. Berkeley: University of California Press.

Horkheimer, M. (1974). *Eclipse of reason*. New York: Oxford University Press.

Horkheimer, M., & Adorno, T. W. (1972). *The dialectic of enlightenment*. New York: Herder and Herder.

Horwitz, A. V. (1982a). Sex-role expectations, power, and psychological distress. *Sex Roles, 8*, 607–623.

Horwitz, A. V. (1982b). *The social control of mental illness*. New York: Academic Press.

Horwitz, A. V. (2002). *Creating mental illness*. Chicago: University of Chicago Press.

Horwitz, A. V., & Mullis, J.S. (1998). Individualism and its discontents: The response to the seriously mentally ill in late twentieth century America. *Sociological Focus, 31*, 119–133.

Karoly, P. (1999). A goal systems – self-regulatory perspective on personality, psychopathology and change. *Review of General Psychology, 3*, 264–291.

Kellner, D. (1989). *Critical theory, Marxism, and modernity*. Baltimore: John Hopkins University Press.

Keyes, C. L. M. (2002a). The mental health continuum: From languishing to flourishing in life. *Journal of Health and Social Behavior, 43*, 207–222.

Keyes, C. L. M. (2002b). "Complete mental health: An agenda for the 21st Century." In C. L. M. Keyes & J. Haidt (Eds.), *Flourishing: Positive psychology and the life well-lived* (pp. 293–312). Washington, D. C.: American Psychological Association.

Kirk, S. A., & Kutchins, H. (1992). *The selling of DSM: The rhetoric of science in psychiatry*. New York: Aldine de Gruyter.

Klerman, G. L. (1978). Affective disorders. In M. Armand & M. D. Nicholi, Jr. (Eds.), *The Harvard guide to modern psychiatry* (pp. 253–281). Cambridge, MA: Belknap Press.

Klerman, G. L., & Weissman, M. M. (1989). Increasing rates of depression. *Journal of the American Medical Association, 261*, 2229–2235.

Laing, R. D. (1960). *The divided self*. London: Tavistock.

Lewinsohn, P., Rohde, P., Seeley, J., & Fischer, S. (1993). Age-cohort changes in the lifetime occurrence of depression and other mental disorders. *Journal of Abnormal Psychology, 102*, 110–120.

Liem, R., & Liem, J. (1978). Social class and mental illness reconsidered: The role of economic stress and social support. *Journal of Health and Social Behavior, 19*, 139–56.

Linville, P. W. (1987). Self-complexity as a cognitive buffer against stress-related illness and depression. *Journal of Personality and Social Psychology 52*, 663–676.

Lunbeck, E. (1994). *The psychiatric persuasion: Knowledge, gender, and power in modern America*. Princeton, NJ: Princeton University Press.

Marcuse, H. (1955). *Eros and civilization*. Boston: Beacon Press.

Marcuse, H. (1964). *One-dimensional man*. Boston: Beacon Press.

Maryanski, A., & Turner, J. (1992). *The social cage: Human nature and the evolution of society*. Stanford, CA: Stanford University Press.

Mayer, K. U. (2001). The paradox of global social change and national path dependencies: Life course patterns in advanced societies. In A. E. Woodward & M. Kohli (Eds.), *Inclusions and exclusions in European societies* (pp. 89–110). London: Routledge.

Mayer, K. U. (2004).Whose lives? How history, societies and institutions define and shape life courses. *Research in Human Development, 1*, 161–187.

McLeod, J. D., & Kessler, R. C. (1990). Socioeconomic status differences in vulnerability to undesirable life events. *Journal of Health and Social Behavior, 31*, 162–172.

Mechanic, D. (1999). Mental health and mental illness: Definitions and perspectives. In A.V. Horwitz & T. L. Scheid (Eds.), *A handbook for the study of mental health* (pp. 12–28). Cambridge: Cambridge University Press.

Mills, C. W. (1959). *The sociological imagination*. New York: Oxford University Press.

Mirowsky, J. (1985). Depression and marital power: An equity model. *American Journal of Sociology, 91*, 557–592.

Mitchell, J. (1974). *Psychoanalysis and feminism*. New York: Pantheon.

Myles, J. 1993. Is there a post-Fordist life course? In W.R. Heinz (Ed.), *Institutions and gatekeeping in the life course* (pp. 171–185). Weinheim: Deutscher Studien-Verlag.

O'Rand, A. M., & Henretta, J. C. (1999). *Age and inequality*. Boulder, CO: Westview Press.

Pearlin, L. I. (1989). The sociological study of stress. *Journal of Health and Social Behavior, 30*, 141–256.

Prilleltensky, I. (1994). *The morals and politics of psychology: Psychological discourse and the status quo*. Albany, NY: State University of New York Press.

Rabinow, P. (1984). *The Foucault reader*. New York: Pantheon Books.

Rose, J. (1983). Femininity and its discontents. *Feminist Review, 14*, 5–21.

Rose, J. (1989). Where does the misery come from? Psychoanalysis, feminism, and the event. In R. Feldstein & J. Roof (Eds.), *Feminism and psychoanalysis*. Ithaca, NY: Cornell University Press.

Rose, N. (1989). *Governing the soul: The shaping of the private self*. London and New York: Routledge.

Rosenau, P. M. (1992). *Postmodernism and the social sciences*. Princeton, NJ: Princeton University Press.

Rosenfield, S. (1999). Gender and mental health: Do women have more psychopathology, men more, or both the same (and why?). In A. V. Horwitz & T. L. Scheid (Eds.), *A handbook for the study of mental health* (pp. 349–360). Cambridge: Cambridge University Press.

Ryff, C. D., & Singer, B. (1998). The contours of positive human health. *Psychological Inquiry, 9*, 1–28.

Scheff, T. (1966). *Being mentally ill: A sociological theory*. Chicago: Aldine.

Scott, W. J. (1990). PTSD in DSM-III: A case in the politics of diagnosis and disease. *Social Problems, 37*, 294–310.

Seligman, M. E. P. (1975). *Helplessness: On depression, development, and death*. San Francisco: Freeman.

Shanahan, M. J. (2000). Pathways to adulthood in changing societies: Variability and mechanisms in life course perspective. *Annual Review of Sociology, 26*, 667–692.

Simmel, G. ([1903]1971). The metropolis and mental life. In D. Levine (Ed.), *Georg Simmel* (pp. 324–339). Chicago: University of Chicago Press.

Simmel, G. ([1907] 1978). *The philosophy of money*. T. Bottomore and D. Frisby (Eds.). London: Routledge and Kegan Paul.

Spielberger, C. D., & Rickman, R. L. 1990. Assessment of state and trait anxiety. In N. Sartorius, V. Andreoli, G. Cassano, L. Eisenberg, P. Kielcolt, P. Pancheri, & G. Racagni (Eds.), *Anxiety: Psychobiological and clinical perspectives* (pp. 69–83). New York: Hemisphere Publishing.

Szasz, T. S. (1961). *The myth of mental illness*. New York: Hoeber-Harper.

Thoits, P. A. (1983). Multiple identities and psychological well-being: A reformulation and test of the social isolation hypothesis. *American Sociological Review, 48*, 174–187.

Thoits, P. A. (1985). Self-labeling processes in mental illness: the role of emotional deviance. *American Journal of Sociology, 91*, 221–249.

Turner, R. J., Wheaton, B., & Lloyd, D. A. (1995). The epidemiology of social stress. *American Sociological Review, 60*, 104–25.

Twenge, J. M. (2000). The age of anxiety? Birth cohort change in anxiety and neuroticism, 1952–1993. *Journal of Personality and Social Psychology, 79*, 1007–1021.

Twenge, J. M. (2002). Birth cohort, social change, and personality: The interplay of dysphoria and individualism in the 20th Century. In D. Cervone & W. Mischel (Eds.), *Advances in personality science* (pp. 196–218). New York: Guilford Press.

Twenge, J. M., & Campbell, W. K. (2001). Age and birth cohort differences in self-esteem: A cross-temporal meta-analysis. *Personality and Social Psychology Review, 5*, 321–244.

Twenge, J. M., Zhang, L., & Charles, I. (2004). It's beyond my control: A cross-temporal meta-analysis of increasing externality in locus of control, 1960–2002. *Personality and Social Psychology Review, 8*, 308–319.

Wachtel, P. (1983). *The poverty of affluence*. New York: Free Press.

Waitzkin, H. (1989). A critical theory of medical discourse: Ideology, social control, and the processing of social context in medical encounters. *Journal of Health and Social Behavior, 30*, 220–239.

Wakefield, J. (1992a). The concept of mental disorder: On the boundary between biological facts and social values. *American Psychologist, 47*, 373–388.

Wakefield, J. (1992b). Disorder as harmful dysfunction: A conceptual critique of DSM-III-R's definition of mental disorder. *Psychological Review, 99*, 232–247.

Wakefield, J. (1999). The measurement of mental disorder. In A. V. Horwitz & T. L. Scheid (Eds.), *A handbook for the study of mental health* (pp. 29–57). Cambridge: Cambridge University Press.

Wheaton, B. (1980). The sociogenesis of psychological disorder: An attributional theory. *Journal of Health and Social Behavior, 24*, 100–24.

Wheaton, B. (1994). Sampling the stress universe. In W. R. Avison & I. H.Gotlib (Eds.),*Stress and mental health: Contemporary issues and prospects for the future* (pp. 77–114). New York: Plenum.

Wheaton, B. (1999). The nature of stressors. In A. V. Horwitz & T. L. Scheid (Eds.), *A handbook for the study of mental health* (pp. 176–197). Cambridge, UK: Cambridge University Press.

Wheaton, B. (1978). The sociogenesis of psychological disorder: Re-examining the causal issues with longitudinal data. *American Sociological Review, 43*, 383–404.

Young, A. (1995). *The harmony of illusions: Inventing post-traumatic stress disorder*. Princeton, NJ: Princeton University Press.

Part III
The Social Origins of Mental Health and Mental Illness

6
Class Relations, Economic Inequality and Mental Health: Why Social Class Matters to the Sociology of Mental Health

Carles Muntaner, Carme Borrell, and Haejoo Chung

Psychiatric epidemiologists were among the first scientists to document that the poor suffer from a higher rate of mental disorders than the affluent. Mental health and, more precisely, psychiatric research have propelled many studies on economic inequality and mental disorders which reflect the humanistic concerns of psychiatrists. These studies are motivated by a desire to improve the living conditions of workers, immigrants, and racial or ethnic minorities (e.g., Blazer, Kessler, McGonagle, & Swartz, 1994; Eaton, Buka, Addington, Bass, Brown, Cherker-zian, Forman-Hoffman, Gilbert, Hayden, Jain, Lehrer, Martin, Mielke, Norberg, Thomas, & Yu, 2004; Jacobi, Wittchen, Hölting, Höfler, Pfister, Müller, & Lieb, 2004; Lahelma, Martikainen, Rahkonen, Roos, & Saastamoinen, 2005; Regier, Boyd, Burke, Rae, Myers, Kramer, Robins, George, Karno, & Locke, 1988; Roberts & Lee, 1993). The absence or poor quality of psychiatric care for poor working class, immigrant, or racial and ethnic minority populations (Alegria, Bijl, Lin, Walters, & Kessler, 2000; Cohen, Houck, Szanto, Dew, Gilman, & Reynolds, 2006; Muntaner, Wolyniec, McGrath, & Pulver, 1995) raise a related set of concerns about the implications of economic inequality for the treatment of mental disorders.

The psychiatric and public health perspective on economic inequality is "pragmatic" (e.g., Asthana, Gibson, Moon, Brigham, & Dicker, 2004). Following the ethos of public health and medical care, the goal is to "act upon the world" to reduce suffering and increase well-being (Navarro & Muntaner, 2004). Mental disorders, which have a major worldwide impact on disability, are the leading cause of disability among women and, by 2020, are expected to become the main cause of years lost to disability (Murray & Lopez, 1996). Overall, the relevance of economic inequality to psychiatry stems from the strength of the association between economic inequality and mental disorders and the severe consequences that economic inequality has for the quality of life of psychiatric patients (Fryers, Melzer, Jenkins, & Brugha, 2005; Melzer, Fryers, Jenkins, Brugha, & McWilliams, 2003; Poulton, Caspi, Milne, Thomson, Taylor, Sears, & Moffitt, 2002; Stansfeld, Head, Fuhrer, Wardle, & Cattell, 2003).

Most psychiatric research is thus grounded in the medical world with its associated materialism and realism. It is within this context of professional pragmatism and applied science that several findings on the relation between economic inequality and mental health have emerged within the last century. This literature can inform sociology because of the clinical relevance of its categories which correspond to the most severe forms of mental disturbances seen by medical doctors. In spite of its narrow conceptualization of stratification, this relatively simple literature on the relations between economic inequality and mental disorders provides important findings that have proved quite robust across time and place. In turn, sociology can inform research on the social origins and determinants of mental disorders by looking beyond simple stratification, such as the urgent need of patients that cannot afford medical care or new drugs, to consider other dimensions of stratification (e.g. Geyer, Haltenhof, & Peter, 2001).

In this chapter we review recent evidence on the relation between social stratification, social class, and mental disorders, arguing for the need to distinguish between the concepts of social stratification and social class in the sociology of mental disorders. Next, we venture into uncharted territories in the study of social class and mental health by introducing the concept of exploitation. We note a paradox of this area of knowledge: sociologists often adopt the role of epidemiologists and social psychologists while epidemiologists take on the role of sociologists. We end by emphasizing the need for greater cross-fertilization between sociology and epidemiology in the study of social inequalities in mental health.

The Association Between Social Stratification and Mental Disorders

There is a strong inverse association between economic inequality—based on conventional rank indicators—and mental disorders (Eaton & Muntaner, 1999; Muntaner, Eaton, Miech, & O'Campo, 2004a). The evidence is particularly strong to support the association between economic inequality, measured in terms of income, educational credentials, or occupational social class, and the most frequent forms of psychiatric illnesses, such as depression, anxiety disorders, and substance use disorders (Eaton & Muntaner, 1999). For example, a comprehensive meta-analysis of prevalence and incidence studies on socioeconomic position and depression indicated that persons with low educational attainment or low income are at higher risk of depression (Lorant, Deliege, Eaton, Robert, Philippot, & Ansseau, 2003). In the United States, individuals with annual household incomes of less than $20,000 per year were found to have a prevalence of major depression in the past month that was twice as high as that for individuals with annual household incomes of $70,000 or more (Blazer et al., 1994). Studies of U.S. metropolitan areas have found even larger differences (with odds ratios of 11 to 16) between high- and low-income respondents' risks of depression (Eaton, 2001). In a 13-year follow-up study that used psychiatric interviews as a method of assessment, poverty was found to increase the risk of depression by 2.5 times (Eaton, Muntaner, Bovasso, & Smith, 2001). In the same study in east Baltimore, respondents who did not receive income from property were 10 times more likely to have an anxiety disorder than were those who obtained some income from property (Muntaner, Eaton, Diala, Kessler, & Sorlie, 1998).

With regard to occupational social class, the prevalence of depression in the past 6 months among those employed in household services was 7 percent, almost three times that of executive professionals (2.4 percent) (Roberts & Lee, 1993). More recent studies show that blue-collar workers are between 1.5 and 2 times as likely to be depressed as white-collar workers (Eaton et al., 2004). Similar risk increases have been reported with a 1-year follow-up period (Eaton et al., 2004). Being born to parents employed in manual labour occupations confers almost twice the risk of depression for women and almost four times the risk of depression for men compared with those born to at least one parent not in the working class (Eaton et al., 2004). In addition to depression, similar two- to three-fold differences in prevalence between high and low occupational strata have been reported in the United States for substance use disorders, alcohol abuse or dependence, antisocial personality disorder, anxiety disorders, and all psychiatric disorders combined (Eaton, 2001; Eaton et al., 2004; Regier et al., 1988). Internationally, even larger differences have been found—up to a four-fold higher current prevalence of common psychiatric disorders among "working-class" respondents compared with their middle-class counterparts (Regier, Farmer, Rae, Myers, Kramer, Robins, George, Karno, & Locke, 1993).

Poverty is also a consistent risk factor for multiple mental disorders, including depression, anxiety disorders, antisocial personality, and substance-use disorders (Eaton et al., 2004; Eaton & Muntaner, 1999). Cross-sectional and longitudinal studies have found consistent associations between area poverty and mental disorders. In addition, most income inequality studies have shown an association between income inequality and high rates of mental disorders (Muntaner et al., 2004a; Wilkinson & Pickett, 2006).

What Can Epidemiology Contribute to the Sociology of Mental Disorders? The Focus on Proximal Determinants

The challenge for epidemiologists and sociologists alike is to use concepts from stratification research to explain these patterns. There is currently a heated controversy on the relative importance of "neo-material" determinants (contemporary physical or biological risk or protective factors) and "psychosocial" determinants, such as perceptions of relative standing in the income distribution, for explaining socioeconomic gradients in health in wealthy countries (Lynch, Smith, Kaplan, & House, 2000; Muntaner, 2004; Pearce & Davey Smith, 2003). In brief "neo-material" scholars claim that most social inequalities in health are determined by "material" (socially determined physical and chemical) risk and protective factors linked to poverty and inequality, such as poor housing, poor diet, drugs, environmental and workplace hazards, injuries, poor transportation, lack of access to quality health care, or physical violence (Lynch et al., 2000). Psychosocial scholars, on the other hand, stress the role of perceptions of inequality, social capital, perceptions of job stress, or social isolation (Wilkinson, 2005). Research supports both types of explanations.

Neo-material indicators of economic inequality, such as owning a car or a house, and indices of deprivation have recently been incorporated into research on the social epidemiology of mental disorders (Lewis, Bebbington, Brugha, Farrell, Gill, Jenkins, & Meltzer, 1998, 2003; Weich & Lewis, 1998). For example, in a national survey of United Kingdom households, an independent association was found between housing tenure and access to a car, on the one hand, and neurotic disorder (including some anxiety disorders) and depression, on the other (Lewis et al., 2003; Weich & Lewis, 1998). Also, an analysis of the British Household Panel Survey found that low material standard of living was associated with risk for depression and anxiety disorders (Lewis et al., 1998). A geographic area deprivation index, including housing tenure and car ownership, has been associated with the prevalence and persistence of risk for depression. Although deprivation indicators suggest that absence of material goods increases the risk of psychiatric disorders, research has yet to uncover the specific mechanisms linking material factors to depression or anxiety (e.g., food insecurity, bad diet; poor housing, fear of being evicted, homelessness; noise, pollution, dirt, physical violence, extreme temperatures at work or in the community; unsafe working conditions, physical overwork, exhaustion, lack of sleep; poor transportation; poor health, chronic diseases; unmet health care needs).

Studies have also provided cross-sectional and prospective evidence of an association between psychosocial factors, such as perceived job demands and perceived financial hardship, on the one hand, and depression, symptoms of depression, or anxiety disorders, on the other (Eaton et al., 2001; Weich & Lewis, 1998). Since the mid-seventies' Whitehall studies, there have been a large number of studies showing that the effects of social stratification on mental health are partially mediated by psychosocial factors such as "job autonomy" or "lack of control" (Marmot, 2004). A substantial amount of this evidence in social epidemiology comes from the Whitehall studies themselves (Marmot, 2004). In addition, in sociology, a large number of studies have shown compatible results. "Material" risk factors and biomedical indicators are less likely to be included in those studies (e.g., Turner, Wheaton, & Lloyd, 1995; see the *Journal of Health and Social Behavior* over the last twenty years), implying that they may overstate the importance of psychosocial factors relative to material factors.

Another common limitation of most "psychosocial" studies is an over-reliance on self-report measures of both psychosocial risk factors and mental health outcomes (including questionnaires and lay-administered diagnostic interviews), coupled with an infrequent use of clinical diagnostic interviews, to assess mental disorders. Such methods produce vulnerability to self-report bias (persons might have a tendency to report both "stress" and "mental disorder" without having either). Even in prospective studies that take into account reverse causation it is difficult to rule out the possibility that features of the material environment (physical and biological exposures) are confounded with a respondent's perceptions (Macleod, Davey Smith, Heslop, Metcalfe, Carroll, & Hart, 2002). Nevertheless, the reported associations of job insecurity or remaining in a downsized organization with symptoms of anxiety and depression suggest that psychosocial exposures can have independent effects on psychiatric disorders (Ferrie, Shipley, Stansfeld, Davey Smith, & Marmot, 2003).

In sum, epidemiology's emphasis on the material and objective as well as on the psychosocial and subjective can help refine both methods and explanations in the sociology of mental disorders. There are two important implications of this ongoing debate for sociological models and methods. First, the potential neglect of material resources in the determination of mental disorders forces a reappraisal of sociological "stress" models; they may underestimate the role of material resources in mental disorders. Second, evidence of self-report bias or confounding encourages more emphasis on objective assessments of exposures, and less emphasis on self-reports.

Social Class Structure and Mental Health

Although there have been relatively few empirical studies on social class, the need to study social class proper has been noted by social epidemiologists and sociologists alike (Krieger, Williams, & Moss, 1997; Muntaner & O'Campo, 1993). While social stratification refers to the ranking of individuals in some economic (e.g., income), political (e.g., power within organizations) or cultural (e.g., education) continuum, social class deals with the social relations (owner, worker, self-employed; manager, supervisor, worker; professional, technician, unskilled worker) that generate economic, political and cultural inequalities in a social system (Muntaner et al., 1998). Most research on social inequalities in mental health relies on indicators of social stratification and does not include any analysis of social class relations (Muntaner & Lynch, 1999). Nevertheless, social class positions based on employment relations (e.g., workers, managers, employers) can be powerful determinants of population health via exposure to risk or protective factors such as social and health services or income (Bartley & Marmot, 2000). In a series of studies (e.g., Burrell, Muntaner, Benach, & Artazcoz, 2004; Muntaner et al., 1995; Muntaner, Burrell, Benach, Pasarin, & Fernandez, 2003; Muntaner et al., 1998; Muntaner & Parsons, 1996), we have examined the relationship between social class and mental health within a Neo-Marxian framework which emphasizes class employment relations (Wright, 2005).[1] To illustrate the conceptual and empirical importance of this approach to class analysis, we underscore the conceptual

---

[1] Most of the measures we have used in our studies do not distinguish the neo-Marxian conceptualization of social class from the neo-Weberian conceptualization, a framework that focuses on class as employment relations but does not contemplate exploitation as a central mechanism. We discuss the importance of adding indicators of exploitation below.

differences between social stratification and class approaches and provide empirical support for the unique relation between class and mental health.

Social stratification usually refers to the ranking of individuals along a continuum of economic attributes such as income or years of education. These rankings are known as "gradient" indicators in epidemiology (Muntaner et al., 2004a). Most researchers use several measures of social stratification simultaneously because single measures have been insufficient to explain social inequalities in the health of populations. There is little doubt that measures of social stratification are important predictors of patterns of morbidity from mental disorders (Eaton et al., 2004; Lynch & Kaplan, 2000). However, despite their usefulness in predicting mental health outcomes, these measures do not reveal the social mechanisms that explain how individuals come to accumulate different levels of economic (and political or cultural) resources (Muntaner & Lynch, 1999).

Class inequality, which includes relations of property and control over the labour process, is also associated with mental illness. Social class, understood as social relations linked to the production of goods and services (Krieger et al., 1997) is conceptually and empirically distinct from social stratification/socioeconomic status (SES). Moreover, social class is associated with mental disorders over and above SES indicators .(Borrell et al., 2004; Muntaner et al., 2003; Muntaner et al., 1998; Wohlfarth, 1997; Wohlfarth & van den Brink, 1998). One study found a small overlap between SES and social class measures, although the association between social class and depression could not be accounted for by SES (Wohlfarth, 1997). Other studies have found initial evidence of a nonlinear relationship between social class and mental health, as would be predicted by social class models but not by SES models (Muntaner et al., 2003; Muntaner et al., 1998). For example, low-level supervisors (who do not have policy-making power but can hire and fire workers) have higher rates of depression and anxiety than both upper-level managers (who have organizational control over policy and personnel) and front-line employees (who have neither). Control over organizational assets is determined by the possibility of influencing company policy (making decisions over number of people employed, products or services delivered, amount of work performed, and size and distribution of budgets) and by sanctioning authority over others in the organization (granting or preventing pay raises or promotions, hiring, and firing or temporally suspending subordinates). The repeated experience of organizational control at work would protect most upper-level managers against mood and anxiety disorders. Low-level supervisors, on the other hand, are subjected to "double exposure": the demands of upper management to discipline the workforce and the antagonism of subordinate workers, while exerting little influence over company policy. This "contradictory class location" (Wright, 1996) may place supervisors at greater risk of depression and anxiety disorders than either upper management or non-supervisory workers. The bottom line is that this finding was predicted by the "contradictory class location" hypothesis but was not predicted or explained by indicators of years of education or income gradients. The gradient ("SES") hypothesis would have led to the expectation that supervisors, because of their higher incomes, would present *lower* rates of anxiety and depression than workers.

According to this example, the theoretical and explanatory power of social class stems from social relations of ownership or control over productive resources (i.e., physical, financial, and organizational). Social class relations have important consequences for the lives of individuals. The extent of an individual's legal right and power to control productive assets determines an individual's ability to acquire income. And income determines in large part the individual's standard of living. Thus the class position of "business owner" compels its members to hire "workers" and extract labor from them, while the "worker" class position compels its members to find employment and perform labor. Social class provides an explicit relational mechanism (property, management) that explains how economic inequalities are generated and how they may affect mental health.

In a recent study we further examined the relationships between measures of social class (Wright's social class indicators, i.e., relationship to productive assets) and indicators of mental health (Borrell et al., 2004). We tested this scheme using the Barcelona Health Interview Survey, a cross-sectional survey of 10,000 residents of the city's non-institutionalized population in 2000. Health-related variables included self-perceived health (tapping mostly mental health), nicotine addiction, eating behaviors, and injuries. Findings revealed that, contrary to conventional wisdom, health indicators are often worse for employers than for managers, and that supervisors often fare more poorly than workers. Our findings highlight the potential health consequences of social class positions defined by relations of control over productive assets. They also confirm that social class taps into parts of the social variation in health that are not captured by conventional measures of social stratification. Property relations, which figure prominently in both Marxian and Weberian traditions, do not, however, exhaust the theoretical spectrum of class concepts. Another untapped notion is that of class exploitation.

Social Class Beyond Property: The Link Between Exploitation and Mental Health

Although property relations might be important predictors of mental disorders (Eaton & Muntaner, 1999; Wohlfarth, 1997), they do not capture the underlying mechanism in the Marxian class tradition, namely exploitation (Wright, 1996). According to that tradition, a measure of social class should not only capture property relations but also the domination of the "exploited" by the "exploiter" and the extraction and appropriation of labour effort (Resnick & Wolff, 1982; Wright, 1996). In fact, most Neo-Marxian measures of social class are exchangeable with Neo-Weberian measures of employment relations because they capture only property relations. That is, both sets of indicators tap into employment relations or labour market exchanges such as "employer" "employee", but do not capture the amount of labour effort extracted from the "employee" by the "employer", which forms the basis of "exploitation" as a social mechanism in the classic Marxian tradition (Muntaner et al., 1998;

Wright, 2005). To follow that tradition more closely, indicators of class exploitation should take into account that: 1) the material welfare of a class causally depends on the material deprivation of another; 2) this causal relation in 1) involves the asymmetrical exclusion of the exploited class from access to certain productive resources (e.g., property rights); and 3) the causal mechanism that translates the exclusion in 2) into differential welfare involves the appropriation of the fruits of labour of the exploited class by those who control the access to productive resources (i.e., the exploiter class) (Wright, 1996). Thus, we can observe that most Neo-Marxian measures of social class measure 1) and 2) in the form of property relations, but do not capture the appropriation of labour effort. In a recent study (Muntaner, Li, Xue, O'Campo, Chung, & Eaton, 2004b; Muntaner, Li, Xue, Thompson, O'Campo, Chung, & Eaton, 2006) we found an association between class exploitation and depression using organizational level indicators that capture both property relations and the extraction of labour effort (for-profit ownership, managerial domination, lack of wage increases). These indicators were strong predictors of depressive symptoms in these studies. They are different from employment relations indicators in that they capture social class exploitation at the organizational level (i.e., the combination of for-profit ownership, managerial pressure, and lack of wage increases taps into high levels of extraction of labour effort and low compensation, or higher exploitation, as compared to the residual category).

In sum, our argument is that there are a number of class constructs that can illuminate the relation between economic inequality and mental health. There a numerous, literally hundreds of measures of mental health in the literature (see Buro's Mental Measurement volumes). In contrast, the sociological part of the equation remains vastly underdeveloped, with researchers using only a handful of measures (income, education, occupation).

The Complex Relation Between the Sociology of Mental Disorders, Psychiatric Epidemiology, and Public Mental Health

In spite of their pragmatic, often non-theoretical approach to social factors, psychiatric epidemiology and public mental health have now and then tackled structural inequalities. A strong concern for social justice and reducing inequalities (race, gender, poverty) could explain the strong interest in social inequalities in health among epidemiologists. The contemporary definition of public health—as organized efforts by society to improve the health of populations—implicitly acknowledges both social determinants and collective responsibility for the public's health (Last, 1995).

Public mental health is thus faced with the obligation to improve the health of groups affected by social inequality—that is, public health officials have the responsibility to improve the mental health of populations that, due to economic, political, or cultural inequalities, have a high rate of mental disorders. In these disciplines it is understood that a society's unequal distribution of economic, political, or cultural resources will generate worse mental health among the relatively poor, powerless, and those with less credentials (Navarro & Muntaner, 2004). Furthermore, it is widely recognized that inequalities in property generate an intergenerational transmission of poverty that has disproportionately affected African-Americans in the U. S. (Conley & Bennett, 2001). Other acknowledged sources of economic inequality involve political inequalities that preclude immigrants from obtaining equal rights while confining them to economic, political, and cultural subordination, and cultural factors such as racism, ideology, or ignorance that can lead to labour market discrimination and residential segregation with negative economic, political, and cultural consequences for people of various races and ethnicities, nationalities, religions, age groups, sexual orientations, gender, diseases or disabilities, and socioeconomic positions.

It is within this public health ethos of reversing disparities associated with the social movements of the sixties and seventies that recent research focuses on the interactions between class, gender, and race/ethnicity when predicting mental health (Artazcoz, Benach, Borrell, & Cortes, 2004; O'Campo, Eaton, & Muntaner, 2004; Outram, Mishra, & Schofield, 2004). Although generalizations are often inaccurate in epidemiology, overall this body of research on the triad of class, gender and race tends to find worse mental health among members of the groups exposed to the three forms of inequality (Krieger, Waterman, Hartman, Bates, Stoddard, Quinn, Sorensen, & Barbeau, 2006) Epidemiologists have also been leaders in topics that overlap with the more structural concerns traditionally associated with sociology such as the study of the mental health effects of new forms of labour market arrangements (Artazcoz, Benach, Borrell, & Cortes, 2005; Kim, Muntaner, Khang, Paek, & Cho, 2006), the effects of social class across the lifespan (Breeze, Fletcher, Leon, Marmot, Clarke, & Shipley, 2001), or the contextual effects of neighbourhood economic inequality on mental disorders (Eibner, Sturn, & Gresenz, 2004; Muntaner et al., 2004a; Muntaner et al., 2004b; Schneiders, Drukker, van der Ende, Verhulst, van Os, & Nicolson, 2003; Stafford & Marmot, 2003; Wainwright & Surtees, 2004). Because these studies are often published outside of the sociological mainstream, their contributions to theories of social inequality remain under-recognized.

There is, moreover, a curious paradox that looms large in the literature on the sociology of mental health. It is not uncommon to observe that: 1) epidemiologists and public health researchers without a PhD in sociology are those who bring a socio-structural perspective to health inequalities (e.g., Krieger et al., 1997; Muntaner et al., 1998); and 2) in spite of some notable exceptions (Kohn & Schooler, 1983), sociologists have been devoted to socio-psychological rather than socio-structural explanations (Pearlin, 1989; Thoits, 2005). Sociologists are leaders in psychiatric epidemiology and public mental health without bringing a particular sociological content to their work (Kessler, McGonagle, Zhao, Nelson, Hughes, Eshleman, Wittchen, & Kendler, 1994). A detailed historical, professional, and institutional analysis (e.g., are health researchers trained to be critical in general so they dare to approach thorny issues such as "class" when they shift to social inquiry? or why did Pearlin's social psychology have more influence on the sociology of mental health than Kohn's socio-structural perspective?), will be needed to sort out the merit of these propositions. They suggest, however, the need for more sustained attention to structural explanations in sociology of mental health research.

Given the soundness of the methods and the robustness of the findings in psychiatric epidemiology and public mental health, one might be tempted to conclude that deeper sociological insights are superfluous to such applied disciplines. Why not just raise the minimum wage or increase welfare assistance to the poor as primary prevention? The answer is not so simple as implicit sociological models permeate both psychiatric epidemiology and public mental health with sharp differences in their policy implications (Muntaner, Eaton, & Diala, 2000).

More specifically, underlying most research on economic inequality and mental health we find competing, implicit, sociological models of what constitutes sound social and mental health policy. Two opposing views of the social inequalities in mental health are prominent (Muntaner et al., 2000). The first is that behaviour is a matter of individual agency or volitional control, accounting for the disproportionate burden of mental illness among workers, women, and minorities. This view holds that most social outcomes, including mental health, reflect personal autonomous choices and that therefore there is little that society, as a whole, is obliged to do for people who are afflicted by mental disorders (Muntaner & Lynch, 1999). In one study (Link, Schwartz, Moore, Phelan, Struening, Stueve, & Colten, 1995), for example, educated "liberals" respected the autonomy and individual rights of homeless persons but felt little obligation to do anything to improve their situation.

In contrast, the "structural" view focuses on social relations of class, race, ethnicity, and gender inequality as determinants of individual behaviour and mental health (Muntaner et al., 2000). The mental health policy implications of this view include a collective responsibility for those whose mental health is negatively affected by class, gender, and racial and ethnic inequalities in access to economic, political, and cultural resources. For example, a recent ethnographic study of African-American and white working-class men concluded that African-American men have a greater sense of collective responsibility and are less prone to use individual responsibility as an explanation for personal outcomes than are their white counterparts (Lamont, 2000). Western European and U.S. whites are more likely to use individualistic attributions for the outcomes of persons in social situations—personal attributes are seen as the cause of personal outcomes, as opposed to the features of the situation (Nisbett, 2003). The implication is that unless we make the social-structural inequalities explicit we cannot use social science to choose between policy perspectives.

Although most studies in social inequalities in mental health (Eaton et al., 2004) use stratification indicators that eschew social structure (i.e., the set of economic, political and cultural relations in a given social system) (Muntaner & Lynch, 1999), there is nowadays sufficient evidence to suggest that class, gender, and racial/ethnic inequalities in mental health stem from social structures, rather than solely from personal choices or individual attributes. Studies using employment relations as indicators of social class have found that they predict mental disorders over and above mere stratification indicators (see review by Muntaner et al., 2004a). The implication is that structural social class measures are useful in the sociology of mental disorders because they are strong predictors of mental disorders (Muntaner et al., 2004a) but also because they provide a social mechanism (e.g., the relation between supervisor and supervisee) for explaining those effects.

Conclusion: The Sociology of Mental Health Can (And Should) be More Structural

The evidence on the inverse association between measures of social stratification such as income and education and common mental disorders is well established. Yet little is known about the relation between the social processes that generate economic inequalities and mental health. Recent research points to the need for sociology of mental health to delve into the social relations that produce social inequalities in mental health, not only into the micro social processes linking social interactions to mental disease (e.g., stress, coping, support, stigma). Social mechanisms generating economic inequalities such as relations of production, property relations, or exploitation are too central to social systems to be addressed exclusively by epidemiologists. Sociological input will be ultimately essential to the advancement of our understanding of the relation between economic inequality and mental health. Greater sociological insight into research on social inequalities in mental health would give sociology more depth (after all, sociology should be the study of social relations); would allow testing of alternative causal models for the production of mental illness, which now are not accessible due to focus on the outcomes of social processes (e.g., income inequalities); and would yield deeper causal models that allow for more effective interventions.

References

Alegria, M., Bijl, R. V., Lin, E., Walters, E. E., & Kessler, R. C. (2000). Income differences in persons seeking outpatient treatment for mental disorders: a comparison of the United States with Ontario and The Netherlands. *Archives of General Psychiatry, 57*, 383–91.

Artazcoz, L., Benach, J., Borrell, C., & Cortes, I. (2004). Unemployment and mental health: Understanding the interactions among gender, family roles, and social class. *American Journal of Public Health, 94*, 82–88.

Artazcoz, L., Benach, J., Borrell, C., & Cortes, I. (2005). Social inequalities in the impact of flexible employment on different domains of psychosocial health. *Journal of Epidemiology and Community Health, 59*, 761–767.

Asthana, S., Gibson, A., Moon, G., Brigham, P., & Dicker, J. (2004). The demographic and social class basis of inequality in self reported morbidity: An exploration using the health survey for England. *Journal of Epidemiology and Community Health, 58*, 303–307.

Bartley, M., & Marmot, M. (2000). Social class and power relations at the workplace. *Occupational Medicine: State of the Art Reviews, 15*, 73–78.

Blazer, D. G., Kessler, R. C., McGonagle, K. A., & Swartz, M. S. (1994). The prevalence and distribution of major depression in a national community sample: The National Comorbidity Survey. *American Journal of Psychiatry,151*, 979–86.

Borrell, C., Muntaner, C., Benach, J., & Artazcoz, L. (2004). Social class and self-reported health status among men and women: What is the role of work organisation, household material standards and household labour? *Social Science and Medicine, 58*, 1869–1887.

Breeze, E., Fletcher, A. E., Leon, D. A., Marmot, M. G., Clarke, R. J., & Shipley, M. J. (2001). Do socioeconomic disadvantages persist into old age? Self-reported morbidity in a 29-year follow-up of the Whitehall study. *American Journal of Public Health, 91*, 277–283.

Cohen A., Houck, P. R., Szanto, K., Dew, M. A., Gilman, S. E., Reynolds, C. F. (2006). Social inequalities in response to antidepressant treatment in older adults. *Archives of General Psychiatry, 63*, 50–6.

Conley, D., & Bennett, N. G. (2001). Birth weight and income: Interactions across generations. *Journal of Health and Social Behavior, 42*, 450–465.

Eaton, W. W. (2001). *The sociology of mental disorders* (3rd ed.). London, UK: Praeger.

Eaton, W. W., Buka, S., Addington, A. M., Bass, J., Brown, S., Cherkerzian, S., Forman-Hoffman, V., Gilbert, S., Hayden, K., Jain, S., Lehrer, J., Martin, L., Mielke, M., Norberg, K., Thomas, C., & Yu, J. (2004,). Risk factors for major mental disorders: A review of the epidemiologic literature. Retrieved January 24th, 2005, from *http://apps1.jhsph.edu/weaton/MDRF/main.html*

Eaton, W. W., & Muntaner, C. (1999). Socioeconomic stratification and mental disorder. In A. V. Horwitz & T. L. Scheid (Eds.), *A handbook for the study of mental health: Social contexts, theories and systems* (pp. 259–283). New York, NY: Cambridge University Press.

Eaton, W. W., Muntaner, C., Bovasso, G., & Smith, C. (2001). Socioeconomic status and depression. *Journal of Health and Social Behavior, 42*, 277–293.

Eibner, C., Sturn, R., & Gresenz, C. R. (2004). Does relative deprivation predict the need for mental health services? *Journal of Mental Health Policy and Economics, 7*, 167–175.

Ferrie, J. E., Shipley, M. J., Stansfeld, S. A., Davey Smith, G., & Marmot, M. (2003). Future uncertainty and socioeconomic inequalities in health: The Whitehall II study. *Social Science and Medicine, 57*, 637–646.

Fryers, T., Melzer, D., Jenkins, R., & Brugha, T. (2005). The distribution of the common mental disorders: Social inequalities in Europe. *Clinical Practice and Epidemiology in Mental Health, 1*, 14.

Geyer, S., Haltenhof, H., & Peter, R. (2001). Social inequality in the utilization of in – and outpatient treatment of non-psychotic/non-organic disorders: A study with health insurance data. *Social Psychiatry and Psychiatric Epidemiology, 36*, 373–380.

Jacobi, F., Wittchen, H. U., Holting, C., Hofler, M., Pfister, H., Muller, N., & Lieb, R. (2004). Prevalence, co-morbidity and correlates of mental disorders in the general population: Results from the German Health Interview and Examination Survey (GHS). *Psychological Medicine, 34*, 597–611.

Kessler, R. C., McGonagle, K. A., Zhao, S., Nelson, C. B., Hughes, M., Eshleman, S., Wittchen, H. V., & Kendler, K. S. (1994). Lifetime and 12-month prevalence of DSM-III-R psychiatric disorders in the United States. *Archives of General Psychiatry, 51*, 8–19.

Kim, I. H., Muntaner, C., Khang, Y. H., Paek, D., & Cho, S. I. (2006). The relationship between nonstandard working and mental health in a representative sample of the South Korean population. *Social Science and Medicine* (in press).

Kohn, M. L., & Schooler, C. (1983). *Work and personality: An inquiry into the impact of social stratification.* Norwood, NJ: Ablex Pub. Corp.

Krieger N., Waterman, P. D., Hartman, C., Bates, L. M., Stoddard, A. M., Quinn, M. M., Sorensen, G., & Barbeau, E. M. (2006). Social hazards on the job: Workplace abuse, sexual harassment, and racial discrimination – a study of Black, Latino, and White low-income women and men workers in the United States. *International Journal of Health Services, 36*, 51–85.

Krieger, N., Williams, D. R., & Moss, N. E. (1997). Measuring social class in U.S. public health research: Concepts, methodologies, and guidelines. *Annual Review of Public Health, 18*, 341–378.

Lahelma, E., Martikainen, P., Rahkonen, O., Roos, E., & Saastamoinen, P. (2005). Occupational class inequalities across key domains of health: Results from the Helsinki Health Study. *European Journal of Public Health, 15*, 504–510.

Lamont, M. (2000). *The dignity of working men.* New York, NY: Russell Sage.

Last, J. (1995). *A dictionary of epidemiology.* New York, NY: Oxford University Press.

Lewis, G., Bebbington, P., Brugha, T., Farrell, M., Gill, B., Jenkins, R., & Meltzer, H. (1998). Socioeconomic status, standard of living, and neurotic disorder. *Lancet, 352*, 605–609.

Lewis, G., Bebbington, P., Brugha, T., Farrell, M., Gill, B., Jenkins, R., *et al.* (2003). Socio-economic status, standard of living, and neurotic disorder. *International Review of Psychiatry, 15*, 91–96.

Link, B. G., Schwartz, S., Moore, R., Phelan, J., Struening, E., Stueve, A., & Colten, M. E. (1995). Public knowledge, attitudes, and beliefs about homeless people: Evidence for compassion fatigue. *American Journal of Community Psychology, 23*, 533–555.

Lorant, V., Deliege, D., Eaton, W., Robert, A., Philippot, P., & Ansseau, M. (2003). Socioeconomic inequalities in depression: A meta-analysis. *American Journal of Epidemiology, 157*, 98–112.

Lynch, J. W., & Kaplan, G. A. (2000). Socioeconomic position. In L. F. Berkman & I. Kawachi (Eds.), *Social epidemiology* (pp. 76–94). New York: NY: Oxford University Press.

Lynch, J. W., Smith, G. D., Kaplan, G. A., & House, J. S. (2000). Income inequality and mortality: Importance to health of individual income, psychosocial environment, or material conditions. *British Medical Journal, 320*, 1200–1204.

Macleod, J., Davey Smith, G., Heslop, P., Metcalfe, C., Carroll, D., & Hart, C. (2002). Psychological stress and cardiovascular disease: Empirical demonstration of bias in a prospective observational study of Scottish men. *British Medical Journal, 324*, 1247–1251.

Marmot, M. (2004). *The status syndrome.* New York: Times Books.

Melzer, D., Fryers, T., Jenkins, R., Brugha, T., & McWilliams, B. (2003). Social position and the common mental disorders with disability: Estimates from the National Psychiatric Survey of Great Britain. *Social Psychiatry and Psychiatric Epidemiology, 38*, 238–243.

Muntaner, C. (2004). Commentary: Social capital, social class, and the slow progress of psychosocial epidemiology. *International Journal of Epidemiology, 33*, 674–680.

Muntaner, C., Borrell, C., Benach, J., Pasarin, M. I., & Fernandez, E. (2003). The associations of social class and social stratification with patterns of general and mental health in a Spanish population. *International Journal of Epidemiology, 32*, 950–958.

Muntaner, C., Eaton, W., & Diala, C. (2000). Socioeconomic inequalities in mental health: A review of concepts and underlying assumptions. *Health, 4*, 89–15.

Muntaner, C., Eaton, W. W., Diala, C., Kessler, R. C., & Sorlie, P. D. (1998). Social class, assets, organizational control and the prevalence of common groups of psychiatric disorders. *Social Science and Medicine, 47*, 2043–2053.

Muntaner, C., Eaton, W. W., Miech, R., & O'Campo, P. (2004a). Socioeconomic position and major mental disorders. *Epidemiologic Reviews, 26*, 53–62.

Muntaner, C., Li, Y., Xue, X., O'Campo, P., Chung, H. J., & Eaton, W. W. (2004b). Work organization, area labor-market characteristics, and depression among U.S. nursing home workers: A cross-classified multilevel analysis. *International Journal of Occupational and Environmental Health, 10*, 392–400.

Muntaner, C., Li, Y., Xue, X., O'Campo, P., Chung, H. J., & Eaton, W. W. (2006). County level socioeconomic position, work organization and depression disorder: A repeated measures cross-classified multilevel analysis of low-income nursing home workers. *Health and Place, 12*, 688–700.

Muntaner, C., & Lynch, J. (1999). Income inequality, social cohesion, and class relations: A critique of Wilkinson's neo-Durkheimian research program. *International Journal of Health Services, 29*, 59–81.

Muntaner, C., & O'Campo, P. J. (1993). A critical appraisal of the demand/control model of the psychosocial work environment: Epistemological, social, behavioral and class considerations. *Social Science and Medicine, 36*, 1509–1517.

Muntaner, C., & Parsons, P. E. (1996). Income, social stratification, class, and private health insurance: A study of the Baltimore metropolitan area. *International Journal of Health Services, 26*, 655–671.

Muntaner, C., Wolyniec, P., McGrath, J., Pulver, A. E. (1995). Differences in social class among psychotic patients at inpatient admission. *Psychiatric Services, 46*, 176–8.

Murray, C. J., & Lopez, A. D. (1996). Evidence-based health policy – lessons from the global burden of disease study. *Science, 274*, 740–743.

Navarro, V., & Muntaner, C. (2004). *Political and economic determinants of population health and well-being: Controversies and developments*. Amityville: The Baywood Publishing Company.

Nisbett, R. E. (2003). *The geography of thought*. New York, NY: The Free Press.

O'Campo, P., Eaton, W. W., & Muntaner, C. (2004). Labor market experience, work organization, gender inequalities and health status: Results from a prospective analysis of U. S. employed women. *Social Science and Medicine, 58*, 585–594.

Outram, S., Mishra, G. D., & Schofield, M. J. (2004). Sociodemographic and health related factors associated with poor mental health in midlife Australian women. *Women's Health, 39*, 97–115.

Pearce, N., & Davey Smith, G. (2003). Is social capital the key to inequalities in health? *American Journal of Public Health, 93*, 122–129.

Pearlin, L. I. (1989). The sociological study of stress. *Journal of Health and Social Behavior, 30*, 241–256.

Poulton, R., Caspi, A., Milne, B. J., Thomson, W. M., Taylor, A., Sears, M. R., & Moffitt, T. E. (2002). Association between children's experience of socioeconomic disadvantage and adult health: A life-course study. *Lancet, 360*, 1640–1645.

Regier, D. A., Boyd, J. H., Burke, J. D., Jr., Rae, D. S., Myers, J. K., Kramer, M., Robins, L. N., George, L. K., Karno, M., & Locke, B. Z. (1988). One-month prevalence of mental disorders in the United States. Based on five epidemiologic catchment area sites. *Archives of General Psychiatry, 45*, 977–986.

Regier, D. A., Farmer, M. E., Rae, D. S., Myers, J. K., Kramer, M., Robins, L. N., George, L. K., Karno, M., & Locke, B. Z. (1993). One-month prevalence of mental disorders in the United States and sociodemographic characteristics: The Epidemiologic Catchment Area study. *Acta Psychiatrica Scandinavia, 88*, 35–47.

Resnick, S., & Wolff, R. D. (1982). Classes in Marxian theory. *Review of Radical Political Economics, 13*, 1–18.

Roberts, R. E., & Lee, E. S. (1993). Occupation and the prevalence of major depression, alcohol, and drug abuse in the United States. *Environmental Research, 61*, 266–278.

Schneiders, J., Drukker, M., van der Ende, J., Verhulst, F. C., van Os, J., & Nicolson, N. A. (2003). Neighbourhood socioeconomic disadvantage and behavioural problems from late childhood into early adolescence. *Journal of Epidemiology and Community Health, 57*, 699–703.

Stafford, M., & Marmot, M. (2003). Neighbourhood deprivation and health: Does it affect us all equally? *International Journal of Epidemiology, 32*, 357–366.

Stansfeld, S. A., Head, J., Fuhrer, R., Wardle, J., & Cattell, V. (2003). Social inequalities in depressive symptoms and physical functioning in the Whitehall II study: Exploring a common cause explanation. *Journal of Epidemiology and Community Health, 57*, 361–367.

Thoits, P. A. (2005). Differential labeling of mental illness by social status: A new look at an old problem. *Journal of Health and Social Behavior, 46*, 102–119.

Turner, R. J., Wheaton, B., & Lloyd, D. (1995). The epidemiology of social stress. *American SociologicalReview, 60*, 104–125

Wainwright, N. W., & Surtees, P. G. (2004). Area and individual circumstances and mood disorder prevalence. *British Journal of Psychiatry, 185*, 227–232.

Weich, S., & Lewis, G. (1998). Material standard of living, social class, and the prevalence of the common mental disorders in Great Britain. *Journal of Epidemiology and Community Health, 52*, 8–14.

Wilkinson, R. (2005). *The impact of inequality*. New York: The New Press.

Wilkinson, R. G., & Pickett, K. E. (2006). Income inequality and population health: A review and explanation of the evidence. *Social Science and Medicine, 62*, 1768–1784.

Wohlfarth, T. (1997). Socioeconomic inequality and psychopathology: Are socioeconomic status and social class interchangeable? *Social Science and Medicine, 45*, 399–410.

Wohlfarth, T., & van den Brink, W. (1998). Social class and substance use disorders: The value of social class as distinct from socioeconomic status. *Social Science and Medicine, 47*, 51–58.

Wright, E. O. (1996). *Class counts*. Cambridge: Cambridge University Press.

Wright, E. O. (2005). *Approaches to class analysis*. Cambridge: Cambridge University Press.

7
Work and the Political Economy of Stress: Recontextualizing the Study of Mental Health/Illness in Sociology

Rudy Fenwick and Mark Tausig

The sociology of mental health has produced an impressive set of findings about the social causes and consequences of mental illness. Yet, to many researchers, it seems that the insights produced by these findings have not penetrated other parts of the discipline or to its core. One irony of this situation is that the earliest sociological expositions (those of Marx, Weber and Durkheim) that established the discipline discussed the psychological consequences of social order, yet the current work of sociologists studying mental health is not seen as contributing to our basic understanding of society.

How has this come to pass? In our view, the answer is partly related to the absence of research that links the unequal distribution of mental health outcomes across individuals and groups in society to more general structural dynamics that routinely produce and reproduce unequal outcomes in the distribution of other social, economic and psychological rewards, such as income, wealth, status, power and cognitive abilities. While we have recognized that social positions such as class, gender and race affect exposure to health risk and access to health-related resources (Link & Phelan, 1995), we have yet to specify exactly the way in which this occurs or how it is related to other socioeconomic processes.

This is largely because, as Schwartz (2002) points out, most sociological mental health research works with outcomes conceived and measured as individual attributes and not as characteristics of social positions. One drawback of this orientation is that it obscures the linkages between social structures and processes and social effects. Indeed, it makes mental health outcomes an anomic or pathological result of "person-environment" misfit rather than a routine result of social organization and inequality.

A strategy for addressing this issue is to elaborate a model that explicitly links these individual outcomes – and their distributions – to socioeconomic structures and processes that operate both on the macro/societal level and the meso/organization level. Such an approach directly inserts mental health research into the research discourse of other sociological subfields and links it to central sociological questions of social organization and social inequality. We suggest that mental health outcomes need to be understood as outcomes of structural dynamics that produce social inequality in general, and not solely in terms of inequalities in the distributions of mental illness.

In this chapter we will describe such a theoretical approach to the study of the relationship between the organization of work and mental health. We propose "contextualizing" or "re-contextualizing" mental health/illness as a fundamental outcome of the organization of work, just as are extrinsic outcomes such as income. We will do so by elaborating the relationship between work and health to show how that relationship is affected by institutional and organization conditions and change using a   model that is common for explaining income inequality.

Structural Labor Markets and the "Political Economy of Stress"

We call this approach the "political economy of stress" because it assigns a central role to economic processes in determining social outcomes (Collins, 1988). This was the perspective that greatly influenced the works of classic nineteenth century social scientists such as Adam Smith, Karl Marx, and to a somewhat lesser extent, Max Weber. More recently, it has been influential in the development of a structural labor market approach to the study of occupational and earnings attainment in the sociological literature on stratification. The overriding theme of this literature has been to specify the structural dynamics that translate general macroeconomic processes, such as changing labor market supply and demand, into individual and aggregate outcomes, such as job earnings and career mobility (DiPrete & Nonnemaker, 1997; Rosenfeld, 1992). This structural approach to labor markets arose in the 1970s and 1980s as a critique of the then-dominant approaches to labor market outcomes in sociology and economics: status attainment and neoclassical supply and demand theories, respectively. It was critical of both the conceptualization of a single, undifferentiated labor market in which all workers compete, and the view that the outcomes of that competition were entirely the result of "supply side" individual "human capital" factors, such as educational level (Beck, Horan & Tolbert, 1978; Stolzenberg, 1978). Instead, the structural approach argued that there were multiple labor markets "segmented" by industry, occupation, and region, as well as by race and gender; and that income and occupational outcomes were determined not only by the characteristics workers brought to their work, but also by the "demand side" characteristics of jobs, firms and industries in which they worked.

The structural labor market perspective has focused on conceptualizing and measuring the structures of jobs and firms that either provide *resources* and opportunities to workers for higher earnings and career advancement (good jobs) or create *risks* for workers by constraining their earnings and mobility (bad jobs). The former, "good" jobs have been characterized by structures such as internal labor markets, job ladders, and vacancy chains that restrict competition for hiring and promotion through rationalized procedures such as on-the-job training and seniority rules. In turn, these job structures have been associated with the need and ability of firms to acquire and maintain highly skilled employees. Firms that offer "good" jobs tend to be larger firms (Stolzenberg, 1978), firms in oligopolistic and capital intensive industries (Beck, Horan and Tolbert, 1978), and firms whose core employees are not easily replaceable, such as professionals (Williamson, 1975). As a result, good jobs provide workers with higher earnings and more mobility.

By contrast, the latter, "bad" jobs have been associated with externalized hiring and the lack of rationalized, or any, promotion procedures. In turn, these job structures have been associated with firms that are labor cost conscious: smaller firms in competitive and labor intensive industries, and who rely on employees with few, easily acquired skills, and thus are easily replaceable. Bad jobs pay lower wages and provide few, if any, mobility opportunities.

Over the past thirty years, the structural labor market literature has been increasingly successful in specifying the "meso" structures of jobs, firms and industries that link the macro dynamics of the political economy to micro economic outcomes such as income and promotions of individual workers. As a result, this perspective has articulated a model that describes how inequalities in earnings and occupational mobility are the normal outcomes of the structural dynamics of the political economy rather than the results of anomic social structures or pathologies that make some individuals and groups less competitive in the labor markets (e.g., "the culture of poverty"). We argue that this perspective applies to the work-mental health relationship as well.

Existing Approaches to Assessing the Work-Mental Health Relationship

Current theoretical developments in the study of the social origins of mental health and illness focus on a very similar problematic in which we realize that individual exposure to stressors and personal coping and support resources (i.e., human capital factors) are not sufficient to explain mental health status attainment; yet we have not fully elaborated and explored empirically a more structural approach that accounts for the aggregate distribution of stressors and coping resources.

Mental health researchers have focused on what is arguably the most significant non-economic outcome of work: "job stress," and have employed both micro and macro level approaches to the problem. Existing research can be categorized into four approaches: (1) micro analyses of the relationships between individual work and employment (or unemployment) experiences and individual mental health outcomes and changes in individual outcomes (e.g., Cobb & Kasl, 1978; French, Caplan & Harrison, 1982; House, 1980; Jahoda, 1982; Karasek, 1979; Karasek & Theorell, 1990; Kasl, 1978; Liem & Rayman, 1982); (2) macro analyses of the relationships between aggregate changes in economic indicators and aggregate changes in the mental and physical health of a population (e.g., Brenner, 1973, 1976, 1984, 1987); (3) macro-micro contextual analyses of the effects of changes in macro economic indicators on individual experiences and the relationships between these experiences and individual outcomes and changes in outcomes (e.g., Catalano & Dooley, 1977, 1979; Catalano, Dooley, & Jackson,

1985; Fenwick & Tausig, 1994; Turner, 1995); and (4) case studies of working conditions and worker mental health in specific organizations (e.g., Kasl & Cobb, 1979; Perrucci, Perrucci, Targ, & Targ, 1988).

From the micro analytic perspective, there is an extensive literature on the relationship between the characteristics or attributes of jobs and the mental, and physical, health of individual workers. This research has examined the potentially stressful characteristics of the physical work environment, organizational properties of work and social relationships with co-workers and supervisors (e.g., House, 1980; Kahn, 1974; Karasek, 1979; 1989a; Kasl, 1978). Two models of the etiology of job stress have developed out of this research. (1) The "person-environment fit" model argues that stress develops out of a discrepancy between characteristics of the work environment and individual characteristics (French, Caplan, & Harrison, 1982). (2) The "job demands-control" model argues that stress arises when there is inadequate structural capacity (control) to meet job demands (Karasek, 1979; Karasek & Theorell, 1990). However, neither of these models has been concerned with the structural origins and dynamics of stressful job conditions. Research at the micro level has measured individual job conditions, such as decision latitude, job demands, and social support, and characteristics, such as level of education, unemployment experience, and perceived insecurity (e.g., the Quality of Employment Surveys; Quinn, Mangione, & Seashore, 1973; Quinn & Staines, 1977). And, in the work of Karasek and his associates these descriptions were aggregated to characterize the conditions of jobs rather than the perceptions of individual workers (Karasek, 1979; Karasek & Theorell, 1990). Thus, the characteristics of "healthy work" could be described, but the organizational and socioeconomic contexts in which "healthy work" occurs were not incorporated.

At the other end, research on work and health that begins at the macro level does so by measuring aggregate indicators of the overall economy based on Census and Labor Department data- at least in the United States (e.g., rates of unemployment, cost of living, etc.) to describe the macro socioeconomic context of work and health (Brenner, 1973, 1995). This approach, derived from the human ecology perspective, argues that changes in macro socioeconomic structures, and in particular labor markets as measured by changes in unemployment rates, directly affect the exposure of the population to health risks, also measured by aggregate rates, e.g., of suicide and hospitalization. The limits of this approach have been in its inability to disaggregate the relationships to explain differences in individual outcomes- the so-called "ecological fallacy." Additionally, while many of the macroeconomic measures can also be disaggregated to the level of industry (e.g., manufacturing, retail, professional services, etc.), they cannot measure variations of organizational characteristics within a given industry that potentially have effects on individual experiences and health outcomes (e.g., profitability, market share, product/service diversity, branch plant versus single plant/headquarters, authority centralization, etc.). Thus, this approach cannot describe the meso organizational context.

Nor, can research that has linked macro and micro work-health relationships (e.g., Catalano & Dooley, 1977, 1979, 1983; Fenwick & Tausig, 1994). As with the purely macro approach, macro-micro research starts with the assumption that the underlying causes of work-related stress outcomes rests with macro structures and processes. But, because this approach measures outcomes at the level of individuals rather than aggregate rates, it is able to describe many of the indirect as well as direct macro effects. Thus, for example, researchers have found that high levels of unemployment affect not just the unemployed, but many of the employed as well. Catalano and Dooley (1977, 1979, 1983) linked employee perceptions of insecurity during economic downturns to employee well-being, while Fenwick and Tausig (1994) and Tausig and Fenwick (1999) specified job restructuring as a link between changing unemployment rates and stress outcomes of individual employed workers. However, because the outcomes are measured via surveys of individual workers, only their immediate knowledge of the characteristics of their employing firms has been ascertainable. This has been usually limited to whether or not they are personally members of a labor union, the number of employees (they think) work at the same worksite, and the type of product and/or service the firm produces (industry). More detailed and independent measures- such as those described in the preceding paragraph- of these important meso structures were not available.

When these organizational structures have been directly measured, it has almost always been done in a case study, as in studies of the effects of plant closings (e.g, Perrucci et al., 1988). Case studies allow for multiple methods and multilevel measurement. Employees can be surveyed, and aspects of their health measured directly; supervisory and management personnel can also be interviewed and organizational documents can be examined to get at structures and practices which are unfamiliar to lower level employees (those most likely to be interviewed in most surveys). However, the choice of organization to be studied is usually made on the basis of convenience, significance, and/or uniqueness. Thus, the generalizability of results is questionable.

This brief review clearly shows that the elements of a general understanding of the way in which work affects mental health have been identified. Each of these approaches has produced valuable insights into the relationship between work and mental health, but each has clear limits and no line of research explicitly links the relationship to core sociological issues, such as those conceptualized and analyzed in structural labor market research. But, by combining the various lines of research on job stress we can begin building a similar conceptual model. We start with the simple premise that macroeconomic context affects labor markets which, in turn, affect the "meso," organizational context and the organizational context affects specific work conditions that affect worker well-being.

The sociological study of health and illness is centered on the observation that morbidity and mortality are inversely related to status. Hence, the proper study of health is to relate positions in social structures (including occupational and organizational structures) to differences in exposure to health-related risk and health-related resources. But there are two matters that have yet to be addressed by this approach; how is standing in a social hierarchy translated into health risk and, what does this tell us about social organization? We argue that positions in social hierarchies, such as occupational and organizational structures, affect health risk and resources through the operation of the labor markets that sort persons into jobs with various levels of health-risky qualities. Second, we argue that labor markets themselves reflect the organization of social stratification and its consequences. In other words, the health consequences of work are a mirror of the way that social systems are organized and how they are maintained. Hence, the study of the relationship between work and health is the study of labor markets, occupational attainment and organizational structure and environment.

The Elements of a Model

The previous discussion can be used to identify the elements of a model that shows expected relationships among constructs at various levels (macro, meso, micro) of analysis. Figure 7.1 shows these elements in relation to worker mental health.

Although we will discuss these elements in more detail, here we will provide a quick overview. According to Gerhardt (1989), ". . . inequality is one of the major sources of suffering in modern society, and that inequality is an expression of covert and overt social conflict" (p. 275). This is another reason we call our model "the *political* economy of stress": ultimately, the work-mental health relationship reflects the conflict between economic organizational interests and individual interests. Our model is intended to reflect this perspective by suggesting that race, SES and gender have "fundamental" effects on structures which are related to worker mental health. Race, SES and gender are related to labor market structures that determine what types of jobs are available to what types of people and they are related directly to work conditions. Macro-economic processes affect labor market conditions directly through such factors as unemployment rates and globalization and they affect organizational structures by causing organizations to restructure in an attempt to adapt to changing economic conditions. Organizations, however, are not infinitely flexible, in part because their forms are constrained by their institutional environment, which itself reflects widely-held cultural notions about the organization of productive labor. Finally, worker mental health as it is related to work is most directly determined by the concrete characteristics of jobs; however, these characteristics are not in themselves "givens." Jobs do not reflect a "natural" fit between task and technology, nor are they an inevitable result of processes of market and/or organizational "rationalization." Rather, jobs are an outcome of macro and meso structural dynamics.

This model also depicts the ways in which the study of worker mental health can be linked to the concerns of other sociologists who study labor markets, stratification, economic sociology, organizations and work.

Work Conditions and Mental Health

Most directly psychological reactions to work come from the day-to-day conditions of that work. Research on the relationship between work and psychological well-being has clearly established that some jobs are "good" and others are "bad" for one's

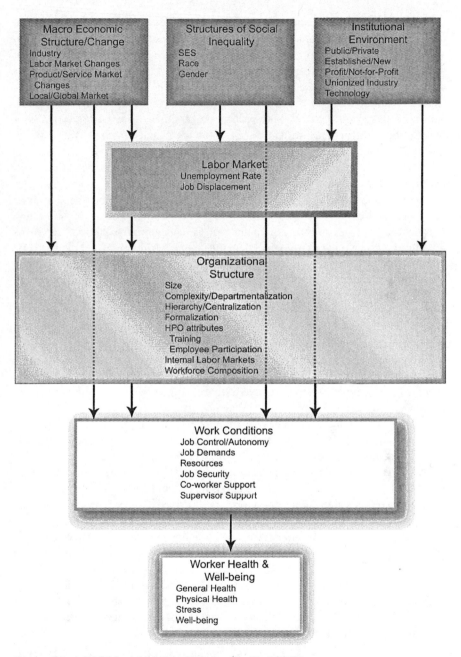

FIGURE 7.1. A Multi-Level Model of Worker Health (MWH).

mental health. Good jobs are substantively complex, they allow workers to utilize their skills, they provide a moderate level of psychological work demands and high levels of decision latitude, schedule control and occupational direction, control and planning (DCP), and they include high levels of co- worker and supervisor support (Fenwick & Tausig, 2001; Karasek & Theorell, 1990; Karasek, Triantis, & Chaudhry, 1982; Kohn & Schooler, 1983; Link, Lennon, & Dohrenwend, 1993). These are characteristics that either reduce workers' risks of exposure to stress or provide them with coping resources. Bad jobs are characterized by the opposite qualities: simple, routine skills, high demands with little control over any aspect of the job, and little support. These are characteristics that increase the risk of stress exposure and reduce the available coping resources.

The job demand/control model (Karasek, 1979) has become the dominant theoretical and empirical approach for relating work structures to job strain and stress. It is a very simple argument that is conceptually familiar to stress researchers. When the psychological demands of the job are high, and the worker's control over those demands (decision latitude) is low, then a condition of strain is created that is linked to outcomes such as fatigue, anxiety, depression and risk of physical illness (especially cardiovascular illness). Support received from supervisors and co-workers can buffer the effects of high demands and low control on stress-related outcomes (Johnson & Hall, 1988). Karasek (1989a) directly equates job demands to stressors and job control to personal control and coping.

Empirical evaluations of the demand/control model (and its variants) suggest that, on balance (and notwithstanding methodological and sampling issues), it successfully accounts for stress related to these work conditions (De Lange, Taris, Kompier, Houtman, & Bongers, 2003; Van Der Doef & Maes, 1999). Although the model proposes an interaction between high job demands and low decision latitude (control), studies also find that these two work conditions can independently affect perceptions of stress (De Lange et al., 2003). Hence, the demand/control model is one way to specify the psychological consequences of work at the individual level, although it does not include all job conditions that are known to affect worker stress.

It is most important to note that work conditions should be viewed as characteristics of the organization and not of the worker (Karasek & Theorell, 1990). The levels of job demands and decision latitude in a particular job are established at the organizational or workplace level as part of the general way that activity at the organization level is coordinated and controlled (Karasek, 1979; Soderfeld, Soderfeldt, Jones, O'Campo, Muntaner, Ohlson, & Warg, 1997). It follows, then, that we need to also understand the ways in which specific jobs come to have the structures that they do by considering the several determinants of organizational structure as specified in our model.

Stratification and the Labor Market

Organizational structures- including jobs- are partially determined by labor market conditions that are themselves affected by macroeconomic, institutional and social stratification conditions. Here we describe the structure of labor markets and the relationship between race and gender and labor market structure to specify how these stratification factors are directly and indirectly associated with job-related mental health outcomes.

Labor markets are defined, "as the arenas in which workers exchange their labor power in return for wages, status, and other job rewards." (Kalleberg & Sørensen, 1979, p. 351). Note that job rewards include psychological benefits such as job satisfaction and job-related well-being. In classic economic models, the labor market is perfectly competitive and workers compete for jobs and job-related rewards on the basis of their human capital including, education, ability and experience. However, models of the labor market based on these assumptions do not match actual patterns. In particular, worker labor market outcomes are also related to gender and race in such a way that the labor market is said to be segmented into at least two parts and there is little mobility between the parts.

Segmented labor markets consist of distinct labor markets, including one or more primary sectors offering jobs with high wages, good working conditions, chances for promotion, job security and job satisfaction; these are contrasted with secondary sectors offering jobs that pay poorly, have poor work conditions, little chance for promotion, low job security and low job satisfaction (Piore, 1975). The presence of a segmented labor market with little mobility from segment to segment suggests that worker satisfaction and well-being are partially determined by this labor market structure and the effect this structure has on the quality of jobs held by particular workers. Workers who compete in primary labor markets compete over good jobs, while workers who compete in the secondary labor markets compete over poor jobs.

Workers who compete in primary and secondary labors markets differ by social position. Specifically, women and minorities as well as those with low education are more likely to compete in secondary labor markets. In this regard labor markets resemble status structures in the larger social system. And, because mobility between segments is low, the segmented labor market maintains these status distinctions. Labor market segmentation reflects gender and racial opportunity structures that in turn affect exposure to stressful work conditions in ways that are consistent with general observations about stratification and mental health.

Macroeconomic Condition, Labor Markets and Organizations

Work conditions that affect mental health are also partially determined by macroeconomic conditions via the effects of the macro-economy on labor markets and organizational structures. Researchers in the sociology of work have addressed these relationships by considering the transformation of the workplace as a function of global changes (in both the geographic and figurative senses) as well as in response to economic cycles.

The most generic way to describe the state of the macro-economy is with respect to the unemployment rate and its effect on occupational mobility. The level of unemployment is not uniform across labor markets. Those in secondary labor markets are more likely to face layoffs and wage reductions (DiPrete &

Nonnemaker, 1997). In addition, Catalano and Dooley (1977, 1979, 1983) linked economic contractions to a general increase in individual exposure to undesirable job and financial events and, hence, to distress.

During recessions a number of economic and social processes are set in motion which can have consequences for well-being. The profitability of firms declines, as does the size of their product markets. These threats to the firm often bring about layoffs and/or job restructuring. Layoffs increase the pool of unemployed workers. Labor markets become more competitive. Employee wages stagnate or decline. Firms also redefine (restructure) job duties to make up for lost employees and to increase productivity. Fenwick and Tausig (1994) have shown that during recessions jobs are often restructured in ways which make them more stressful. Employers react to reductions in economic activity by increasing the level of job demands and decreasing levels of decision latitude for remaining workers. In turn, these job conditions are associated with increased distress.

In the sociology of work, however, recent research has focused on the restructuring of the workplace as a consequence of global competition, technological change, downsizing, the use of contingent labor and environmental uncertainty (Cornfield, Campbell, & McCammon, 2001; Smith, 1997). Many work organizations have adopted structures with flatter hierarchies of authority and "devolved" decision-making to make organizations more flexible and competitive in response to changed macro structural conditions. In these high performance organizations (HPOs) there is greater emphasis on "lean" productivity and productivity incentives, greater reliance on training and greater emphasis on teamwork (Cappelli, Bassi, Katz, Knoke, Osterman, & Useem, 1997). One of the core interests among sociologists studying these new forms of work is the extent to which the restructuring of work results in a shift in the locus of control from employers to employees (i.e., employees have more decision responsibility and latitude). Research, however, suggests that these new work structures generally intensify work (increase job demands) and do not radically alter organizational control systems (Smith, 1997).

These studies have largely been concerned with understanding the implications of macro-economic change on the traditional employment contract (including; productivity, relationships between "core" workers and "temps", job stability and careers, and changes in the authority structures found in the workplace) (Hirsch & Naquin, 2001; Kalleberg, 2001). But it is also clear that job restructuring that results from organizational responses to increased competition and the need for flexibility centers on changes in the work load and issues of work control that are important to the way we understand work-related mental health outcomes.

Institutional Environments, Labor Markets and Organizations

Labor markets and organizations are also embedded in institutional structures that affect organizational approaches to work design. Organizations often arrange their core activities according to accepted models in their fields (D'Aunno, Succi, & Alexander, 2000; DiMaggio & Powell, 1983). Organizations are also sensitive to local conditions that affect the size and quality of labor markets and product demand.

Institutional theorists argue that organizational structures come to resemble one another, in part, because there exists a common "rational" model for organizing activity that is culturally and socially legitimate and which, in turn, legitimates organizational forms. Hence, even in light of macro-economic change, organizations are slow to change fundamental structural conditions. The transformation of work conditions described above, however, suggests a new organizational form that alters the traditional relationship between employers and employees and that, therefore, could alter the stressfulness of particular working conditions (Smith, 1997).

The arch typical model of bureaucratic organization relies on elaborate rules and direct ("close") supervision to accomplish the organizational objective of coordination and control (Edwards, 1975). In turn, it is through rules and supervision that the levels of demand and control found within particular jobs are determined, which, in turn, determines levels of job-related distress. But, it has been suggested that new forms of organization necessitated by macro-economic change, in particular the invention of the high performance organization (HPO), represent a shift away from this traditional bureaucratic structure. HPOs are characterized by a flatter authority structure- less direct supervision- and more decision-making responsibility at lower levels of the organization- fewer job specific rules (Cornfield, Campbell & McCammon, 2001). The implications of these changes have implications have implications for the stressfulness of work, especially by increasing decision latitude.

Existing research, however, suggests that HPOs and similar organizational forms do not, in reality, meaningfully reallocate authority from bureaucratic control models (Barker, 1993; Prechel, 1994; Taplin, 1995; Vallas & Beck, 1996). However, it is clear that our model of the stress process needs to account for the role that institutional and transformative institutional forces have for the way that work is structured.

The Political Economy of Stress

The "sociological" study of the stress process (Pearlin, 1989) examines the ways in which, ". . .the various structural arrangements in which individuals are embedded determine the stressors they encounter. . ." (Aneshensel, Rutter, & Lachnenbruch, 1991, p. 167). Our theoretical approach, "the political economy of stress", links the research literature on the direct relationship between macro-economic structure and distress with the literature on work and distress by suggesting that work structures, themselves, are a consequence of macro-economic structure and change. Further, we suggest that individual placement in specific work structures is a consequence of position in social stratification systems (such as gender, race and SES) and resulting positions in labor markets. Thus, exposure and vulnerability to stressors can be linked to the structural arrangements in which individuals are embedded (to wit, the economy, stratification systems and labor markets). In this manner, our approach describes how a political economy perspective can be applied to the sociology of mental health.

We argue that work roles are not just technologically-determined "givens" of the production and labor processes, but rather are part of the "contested terrain" of the workplace, i.e., the relative power of workers and their employers vis-à-vis each other. As such, the structure of the organization, how work is coordinated and controlled, must also be considered. This argument is not new; it is one that has been made with respect to other aspects of work, both extrinsic and intrinsic: e.g., income, job commitment and satisfaction, or "fulfillment" (see Kalleberg & Griffin, 1980; Kalleberg, Wallace & Althauser, 1981; Lincoln & Kalleberg, 1985; Spaeth, 1985). The logic of this research clearly implies similar relationships for stress-related aspects of work structures: power implies the ability to resist, avoid, and/or impose stressful work tasks.

We also argue that the relative power of workers and their employers are products of the political economy: i.e., capital, resource, product and labor markets, as well as public policies which affect these markets. In keeping with the focus of much of the previous macro-economy stress research we emphasize the importance of labor markets and their segmentation. This emphasis is consistent with a basic assumption in much of the literature on work and inequality – that it is through labor markets that the other aspects of the political economy have their effects on the job structures and rewards of individual workers (Kalleberg, 1989; Kalleberg & Berg, 1987, p. 8–9).

Economic theories ranging from neoclassical to Marxist assume the fundamental importance of labor market position in determining the economic power of workers. According to the implicit logic of neoclassical theory (Becker, 1975; Friedman, 1953; Smith, 1990), an oversupply of workers with appropriate qualifications to fill particular jobs relative to demand limits workers' employment choices, thus reducing their control over the conditions of their employment. Marxist theory is more explicit. For Marx, unemployment has a "disciplinary" effect on workers in that fear of unemployment causes them to work harder and demand less (fewer resources and rewards) from their employers. This fear is enhanced by the existence of a "reserve army" of unemployed persons which employers can use as an alternative source of cheaper labor if their employees do not "discipline" themselves (Marx, 1978, pp. 592–601; Starrin, Lunberg, Angelow, & Wall, 1989). In both theories stress is an outcome of the actual or potential "life event" of unemployment *per se*, and also of the workers' reduced abilities to exercise control over work (job conditions), and thus to resist stressful work demands. "The analysis of labor markets...permits an understanding of the way macro forces associated with the economy of a society and elements of social structure impinge on the microrelations between employers and workers in determining various forms of inequality" (Kalleberg & Sorensen, 1979, p. 351).

Workers' labor market position, however, is not the only aspect of the political economy affecting the stressfulness of work roles. The economic power of employers is also crucial. For example, the literature on industrial sectors and labor market segmentation emphasizes how jobs are structured by the market situation of firms and industries (Beck, Horan, & Tolbert, 1978; Hodson, 1978; Lincoln & Kalleberg, 1985). Those firms and industries whose market position is precarious (i.e., in highly unstable, competitive, low profit markets) structure jobs to be unstable, with few resources and rewards provided to workers. The literature's description of these jobs is consistent with those characteristics of work which have been found to produce stress, including unsafe working conditions, lack of autonomy, skill underutilization, demand overload, inadequate information for task performance, etc. (Edwards, 1979; Lincoln & Kalleberg, 1985). In contrast, industries and firms in more stable, protected market situations develop job structures such as internal labor markets and job ladders, that are thought to reduce work stress (Edwards, 1979).

Aside from market position, the overall structure of work organizations will affect the structure of particular jobs and the likelihood that they will produce stress. Of all organizational characteristics, the level of bureaucratization is the most important in this regard, even if its conceptual link to job stress appears at first to be somewhat ambiguous. On the one hand, bureaucratization means elaboration of formal job rules and procedures that can protect workers from arbitrary and stress-producing work tasks (Edwards, 1979; Lincoln & Kalleberg, 1985). This is especially true where unions have initiated bureaucratization in the form of labor management contracts (Kochan, Katz, & McKersie, 1986). However, bureaucratization also concentrates authority within top organizational positions (management) and increases job differentiation among lower positions (Blauner, 1964; Spenner, 1983; Weber, 1946). The result is loss of workers' control over their jobs, an outcome that should make these jobs more stressful. Overall, bureaucratization is determined mainly by organizational size, and especially the number of employees (Stolzenberg, 1978), as are its stress-producing consequences along with high levels of worker dissatisfaction and conflict (Lincoln, 1978).

These arguments have an obvious longitudinal dimension, in that changes in the market positions of workers and firms increase or reduce the stressful characteristics of jobs. Most significantly, economic downturns (recessions) lead to deterioration of market situations for both. In these situations the survival of firms may be threatened, forcing them to reduce production costs by laying-off some workers and restructuring the jobs of their remaining workers in order to maintain levels of productivity and profits (Marx, 1978; Starrin, et al., 1989). Such restructuring may include speed-ups or work overload due to reduced staffing, reduced margins of error in output, and relaxation of rules governing worker safety and health (Brenner & Mooney, 1983). In general, this restructuring is designed to pass the increased vulnerability of the firm on to their workers. With higher unemployment rates, and thus in a weaker market position, workers lack the power to resist restructuring (Marx, 1972, 1978). For these workers restructuring means jobs with increasingly stress-producing characteristics.

Increased bureaucratization among firms also appears to be a consequence of economic downturns. One reason for this is suggested by the discussion of restructuring. Typically, organizations - and indeed, all social groups- tend to respond to crisis situations by centralizing authority (Simmel, 1955). This centralization is, in turn, a response to the need to limit internal conflicts and dissension (Crozier, 1964) and provide a more "efficient" means of allocating increasingly scarce resources. A second reason is that economic downturns almost always result in increasing economic concentration within industries. Because of their "economies of scale," larger firms are those most likely to survive the downturns, and they tend to grow larger as they acquire the market share of small firms that did not survive (Edwards, 1979; Marx, 1972, 1978). Again, the result would be a more bureaucratic structure with increasingly stress-producing job structures.

Organizational structures also change to reflect the general economic environment. Work organizations have adopted structures with flatter hierarchies of authority and "devolved" decision-making to make organizations more flexible and competitive in response to changed macro structural conditions (globalization, downsizing, temporary labor).

Social Stratification and the Political Economy of Stress

The discussion of the political economy of stress above describes the root process that we believe explains the dynamic relationships between a central context of individual adult social life (employment), as well as the macro-structural processes and the meso-organizational conditions that create this context, on the one hand, and the outcome of individual distress, on the other. The contextualization of the stress process also includes a consideration of the way that social stratification affects worker experience.

Stratification systems reflect distributions of valued social resources. As such they affect and are affected by the political economic distribution of power. In turn, these effects will be related to the health and well-being of individuals as described them above. An individual's position in a stratification system (e.g. gender, race or SES) affects access to resources (by definition) which affect the ability to resist the demands of others. Thus, position in a stratification system affects one's vulnerability to the effects of stressors encountered in that position. Moreover, position affects exposure to stressors as well by influencing the likelihood that changes in conditions (in the political economy, for example) will result in changes in work conditions or work status. Indeed, the ability to trace the direct and indirect consequences of macro-economic structure and change as they are affected by position in stratification systems is precisely what we define as the sociological study of the stress process.

Because the political economy of stress argument relies on the relative power of workers and employers, it stands to reason that those workers with the least power will also be those who experience the greatest effects of macroeconomic and job structure change. Persons in peripheral industries, those employed in smaller firms with low-level occupations, those who do not own capital or control the labor of others, and those with little experience are most likely to be exposed to both macro-economically induced change and to work-related stressors that follow from macro-economic change (Bibb & Form, 1977). Those in relatively low power positions will have less ability to resist the way in which their work is organized and hence, the degree to which their work is stressful.

Workplace Control and the Political Economy of Stress

Workplace control theory also asserts that work practices – how work is organized and regulated – reflect the outcome of a "political" relationship between workers and owners or managers (see for example, Hodson, 1999). This perspective is most directly concerned with understanding the struggle between workers and management over control of the workplace and only indirectly concerned with psychological outcomes in the workplace (i.e., job satisfaction). We argue that the outcome, workplace control, can be conceptualized at the individual level as the work conditions of decision latitude and job demands (i.e., work practices).

According to Hodson (1999), students of workplace control regard specific organizational structures as "strategic moves by management to ensure its control of the labor process" (p. 293). However, organizations cannot simply impose these structures on workers because worker's labor power gives them the ability to resist (at some level) the will of management. It is the outcome of this struggle that determines the level of workplace control realized by workers and management. Since workplace control accounts for both the amount of worker autonomy (latitude) and job content (demands), the perspective can be used to predict the components of the demand/control model. Theoretically we are conceptualizing the outcome of the political process reflected in the notion of workplace control in terms of the concrete work conditions of job demands and decision latitude.

From a management perspective, the organization of the workplace accomplishes two things: coordination and control. Coordination involves structuring activities via some degree of standardization and specialization to reach organizational objectives. Control involves the concentration of authority via some degree of centralization, formalization and supervision. Modern organizations use bureaucratic structures to accomplish these objectives (Edwards, 1979). Workers then experience the consequences of management structures that define coordination and control in the bureaucratic organization as work conditions that include job demands and decision latitude. Hence we can specify the psychological consequences of bureaucratic control in relation to job demands and decision latitude as they are determined by organizational size, formalization, departmentalization and hierarchy- standard measures of organizational structure in bureaucracies. These features of organizational structure represent the way that managers attempt to coordinate productive activity and exert control in the workplace.

Summary

The "Political Economy of Stress" model represents an attempt to account for the work-mental health relationship by systematically incorporating relevant structural factors into a consistent, cross-level sociological argument. In doing so, the model utilizes relevant existing sociological literature, in particular that developed from the structural labor market perspective. The result of this approach is that work-related stress can now be seen as an outcome of the same processes that determine wages and occupational attainment.

The core assumption of the model is that social conflict as manifested in social stratification, institutional processes, labor market structure and, organizational structure determines specific job conditions and hence, psychological well-being. At each analytic level the same issue of conflict/control underlies the explanation for the particular structures observed and the role such structures play in affecting psychological well-being. This unifying theme allows us to understand how conditions at one level affect relevant conditions at other levels.

At the individual worker level, the "balance" between job demands and decision latitude (autonomy) affects worker well-being. At the organizational level, the conflict between workers and employer preferences determines the level of demand and decision latitude experienced by a given employee. Macroeconomic conditions directly affect labor markets that represent one means by which the interests of workers and employers are regulated. Further, macroeconomic conditions affect the relative power of employees and employers in specific organizations. Access to labor market opportunities is similarly conditioned by social stratification that, itself, represents the outcome of conflict processes. Hence, at all levels, the "political" relationships between actors or strata determines the distribution of valued social resources (broadly, economic resources) and the psychological well-being of workers.

Research Design Considerations

The conceptual scheme described above is clearly multilevel, and thus its ultimate evaluation is dependent upon obtaining, measuring, and testing relations among data at multiple levels: (1) "macro" socioeconomic; (2) "meso" organization; and (3) "micro" individual. As the discussion above suggested, both "macro" level and "micro" level data have long been available to mental health researchers in the forms of Census and Labor Department indicators and social surveys, respectively. What has been missing until recently has been direct, independent, and representative "meso" level data on organizational structures. Indeed, this is likely the greatest reason that the "meso" level, and particularly organizational structure, has been the most conceptually "underdeveloped" area in job stress research and why a political economy of stress perspective has not been developed and tested.

This was recognized as such by the National Institute of Occupational Safety and Health (NIOSH) in its 1996 National Occupational Research Agenda. This report specified the greatest occupational health research problems as: (1) the need to accurately describe and measure significant organizational structures and practices that affect the health and safety of workers – both directly and indirectly by mediating the effects of macroeconomic and social processes; and (2) to do so for a representative sample of workers and organizations, so that the prevalence of these effects become known and so that policies can be developed that have general applicability to all types of organizations and all workers (USDHHS, 1996).

This problem was also recognized by structural labor market researchers during the 1980s as they increasingly focused on the organizational determinants of income and occupational mobility. In response to this need, the National Science Foundation funded a number of pilot studies to develop a methodology for collecting multilevel data which would be representative of both individual workers and of employing firms. Based on "hyper-network," or "multiplicity sampling" techniques, a multistage sampling strategy of "going up the ladder" was developed (Spaeth & O'Rourke, 1996). In the first stage, individual respondents in a probability sample provided information on characteristics of their jobs *and* they identified the establishment where they worked by name, address, and telephone number. This information was then used to contact organizational members who were in positions to be knowledgeable about relevant structural characteristics of the work establishment. In principle, this procedure yielded a probability sample of all work establishments in the United States, with the probability of selection being proportionate to establishment size (number of employees). (Spaeth & O'Rourke, 1996). This project culminated in a National Organizational Study that was then linked to a "work" module in the 1991 General Social Survey (Spaeth & O'Rourke, 1996).

While this project yielded impressive results by linking information of individual workers to that provided by their work establishments, the 1991 GSS-NOS study concentrated on issues of job training and promotional structures (matters of interest to structural labor market researchers), but provided no data on either the health of workers or health-relevant organizational structures. However, in 2002 NIOSH sponsored a similar GSS-NOS project that included a "quality of work life" module was included in the 2002 GSS in which respondents were asked about work health and safety and related job characteristics, such as work demand and autonomy. They were also asked to provide contact information on the work establishments. Informants within the establishments were then contacted and asked to provide information on health/safety relevant structures and benefits programs. The 2002 GSS-NOS provides a template for future job stress research that will allow testing of multilevel conceptual models such as our political economy of stress model. The advantage of this type of data structure where there is one respondent per organization is that ordinary least squares regression techniques can be applied without misestimating standard errors. However, it does not allow researchers to distinguish within-context from between-context variance. In this sense analyses will be multi-level but not contextual. Most importantly data collected using this design can be collected for representative samples of workers employed in a representative sample of organizations.

With such a linked dataset it is possible to investigate more completely the relationships depicted in Figure 1 that are of interest both to health researchers and organizational researchers. For example, we have suggested that firms respond to macroeconomic changes such as recessions not only by laying off workers (labor market changes) but also by restructuring the positions and activities of retained employees (work conditions), such as increasing job demands and job insecurity and reducing decision latitude (Fenwick & Tausig, 1994). Because other firms follow similar strategies, workers have fewer employment alternatives (labor market changes) and thus are less able to resist restructuring. The result is more stressful work.

With data sets such as the GSS-NOS that contain direct measures of organizational structures and their links to individual level job conditions we can examine the specific organizational characteristics that are affected by macroeconomic changes and that, in turn, lead to restructuring of individual level positions and activities. With organizational level measures available we can also track how differences in organizations' institutional environments affect stressful work conditions. For example, it has been suggested that the emergence of high performance organizations (HPOs) has led to an increase in both decision latitude and job demands of individual employees as job authority and responsibility have been dispersed downward in these flatter organizational hierarchies (Cappelli et al., 1997). The growth of this organizational form has been traced not to cyclical changes in macroeconomic markets, but to the emergence of new industries, such as software and microelectronics that are relatively unconstrained by history and convention (institutional isomorphism) in the organizational forms they develop (Cappelli et al., 1997). Thus, using the GSS-NOS data we could test a hypothesis that predicts health outcomes while we could also test propositions developed by organizational researchers about earnings and occupational mobility. Because this research design was originally developed to test the structural labor perspective, there is now a direct sense in which political economy and mental health research use the same "language." This increases the likelihood that findings from either perspective will influence the other, as we outline below.

The model we propose is ultimately longitudinal so it is essential that more surveys in the future utilize the GSS-NOS linked format. Longitudinal data would provide crucial information on how the structural dynamics of the political economy at both the macro and meso levels expose workers to varying levels of job stress over their careers. This information would enable researchers to test how a multi-level job stress process contributes to the cumulative advantage/ disadvantage in health based on status inequality over the life course (Pearlin, Schieman, Fazio, & Meersman, 2005). For example, Ross and Wu (1996) found that the health gap between individuals with higher versus lower educational attainment increases over the life course; but, the gap was not explained by differences in income attainment attributable to differences in educational levels. An alternative explanation that could be tested with the above data is that educational attainment is related to the stressfulness of the jobs available to workers both upon completion of their education as well as the likelihood of later upward job mobility into jobs with less stress. For example, the availability of jobs with characteristics that reduce job stress, such as high decision latitude and abundant job resources, increases with educational level, and is highest among occupations that require the highest educational levels: professionals and managers. These are also the occupations that allow for the greatest upward mobility. Conversely, jobs with more stressful characteristics- low decision latitude and few resources- are more prevalent outcomes of low educational attainment. When experienced routinely (day to day) this stress likely has cumulative mental and physical health consequences, from anxiety and depression to cardiovascular illnesses. These jobs are also more likely to be "dead end" jobs with few chances of upward mobility, and their occupants are more likely to experience employment disruptions – layoffs and permanent unemployment – stressful events that "proliferate" over time (Pearlin et al., 2005).

Longitudinal data on the stress process thus would enable sociologists to test another important connection between the status attainment process and health disparities over the life course. And, conversely, this model would enable us to test the link between the stress process and its cumulative health consequences and the status attainment process itself, thus informing researchers in the field of work and social inequality. By extending the model presented in Figure 1, the outcomes that could be studied would include occupational (or even income) attainment. Questions to be answered would include: Is stress experience at time 1 related to occupational status at time 2? To what extent does exposure to stress in lower status jobs limit the potential for occupational mobility, while the lack of exposure in higher status jobs enables individuals to take advantage of mobility opportunities? And, beyond the issue of individual mobility, the model would provide data on the extent to which macro and meso processes increase or decrease the overall levels of mobility. By producing more or less stressful work, to what extent do changes in macro economic markets and organizational structures limit or enable mobility?

Beyond this contribution, however, a multilevel model of the job stress process could help synthesize the contemporary view of workers as "economic man" (woman) pictured in much of the structural labor market research with that of "social man" (woman) presented in the more traditional sociology of work literature. In her critique of structural labor market research, Simpson (1989) argued that researchers using the economic perspective tended to see workers narrowly in terms of their economic attainment- primarily income- and, in turn, their jobs and employers were evaluated in terms of the characteristics that generated differences in economic outcomes, such as internal labor markets, job ladders and vacancy chains. Left out of this model was the older sociological concern with the non-economic attitudes and behaviors of workers, such as their attempts to create meaning from their work (issues of alienation) or community among their fellow workers (solidarity), such as seen in the "human relations" approach (Mayo 1933) as well as the work of Whyte (1948), Roy (1952), Gouldner (1954), or Blauner (1964).

In his response to Simpson's critique, Kalleberg (1989) suggested, that while the earliest structural labor market theories had indeed focused on economic outcomes, the perspective was capable of explaining more "social" outcomes, such as worker commitment. Additionally, this perspective was capable of explicitly linking macro, meso, and micro analysis, while traditional research on work had focused only on micro level processes. However, while later developments, especially the original 1991 National Organizational Study, did begin to focus on issues of worker commitment, the conceptualization of job structures at the individual and organizational levels remains primarily economic, focusing on job training program, internal job ladders, etc.

While we have included such structures in the model presented in Figure 1, we also included those that could be characterized as "social" in that they are primarily concerned with social relations on the job rather than their ability to facilitate economic attainment: e.g., decision latitude, job demands and co-worker support. These are structures that have been central to the study of job stress for the last generation, that measure what Karasek (1989b) called the "psychosocial class structure." By including these as well as economic job structures the above model provides a general way of linking the processes that produce and reproduce both psychosocial and economic classes.

Discussion

Sociologists who study mental health/illness increasingly link mental health to social structures of inequality. Despite this perspective, there is a sense that other parts of the sociological discipline that also study social structures do not see the connection between the subject matters they study and mental health. Apart from its frequent focus on individual mental health outcomes, we have suggested that this may also arise from the lack of theoretical articulation between the study of mental health outcomes and the study of other sociologically important outcomes.

For example, Kalleberg and Sorenson (1979) have argued that, "(s)ince the majority of people in industrial society obtain income and other rewards in exchange for work, labor market processes form the central mechanisms of social distribution in industrial society" (p. 351). By suggesting that "other rewards" include psychological well-being, we propose to link the study of work to the study of mental health and by doing so, to the central mechanism of social distribution that interests the wider sociological discipline.

The purposes of our proposed model, then, are 1) to extend the way sociologists of mental health think about the social causes of psychological disorder and, 2) to extend the way sociologists of work, organizations, and labor economics think about the outcomes of work (i.e., to include health/mental health outcomes as output values from work).

By bringing macroeconomic, institutional, labor market and meso-level organizational structures (back) into the study of the relationship between social structure and mental health, we (re)contextualize the study of the sociology of mental health. It is one thing to note that positions in social structures affect health risks and resources and another to connect this observation to the political economic explanations that have been developed by other sociologists to explain the same general phenomenon, the unequal distribution of rewards in society. But, now, having done so, the prospect that the sociology of mental health will be seen to address core issues of the discipline is improved. Research will be better able to provide a social mirror by which we can reflect on the consequences of the organization of social life. This brings the study of the work-mental health relationship back to formative questions (Marx, Durkheim, and Weber) about the psychological impact of social organization. It also provides a way to understand social organization itself.

References

Aneshensel, C. S., Rutter, C., & Lachenbruch, P. (1991). Social structure, stress and mental health. *American Sociological Review, 56*, 166–178.

Barker, J. R. (1993). Tightening the iron cage: Concertive control in self-managing teams. *Administrative Science Quarterly, 38*, 408–37.

Beck, E. M., Horan, P.M., & Tolbert, C., II. (1978). Stratification in a dual economy: A sectoral model of earnings determination. *American Sociological Review, 43*, 704–20.

Becker, G. S. (1975). *Human capital: A theoretical and empirical analysis with special reference to education, second edition*. Chicago: University of Chicago Press.

Bibb, R., & Form, W.H. (1977). The effects of industrial, occupational, and sex stratification on wages in blue-collar markets." *Social Forces, 55*, 974–996.

Blauner, R. (1964). *Alienation and freedom: The factory worker and his industry*. Chicago: University of Chicago Press.

Brenner, M. H. (1973). *Mental illness and the economy*. Cambridge, MA: Harvard University Press.

Brenner, M. H. (1976). *Estimating the social costs of economic policy: Implications for mental and physical health, and criminal aggression*. Report to the Congressional Research Service of the Library of Congress Joint Economic Committee of Congress. Washington, D.C.

Brenner, M. H. (1984). Estimating the effect of economic change on national mental health and social well-being." Prepared by the Subcommittee on Economic Goals and Intergovernmental Policy of the Joint Economic Committee, U.S. Congress.

Brenner, M. H. (1987). Relation of economic change to Swedish health and social well-being, 1950–1980. *Social Science and Medicine, 25*, 183–95.

Brenner, M. H. (1995). Political economy and health. In, B.C. Amick, III, S. Levine, A. R. Tarlov, & D.C. Walsh (Eds.), *Society and Health* (pp. 211–246). New York: Oxford University Press.

Brenner, M. H., & Mooney, A. (1983). Unemployment and health in the context of economic change. *Social Science and Medicine, 17*, 1125–1138.

Cappelli, P., Bassi, L., Katz, H., Knoke, D., Osterman, P., & Useem, M. (1997). *Change at work*. New York: Oxford University Press.

Catalano, R., & Dooley, D. (1977). Economic predictors of depressed mood and stressful life events. *Journal of Health and Social Behavior, 18*, 292–307.

Catalano, R., & Dooley, D. (1979). The economy as stressor: A sectoral analysis. *Review of Social Economy 37*, 75–187.

Catalano, R., & Dooley, D. (1983). Health effects of economic instability: A test of the economic stress hypothesis. *Journal of Health and Social Behavior, 24*, 46–60.

Catalano, R., Dooley, D., & Jackson, R. (1985). Economic antecedents of help-seeking: Reformulation of time-series tests. *Journal of Health and Social Behavior, 26*, 141–52.

Cobb, S., & Kasl, S. V. (1977). *Termination: The consequences of job loss*. Cincinnati: National Institute of Occupational Safety and Health.

Collins, R. (1988). *Theoretical sociology*. San Diego: Harcourt Brace Jovanovich.

Cornfield, D., B., Campbell, K. E., & McCammon, H. J. (2001). Working in restructured workplaces: An introduction. In D. B. Cornfield, K. E. Campbell & H. J. Mccammon (Eds.), *Working in restructured workplaces: Challenges and new directions for the sociology of work*.(pp. xi–xxii). Thousand Oaks, California: Sage.

Crozier, M. (1964). *The bureaucratic phenomenon*. Chicago: University of Chicago Press.

D'Aunno, T., Succi, M., & Alexander, J. A. (2000). The role of institutional and market forces in divergent organizational change. *Administrative Science Quarterly, 45*, 679–703.

de Lange, A. H., Taris, T. W., Kompier, M., Houtman, I. L. D., & Bongers, P. M. (2003). The *very* best of the millennium: Longitudinal research and the demand-control-(support) model." *Journal of Occupational Health Psychology, 8*, 282–305.

DiMaggio, P. J., & Powell, W. W. (1983). The iron cage revisited: Institutional isomorphism and collective rationality in organizational fields. *American Sociological Review, 48*, 147–160.

DiPrete, T. A., & Nonnemaker, L. K. (1997). Structural change, labor market turbulence, and labor market outcomes. *American Sociological Review, 62*, 386–404.

Edwards, R. (1979). *Contested terrain: The transformation of the workplace in the twentieth century*. New York: Basic Books.

Fenwick, R. & Tausig, M. (1994). The macroeconomic context of job stress. *Journal of Health and Social Behavior, 35*, 266–282.

Fenwick, R. & Tausig, M. (2001). Scheduling stress: Family and health outcomes of shift work and schedule control. *American Behavioral Scientist, 44*, 1179–1198.

French, J. R. P. Jr., Caplan, R. D., & Van Harrison, R. (1982). *The mechanisms of job stress and strain*. New York: John Wiley & Sons.

Friedman, M. (1953). *Essays in positive economics*. Chicago: University of Chicago Press.

Gerhardt, U. (1989). *Ideas about illness: An intellectual and political history of medical sociology*. New York: New York University Press.

Gouldner, A. (1954). *Wildcat strike*. Yellow Springs, OH: Antioch Press.

Hirsch, P. M., & Naquin, C. E. (2001). The changing sociology of work and the reshaping of careers. In Cornfield, D. B.,Campbell, K. E. and McCammon H. J. (Eds.) *Working in restructured workplaces: Challenges and new directions for the sociology of work.* (pp. 427–435). Thousand Oaks, CA: Sage.

Hodson, R. D. (1978). Labor in monopoly, competitive and state sectors of production." *Politics and Society, 8*, 429–80.

Hodson, R. D. (1999). Organizational anomie and worker consent. *Work and Occupations, 26*, 292–323.

House, J. S. (1980). *Occupational stress and the mental and physical health of factory workers*. Ann Arbor, MI: Institute for Social Research Report.

Jahoda, M. (1982). *Employment and unemployment: A social psychological analysis*. New York: Cambridge University Press.

Johnson, J. V., & Hall, E. M. (1988). Job strain, workplace social support, and cardiovascular disease: A cross-sectional study of a random sample of the Swedish working population. *American Journal of Public Health, 78*, 1336–1342.

Kahn, R. L. (1974). Conflict, ambiguity, and overload: Three elements of job stress." Pp. 47–61 in A. McLean (Ed.), *Occcupational stress* (pp. 47–61). Springfield, IL: Thomas.

Kalleberg, A. (1989). Linking macro and micro levels: Bringing the workers back into the sociology of work. *Social Forces, 67*, 582–92.

Kalleberg, A. (2001). The advent of the flexible workplace: Implications for theory and research. In Cornfield, D. B.,Campbell, K. E., & McCammon, H. J. (Eds.) *Working in restructured workplaces: Challenges and new directions for the sociology of wok.* (pp. 437–453). Thousand Oaks, California: Sage.

Kalleberg, A., & Berg, I. (1987). *Work and industry: Structures, markets, and processes*. New York: Plenum.

Kalleberg, A., & Griffin, L. J. (1980). Class, occupation, and inequality in job rewards. *American Journal of Sociology, 85*, 731–768.

Kalleberg, A., & Sorensen, A. B. (1979). The sociology of labor markets. *Annual Review of Sociology, 5*, 351–379.

Kalleberg, A., Wallace, M., & Althauser, R. P. (1981). Economic segmentation, worker power, and income attainment. *American Journal of Sociology, 87*, 651–683.

Karasek, R. A. (1979). Job demands, job decision latitude and mental strain: Implications for job redesign. *Administrative Science Quarterly, 24*, 285–307.

Karasek, R. A. (1989a). Control in the workplace and its health-related aspects. In S. L. Sauter, J. J. Hurrell, and C. L. Cooper (Eds.). *Job control and worker health* (pp. 129–160), Chichester: Wiley.

Karasek, R. A. (1989b). The political implications of psychosocial work redesign: A model of the psychosocial class structure. *International Journal of Health Services, 19*, 481–508.

Karasek, R. A., & Theorell, T. (1989). *Healthy work: Stress, productivity, and the reconstruction of working life*. New York: Basic.

Karasek, R. A., Triandas, K. P., & Chandry, S.S. (1982). Co-worker and supervisor support as moderators of association between task characteristics and mental strain. *Journal of Occupational Behaviour, 3*, 181–200.

Kasl, S. V. (1978). Epidemiological contributions to the study of work stress. In C. L. Cooper and R. Payne (Eds.), *Stress at Work* (pp. 3–48). New York: Wiley-Interscience.

Kasl, S. V., & Cobb, S. (1979). Some mental health consequences of plant closings and job loss. In L. A. Ferman and J.P. Gordus (Eds.), *Mental Health and the Economy* (pp. 255–99). Kalamazoo, MI: W. E. Upjohn Institute for Employment Research.

Kochan, T. A., Katz, H. C., & McKersie, R. B. (1986). *The transformation of American industrial relations*. New York: Basic Books.

Kohn, M., & Schooler, C. (1983). *Work and personality: An inquiry into the impact of social stratification* Norwood, NJ: Ablex.

Liem, R., & Rayman. P. (1982). Health and social costs of unemployment: Research and policy considerations. *American Psychologist, 37*, 1116–23.

Lincoln, J. R. (1978). Community structure and industrial conflict: An analysis of strike activity in SMSA's. *American Sociological Review, 43*, 199–220.

Lincoln, J. R., & Kalleberg, A. L. (1985). Work organization and work commitment: A study of plants and employees in the US and Japan. *American Sociological Review, 50*, 738–60.

Link, B. G., & Phelan, J. (1995). Social conditions as fundamental causes of disease. *Journal of Health and Social Behavior* (Extra Issue) 80–94.

Link, B. G., Lennon, M. C., & Dohrenwend, B. (1993). Socioeconomic status and depression: The role of occupations involving direction, control, and planning. *American Journal of Sociology, 98*, 1351–87.

Marx, K. (1972). The economic and philosophical manuscripts of 1844. In R. C. Tucker, (Ed.), *The Marx-Engels reader*. New York: W.W. Norton.

Marx, K. (1978). *Capital Volume 1*. Moscow: Progress Publishers.

Mayo, E. (1933). *The human problems of an industrial civilization*. New York: Macmillan.

Pearlin, L. I. (1989). The sociological study of stress. *Journal of Health and Social Behavior, 30*, 241–256.

Pearlin, L. I., Schieman, S., Fazio, E. M., & Meersman, S. C. (2005). Stress, health, and the life course: Some conceptual perspectives. *Journal of Health and Social Behavior, 46*, 205–219.

Perrucci, C. C., Perrucci, R., Targ, D. B., & Targ, H. R. (1988). *Plant closings*. Hawthorne, NY: Aldine.

Piore, M. J. (1975). Notes for a theory of labor market stratification. In Edwards, Richard.C., Reich, Michael & Gordon, David M. (Eds.). *Labor Market Segmentation* (pp. 125–150), Lexington, MA: Heath.

Prechel, H. (1994). Economic crisis and the centralization of control over the managerial process: Corporate restructuring and neo-Fordist decision making. *American Sociological Review, 59*, 723–45.

Quinn, R. P., Mangione, T. W., & Seashore, S. E. (1973). *1972–73 Quality of employment survey.* Ann Arbor, MI: Survey Research Center, Institute for Social Research, University of Michigan.

Quinn, R. P., & Staines, G. (1977). *Quality of employment survey, 1977.* Ann Arbor, MI: Survey Research Center, Institute for Social Research, University of Michigan.

Rosenfeld, R. A. (1992). Mobility and career processes. *Annual Review of Sociology, 18*, 39–61.

Ross, C. E., & Wu, C-L. (1996). Education, age, and the cumulative advantage in health. *Journal of Health and Social Behavior, 37*, 104–120.

Roy, D. (1952). Quota restriction and goldbricking in a machine shop. *American Journal of Sociology, 57*, 427–442.

Schwartz, S. (2002). Outcomes for the sociology of mental health: Are we meeting our goals? *Journal of Health and Social Behavior, 43*, 223–235.

Simmel, G. (1955). *Conflict*, translated by Kurt H. Wolff. *The Web of Group-affiliations*, translated by Reinhard Bendix. Glencoe, Ill., Free Press.

Simpson, I. (1989). The sociology of work: Where have the workers gone? *Social Forces, 67*, 563–581.

Smith, M. R. (1990). What is new in 'new structuralist' analyses of earnings? *American Sociological Review, 55*, 827–841.

Smith, V. (1997). New forms of work organization. *Annual Review of Sociology, 23*, 315–339.

Soderfeldt, B., Soderfeldt, M., Jones, K., O'Campo, P., Muntaner, C., Ohlson, C. -G., & Warg, L. -E. (1997). Does organization matter? A multilevel analysis of the demand-control model applied to human services. *Social Science and Medicine, 44*, 527–534.

Spaeth, J. L. (1985). Job power and earnings. *American Sociological Review, 50*, 603–617.

Spaeth, J. L., & O'Rourke D. P. (1996). Design of the National Organizations Study. In Kalleberg, A. L., Knoke, D., Marsden, P. V. & Spaeth, J. L. (Eds.). *Organizations in America: Analyzing their structures and human resource practices* (pp. 23–44). Thousand Oaks, CA: Sage.

Spenner, K. (1983). Deciphering Prometheus: Temporal change in the skill level of work. *American Sociological Review, 48*, 824–37.

Starrin, B., Lunberg, B., Angelow, B. B., & Wall, H. (1989). Unemployment, overtime work and work intensity. In B. Starrin, P. -G. Svensson & H. Wintersberger (Eds.). *Unemployment, poverty and quality of working life: Some European experiences* (pp. 261–75). Berlin: World Health Organization, European Regional Office and the European Center for Social Welfare Training and Research, Education Service.

Stolzenberg, R. M. (1978). Bringing the boss back in: Employer size, employee schooling and socioeconomic achievement. *American Sociological Review, 43*, 813–28.

Taplin, I. M. (1995). Flexible production, rigid jobs: Lessons from the clothing industry. *Work and Occupations, 22*, 412–438.

Tausig, M., & Fenwick, R. (1999). Recession and well-being. *Journal of Health and Social Behavior, 40*, 1–16.

Turner, J. B. (1995). Economic context and the health effects of unemployment. *Journal of Health and Social Behavior, 36*, 213–229.

U.S. Department of Health and Human Services (USDHHS). (1996). *The national occupational research agenda*. Washington, D.C.: Public Health Service. Centers for Disease Control and Prevention National Institute for Occupational Safety and Health.

Vallas, S. P., & Beck, J. P. (1996). The transformation of work revisited: The limits of flexibility in American manufacturing. *Social Problems, 43*, 339–361.

Van Der Doef, M., & Maes, S. (1999). The job demand-control (-support) model and psychological well-being: A review of 20 years of empirical research. *Work and Stress, 13*, 87–114.

Weber, M. (1946). *From Max Weber: Essays in Sociology*. Translated, edited, and with an introduction, by H. H. Gerth & C. W. Mills. New York: Oxford University Press.

Whyte, W. F. (1948). *Human relations in the restaurant industry*. New York: McGraw-Hill.

Williamson, O. E. (1975). *Markets and hierarchies, analysis and antitrust implications: A study in the economies of internal organization*. New York: Free Press.

8
Race and Mental Health: Past Debates, New Opportunities

Teresa Evans-Campbell, Karen D. Lincoln, and David T. Takeuchi

Given its pervasiveness in American social life, race as a construct and topic has a long history of scholarship and debate in sociology and a corresponding research literature, albeit not as extensive, in the sociology of mental health. We argue that inquiries about race and its consequences tend to reflect existing attitudes during different time points. In this chapter, we examine some of the key frameworks used in sociology to study race and mental health. Rather than focusing on specific research contributions, we discuss the general themes that highlight how sociology contributes to the study of race and mental health and vice versa. A second purpose of this chapter is to focus on some directions that may help to advance the sociology of mental health.

Sociology and the Study of Race and Mental Health

Sociology provides some of the theoretical underpinnings on which race and mental health research is constructed. In turn, the sociology of mental health contributes to the discipline by providing theoretical refinements and empirical evidence about how race is linked to psychological and emotional states such as through traumatic events, discrimination, and treatment biases. This reciprocity between the sociology of mental health and the larger body of sociological work is evidenced in some of the common frameworks we outline below that have been used, over time, to study race and mental health. Our review also serves as a reminder that current studies on mental health are influenced by the social and political realities that frame discussions and conversations about race. Past debates have usually reinforced, often unintentionally, the social positions of racial groups rather than contesting the inequities found among racial groups. Support for one theoretical frame over another become solidified into ideological positions about the nature of race, inequality and appropriate policy solutions (Takeuchi & Gage, 2003).

The Early Biological View

Biological determinism or essentialism categorizes people into unequivocal groups based on certain traits such as skin color and phenotypes. These racial characteristics are assumed to be fixed and constant over time. Essentialism, which dominated scientific thinking in the 19th and early 20th centuries, promotes the notion that race is interwoven with physical, moral, and mental traits (Harris & Sim, 2001). Racial groups, accordingly, can be systematically arranged by prized traits (e.g., intelligence, personality) with whites at the top of the hierarchy. Scientific studies during that time, including those in the social sciences, did not contest the existing racial stratification system but tended to explicitly or implicitly maintain it (McKee, 1993).

Of course, essentialism was not uniformly accepted in the social sciences. DuBois (1903) and Boas (1927), among a few, argued that the status of racial groups was not due to the lack of intelligence or motivation, but rather the consequence of inadequate opportunities. Despite these and related arguments, race as an important determinant of intelligence and other valued traits was popular in the general public and scientific papers, principally because it helped justify the treatment of racial groups during this period.

Enter Cultural Theories

In the early 1920s, culture began to replace biological theories of race. The University of Chicago's Sociology of Race Relations program formulated a new theory of race relations that emphasized how people of diverse races assimilated into the established culture. In their theories of assimilation, racial conflict and its resolution involved a linear process of competition, conflict, accommodation, and assimilation. Further, assimilation of racial minority groups would improve race relations among groups (Yu, 2001). Much of this interest was spurred by the immigration of people from Europe, Asia, and Canada. The incorporation of white ethnic groups into the American mainstream, although not without protest, provided positive evidence of the assimilation hypothesis. African Americans and Asian immigrants, however, posed unique challenges for the Chicago School theorists which remain to this day (Alba & Nee, 2003; Tuan, 1998). Would American society overlook physical differences to allow non-whites to assimilate? Could Asian immigrants assimilate and break their ties with their home countries (Yu, 2001)? African Americans and Asian immigrants shared one major difference with white immigrants—they could not easily enter social settings without being identified as phenotypically different from white residents.

Theories of Racism

During the 1950s and leading into the 1960s, the civil rights movement marshaled in fundamental changes in approaching policies and programs to resolve racial inequalities in American society. Racist ideologies were seen as only part of the problem in eliminating racism; the focus was on the larger context of racialized social structure (Bonilla-Silva, 1997). Scholars and activists argued that without attending to racism as a fundamental component of the American social structure, it would not be possible to eliminate the root causes of discriminatory behavior against minority groups.

Accordingly, the social and public policies of the 1960s and early 1970s advanced issues of racial and economic justice in education, employment, and social services. The mental health field, which tends to move at a more conservative pace, also included studies and reforms intended to address institutional forms of racial bias. Some of the first studies of the use of mental health services among racial groups begin in the 1970s and investigated institutional biases and their effects on the mental health status and mental health care of racial and ethnic groups. For example, in their classic study, Sue, McKinney, Allen, and Hall (1974) showed that the existing mental health system was incompatible with the mental health needs of racial and ethnic minorities. This study led to a number of recommendations to reduce the biases against racial groups inherent within the mental health system. Despite the thrust of this early work, the political landscape began to change in the middle 1970s and refocused the discourse and scholarship on race from institutional analyses to one centered more on other social and individual factors.

Theories of Socio-economic Status

In the 1980s and extending through the 1990s, racial bias, institutional racism, prejudice, and discrimination lost momentum as explanations for inequities between racial groups in social, economic, and health indicators. Instead, socioeconomic status, or SES (also social class), grew in popularity as an explanation for racial differences. Since socioeconomic status is one of the strongest determinants of variations in health status (Krieger, 2001), much of the research over the past two decades argued that race effects will be reduced or disappear once SES is considered. SES refers to people's structural location within society based on representations of income, wealth, education, and occupational status (Krieger, Williams, & Moss, 1997). While researchers argue that race and socioeconomic position intersect to explain mental health problems (Neighbors, 1990), still others argue that SES may be part of the causal path that links race and health through economic discrimination (Cooper & David, 1986; Krieger et al., 1997). Some researchers focus less on race and more on the "fundamental causes of health disparities" that are rooted in SES-related resources like money, power and access to knowledge (Link & Phelan, 1995).

SES became a common explanation for race differences for several reasons. First, if race differences are found, social phenomena such as SES, and not biology, explain these differences. Second, social scientists became sensitive about making inferences concerning race that can be construed as "blaming the victim" after Daniel Moynihan was criticized for making inferences about African American families (Wilson, 1987). Third, researchers had difficulty in fitting racial paradigms into the social, political, and health circumstances of Asian and Latino immigrants whose history in the U.S. varied substantially from that of African Americans. Race was seen as a "black and white" issue. Fourth, some social scientists and policy makers saw programs and policies to benefit poor people as having a wider appeal than those that promote racial justice. Fifth, and perhaps most importantly, the social and political climate had changed dramatically from the 1960s to the 1980s. Enthusiasm for the role of the federal government to promote large-scale social change was tempered and issues of race and racial justice were no longer prominent on the national agenda.

Beyond SES

Over the past decade, there has been a renewed interest in studying race as more than a proxy for socioeconomic status. This revitalization was triggered by developments on at least two fronts. On one front, geneticists and social scientists agree that race as a biological measure lacks empirical support. For example, a recent study demonstrates that within a population, differences account for up to 95% of the genetic variation among individuals (Rosenberg, Pritchard, Weber, Cann, Kidd, Zhivotovsky, & Feldman, 2002). Contemporary social scientists also challenge essentialist notions of race by arguing that people make attributions about groups based on stereotypes and prejudices that are tied to some physical traits (Omi & Winant, 1994). That is, race is socially constructed and conceptions of race change over time and place and are shaped by political and social needs. Racial categories carry with them implicit and explicit images and beliefs about racial groups that form the basis and rationale for treatment of group members. Race is particularly meaningful when members of a group are given limited power and denied access to desired goods and resources based on their social membership within that group (Winant, 2000).

While this review is not exhaustive, it does provide a glimpse of the major frames about race that have been influential in the sociology of mental health. While all conceptions of race, even essentialist notions, are still operative at some level, debates are often driven by a prevailing paradigm and an alternative framework that contests it. As indicated earlier, race versus SES discussions consumed much of the research on race and mental health in the 1980s and 1990s. While these inquiries have been healthy for the discipline, they can also become ideological when taken to the extreme and actually constrain research (Massey, 1995). For example, much of policy research on race puts race in the background rather than the foreground of empirical studies because they focus on SES (Myers, 2002). Conversely, race scholars seldom incorporate policy issues into their analyses. The result is a parallel set of empirical and theoretical literatures that seldom merge. Further, scholarship is not external to the everyday realities of race in society. Different theories and research on race can serve to, directly or indirectly, reinforce existing stereotypes, provide justifications for treatment of racial categories, or reinforce the positions of racial groups. Finally, our review suggests that the study of race is often limited to African Americans and whites; few studies address how race impacts the lives of Latinos, American Indians and Alaska Natives, and Asian Americans.

New Opportunities, New Challenges

In this section, we address directions that may help explain the association between race and mental health. Since a number of excellent reviews of race and health have been written (see for example, Brown, Sellers, Brown, & Jackson, 1999;

Ihara & Takeuchi, 2004; U.S. Department of Health and Human Services, 2001), we focus on some different challenges and opportunities that may prove helpful in the near future. We identify three critical gaps or issues in the literature on race and mental health: (1) the omission of analyses of historical events that shape race relations, and specifically the intergenerational transmission of past traumas; (2) the assumption that social psychological processes are similar across racial groups; and (3) the inclusion of geographic contexts in understanding race and mental health.

Historical Trauma

An emerging area in race and mental health is a focus on inter-generational, community-specific trauma such as genocide, slavery, forced relocation, internments, segregation, and political oppression. Clinicians and some researchers have explored the effects of these traumatic assaults through diagnostic categories such as posttraumatic stress disorder (PTSD), anxiety disorders, and adjustment disorders (Evans-Campbell & Walters, 2006). Although these categories may encompass some of the symptoms related to such traumatic events, they fall short of capturing the extreme nature of the resulting distress or its collective and intergenerational impact. Moreover, these diagnostic categories offer little insight into the interplay between historical and current trauma responses.

One attempt to understand these assaults and their impacts is the scholarship on *historical trauma*, defined as the trauma that arises in response to numerous traumatic events experienced by a community over several generations (Brave Heart, 1999b). The trauma is based on events that are profoundly destructive and experienced by many members of a community (Brave Heart, 1999b). Historical trauma is conceptualized as collective in that it impacts a significant portion of the community and as compounding in so much as multiple events occurring over many years come to be seen as parts of a single, overarching traumatic legacy. A key facet of historical trauma is that it is passed on from one generation to the next, as descendents continue to emotionally identify with their ancestral suffering and pain (Brave Heart, 1999a). Indeed, research among diverse populations shows that children and grandchildren of survivors of historically traumatic events have high levels of current interest in ancestral trauma (Danieli, 1998; Nagata, 1991; Whitbeck, Adams, Hoyt, & Chen, 2004). The psychological responses to such historical trauma may include guilt, anxiety, unresolved grief and mourning, and suicidality (Brave Heart, 2000).

According to Simon and Eppert (in press), traumatic historical events share two important characteristics: they are human-initiated and they evoke particular behavioral dynamics. Most notably, they elicit a need to simultaneously remember and forget. That is, while the public is drawn to recount and belatedly "witness" these events, the feelings evoked are so overwhelming that people are prone to shut them out of their psyches. These events may target communities or families directly, as in the case of internment or slavery, or indirectly when aimed at the environment in which people live. Environmental historical traumas include radioactive dumping on tribal lands, flooding of homelands, and the introduction of diseases into communities. Historical trauma can also result from the inability to complete cultural and spiritual ceremonies (Evans-Campbell & Walters, 2006).

The intergenerational impact of historical trauma can be seen on at least two levels, the communal and the interpersonal. On a communal level, the response to an event may include immense and multifaceted losses such as the elimination of a "way of life" after slavery, internment, or relocation. The literature on historical trauma points to a number of similar losses including the loss of traditional spiritual practices or the loss of traditional role models for youth (Evans-Campbell & Walters, 2006). Emerging research illustrates the intergenerational response to such losses. For example, Whitbeck and colleagues (2004) interviewed Native elders in two reservation communities and found that although these individuals were generations removed from many historically traumatic events, ancestral losses were still part of their emotional lives.

Communal level impacts may also include second-order effects related to traumatic events. In a community that has suffered multiple losses, for example, a significant portion of the population might be more susceptible to substance abuse problems or family violence. In this way, the trauma continues to impact subsequent generations, leaving an increasing array of effects. Although the initial perpetrating event may fade into the distance of history, left unchecked by healing processes, the secondary effects of that event can actually amplify with each generation making historical trauma, as a type of trauma, particularly devastating and critical to understand.

At an individual level, the complexities of historical trauma make it difficult to distinguish the exact mechanisms of transmission, but traumatologists speculate that intergenerational transmission can occur through direct and indirect means. In the case of direct transmission, children may hear stories about events experienced by their parents or grandparents and, consequently, experience vicarious trauma (Auerhahn & Laub, 1998). In the case of indirect transmission, traumatic events may lead to poor parenting styles which, in turn, may increase stress in children (Auerhahn & Laub, 1998). Family dynamics may also unconsciously foster indirect transmission. For example, Felsen (1998) found that some children of Holocaust survivors felt they were expected to fulfill "missions" for their parents such as the need to comfort parents, restore lost love objects, act out parental anger, and demonstrate the continued vitality of their community. Notably, these family dynamics are both a result of historical trauma and a mechanism of transmission.

Experiences of traumatic events among historically oppressed people are often varied and heterogeneous. However, some generalizable symptoms among descendents are evident. Much of what we know is based on research with survivors of the Jewish Holocaust and their descendents. Early work in this area documented and explored a constellation of psychological symptoms sometimes collectively dubbed the "survivor syndrome" among survivors of the Jewish Holocaust. These symptoms include denial, agitation, anxiety, guilt, depression, intrusive thoughts, nightmares, psychic numbing, and survivor guilt (Barocas & Barocas, 1980; Eitinger & Strom, 1973; Neiderland, 1968, 1981). Among descendants of these survivors, however, symptoms often take a somewhat different form. The research here suggests that while higher rates of pathology in descendents are not common – rates of mental disorders among children of survivors generally fall within the normal range (Felsen & Ehrlich, 1990; Sigal & Weinfeld, 1989) – patterns of stress-vulnerability are. That is, when survivor children experience contemporary traumatic events, they are significantly more likely than controls to develop PTSD or sub-threshold PTSD (Yehuda, 1999). Moreover, although their symptoms do not meet the criteria for mental disorder, descendents are more likely to experience symptoms of depression, higher levels of anxiety, mistrust, guilt, difficulty handling anger, and somatization over their lifetime compared to others (Bar-On, Eland, Kleber, Krell, Moore, Sagi, Soriano, Suedfeld, van der Velden, & van Ijzendoorn, 1998; Barocas & Barocas, 1980). Notably, while an emerging literature on descendents shows areas of resilience and good adjustment among descendent populations (e.g., Kahana, Harel, & Kahana, 1988; Solomon, Kotler, & Milkulincer, 1988), research continues to demonstrate their vulnerability to traumatic stress (Danieli, 1998).

Similar transgenerational effects have been documented in other populations including among Japanese-Americans after internment (Nagata, 1991), American Indians in response to relocation and cultural genocide (Robin, Chester, & Goldman, 1996) and victims of the Pol Pot regime in Cambodia (Kinzie, Boehnlein, & Sack, 1998). In their research with the Lakota people, Maria Yellow Horse Brave Heart and her collaborators explored mental health and wellness after numerous collective, compounding historically traumatic events. They identified a collection of outcomes among the Lakota which they term "historical trauma response." This response is likened to the *survivor syndrome* and other symptoms common to Holocaust survivors and their descendents and includes: obsessive rumination about dead ancestors; continually reliving the past with a primary life focus on ancestor suffering; survivor guilt; unresolved mourning; depression; intrusive dreams and thoughts; use of coping fantasies that project oneself into the past (Brave Heart, 1999a, 1999b, 2000).

A host of factors can influence the level of distress among descendents in diverse communities. Arguably, the most critical factor affecting intergenerational transmission of massive trauma is communication around the events, particularly silence around the events or guilt-inducing communication (Bar-On et al., 1998; Felsen, 1998; Nagata, Trierweiler, & Talbot, 1999). Not surprisingly, many survivors of traumatic events avoid talking about their experiences and related feelings (Nagata et al., 1999), particularly to their children. For parents, keeping silent about past atrocities may seem protective, but among children, silence can serve to shroud the past in mystery and misunderstanding. Children may feel anger and resentment over their parents' unwillingness to share information, feeling it signals a lack of empathy with their own psychological need for information (Bar-On et al., 1998; Nagata et al., 1999). Indeed, avoidance of and indirect communication around massive trauma are significantly related to poor mental health outcomes in descendents of survivors including paranoia, hypochondria, anxiety, and low self-esteem (Lichtman, 1984). That said, the impact of communication on transmission may be unique to different racial and ethnic groups. In communities where indirect communication is a cultural norm, for example, these mechanisms may work differently, making them particularly challenging to identify.

In addition, societal reactions have an important effect on individual and communal post-trauma adaptation and healing. Danieli (1998) has looked extensively at this phenomenon in relation to Holocaust survivors. In what he terms the "conspiracy of silence," Danieli describes a social context in which those who were not survivors were unable to contemplate the horrific nature of survivor experiences and, moreover, did not want to listen. As a result, survivors remained silent about their experiences leading, in turn, to an increased sense of isolation, loneliness, and high levels of mistrust (Danieli, 1998). In the U.S., acknowledgements of traumatic assaults perpetrated on cultural and ethnic groups are limited and, not surprisingly, people from historically oppressed communities routinely encounter societal reactions such as indifference, disbelief, and avoidance. While there is little discussion in the literature regarding societal reactions to historically traumatic assaults in the U.S., it seems likely that many people are impacted by the tendency to ignore their painful histories.

Research Implications. Critical assessments are needed surrounding the concept of historical trauma, the factors that influence it, and its impact on contemporary mental health in diverse communities. Preliminary scholarship in this area provides a base for rethinking the way trauma impacts historically oppressed communities over time. Yet as scholars begin to grapple with the challenges inherent in conceptualizing historical trauma, it is important to note that the concepts involved are complex, multifaceted, and often interrelated; as such, they do not easily lend themselves to clear answers. Indeed, only limited attempts have been made to operationalize and measure historical trauma. We need to understand the characteristics of historical trauma, how it is transmitted, and how it may manifest in different cultural settings. And perhaps most importantly, given that people from historically oppressed groups continue to experience high levels of trauma, we must begin to explore the cumulative and interwoven nature of historical and contemporary traumas.

One of the most promising areas of future research in this area focuses on the strengths borne out of enduring traumas. Although historical trauma has had negative impacts, affected communities have been quite resilient. For example, Cross (1998) notes that ex-slaves and their descendents emerged from the trauma of slavery with strong family bonds and a communal commitment to education. Evans-Campbell (under review) found that American Indians who had attended boarding school as children had higher levels of enculturation compared to others. These outcomes are not directly associated with mental health; however, they may serve as cultural buffers between trauma and wellness. Research with diverse communities is needed to identify culturally specific responses to historical trauma as well as the strengths and resiliencies that may buffer such trauma among diverse populations.

Race, Social and Psychological Processes and Mental Health

Findings in race and mental health are far from consistent, with some studies reporting more symptoms of psychological distress for racial and ethnic minorities, and others reporting no differences (Brown, Sellers, & Gomez, 1999; Vega &

Rumbaut, 1991). While we have recognized that social positions such as race, socioeconomic status, gender and age affect exposure to health risk and access to health-related resources, we have yet to specify exactly the *way* in which this occurs or how it is related to other social or psychological processes.

The next level of research in this area should go beyond the more simple debates about race versus socioeconomic status (Takeuchi & Williams, 2003). One strategy is to identify the mechanisms and processes by which race is linked to mental health by conducting race-specific analyses. This would go past a simple mediational strategy to think through and tailor theorizing and research about *process* to the social, economic and cultural challenges each race and ethnic group confront. This approach is paramount in understanding mental health inequalities. An examination of the underlying mechanisms and processes involved within racial and ethnic groups is a different strategy than that currently used in much of the traditional racial comparative studies in the social and behavioral sciences. Instead of "explaining away" differences or "controlling for" those factors that might account for observed differences in mental health (the most common strategy used to identify factors that may account for racial differences in health outcomes), this approach explores whether social and psychological factors operate differently within specific racial groups and lead to divergent mental health trajectories and heterogeneity within groups (Kerckoff, 1993; O'Rand & Henretta, 1999).

Social Structure and the Individual

Social causation explanations have been offered to explain the persistent disparities in health outcomes among racial and ethnic groups (House, Kessler, Herzog, Mero, Kenney, & Breslow, 1990; Lieberman, 1985). More recently, a theory of fundamental social causes of health disparities has been offered (Link & Phelan, 1995), which highlights the role of socioeconomic status in observed health inequality and dims the light on "proximal risk factors" (e.g., environmental and behavioral risk factors) that link social location to health. This perspective posits that if proximal factors were eliminated from causal models, the SES-health relationship remains due to the reproduction of the SES-health link through resources such as money, power, social networks, and prestige. While this framework acknowledges the impact of social positions on more proximal factors, such as neighborhoods, social networks and health behaviors, it offers much less in helping us understand the experience of illness or the role that social actors play in influencing outcomes. To advance our understanding of causal processes, we must understand the social and psychological processes through which structural positions influence the individual. Even if changes in social policy, designed to ameliorate particular environmental and social risk factors (e.g., access to resources, attitudes, health behaviors, neighborhood quality), were to be effective, the relationship between social position and health might not be eradicated because it operates in so many diverse ways (Williams, 1990).

For example, some scholars might accept a wide variety of explanations of the "fundamental social causes of health disparities" that are embedded in the larger social structure, yet not accept a social psychological approach to understanding a person's experience and meaning of illness, and consequently, the coping responses across and within racial and ethnic groups. It may be these differential pathways that can lead to differential outcomes. The interplay between social structure and social and psychological processes is not a new idea for sociology. The social structure and personality framework (House, 1977, 1981; McLeod & Lively, 2004) links society to the individual through various social and psychological processes that shift the attention away from stable norms and values toward more changeable, continually readjusting social processes. Symbolic interactionism (Hollander & Howard, 2000; Stryker, 1987) further contextualizes the relationship between the individual and society by focusing on how the *meaning* of an event or situation is constructed through the process of interaction of individuals with their environment. It is this interaction that also allows for shifts, flexibility and variation in meaning and appraisal and, consequently, the differential impact of these experiences on individual health.

These mediating processes are certainly influenced by one's location in the social structure. For example, social and psychological resources are unevenly distributed by social status (Mirowsky & Hu, 1996; Turner & Lloyd, 1999). There are, in fact, racial differences in social psychological processes and the determinants of beliefs and attitudes. Race also has implications for numerous subjective states, such as self-esteem and self-efficacy (Hughes & Demo, 1989). Consequently, individuals with access to the same resources do not share the same experiences that may either affect their mental health or their response to it. Further, resources may reinforce current effects of advantage or disadvantage in some instances and not others. Therefore, we should expect race, as a major structural parameter of social life, to matter in basic social processes that contemporary sociologists usually explore. Failure to attend to those processes that are influenced by race may result in knowledge that reflects a primarily "white" experience of the world (Hunt, Jackson, Powell, & Steelman, 2000). Indeed, the ability to trace the direct and indirect consequences of social structural factors as they are affected by social and psychological processes is consistent with a sociological examination of mental health disparities.

Empirical evidence lends strong support for social and psychological factors such as social support, negative social interactions (e.g., conflict, demands and broken promises) and mastery, as constructs that link social statuses to mental health. Social and psychological resources are thought to increase the likelihood of effective coping and positive health behaviors and potentially buffer or moderate the impact of adverse conditions on mental health outcomes. One hundred years ago, Durkheim's (1897/1951) study of suicide made a significant contribution to the field of sociology. He found that suicides were more prevalent among those with fewer social ties, which in turn, produced a loss of social resources, a reduction in social constraints (based on defined norms and social roles), and ultimately resulted in poor psychological outcomes and increased risk of suicide. Extant reviews of the social support literature since (Cohen & Wills, 1985; House, Umberson, & Landis, 1988; Thoits, 1995) conclude that social support, regardless of the way in which it is measured, has the potential to alleviate the deleterious effects of stress and other undesirable situations on physical, mental, and social outcomes.

A growing body of research also focuses on perceptions of mastery or personal control as important factors influencing mental health. Feelings of mastery have been associated with less psychological distress (Lincoln, Chatters, & Taylor, 2003) and lower rates of depression (e.g., Mirowsky, 1995; Pearlin, Lieberman, Menaghan, & Mullan, 1981) independently and interdependently with social resources like social support. For example, social support theorists (e.g., Thoits, 1985, 1995) maintain that social support can serve to enhance adjustment by increasing one's sense of mastery and involving the individual in active problem-solving. Individuals also maintain a sense of mastery by meeting responsibilities to people in their social network and by receiving assistance from them.

A study by Lincoln and colleagues (2003) is an example of racial differences in social and psychological processes and mental health. Findings from their study reveal divergent predictive models for African Americans and whites. Specifically, social support from relatives indirectly reduced psychological distress by bolstering feelings of personal control among whites. This pattern of relationships did not emerge for African Americans. However, negative interactions with relatives increased psychological distress by eroding feeling of personal control for African Americans; this was not the case for whites. This set of findings not only reveals the distinctive nature of social and psychological processes by race, but also calls into question prior research (within primarily majority samples) which is based on the assumption that the relationships among these factors are similar across racial and ethnic groups.

Research Implications. A structural perspective on the social causes of health disparities recognizes the link between mastery and differential access to power. Despite the recognition that macrolevel factors (e.g., racism, the economy) influence microlevel experiences (e.g., powerlessness, lack of control), few investigators have attempted to examine these links. It may be because microlevel experiences are within the domain of social psychology and less a part of mainstream sociology (Schnittker & McLeod, 2005). However, the issue of structural constraints and their impact on available coping resources is of particular importance for both identifying those life exigencies that are resistant to coping efforts and for understanding the various processes that link race to differential health outcomes.

A new and promising direction in the study of race and mental health disparities examines the negative side of social relationships (Lincoln et al., 2003). Negative interaction refers to unpleasant social exchanges between individuals that are perceived by the recipient as unsupportive, critical, manipulative, demanding, or otherwise inconsequential to their needs. Research on social relationships and mental health suggests that social support and negative interactions are distinct dimensions of social relationships that appear to increase the probability of maladaptive mental health outcomes (Lincoln et al., 2003; Okun & Keith, 1998; Rook,

1984). The majority of studies indicate that, across a variety of samples and indicators, negative social interactions exert a greater effect on mental health than do measures of social support. Evidence suggests that although negative interactions occur less frequently relative to supportive interactions, negative encounters with social network members have the potential to cause emotional distress and to severely increase existing levels of stress (Krause & Jay, 1991). Moreover, the deleterious effects of negative interactions often occur despite the presence of supportive exchanges within an individual's social network.

In sum, to the extent that we are able to decrease negative interactions, enhance supportive relationships and levels of mastery, especially among disadvantaged groups, we should consequently reduce racial and ethnic disparities in health. However, it is important to recognize the limitations of such an approach as well as highlight its strengths. First, modifying any social or psychological resource is a difficult process. Second, the mechanisms that link race to mental health are not the same across all disadvantaged groups. Finally, the mechanisms that currently link race to health are different than they were in the past and will be different in the future – that is, they are moving targets. Improved access to mental health care and advances in treatment are just a couple of examples of the more recent advances that may differentially impact individuals from diverse racial and ethnic groups.

In addition to providing a more complete view of the dynamics of social status and mental health, recent findings present challenges to traditional ways of thinking about racial differences as well as opportunities to broaden our conceptualization and measurement of these constructs. Studies of mastery, for example, suggest that African Americans may ascribe a different meaning to items that suggest personal control, compared to their white counterparts, because of their higher religiosity (Shaw & Krause, 2001). Within a religious context, then, items suggesting that an individual, rather than a higher power, is primarily responsible for what happens to them may have different meanings and consequently, elicit different responses.

Geographic and Social Places

The past decade has been marked by a resurgence of interest in "place" as a social context for framing analyses of race and health. The attention to social contexts is, in some respects, linked to the development of analytic tools that allow for the assessment of multiple hierarchical forms of statistical associations. For the most part, however, studies supposedly about the effects of place have actually been based on the aggregated characteristics of individuals as measured in censuses or other surveys (Gieryn, 2000). Typically, the proportion of variance in health behaviors explained by these operationalizations of place have been relatively small, prompting some to suggest that place has only a limited effect on individual behavior. Alternatively, Macintyre, Ellaway and Cummins (2002) and others suggest that weak effects are more likely due to inadequate conceptualization, operationalization, and measurement of place effects. Based on their reviews of theoretical works and empirical analyses, Gieryn (2000) and Macintyre et al. (2002) suggest the need to move to multifaceted conceptions of "place" encompassing geographic location, material form and infrastructure, and meaning.

Place is defined as a geographically located aggregate of people, practices, and built or natural objects that are invested with meaning and value. Place is treated neither as a spatial backdrop for social interaction nor as a proxy for neighborhood variables. Instead, place is viewed as a socio-ecological force with detectable and independent effects on social life and individual well-being (Werlen, 1993). Places reflect and reinforce social advantages and disadvantages by extending or denying life-chances to groups located in salutary or detrimental locales (Gieryn, 2000). Social processes (e.g., segregation, marginalization, collective action) happen through the intervening mechanism of place (Habraken, 1998) with important effects on health and well-being. Massey (2003), for example, argues that inner city racial segregation produces a high allostatic load among African Americans which leads, in turn, to a variety of deleterious health, cognitive, and emotional outcomes. In another vein, reviews of treatment efficacy studies reveal that interventions often do not have the same effects when moved from the clinic to naturalistic social settings (U.S. Department of Health and Human Services, 2001). Such conclusions suggest that treatment effectiveness studies must take very seriously the effects of place on the implementation and outcomes of clinical activity.

The effects of place on health and health behaviors are far from uniform across population groups and health outcomes. Studies of race and place effects need to move toward more nuanced theorizing about the effects of place on health, and toward creating more integrated theories on how place influences health. Accordingly, more theoretical and empirical work is warranted toward understanding specifically how "places" promote social engagement or social estrangement, stress or security, and health or illness within and across racial minority groups.

If place attachments can facilitate social engagement and a sense of security and well-being, the loss of place can have devastating implications for psychological well-being – particularly for members of racial minority populations (Fullilove, 1996). Understanding place – and related constructs of displacement and emplacement – is critical for understanding the role of race, ethnicity, and racial inequalities in society. Displacement occurs when populations are forced by "push" or "pull" factors to leave places of origin (e.g., immigrants, refugees), place-bound (e.g., prisoners, children in foster care), entrapped in places that become unhealthy over time (e.g., place-bound residents of some central cities) or "without place" (e.g., homeless adults and children). Displacement or dislocation is one of the major sources of poor mental health globally (Mollica, 2000). Racial minority groups are disproportionately represented in different types of displaced groups such as immigrants and refugees, residents in juvenile and adult corrections, homeless populations, and foster care (U.S. Department of Health and Human Services, 2001). Each racial and ethnic group has a different history of displacement, with some groups indigenous to this country and displaced from their homelands, some brought in as slaves, others migrate to the U.S. of their own volition, and still others seek refuge to avoid genocide, wars, and political persecution.

Over the past three decades, the social, behavioral and medical sciences have documented and described displacement and its consequences among racial groups. Researchers have been less successful in shedding light on how people who have been displaced become emplaced in a new geographic location. While we know, for example, that neighborhoods that have a collective sense of efficacy (Earls & Carlson, 2001), social positions based on income, education or occupation (Krieger, 2001), and positive social relationships can all be factors that help emplace individuals (Pescosolido, 1992), we lack a large body of theoretical and empirical studies that investigates whether they operate in different racial groups in the same way. Equally important, researchers have not adequately investigated the mechanisms unique to different racial groups that help individuals become emplaced in social locations. Moreover, the construct of place has been used primarily in urban settings and to study limited racial and ethnic groups. Considering place as more than geographic location allows social scientists and policy makers to consider the distribution of material resources, political power and control, and social differentiation and exclusion (Poland, Lehoux, Holmes, & Andrews, 2005).

Research Implications. Places reflect and reinforce social advantages and disadvantages by extending or denying life-chances to groups located in salutary or detrimental locales (Kelly, 2003). More basic theoretical and empirical work can identify the important elements of place that are enhancing and constraining for racial groups. Race likely influences the dimensions important for creating a sense of belonging and identity with a particular geographic space. Conversely, race can be a potent factor in determining dimensions of place that are alienating, exclusionary, and toxic. Indigenous groups, such as American Indians or Native Hawaiians, have histories of displacement from the spiritual resources of their land. Other racial groups were forced to come to the U.S. as slaves or laborers and have endured the legacy of this struggle. Still others, including immigrants and refugees, have often been labeled as "alien" or "foreign" in ways that cast them apart from the "American" identity. Given these unique histories, race may influence the facets that most matter in the meaning of place. To some indigenous groups, for example, a land base to establish spiritual connections with ancestors may be a critical component in influencing connections with a location. A better understanding about these critical factors will help refine theories of place and develop measures that are congruent with how racial groups find meaning in geographic locations.

Some studies suggest that immigrants tend to have low rates of mental health problems and, over time, their rates increase to levels similar to their native-born counterparts (Ihara & Takeuchi, 2004; Vega & Rumbaut, 1991). While this finding has not been replicated across a wide range of racial and ethnic groups, some intriguing questions are raised about the effects of place on this pattern. On the one hand, since many immigrants may initially settle in racial and ethnic communities, it is possible that residential patterns have a salutary effect on mental health that erodes as immigrants disperse and become more integrated into the mainstream. On the other hand, it is equally plausible that, for immigrants, finding place in the mainstream may include more opportunities to engage in risky behaviors linked to substance use, exposure to stressors such as racial discrimination, and the adoption of western expressions of distress. Since immigration has changed the racial composition of the U.S., studies of place will help us better understand the processes associated with adaptation, adjustment, and integration and various mental health outcomes.

Over 40 years ago, Erving Goffman made profound observations about how place affects the mental health and treatment of individuals. He noted that people with a serious mental illness have lost contact with their place in society and slowly become divorced from the rituals and interactions that sustain their lives (Goffman, 1971). Detachment from one's place is often associated with alienation, demoralization, and distress (Mirowsky & Ross, 1986). When people with a serious mental illness seek treatment, the treatment setting may serve to reinforce their disconnection with their place in society. Goffman's observations are still insightful for contemporary times and consistent with the personal accounts of people who suffer from mental illness (Holley, 1998; Kaysen, 1994; Sheehan, 1982; Shiller, 1996).

Despite Goffman's early observations, we show little progress in turning his insights into an explicit research agenda on place. We lack systematic investigations about how settings such as clinics and hospitals create places for mental health treatment, especially for different racial groups. Moreover, fewer studies exist about how treatment places are linked to negative or successful treatment outcomes. In our view, studies of treatment places are different from past calls to make mental health treatment culturally-sensitive, -appropriate, or –competent. The focus on cultural issues has largely identified attitudes and beliefs of clinicians as major points of intervention (Vega, 2005). Place studies can move beyond attitudes and beliefs by examining the architecture of facilities and how these physical spaces enhance access into treatment and participation in treatment among people with a serious mental illness and their families. While some physical structures are modified to accommodate different groups of people, for example the use of animal caricatures in pediatric clinics or translated signs in hospitals, many of these attempts lack a theoretical or evidentiary basis and few studies examine their impact on access, participation, and treatment outcomes. Since other disciplines and professions such as geography, anthropology, psychology, psychiatry, social work, nursing, and medicine are interested in the construct of place, the possibilities for sociology to cross disciplinary lines to advance the treatment of mental illness for different racial groups is unlimited.

Concluding Comments

A major contribution of the sociology of mental health to sociology is often neglected; principally because it has more to do with the education and training of sociologists from racial and ethnic minority groups than with more substantive contributions to theory and methods. However, the training program, the Minority Fellowship Program (MFP), has contributed immensely to the development of sociology and to the study of race and mental health. The MFP was started in 1974 with seed funding from the National Institute of Mental Health (NIMH). The program was similar to training efforts started in other disciplines and professions like psychology, nursing, and social work. The program was developed to bring in more predoctoral students from racial and ethnic minority groups which would eventually make sociology as a discipline more diverse. By the 2004–05 program year, the MFP had given 1,257 awards to a diverse group of graduate students: 216 African Americans, 120 Latinos, 28 Native Americans, and 81 Asian Americans. While NIMH intended that the funds would increase the number of minority scholars studying mental health issues, it also had the indirect effect of increasing the number of minority sociologists who went into other fields. A number of MFP students did not focus on mental health issues, but eventually went on to make contributions to sociology and the scholarship on race. Larry Bobo and Michael Omi are two examples of sociologists who received MFP funding and have been influential in developing general sociological work on race that holds important insights, not always recognized, for the study of race and mental health. More directly, the work of David Williams, and a score of other past MFP fellows have been critical to bringing issues of race and ethnicity to the forefront of mental health research. Contemporary sociology of race and mental health provides ample opportunities to build from the past or to investigate alternative directions that best explain how these constructs are linked. But, as in the past, the political and social climate will help to shape whether these investigations will prosper in the near future. Sociologists will also have a lot to say by contesting attempts to constrain research on race and mental health. The social mirror provides the metaphor about how we can reflect on our biases and prejudices to make changes in how the study of race is valued and, more importantly, how we make meaningful changes in the racial hierarchy in society. Christopher Edley, Jr. (2001) best captures this spirit:

Race is not rocket science; it is harder than rocket science. Race demands an intellectual investment equal to the task. It also demands relentlessness in research and teaching that will overwhelm the human tendency to let our differences trigger the worst in our natures (p. ix).

Acknowledgments. Authors are listed alphabetically and contributed equally to the writing of this chapter. This chapter is supported by the University of Washington Native Wellness Center (Evans-Campbell), grants from the Hartford Foundation (Lincoln), K01-MH69923 (Lincoln), U01 MH62207 (Takeuchi), and R01 HD049142 (Takeuchi and Lincoln).

References

Alba, R., & Nee, V. (2003). Remaking the American mainstream: Assimilation and contemporary immigration. Boston: Harvard University Press.

Auerhahn, N., & Laub, D. (1998). Intergenerational memory of the Holocaust. In Y. Danieli (Ed), *International handbook of multigenerational legacies of trauma* (pp. 341–354). New York: Plenum Press.

Bar-On, D., Eland, J., Kleber, R., Krell, R., Moore, Yl, Sagi, A., Soriano, El., Suedfeld, P., van der Velden, P., & van Ijzendoorn, M. (1998). Multigenerational perspectives on coping with Holocaust experience: An attachment perspective for understanding the developmental sequelae of trauma across generations. *International Journal of Behavioral Development, 22*, 315–338.

Boas, F. (1927). Fallacies of racial inferiority. *Current History, 25*, 676–682.

Barocas, H., & Barocas, C. (1980). Separation and individuation conflict in children of Holocaust survivors. *Journal of Contemporary Psychology, 38*, 417–452.

Bonilla-Silva, E. (1997). Rethinking racism: Toward a structural interpretation. *American Sociological Review, 62*, 465–480.

Brave Heart, M. Y. H. (1999a). Oyate Ptayela: Rebuilding the Lakota Nation through addressing historical trauma among Lakota parents. *Journal of Human Behavior in the Social Environment, 2*, 109–126.

Brave Heart, M. Y. H. (1999b). Gender differences in the historical trauma response among the Lakota. *Journal of Health and Social Policy, 10*, 1–21.

Brave Heart, M. Y. H. (2000). Wakiksuyapi: Carrying the historical trauma of the Lakota. *Tulane Studies in Social Welfare, 21–22*, 245–266.

Brown, T. N., Sellers, S. L., Brown, K. T., & Jackson, J. S. (1999) Race, ethnicity and culture in the sociology of mental health. In C. S. Aneshensel & J. C. Phelan (Eds), *Handbook of the sociology of mental health* (pp 167–182). New York: Kluwer Academic/Plenum Publishers.

Brown, T. N., Sellers, S. L., & Gomez, J. P. (1999). The relationship between internalization and self-esteem among Black adults. *Social Focus, 35*, 55–71.

Cohen, S. & Wills, T. A. (1985). Stress, social support and the buffering hypothesis. *Psychological Bulletin, 98*, 310–357.

Cooper, R., & David, R. (1986). The biological concept of race and its application to public health and epidemiology. *Journal of Health, Politics, Policy and Law, 11*, 97–116.

Cross, W. (1998). Black psychological functioning and the legacy of slavery: myths and realities. In Y. Danieli (Ed), *International handbook of multigenerational legacies of trauma* (pp. 387–402). New York: Plenum Press.

Danieli, Y. (Ed.). (1998). *International handbook of multigenerational legacies of trauma.* New York, NY: Plenum Press.

DuBois, W. E. B. (1903). *Souls of Black folks.* Chicago: A.C. McClurg & Co.

Durkheim, E. (1897/1951) *Suicide.* New York: Free Press.

Earls, F., & Carlson, M. (2001). The social ecology of child health and well-being. *Annual Review of Public Health, 22*, 143–166.

Edley, C. Jr. (2001). Foreward. In N. Smelser, W. J. Wilson, & F. Mitchell (Eds.), *America becoming: Racial trends and their consequences* (pp. ix). Washington D. C.: National Research Council.

Eitinger, L., & Strom, A. (1973). *Mortality and morbidity after excessive stress: A follow-up investigation of Norwegian concentration camp survivors.* New York: Humanities Press.

Evans-Campbell, T. (Under Review). Far from home: The impact of Indian boarding school attendance on mental health and wellness among urban American Indians/Alaska Natives. *Cultural Diversity and Ethnic Minority Psychology.*

Evans-Campbell, T., & Walters, K. L. (2006). Indigenist practice competencies in child welfare practice: A decolonization framework to address family violence and substance abuse among First Nations peoples. In R. Fong, R. McRoy, & C. Ortiz Hendricks (Eds.), *Intersecting child welfare, substance abuse, and family violence: Culturally competent approaches.* Washington, DC: CSWE Press.

Felsen, I. (1998). Transgenerational transmission of effects of the Holocaust. In Y. Danieli (Ed), *International handbook of multigenerational legacies of trauma* (pp. 43–68). New York: Plenum Press.

Felsen, I., & Erlich, H. (1990). Identification patterns of offspring of Holocaust survivors with their parents. *American Journal of Orthopsychiatry, 60*, 506–520.

Fullilove, M. (1996). Psychiatric implications of displacement: Contributions from the psychology of place. *American Journal of Psychiatry, 153*, 1516–1523.

Gieryn, T. (2000). A space for place in sociology. *Annual Review of Sociology, 26*, 463–496.

Goffman, E. (1971). *Relations in public*. London: Allen Lane.

Habraken, J. (1998). *The structure of the ordinary: Form and control in the built environment*. Cambridge, MA: MIT Press.

Harris, D. R., & Sim, J. J. (2001). An empirical look at the social construction of race: The case of multiracial adolescents. Population Studies Center Research Report 00–452. Ann Arbor: University of Michigan.

Hollander, J. A., & Howard, J. A. (2000). Social psychological theories on social inequalities. *Social Psychology Quarterly, 63*, 338–351.

Holley, T. E. (1998). My mother's keeper: A daughter's memoir of growing up in the shadow of schizophrenia. New York: William Morrow.

House, J. S. (1977). The three faces of social psychology. *Sociometry, 40*, 161–177.

House, J. S. (1981). *Work stress and social support*. Reading, MA: Addison-Wesley.

House, J. S., Kessler, R. C., Herzog, A. R., Mero, R. P., Kinnery, A. M., & Breslow, M. J. (1990). Age, socioeconomic status, and health. *Milbank Quarterly, 68*, 345–383.

House, J. S., Umberson, D., & Landis, K. R. (1988). Structures and processes of social support. *Annual Review of Sociology, 14*, 293–318.

Hughes, M., & Demo, D. H. (1989). Self-perceptions of Black Americans: Self-esteem and personal efficacy. *American Journal of Sociology, 95*, 132–159.

Hunt, M. O., Jackson, P. B., Powell, B., & Steelman, L. C. (2000). Color-blind: The treatment of race and ethnicity in social psychology. *Social Psychology Quarterly, 63*, 352–364.

Ihara, E. & Takeuchi, D. (2004). Ethnic minority mental health services. In B. Lubotsky Levin & J. Petrila (Eds.), *Mental health services: A public health perspective*. London: Oxford Press.

Kahana, B., Harel, Z., & Kahana, E. (1988). Predictors of psychological well-being among survivors of the Holocaust. In J. P. Wilson, Z. Harel, & B. Kahana (Eds.), *Human adaptation to extreme stress: From Holocaust to Vietnam* (pp. 171–192). New York: Plenum Press.

Kaysen, S. (1994). *Girl interrupted*. New York: Vintage Books.

Kelly, S. E. (2003). Bioethics and rural health: Theorizing place, space, and subjects. *Social Science and Medicine, 56*, 2277–2288.

Kerckoff, A. (1993). *Diverging pathways: Social structure and career deflections*. New York: Cambridge University Press.

Kinzie, J., Boehnlein, J., & Sack, W. (1998). The effects of massive trauma on Cambodian parents and children. In Y. Danieli (Ed), *International handbook of multigenerational legacies of trauma* (pp. 211–221). New York: Plenum Press.

Krause, N., & Jay, G. (1991). Stress, social support, and negative interaction in later life. *Research on Aging, 13*, 333–363.

Krieger, N. (2001). Historical roots of social epidemiology: Socioeconomic gradients in health and contextual analysis. *International Journal of Epidemiology, 30*, 899–900.

Krieger, N., Williams, D. R., & Moss, N. E. (1997). Measuring social class in U.S. public health research: Concepts, methodologies, and guidelines. *Annual Review of Public Health, 18*, 341–389.

Lichtman, H. (1984). Parental communication of Holocaust experiences and personality characteristics among second-generation survivors. *Journal of Clinical Psychology, 40*, 914–924.

Lieberman, S. (1985). *Making it count*. Berkeley: University of California Press.

Lincoln, K. D., Chatters, L. M., & Taylor, R. J. (2003). Psychological distress among Black and white Americans: Differential effects of social support, negative interaction and personal control. *Journal of Health and Social Behavior, 44*, 390–407.

Link, B. G., & Phelan, J. C. (1995). Social conditions as fundamental causes of disease. *Journal of Health and Social Behavior, 35*, 80–94.

Macintyre, S., Ellaway, A., & Cummins, S. (2002). Place effects on health: How can we conceptualize, operationalize, and measure them? *Social Science and Medicine, 55*, 125–139.

Massey, D. S. (1995). The bell curve: Intelligence and class structure in American life. *American Journal of Sociology, 101*, 747–753.

Massey, D. (2003). Segregation and stratification: A biosocial perspective. *Dubois Review, 1*, 7–25.

McKee, J. B. (1993). *Sociology and the race problem: The failure of a perspective.* Chicago: University of Illinois Press.

McLeod, J. D., & Lively, K. J. (2004). Social structure and personality. In J. D. Delamater (Ed.), *Handbook of social psychology* (pp. 77–102). New York: Kluwer/Plenum.

Mirowsky, J. (1995). Age and the sense of control. *Social Psychology Quarterly, 58*, 31–43.

Mirowsky, J., & Hu, P. (1996). Physical impairment and the diminishing effects of income. *Social Forces, 74*, 1073–1096.

Mirowsky, J., & Ross, C. (1986). Social patterns of distress. *Annual Review of Sociology, 12*, 23–45.

Mollica, R. F. (2000). Waging a new kind of war. *Scientific American, 282*, 54–57.

Myers, S. L., Jr. (2002). Presidential address: Analysis of race as policy analysis. *Journal of Policy Analysis and Management, 21*, 169–190.

Nagata, D. (1991). Intergenerational effects of the Japanese American internment. Clinical issues in working with children of former internees. *Psychotherapy, 28*, 121–128.

Nagata, D., Trierweiler, S, & Talbot, R. (1999). Long-term effects of internment during early childhood in third generation Japanese Americans. *American Journal of Orthopsychiatry, 69*, 19–29.

Neiderland, W. G. (1968). Clinical observations on the "Survivor Syndrome." *International Journal of Psychoanalysis, 49*, 313–315.

Neiderland, W. G. (1981). The survivor syndrome: Further observations and dimensions. *Journal of American Psychoanalytic Association, 29*, 413–425.

Neighbors, H. W. (1990). The prevention of psychopathology in African Americans: An epidemiological perspective. *Community Mental Health Journal, 26*, 167–179.

Okun, M. A., & Keith, V. M. (1998). Effects of positive and negative social exchanges with various sources on depressive symptoms in younger and older adults. *Journals of Gerontology: Psychological Sciences, 53B*, P4–P20.

Omi, M., & Winant, H. (1994). *Racial formation in the United States: From the 1960s to the 1990s.* New York: Routledge.

O'Rand, A., & Henretta, J. (1999). *Age and inequality: Diverse pathways through later life.* Boulder, CO: Westview Press.

Pearlin, L. I., Lieberman, M. A., Menaghan, E. G., & Mullan, J. T. (1981). The stress process. *Journal of Health and Social Behavior, 22*, 337–356.

Pescosolido, B. A. (1992). Beyond rational choice: The social dynamics of how people seek help. *American Journal of Sociology, 97*, 1096–1138.

Poland, B., Lehoux, P., Holmes, D., & Andrews, G. (2004). How place matters: Unpacking technology and power in health and social care. *Health and Social Care in the Community, 13*, 170–180.

Robin, R. W., Chester, B., & Goldman, D. (1996). Cumulative trauma and PTSD in American Indian communities. In A. Marsella, M. Friedman, E. Gerrity, & Scurfield (Eds.), *Ethnocultural aspects of posttraumatic Stress disorder* (pp. 239–253). Washington, DC: American Psychological Association.

Rook, K. S. (1984). The negative side of social interaction: Impact on psychological well-being. *Journal of Personality and Social Psychology, 46*, 1097–1108.

Rosenberg, N. A., Pritchard, J. K., Weber, J. L, Cann, H. M., Kidd, K. K., Zhivotovsky, L. A., & Feldman, M. (2002). Genetic structure of human populations. *Science, 298*, 2381–2385.

Schnittker, J., & McLeod, J. D. (2005). The social psychology of health disparities. *Annual Review of Sociology, 31*, 75–103.

Shaw, B., & Krause, N. (2001). Exploring race variations in aging and personal control. *Journal of Gerontology: Social Sciences, 56B*, S119–S124.

Sheehan, S. (1982). *Is there no place on earth for me?* Boston: Houghton Mifflin.

Shiller, L. (1996). *The quiet room: A journey out of treatment of madness.* New York: Warner Books.

Sigal, J., & Weinfeld, M. (1989). *Trauma and rebirth: Intergenerational effects of the Holocaust.* New York: Praeger.

Simon, R. I., & Eppert, C. (In press). Remembering obligation: Pedagogy and the witnessing of testimony and historical trauma. *Canadian Journal of Education.*

Solomon, Z., Kother, M., & Mikulincer, M. (1988). Combat-related PSTD among second generation Holocaust survivors: Preliminary findings. *American Journal of Psychiatry, 145*, 865–868.

Stryker, S. (1987). The vitalization of symbolic interactionism. *Social Psychology Quarterly, 50*, 83–94.

Sue, S., McKinney, H., Allen, D., & Hall, J. (1974). Delivery of community mental health services to black and white clients. *Journal of Counseling and Clinical Psychology, 42*, 794–801.

Takeuchi, D., & Gage, S. (2003). What to do with race: Changing notions of race in the social sciences. *Culture, Medicine and Psychiatry, 27*, 435–445.

Takeuchi, D. T., & Williams, D. R. (2003). Race, ethnicity and mental health: Introduction to the special issue. *Journal of Health and Social Behavior, 44*, 233–236.

Thoits, P. (1985). Social support and psychological well-being: Theoretical possibilities. In I. G. Sarason & B. Sarason (Eds.), *Social support: Theory, research, and application* (pp. 51–72). Boston: Kluwer.

Thoits, P. A. (1995). Stress, coping, and social support process: Where are we? What next? *Journal of Health and Social Behavior, 35*, 53–79.

Tuan, M. (1998). *Forever foreigners or honorary whites: The contemporary Asian American experience.* New Jersey: Rutgers University Press.

Turner, R. J., & Lloyd, D. A. (1999). The stress process and the social distribution of depression. *Journal of Health and Social Behavior, 42*, 310–325.

U.S. Department of Health and Human Services. (2001). *Mental health: Culture, race, and ethnicity. A supplement to mental health: A report of the Surgeon General.* Rockville, MD: U.S. Department of Health and Human Services, Substance Abuse and Mental Health Services Administration, Center for Mental Health Services.

Vega, W. A. (2005). Higher stakes ahead for cultural competence. *General Hospital Psychiatry, 27*, 446–450.

Vega, W. A., & Rumbaut, R. G. (1991). Ethnic minorities and mental health. *Annual Review of Sociology, 17*, 351–383.

Werlen, B. (1993). *Society, action, and space: An alternative to human geography.* London: Routledge.

Whitbeck, L., Adams, G., Hoyt, D., & Chen, X. (2004). Conceptualizing and measuring historical trauma among American Indian people. *American Journal of Community Psychology, 33*, 119–130.

Williams, D. R. (1990). Socioeconomic differentials in health: A review and redirection. *Social Psychology Quarterly, 53*, 81–99.

Williams, D. R., & Collins, C. (1995). U.S. socioeconomic and racial differences in health: Patterns and explanations. *Annual Review of Sociology, 21*, 349–386.

Wilson, W. J. (1987). *The truly disadvantaged: The inner city, the underclass and public policy*. Chicago: University of Chicago Press.

Winant, H. (2000). Race and race theory. *Annual Review of Sociology, 26*, 169–185.

Yehuda, R. (1999). *Risk factors for posttraumatic stress disorder*. Washington, DC: American Psychiatric Press.

Yu, H. (2001). *Thinking Orientals: Migration, contact, exoticism in modern America*. Oxford: University Press.

9
Life Course Perspectives on Social Factors and Mental Illness

Linda K. George

Virtually all major issues in the study of mental health involve conceptualizing and modeling change. Social selection and social causation, estimating the effects of stress, identifying other antecedents of mental illness, examining the consequences of mental illness – these and many other topics require conceptualization of processes and analysis of longitudinal data. Despite the centrality of dynamic processes to our understanding of mental health and illness, most longitudinal studies span relatively short periods of time and focus on temporality as a prerequisite for causal inference.

Life course perspectives offer a complementary way of conceptualizing and modeling stability and change. The most obvious characteristic of life course research is the focus on longer periods of time than are characteristic of most longitudinal studies. Equally important, in life course research, temporality is the conceptual focus rather than primarily a methodological issue. A prime illustration of the difference in focus between most longitudinal studies and life course studies of mental illness is the issue of social causation and selection. A substantial body of research has focused on the extent to which social factors are causes or consequences of mental illness (e.g., Johnson, 1991; Ross & Mirowsky, 1995). Life course theorists, in contrast, rarely think in those terms. Rather, they are interested in the dynamic interplay between social factors and illness, typically seeking to trace temporal pathways. The pathways or trajectories often include lagged effects, reciprocal effects, and/or cyclical effects – temporal patterns that cannot easily be categorized as selection or causation effects.

The purpose of this chapter is to consider the cross-fertilization of life course research and the sociology of mental health and mental illness. The chapter begins with a brief review of the four major principles that underlie life course perspectives. Few empirical studies include attention to all four of these principles – but all life course studies focus on at least one of them. Most of the chapter is devoted to three major themes regarding temporality, social factors, and mental health or illness. The first, and most complex, focuses on the relationships between social factors and mental health over long periods of time and several specific research topics are reviewed. The second major theme is the dynamics of recovery and recurrence among the mentally ill. The third area is the social transmission of mental health problems across generations. For each of these themes, the potential contributions of life course perspectives are highlighted, as are the ways that mental health research serves as a strategic site for applying and empirically testing life course principles. The chapter ends with a short section on a critical issue for future research.

It is prudent to note how the terms "mental health" and "mental illness" are used in this chapter. Although this field is typically referred to as social factors and mental health, almost all research focuses on mental health problems. Mental health problems are conceptualized and measured in a variety of ways, ranging from distress, to symptom scales that correspond to diagnostic entities (e.g., depression symptoms), to specific psychiatric disorders. There have been lively debates about the extent to which diagnostic categories are valid, discrete, and meaningful (e.g., Kessler, 2002; Mirowsky & Ross, 1989). This review covers research using the broad range of measures of mental health problems – discrete as well as continuous measures, diagnostic categories as well as distress. As discussed below, the use of diagnostic or other dichotomous measures of mental health problems is especially relevant for research that incorporates life course principles.

Life Course Perspectives: Key Principles

There is no unified theory of the life course – nor, as I have argued elsewhere, should there be. Life course perspectives can best to be used in conjunction with specific theories (George, 2003). That is, life course perspectives are best tested in the context of specific topics – topics for which the importance of long-term processes has been recognized and which offer theories with which life course principles can be integrated. As I argue throughout this chapter, research on mental health and mental illness is ideally positioned to profit from incorporation of life course principles and provides research questions and theories that are superbly suited for testing life course principles.

Although life course perspectives do not comprise an integrated theory, they share four core principles, each of which can augment our understanding of mental health.

Long-term Temporal Patterns. The first and most fundamental principle of life course perspectives is the need to examine temporality over long periods of time (Elder, Johnson, & Crosnoe, 2003). Indeed, although few studies can or should incorporate all four key life course principles, a focus on long-term temporal patterns is the defining characteristic of life course research.

Life course perspectives take a long view of biography, often covering decades or longer. Key assumptions of life course perspectives are that lives unfold over time in long-term pathways or trajectories; that the present cannot be understood without knowledge of the past, including the distant past; and that, in addition to the *content* of trajectories (e.g., marital histories, occupational careers), their temporal characteristics also are important (Settersten, 2006). Potentially important temporal characteristics include *length of exposure* (i.e., the extent to which time in a given state affects outcomes of interest), *sequencing* (i.e., the extent to which the order in which events or exposures occur affects outcomes of interest), and *duration dependence* (i.e., the extent to which time in a given state alters the probability of movement to another state) (Alwin, Hofer, & McCammon, 2006).

Two primary types of data are used in life course research. Multiple measurements over long periods of time are, of course, preferred. Because of the large investments of time, money, and effort required for longitudinal studies that span large proportions of the life course, retrospective data also are frequently used. Retrospective data are inferior to prospective data in multiple ways (e.g., memory problems, "rewriting" the past). Nonetheless, techniques such as life history calendars (e.g., Scott & Alwin, 1998) can yield rich data about life course patterns. Also, the more objective (e.g., recall of dates of earlier marriages vs. recall of the quality of earlier marriages) and vivid (i.e., recall of sexual assault vs. recall of first kiss) the information sought, the more accurate the retrospective data.

A variety of modeling techniques are used to examine life course patterns: regression techniques in which factors measured at one point in time are used to predict outcomes observed later in time, path models that posit complex combinations of direct and indirect effects, survival or event history models that estimate "time till" transitions or other discrete outcomes, and growth curve models in which trajectories are the independent and/or dependent variables (e.g., trajectories of social support predicting trajectories of depressive symptoms).

As described in more detail in the next section of this chapter, there is substantial evidence that the cross-fertilization of this life course principle with key research questions in the sociology of mental health has considerable payoff. One of the most useful outcomes of this cross-fertilization has been a reframing of some key theories of mental health. For example, taking a long-term perspective renders the social selection versus social causation debate essentially moot. Rather than focusing on reapportioning variance to selection and causation factors, the principle of temporality focuses attention of delineating the multiple pathways that do and do not result in mental health problems (for a more detailed discussion, see George, 2003). The stress exposure versus stress vulnerability debate can also be reframed when viewed from the perspective of the rates of growth in both stressors and mental health outcomes (George & Lynch, 2003).

The Intersection of Biography and History. Life course perspectives attend to elements of context that are often ignored or underemphasized by other conceptual frameworks. One of those is historical context. Elder's seminal *Children of the Great Depression* (1974), generally recognized as the work that first articulated life course perspectives, examined the effects of an historical event on lives in the short- and long-term, including the risk of mental health problems. Historical context takes multiple forms – not only highly visible events such as the Great Depression and wars, but also historical trends (e.g., increasing divorce rates) and changes in public policy (e.g., the deinstitutionalization of mental patients during the 1970s and 1980s). Not all life course studies focus specifically on historical context. Nonetheless, this principle is intended to remind all investigators that their data are historically embedded and that societal norms and conditions provide opportunities and constraints that differ across historical time.

A variety of important issues in mental health research provide opportunities to test hypotheses about the effects of historical context. One example is possible historical changes in the nature or strength of the relationships between marital status and mental health. There have been dramatic changes in the average age of first marriage, the risk of divorce, and family structure during the past half century. Whether these changes have altered the relationships among marital status, marital dissolution, and mental well-being have not been adequately explored. Similarly, the labor market has been dramatically restructured as a result of globalization, the demise of the working class in the U.S., the changing social contract between employers and employees, and the transition to a post-industrialized service economy. It has long been known that stable employment, especially in jobs on the high end of the occupational hierarchy, is a positive predictor of mental health. It is not known whether the structural transformations of the labor market have affected rates of mental health problems (albeit, see Dooley, Prause, & Ham-Rowbottom, 2000, for a study of the effects of underemployment – which has reached previously unparalleled levels – on mental health).

Linked Lives. A third principle of life course perspectives is awareness that individual lives are interdependent and socially embedded. Although much sociological research focuses on social relationships, life course perspectives typically view social ties in broader terms. Put simply, life course perspectives contend that there is virtually no outcome of interest (e.g., health, SES) that is *not* affected by the social networks within which individuals are embedded. Life course scholars also argue against investigations in which social relationships are restricted to those in a given domain (e.g. restricting studies of occupations to social relationships on the job). As is true for historical context, social relationships underlie and affect all areas of life, providing both opportunities for and constraints on individuals.

The focus on linked lives meshes nicely with several key issues in the sociology of mental health. Examples include the importance of social support as a buffer of stressful experiences, the caregiving role that family members must frequently play when loved ones are mentally ill, and the mental health consequences of loss of significant others via death or estrangement and conflicted relationships.

Human Agency. A final life course principle focuses on human agency – on the long-term consequences of individual decisions and actions. Social science disciplines, of course, recognize the need to understand the relative roles of social determinism and human agency – and the formidable challenges in making such determinations. Life course perspectives add some subtle facets to this quest. First, life course perspectives focus more on within-person changes over time than do most sub-fields in the social sciences. Life course studies typically examine between-person patterns as well, but the emphasis on long-term patterns and trajectories highlights alternate pathways that are shaped by individual choices as well as by contextual opportunities and constraints. One important element of this principle is determining how choices made earlier in life (e.g., whether to attend college, whether to marry) have long-term consequences. Second, as noted above, life course scholars typically avoid the terms selection and causation, focusing instead on the dynamic interplay of social factors. Both "selection" and "causation" connote processes outside the individual's control, thus underemphasizing the role of human agency (e.g., social scientists talk about being *"selected"* into marriage or a specific occupation – not about individuals *deciding* to marry or pursue a specific career). Finally, although the effects of human agency and social determinism cannot be definitively established, simply highlighting human agency as a core principle alters investigators' interpretation of research findings.

Relatively little research to date has examined the effects of long-term patterns of human agency on mental health outcomes. An example of life course research that examines the impact of individual decision-making on mental health outcomes is Elder's studies of individuals who made the transition to adulthood during World War II. The decision of World War II veterans to use the GI Bill to obtain advanced education proved to be a milestone in terms of both socioeconomic achievements and mental health throughout adulthood (e.g., Laub & Sampson, 2005). Clearly, however, this is a component of the cross-fertilization of life course and mental health research that merits increased attention.

Mental Illness: Taking the Long View

As noted above, the defining characteristics of life course research are (a) examining long-term patterns of change and stability and (b) paying explicit attention to temporal characteristics. The greatest volume of research on mental health problems that incorporates and/or speaks to life course perspectives focuses on long-term patterns of social risk factors and their impact on mental health outcomes. In this section, three topics that take the long-view in understanding mental health are examined.

Mental Health Across the Life Course

Ideally, one would like to begin with an overview of patterns of mental health problems across the life course. Confident conclusions about such patterns would require prospective data that span the life course. In addition, because historical context is likely to affect rates of mental health problems and, perhaps, their timing within the life course, long-term prospective data for multiple cohorts would be required. Unfortunately, such data do not exist. Findings from two long-term longitudinal studies are reviewed below. The quality of these studies, however, does not permit confident or generalizeable conclusions. Beyond those studies are two alternatives: (1) postponing consideration of this issue until adequate data are available or (2) examining age differences (which confound age and cohort) in mental health problems, keeping in mind the limitations of cross-sectional comparisons. On the assumption that cross-sectional data are, at minimum, a source of hypotheses to be tested on longitudinal data, age differences in mental health problems also are reviewed.

Long-term Longitudinal Studies. Elder, Clipp, and colleagues used data from the Terman Study of men to examine the short- and long-term consequences of World War II combat experience (compared to non-combat experience and non-military service) on physical and mental health (Clipp, Pavalko, & Elder, 1992; Elder, Shanahan, & Clipp, 1994). The Terman Study began in 1921–22, recruiting boys and girls with high IQ scores who were age 3–19 at baseline. Data were collected at 13 irregular intervals using multiple modes of inquiry; the last time of measurement was 1991–1992. Clipp et al. (1992) identified six trajectories of mental health over the course of adulthood: stable high mental health, stable low mental health, increasing mental health over time, decreasing mental health over time, decreasing mental health followed by increasing mental health, and a highly fluctuating pattern. The most prevalent pattern was stable high mental health, followed by increasing mental health over time. Although these life course patterns and their distributions accurately describe the sample, the findings cannot be generalized to the population because they applied only to men and the sample was non-representative in intellectual abilities. In addition, measurement of mental health varied over time; Clipp et al. developed their trajectories using ratings based on review of information that varied widely across times of measurement. Demonstrating that multiple trajectories are needed to adequately describe long-term patterns of mental health is the major contribution of this study.

Vaillant and colleagues also examined the long-term consequences of combat exposure on the mental health of male World War II veterans, relative to peers who had not experienced combat. Data for this study were from a study of male Harvard undergraduates that began in 1940–41. Data were collected annually through 1946 and then biennially every two years for 50 years or until death, typically by mail survey. For the sample as a whole, mental health problems were relatively rare with the exception of alcoholism (Cui & Vaillant, 1996). Compared to their peers, men who experienced combat reported much higher rates of PTSD symptoms, both immediately after the war and throughout old age (Lee, Vaillant, Torrey, & Elder, 1995). PTSD symptoms were especially likely among men who experienced combat and had pre-military mental health problems. This study has the same limitations as those based on the Terman men: all male, non-representative sample and methodologically questionable assessments of mental health problems. It also highlights some of the complexities of social selection and causation in that it is difficult to untangle the independent effects of pre-military mental health problems and combat exposure on subsequent mental health.

Age Differences in Mental Health Problems. Two studies examined age differences in depressive symptoms during adulthood in substantial detail (Mirowsky & Ross, 1992; Schieman, Van Gundy, & Taylor, 2002). Both studies are based on representative data from community samples. Findings are both congruent and discrepant across the two studies. Mirowsky and Ross (1992) report that middle-aged adults report fewer depressive symptoms, on average, than young and old adults. Schieman et al. (2002) report that average levels of depressive symptoms decrease across age groups and are lowest among older adults.

Both studies include detailed analyses to identify the extent to which differences across age groups are due to compositional differences on social factors known to predict depression. Mirowksy and Ross report that the lower level of depressive symptoms among middle-aged adults is largely explained by the fact that, compared to their younger and older counterparts, middle-aged people are more economically advantaged, are more likely to have stable marriages and jobs, are relatively free of physical health problems, and have higher levels of perceived personal control. They conclude that sense of control is the major proximal predictor of depressive symptoms. Schieman et al. report that the lower levels of depression reported by older adults primarily reflect the fact that older adults report fewer economic hardships, fewer interpersonal conflicts, and greater religiosity than young and middle-aged adults. Similar to Mirowsky and Ross, Schieman et al. found levels of mastery to be lowest among the oldest age group, pointing out that the inverse relationship between age and depression is somewhat suppressed by sense of mastery. Without longitudinal data across the life course, it is difficult to reconcile the age differences reported by Mirowsky and Ross and Schieman et al. Note, however, that these are bivariate differences. The compositional factors that *explained* observed age differences in levels of depression were remarkably similar across the two studies.

Epidemiologic data on age differences in psychiatric diagnoses is available from two primary sources: The National Comorbidity Survey (NCS) (e.g., Kessler, McGonagle, Zhao, Nelson, Hughes, et al., 1994) and the Epidemiologic Catchment Area (ECA) studies (e.g., Robins & Regier, 1991). The NCS has two advantages over the ECA: the data are more recent and are based on a nationally representative sample. ECA data are from five locally representative areas and have been extrapolated to generate national estimates. Unfortunately, however, the NCS sampled only adults age 18–64 at baseline. Therefore, age differences in psychiatric disorder observed in the ECA are reviewed here. Although there are small differences across diagnoses, the general pattern for Axis I psychiatric disorders is a linear decrease across age groups (Robins & Regier, 1991). That is, the prevalence of mental illness peaks during young adulthood and is lowest among older adults. Although this pattern is only partially compatible with age distributions of social resources (especially income and physical health), it is congruent with selective mortality. Mental illness is a risk factor for mortality. Consequently, to the extent that the most severely mentally ill die before old age, it is not surprising to find a relatively healthy group of late life survivors. Mortality selection also is more compatible with the age differences in depressive symptoms reported by Schieman et al. than those observed by Mirowsky and Ross.

Life course patterns of mental health is an ideal topic for the cross-fertilization of life course perspectives and the sociology of mental health. The latter focuses attention on the distributions of stressors and resources that either protect individuals or put them at increased risk for mental illness. Life course perspectives remind us that these risk and protective factors are not consistent across the life course and that age changes in mental health may reflect these temporal patterns.

The Persisting Effects of Early Traumas and Adversities

The effects of traumas and adversities experienced early in the life course on mental health at later ages is arguably the most important contribution of life course perspectives to mental health research – certainly the sheer volume of studies is largest for this topic. Two related, but distinct bodies of research have emerged. One focuses on childhood traumas; the other on late adolescence and early adulthood.

Childhood Traumas and Adversities. A variety of childhood traumas and adversities substantially increase the risk of later mental health problems. Childhood traumas are typically defined as occurring before the age of 11, but some investigators set the boundaries a year or two earlier or later. Childhood traumas significantly related to mental health problems in middle and later adulthood include parental death, parental divorce, physical abuse, and sexual abuse. There is strong and consistent evidence that parental divorce during childhood is associated with a variety of mental health outcomes, including general distress, depressive symptoms and disorder, and anxiety symptoms and disorders (e.g., Cherlin, Chase-Lansdale, & McRae, 1998; Harris, Brown, & Bifulco, 1990; McLeod, 1991; O'Connor, Thorpe, Dunn, & Golding, 1999; Ross & Mirowsky, 1999). Evidence for parental death, however, is mixed. Some studies report that parental death at an early age is associated with increased risk for mental health problems in adulthood (e.g., Hallstrom, 1987; Harris et al., 1990); other studies fail to observe a relationship between parental death and adult mental health (e.g., Tweed, Schoenbach, George, & Blazer, 1989).

Childhood abuse/neglect also is associated with mental health problems during adulthood (e.g., Horwitz, Widom, McLaughlin, & White, 2001; Kessler & Magee, 1994). Childhood sexual assault is an especially potent harbinger of mental health problems, usually PTSD and/or depression, both immediately after the assault and throughout adulthood (e.g., Roberts, O'Connor, Dunn, & Golding, 2004; Winfield, George, Swartz, & Blazer, 1990; Yama, Tovey, & Forgas, 1993). Indeed, even if children are not victims of abuse or assault, witnessing such aggression has persisting effects on adult mental health (e.g., Kessler & Magee, 1994; Shaw & Krause, 2002 – the latter demonstrates that effects persist 70 years after witnessing the violence).

The effects of childhood poverty/low SES on adult mental health also have been examined. Most, but not all, studies report the childhood economic deprivation is a risk factor for adult mental illness (e.g., Gilman, Kawachi, Fitzmaurice, & Buka, 2003; Hallstrom, 1987; Landerman, George, & Blazer, 1991), but the magnitudes of these relationships are smaller than those for childhood traumas. Recent studies also report that residential instability and living in unstable, poor, and disorganized neighborhoods during childhood increase the odds of mental health problems in adulthood (Gilman et al., 2003; Wheaton & Clarke, 2003).

For life course scholars, establishing relationships between childhood events and later mental health problems is only the first step. Equally, if not more, important is identification of the pathways and mechanisms that account for the persisting effects of childhood adversities – and that result in subsequent mental health problems for some, but not all, who experience such adversities. Much has been learned about the pathways by which childhood traumas increase vulnerability to mental health problems decades later. Childhood traumas and adversities substantially reduce individuals' socioeconomic achievements and ability to develop and sustain high-quality social relationships (e.g., Harris et al., 1990; McLeod, 1991; O'Connor et al., 1999; Ross & Mirowsky, 1999; Shaw & Krause, 2002) which, in turn, increase vulnerability to mental health problems. Another pathway is between childhood adversities and higher exposure to stressful life events during adulthood (e.g., Horwitz et al., 2001; O'Connor et al., 1999). The mechanisms by which early stress produces high levels of stress decades later remain unidentified, but the relationship is a strong one.

It should be noted that appropriate resources can short-circuit the relationships between early adversities and later mental health problems. The potential negative effects of parental divorce, for example, can be prevented if parent-child relationships remain good after the divorce, if the child receives adequate parental supervision, and if the custodial parent is not severely economically deprived (e.g., Harris et al, 1990; Landerman et al., 1991).

Research on the persisting effects of childhood traumas reviewed thus far focused on the "main effects" or "direct effects" of early adversities on subsequent mental health. There is another way in which childhood traumas operate to increase the risk of mental health problems later in life. Several investigators report that severe childhood stressors interact with recent life stress to multiplicatively increase the likelihood of psychiatric symptoms and disorders (Kraaij & Wilde, 2001; Landerman et al., 1991; O'Neil, Lancee, & Freeman, 1987). In a related but distinct vein, Davies, Avison, and McAlpine (1997) found that higher rates of depression among single mothers than married mothers were partially explained by single mothers' higher levels of childhood adversity. These results suggest that the early experience of severe stress may create a lifelong vulnerability to stress, such that lower levels of adult stress will trigger mental health problems.

Adult Traumas. Traumas experienced after childhood also can be potent risk factors for mental health problems both immediately after the trauma and many years later. The most frequently studied adult trauma is combat exposure during war. By now, veterans of three major wars have been studied over varying lengths of time: World War II, Korea, and Vietnam. There is strong and consistent evidence linking combat exposure to subsequent mental health problems, including PTSD, depression, anxiety, and substance abuse problems (Clipp et al., 1992; Cui & Vaillant, 1996; Elder et al., 1994; Kulka, Schlenger, Fairbank, Hough, Jordan, Marmar, & Weiss, 1990; Lee et al., 1995). Moreover, the increased risk of mental health problems among combat veterans remains as much as 50–60 years later.

Pathways between combat exposure and subsequent mental health problems have been identified. Conditions after discharge from the military are consequential. Veterans who are able to find employment quickly, who obtain higher status jobs, and who marry adjust more quickly to civilian life and are at lower risk of mental health problems (e.g., Elder et al., 1994; Kulka et al., 1990). In addition, the accumulation of social resources over time lessens the risk mental distress and disorder during the decades following combat exposure. In addition to social bonds with family and friends, Elder and Clipp (1988) report that continued postwar contact with the "comrades" with whom combat was shared also decreases the risk of postwar mental illness. There also is evidence of "selection effects:" men who experienced mental health problems prior to combat exposure were at especially high risk of psychiatric symptoms and disorder both immediately after the war and decades later (Elder et al., 1994; Lee et al., 1995). Other selection effects influence risk of combat exposure. Men with lower levels of education and with pre-existing psychiatric symptoms and/or adjustment problems were more likely than their advantaged peers to experience combat. Thus, men with the fewest resources with which to cope with combat trauma were the most likely to experience it.

It should be noted that military experience also brought life course advantages to some veterans. In particular, men for whom military service interrupted long-term patterns of deviance (Laub & Sampson, 2005) and those who took advantage of the GI Bill to obtain higher education that was otherwise unavailable to them (Elder et al., 1994; Laub & Sampson, 2005) experienced fewer psychiatric problems than men who did not use their military experience to accumulate economic and social resources. Note, however, that all veterans, whether or not they were exposed to combat, were eligible for the GI Bill. The proportion of veterans who reaped advantages from military service and also experienced combat is unknown.

Stress Accumulation. Recently, the conceptualization and measurement of stress has broadened beyond stressful life events and chronic stressors to incorporate the individual's stress history. Cumulative stress or adversity (Turner & Lloyd, 1995), lifetime history of stress (Wheaton, 1996), and operant stress (Turner & Avison, 1992) all broaden the scope of stress measurement and include major lifetime traumas regardless of their recency. These more comprehensive stress measures are (a) more strongly related to mental health outcomes and (b) better able to explain status differences in mental health problems than are measures restricted to the present and recent past (e.g., Turner & Avison, 2003; Turner & Lloyd, 1999). Note, however, that summing lifetime traumas does not permit fine-grained analyses of the impact of timing, sequencing, and other specific temporal patterns.

Another method of assessing stress accumulation is to use growth curve models to examine the effects of "growth" of stress over time on the "growth" of mental health problems. In previous studies, Scott Lynch and I were able to demonstrate that (a) growth in loss-related stressors predicted growth in depressive symptoms in a sample of older adults (Lynch & George, 2000), (b) that the usual social factors used as controls in stress research (e.g., SES, demographic characteristics) predicted baseline levels of stress and depression but did not predict growth in either (George & Lynch, 2003; Lynch & George, 2000), and (c) that African Americans reported greater levels of growth in both stress and depression than whites (George & Lynch, 2003). We also discuss the implications of using growth curve models for reframing the issue of the differential effects of stress exposure and stress vulnerability.

Stress accumulation also is an ideal site for the cross-fertilization of mental health theory and life course perspectives. The concept of cumulative stress or adversity is highly compatible with the theory of cumulative advantage/disadvantage, which has become a staple of life course research (e.g., Dannefer, 2003; O'Rand, 2002). Overall, the stress paradigm has proven to be an especially useful and straightforward theoretical framework for incorporating life course principles.

Life Course Milestones and Turning Points

Most of the statistical techniques used in the social and behavioral sciences estimate the linear relationships between variables. These techniques often accurately model hypothesized relationships (e.g., a "dose-response" relationship between stress and depression). But not all research questions imply linear relationships and caution is needed to insure that linear models are not estimated in a pro forma way.

Some individuals experience events or conditions that are milestones or turning points in the life course. Conceptually this implies that certain events or conditions literally change the direction of life course pathways (Nagin, Pagani, Tremblay, & Vitaro, 2003; Ronka, Oravala, & Pulkkinen, 2003). Statistically, milestones and turning points are observed as deflections which change either the direction or rate of change in trajectories (Haviland & Nagin, 2005; Seidman & French, 2004).

Mental health problems experienced early in the life course can be milestones or turning points, resulting in a variety of alterations in the life course. This is another topic for which dichotomous measures of mental illness are especially salient. A milestone implies a discrete change in status or direction. The only way to study mental illness as a life course milestone is to identify the times at which individuals transition into mental illness and trace subsequent alterations in their lives. Two primary types of turning points have been studied to date.

The Consequences of Early Mental Illness for Adult Achievements. There is substantial evidence that mental health problems during childhood, adolescence, and/or early adulthood are associated with poor social and economic achievements in later adulthood. Early onset mental health problems predict lower educational attainment (e.g., Chen & Kaplan, 2003; Gore & Aseltine, 2003; Woodward & Fergusson, 2001) and lower occupational status and income (Chen & Kaplan, 2003; Wiesner, Vondracek, Capuldi, & Porfeli, 2003). Adult social bonds also are negatively affected; early onset psychiatric disorder predicts decreased likelihood of marriage, especially for persons with psychotic disorders (e.g., Walkup & Gallagher, 1999); earlier age of marriage for persons with affective and substance abuse disorders (e.g. Forthhofer, Kessler, Story, & Gottlib, 1996), earlier parenthood (e.g., Woodward & Fergusson, 2001), and higher rates of divorce (e.g., Wade & Pevalin, 2004).

The findings cited above are primarily from longitudinal studies that followed samples from adolescence through early to mid-adulthood. Although important, these studies cannot inform us about whether later onset of mental illness has similar effects on life course accomplishments. Logically, earlier onset would be more likely to decrease later achievements because both socioeconomic achievements, especially educational attainment, and family formation are typically established during young adulthood. Turnbull and colleagues compared individuals who experienced early (age 25 and younger) and later (age 26 and older) onset. They found that SES and family characteristics among those with late onset were no different from age peers who had no history of psychiatric disorder. Those with early onset, however, had significantly lower levels of SES and poorer family outcomes than their age peers who had no history of psychiatric disorder (Turnbull, George, Landerman, Swartz, & Blazer, 1990). Freud is credited with saying that the major tasks of adulthood are to love and to work. Clearly, early onset of mental health problems places successful fulfillment of those tasks at risk and can be a turning point in the life course.

The Consequences of Early Mental Illness for Adult Mental Health. Early onset of mental health problems also is a powerful predictor of recurrent mental health problems throughout adulthood. For example, Woodward and Fergusson (2001) report that anxiety disorder during adolescence is the strongest predictor of anxiety disorder in early adulthood. Similarly, Kim-Cohen and colleagues (Kim-Cohen, Caspi, Moffitt, Harrington, Milne, & Poulton, 2003), using data from a 15 year longitudinal study, report that 75% of the adults who experienced psychiatric disorders had also experienced mental illness as adolescents. Using data from the long-term study of Harvard undergraduate men, Vaillant and colleagues report that depression and excessive alcohol use during young adulthood are associated with increased risk of depression at ages 47 (Long & Vaillant, 1985) and 65 (Vaillant & Vaillant, 1990).

Delinquency during adolescence also increases the risk of multiple psychiatric disorders during adulthood. Using data from a sample of British women who were followed from birth though age 52, Kuh, Hardy, Rodgers, and Wadsworth (2002) report that adolescent delinquency predicted major depressive disorder in middle age. Similarly, Hagan and Foster (2003) report strong associations between adolescent delinquency and adult depression for both men and women and alcoholism for men. In both studies, the effects of juvenile delinquency were estimated with a wide variety of other predictors of mental health problems statistically controlled (e.g., educational attainment, adult SES, marital status). These authors posit that juvenile delinquency is a stronger predictor of depression and substance abuse than of antisocial personality, suggesting that what is called "conduct disorder" in psychiatric nomenclature is a generalized risk factor for a variety of mental health problems during adulthood.

There are undoubtedly multiple reasons for the strong relationships between early and later psychiatric problems. Genetics may play a role, although the often-observed shift from juvenile delinquency to affective or substance use disorders during adulthood seems to contradict the theory that specific genes lead to family histories of specific disorders. Unmeasured social factors may partially account for the strength of these associations. Obvious social risk factors (e.g., SES, demographic characteristics) have been controlled in the studies cited above, but those risk factors were measured at a single point. It is possible that more fine-grained patterns of change and stability would partially explain the pathways from early to subsequent mental health problems. Other scholars hypothesize that both early onset psychiatric problems and other adversities experienced early in life change brain anatomy and chemistry in ways that sustain vulnerability to mental health problems over time (e.g., Schulenberg, Sameroff, & Cicchetti, 2004).

It also is important to recognize that early adjustment problems, especially juvenile delinquency, often do not lead to mental health problems during adulthood. Two studies demonstrate this particularly well. In a series of research papers (e.g., Laub, Nagin, & Sampson, 1998; Sampson & Laub, 1990) and a book (Laub & Sampson, 2003) based on a sample of delinquent males born in the 1920s who were studied intermittently until age 70, Sampson and Laub demonstrate that the accumulation of social resources, especially stable jobs and supportive marriages, inhibit adult crime, psychiatric symptoms, and substance abuse/dependence. Long and Vaillant (1985) studied a sample of inner-city men from the time they were children until they were age 47. During childhood, boys from unstable homes exhibited substantially higher rates of delinquent behavior and psychiatric symptoms than boys in stable homes. By age 47, however, psychiatric and substance use symptoms were unrelated to childhood family stability. Both studies were based on high-risk samples where elevated rates of psychiatric problems during adulthood would be expected as a result of socioeconomic deprivations and high rates of delinquency. In both samples, however, surprisingly high proportions of study participants were able to overcome their early adversities and be productive and healthy adults. Thus, multiple trajectories describe both samples, with some pathways associated with continued psychiatric vulnerability during adulthood and other pathways demonstrating impressive resilience. Although early onset of psychiatric problems is a far from perfect predictor of mental health problems later in the life course, it is clear that early onset can be a milestone or turning point associated with chronic or recurrent psychiatric problems across adulthood.

The cross-fertilization of life course perspectives and the sociology of mental health is ripe for furthering our understanding of the conditions under which mental illness does and does not become a life course milestone. Although life course perspectives assume a link between past and current statuses, mental health theory informs us about the most likely pathways linking early mental illness to later achievements and mental health.

The Dynamics of Recovery and Recurrence of Mental Illness

Social scientists have paid little attention to the role of social factors in recovery from and recurrence of psychiatric disorder. A primary reason for this is that, as described above, recovery and recurrence necessitate conceptualizing mental health problems in terms of discrete categories representing the presence or absence of illness. Nonetheless, two social factors are strongly implicated in patterns of recovery from and recurrence of psychiatric disorders.

Most research examining recovery and recurrence of mental illness has focused on major depressive disorder (MDD). MDD is largely a chronic or episodic disease. Some individuals experience a single episode of MDD, recover, and never experience a recurrence, but this is rare – and is especially rare in the absence of sustaining a maintenance level of psychotropic medication (Geddes, Carney, Davies, Furuhawa, Kupfer, Frank, & Goodwin, 2003). Recovery from MDD exhibits a clear pattern of duration dependence. Specifically, for approximately one year after the onset of MDD, the odds of recovery increase. After a year, the odds of recovery steadily decrease, signaling a pattern of chronic depressive disorder. Evidence is quite consistent: 50% or fewer of MDD patients will recover within a year (e.g., Bosworth, Hays, George, & Steffens, 2002; Keller, Shapiro, & Lavori, 1982). Most people who recover from MDD will experience a recurrence. Recurrence also exhibits a pattern of duration dependence, although it is more variable than the pattern for recovery. Research evidence suggests that between one-third and one-half of recovered MDD patients will experience recurrence within two years and fully 85% will experience recurrence within 15 years (Mueller, Leon, Keller, Solomon, Endicott, Coryell, Warshaw, & Maser, 1999).

Two issues merit mention at this point. First, the vast majority of studies examining recovery from and recurrence of MDD are based on clinical samples. But evidence suggests that only about half of the people who experience MDD receive treatment for it (e.g., Kessler et al., 1994). Recovery rates in the three community-based studies available are generally consistent with those reported in clinical samples (Honkalampi, Hintikka, Haatainer, Koivamma-Honkanen, Tanshanen, & Vinamaki, 2005; McLeod, Kessler, & Landis, 1992; Pevalin & Goldberg, 2003). Recurrence rates were examined in two of these studies and varied widely Honkalampi et al., 2005; Pevaline & Goldberg, 2003). Overall, however, almost all that is known about the "natural history" of MDD is based on clinical samples and may not apply to untreated cases.

Second, most studies of the course and outcome of MDD (and other psychiatric disorders) cover relatively short periods of time (from 6 months to four years), although a few studies are based on data covering decades. The question arises: Should relatively short-term studies of recovery and recurrence be viewed as life course research? Technically, of course, the answer is no. Because both complex temporal processes and the effects of social factors are so prominent, however, these studies demonstrate much of the logic of life course research despite their shorter than desirable time frames.

The Role of Social Support in Recovery and Recurrence

George and colleagues were among the first to demonstrate that social support is a potent predictor of recovery from MDD in a clinical sample (George, Blazer, Hughes, & Fowler, 1989). Since then, a myriad of clinical studies, in the U.S. and other countries, and covering intervals ranging from three months to five years have reported that high levels of social support predict higher odds of recovery from MDD and shorter time until recovery (e.g., Bosworth et al., 2002; Bosworth, McQuoid, George, & Steffens, 2002; Lara, Leader, & Klein, 1997; Nasser & Overholser, 2005; Steffens, Pieper, Bosworth, MacFall, Provenzale, Payne, Carroll, George, & Krishnan, 2005). Social support also increased the odds of recovery from MDD in three community studies: a British study spanning 8 years (Pevalin & Goldberg, 2003), a one-year U.S. study (McLeod et al., 1992, and a two-year longitudinal study of women in New Zealand (Honkalampi et al., 2005).

Social support is a multidimensional construct and there are multiple conceptualizations of its relevant dimensions. Most investigators, however, concur that two major dimensions are perceived social support and instrumental support. Perceived social support refers to the individual's subjective assessment of the adequacy of the quantity and quality of support available. Instrumental support refers to tangible (e.g., help with shopping or housework) and intangible (e.g., provision of advice) forms of assistance received from family and friends. Research on the role of social support in recovery from MDD consistently finds that perceived social support has the strongest effects on recovery (e.g., George et al., 1989; Lara et al., 1997; Nasser & Overholser, 2005; Steffens et al., 2005) results for instrumental support are mixed (e.g., George et al., 1989; Hays, Steffens, Flint, Bosworth, & George, 2001).

The strong relationships between perceived social support and recovery from MDD pose a methodological challenge. The general assumption is that social support is independent of MDD and, thus, is a resource that facilitates recovery. An alternate hypothesis, however, is that depression causes negative perceptions of life in general and social support in particular, confounding the two phenomena. A number of studies tackled this issue directly, using a variety of methods including time series analysis and patterns of interaction (Blazer & Hughes, 1991; George et al., 1989; Steffens et al., 2005). Results indicate that perceived social support is distinct from depressive cognitions, permitting confident conclusions that high levels of perceived social support facilitate recovery from MDD.

It is reasonable to hypothesize that loss of or reductions in social support might also predict recurrence of MDD. Unfortunately, I am aware of no studies that have tested this hypothesis—largely, I suspect, because loss of significant others is studied as a stressor rather than as a loss of social support. This is an important topic for future research, in part because there is some evidence that chronic and recurrent depression leads, over time, to reductions in social support from family and friends (e.g., Holmes-Eber & Riger, 1990).

Another neglected dimension of the effects of social relationships on recovery and recurrence of MDD and other psychiatric disorders is conflict and negative interactions with significant others. Negative interactions with significant others are significant predictors of a variety of health outcomes in non-clinical studies: physical symptoms (Edwards, Hershberger, Russell, & Markert, 2001), incidence of the common cold (Cohen, 2004), subjective well-being (Rook, 1984), psychological distress (Newsom, Rook, Nishishiba, Sorkin, & Mahan, 2005), and depressive symptoms (Krause & Rook, 2003). I am aware of only one study, however, that examined the effects of negative social interaction on recovery from MDD. McLeod and colleagues (1992) found that both conflicted relationships with friends and negative reactions from one's spouse significantly increased time to recovery from MDD. In a similar vein, George et al. (1989) found that perceived social support was a strong predictor of recovery from MDD, but married MDD patients were less likely to recover than unmarried patients. We speculated that the marriages of depressed patients were more a source of stress than of support.

Sociologists who study mental health have much to offer to our understanding of the factors associated with recovery and recurrence of mental illness. The sociology of mental health offers a broad range of potential risk and protective factors that have not yet been adequately examined in relation to the dynamics of mental illness. Because the "natural history" of MDD and other psychiatric disorders spans long periods of time, life course principles also should be incorporated. This important opportunity for cross-fertilization will remain unfulfilled, however, unless sociologists are willing to employ dichotomous measures of being "in" and "out" of illness episodes.

The Role of Stress in Recovery and Recurrence

Research evidence concerning the role of stress in recovery from and recurrence of MDD is inconsistent. I am aware of only two studies in which stressful life events were observed to delay recovery from MDD. Bosworth and colleagues followed patients with coronary artery disease for a year. They report that stressful life events over that interval predicted both the onset of MDD and decreased rates of recovery among those with MDD (Bosworth, Steffens, Kuchibhatla, Jiang, Arias, O'Connor, & Krishnan, 2000). Similarly, Pevalin and Goldberg (2003) reported that, over 8 years, stressful life events reduced the odds of recovery from MDD in their British community-based study. In contrast, George and colleagues (1989) report that negative life events were unrelated to the odds of recovery in their clinical sample. Clearly this issue merits additional research.

Research on the role of stressors (typically stressful life events) in recurrence of MDD has sparked considerable controversy. First, evidence has been mixed, with some studies reporting that stress significantly increases the likelihood of recurrence (e.g., Daley, Hammen, & Rao, 2000; Frank, Tu, Anderson, & Reynolds, 1996), and other studies reporting no significant relationship between stressors and recurrence (e.g., Kendler, Thornton, & Gardner, 2000; Lewinsohn, Allen, Seeley, & Gotlib, 1999).

Additional complexities emerge when investigators examine whether stress is *differentially important* for the onset of first vs. recurrent episodes. Recently, the "kindling hypothesis," which had been observed in neurological investigations, primarily animal studies, caught the attention of psychiatrists and psychologists (Post, 1992). In essence, the kindling hypothesis posits that powerful predictors of the onset of a chronic or episodic illness will be less potent predictors of recurrences and/or increasing severity of illness (Hlastala, Frank, Kowalski, Sherrill, Tu, et al.,

2000; Segal, Williams, Teasdale, & Gemar, 1996). A couple dozen studies have examined whether the relationship between stress and depression exhibits a kindling pattern – that is, whether stress is a more powerful predictor of first-episode MDD than of recurrences of MDD. Most studies are between-persons designs in which risk factors are compared across groups of first-episode and recurrent-episode MDD patients. Kendler and colleagues, however, followed nearly 2,400 female twin pairs for nine years and were able to perform within-person analyses of first and recurrent episodes of MDD (Kendler et al., 2000) – indeed, they observed as many as nine recurrences. Regardless of research design, findings demonstrate that stressors are stronger predictors of first-episode MDD than of recurrent MDD (see Mazure, 1998 and, especially, Monroe & Harkness, 2005, for superb reviews).

Given the consistency of findings, controversy about the kindling hypothesis is not based on empirical evidence; rather, it is interpretation of the findings that is disputed. In essence, two positions have emerged. One group of scholars interprets the weaker effects of stress on recurrent than first-episode MDD as evidence that major depression usually originates (i.e., first episode) when external demands overwhelm the instrumental, cognitive, and affective capacities of the individual. Recurrent episodes, in contrast, are generally triggered by internal dysfunction. In essence, over time, MDD becomes a more autonomous and self-starting disease (e.g., Farmer, Harris, Redman, Sadler, Mahmood, & McGuffin, 2000; Kendler et al., 2000; Lewinsohn et al., 1999). Monroe and Harkness (2005) label this the *stress autonomy model*. Another group of investigators interpret the evidence much differently, hypothesizing that individuals become more vulnerable to recurrence with increasing numbers of previous episodes. They interpret the weaker associations between stress and recurrent as compared to first-episode depression as evidence that, as recurrences cumulate, lower levels of stress are required to trigger recurrence (e.g., Brilman & Ormel, 2001; Hammen, Henry, & Daley, 2000). Monroe and Harkness term this the *stress sensitization model*. It is interesting to note that the authors of both systematic reviews of the kindling hypothesis and MDD favor the stress sensitization model, although they also acknowledge that research to date cannot adjudicate between the two models (Mazure, 1998; Monroe & Harkness, 2005).

Two implications of the kindling hypothesis debate are especially relevant. First, the question of whether individuals become increasingly sensitive to lower levels of stress over time is a life course question. Social scientists are already working with concepts such as cumulative stress to estimate the effects of lifetime stress on mental health. It also would be useful to determine whether, as stress cumulates over the life course, less severe forms of stress are sufficient to trigger mental distress and/or illness. Evidence generated by studies that had nothing to do with stress sensitization is compatible with that interpretation. Both the often-observed (a) persisting effects of early traumas and (b) interactive effects of childhood traumas and recent stress on adult mental health may reflect stress sensitizing processes. Second, most research on the kindling hypothesis is based on clinical samples and/or between-persons designs. Studies based on representative community-based samples and that follow the same individuals for long periods of time are needed to produce stronger evidence. Addressing this issue through the integration of stress theory and life course principles would shed new light on the kindling hypothesis.

Linked Lives: Intergenerational Transmission of Mental Health Problems

The concept of linked lives reminds us that mental health is a function of not only personal assets and liabilities, but also the nature and quality of our connections to significant others. The powerful role of social support has been described in other sections of this chapter. This section focuses on another facet of linked lives: evidence about the intergenerational transmission of mental illness. Genetic determinants of mental illness are beyond the scope of this review; rather, the emphasis here is on the extent to which the children of mentally ill parents exhibit mental health problems and what is known about the pathways by which transmission of mental health problems across generations occurs.

Evidence for the Intergenerational Transmission of Mental Health Problems

Evidence that mental illness is reproduced across familial generations is both plentiful and consistent (Downey & Coyne, 1990; Goodman & Gotlib, 1999). This evidence rests on two research designs: cross-sectional studies that compare rates of mental health problems among the offspring of mentally ill and non-mentally ill parents and longitudinal studies that follow both parents and children over time. The latter, of course, are methodologically superior – not only because changes in psychiatric symptoms and disorders can be traced over time, but also because the effects of children's length of exposure to parental mental illness can be measured.

Children's mental health has been measured in terms of psychiatric disorder and behavioral problems. The primary determinant of the measurement approach used is the age of the children. Standard psychiatric diagnostic systems are feasible for adolescents and young adults. For younger children, behavioral problems are better indicators of adjustment (Goodman & Gotlib, 1999).

Although both mothers and fathers have the potential to transmit mental health problems to their offspring, (non-genetic) research to date has focused virtually exclusively on mothers. Few investigators offer a rationale for restricting the parental generation to mothers, but it is apparently assumed that mothers interact more with their children, are more likely to co-reside with their children, and have closer relationships with their children than fathers. Type of maternal psychiatric disorder might be expected to affect the likelihood of intergenerational transmission, but the vast majority of studies to date focus on mothers suffering from affective disorders in general and either depression or anxiety disorder in particular.

Evidence to date documents strong relationships between mothers' mental illness and mental health problems among their children (e.g., Andrews, Brown, & Creasey, 1990; Bifulco, Moran, Ball, Jacobs, Baines, Bunn, & Cavagin, 2002; Ellenbogen & Hodgins, 2004; Hammen, Brennan, & Shih, 2004). Indeed, I could not locate any study that failed to report a significant relationship between mothers' and children's mental health. In arguably the best study to date, which followed mentally ill and non-mentally ill mothers and their children for 10 years (until the children were in their late teens or early adulthood), the children of mentally ill mothers were four times more likely than the children of non-mentally ill mothers to qualify for a diagnosis of affective disorder (Bifulco et al., 2002).

Pathways from Mothers' to Children's Mental Health

Most investigators take the position that mothers' mental health *per se* cannot account for the observed patterns of intergenerational transmission. Instead, there must be pathways or mechanisms by which mental health problems traverse generations. Moreover, mentally ill mothers differ from non-mentally ill mothers in numerous ways, necessitating that intergenerational transmission be examined with a broad range of variables statistically controlled (e.g., SES, maternal marital status). Some investigators report identifying the pathways by which maternal mental illness reproduces mental health problems in their children. For example, Bifulco and colleagues (2002) report that the effects of maternal major depressive disorder on their adolescent/young adult children's mental health were totally mediated by childhood abuse and/or neglect. More commonly, partial mediating effects are reported – e.g., Hammen, Shih, and Brennan (2004) reported that most of the relationship between mothers' MDD and depression in their offspring was mediated by children's interpersonal distress (poor relationships with both peers and family members). Similarly, Ellenbogen and Hodgins (2004) report that poor parenting mediated most of the relationship between maternal MDD and their children's behavior problems. In contrast, Andrews and colleagues (1990), in a study of depressed mothers and their young adult daughters, report that maternal depression, poor parenting by the mother, and abuse/neglect of the children were independent predictors of MDD among the daughters.

It also appears that maternal mental illness can interact with a variety of factors to affect the odds of children's mental health problems. Hammen, Brennan, and Shih (2004), for example, report that maternal depression had only modest direct effects on children's depression, but that the interaction of family discord and maternal depression greatly increased the likelihood of MDD among children (the direct effects of family discord also were modest). In a somewhat different vein, Brennan, Le Brocque, & Hammen (2003) examined the interactive effects of maternal depression on children's MDD in an attempt to understand the conditions under which maternal depression did *not* increase the risk of their children's depression. They identified three factors that interacted with maternal depression to *protect* their children from depressive disorder: the mother exerted low levels of parental control, high maternal warmth, and low levels of maternal over-involvement with her children.

Much remains to be learned about the conditions under which parental mental illness—both mothers' and fathers'—reproduce mental health problems in their children. Research to date has not been fine-grained—for example, I was unable to locate any studies that determined whether the effects of maternal depression differed for sons and daughters. Applying a life course perspective to this issue also raises a myriad of questions. Two obvious examples are: To what extent do duration and severity of parental mental illness affect their children's mental health? Once children leave the parental home, do the negative effects of parental mental illness dissipate or is parental mental illness a form of childhood trauma that persists across the children's life course?

Looking to the Future

Several years ago, I wrote my first (and only other) review of what life course perspectives offer the sociological study of mental health and mental illness. At that time, I stated, "Of necessity, discussion will focus more on the *potential* of life course perspectives to inform us about the antecedents and consequences of mental health than about its demonstrated utility" (George, 1999, p. 565). Since then, the volume and quality of life course research on mental health and illness has increased dramatically. Approximately half of the research cited in this review was published in 2000 or later. This research did not exist when I first reviewed this topic and speaks to the increased cross-fertilization of the sociology of mental health and life course perspectives.

Despite the very real gains in applying life course principles to issues concerning mental distress and disorder, many important issues remain unaddressed or under-addressed. I have attempted to identify issues that merit attention in future research throughout this chapter. In this section, I address two issues that I believe are critical to future incorporation of life course principles into social research on mental illness.

Enhancing Data Collection

The ideal research design for life course studies is of course longitudinal data that spans decades. A few studies meet or almost live up to this ideal and others will undoubtedly do so in the future. There are, however, relatively inexpensive ways that studies spanning briefer periods of time could collect data that enhance their appropriateness for life course research.

As described above, techniques that increase our ability to collect reliable and valid retrospective data (e.g., life history calendars) are now available. To the extent possible, the field should incorporate retrospective histories of important domains of life experience. Examples of potentially important personal histories that can be collected include occupational histories, marital histories, military histories, medical histories, and histories of religious and organizational involvement. Mental health researchers have already demonstrated the ability to collect data about early traumas/adversities and major lifetime stresses—and demonstrated that these temporally-expanded measures of stress contribute to current mental health. Many research topics in the sociology of mental health have the potential to be better understood by combining retrospective and contemporaneous data.

Another method of enhancing the ability to perform fine-grained analyses of temporal issues related to mental health is to ask research participants to date the occurrence of relevant changes in their lives. The typical panel study has intervals ranging from 2–5 years between measurements. Participants' lives can change in numerous ways between measurements – and investigators often desire to examine how those changes affect outcomes of interest. Simply asking participants exactly when these changes occurred opens the door to a set of analysis techniques that permit temporal analyses otherwise not possible.

In short, the field will be advanced if investigators pay more attention to issues of timing and are more attentive to including temporal issues in their research designs.

The Need to Study Both Psychiatric Symptoms and Psychiatric Disorders

Throughout this chapter, I have noted important research topics in the sociology of mental illness that cannot be addressed unless investigators are willing to investigate dichotomous measures of mental illness as well as continuous measures of psychiatric symptoms. In my final comments, I will make a last plea for the study of mental illnesses as defined in psychiatric nomenclature and which can be ascertained using structured interviews.

The sociological study of specific mental illnesses is important for both scientific and policy reasons. Scientifically, failure to study psychiatric disorders results in a poorer sociological understanding of human lives. Research to date suggests that the same social factors that generate milder forms of distress also predict the onset of mental illnesses. Beyond those similarities, however, are a range of social consequences that are unique to mental illness. Although milder forms of distress have negative consequences, the consequences of mental illness can be devastating. Stigma is an issue for people who experience recurrent episodes of mental illness, with symptoms that often preclude self-care, let alone living up to their work and family responsibilities; it is not an issue for psychological distress. A mild, temporary increase in distress is more prevalent among the population than the onset of a psychiatric disorder, but it is the latter that has the potential to truncate educational and occupational achievements, to tear families apart, and to place individuals' children at risk of reproducing the same dysfunctional syndromes. Social rejection, downward social mobility, and family dissolution – these are issues of primary interest to social scientists. These issues are affected by mental illness, not mild levels of distress.

Social scientists also need to understand that policy makers and practitioners are interested in what they can contribute to knowledge about preventing, identifying, and treating mental illnesses. They are not interested in results showing that a social factor increases average scores on a psychiatric symptom scale two-thirds of a standard deviation. Mental health professionals are interested in what we can contribute to their understanding of individuals suffering large number of symptoms that severely compromise their ability to function. They are interested in the social antecedents and the social consequences of mental illness. And we have much to offer them.

I am not suggesting that social scientists adopt psychiatric nomenclature in a thoughtless way. Nor am I advocating that social scientists throw out continuous measures of psychological distress or symptoms. I am arguing for an eclectic approach in which, depending on the research questions and the intended audience, psychiatric disorder, psychological distress, or both are acceptable tools of the trade.

The cross-fertilization of the sociology of mental illness and life course principles is alive and well, with great opportunities for continuing contributions. If social scientists are willing to study psychiatric disorder, as well as psychological distress, much will be learned about the social antecedents and consequences of mental illness and the profound effects of mental illness, not only in the present, but also in the long term. If social scientists are willing to study long-term patterns of social resources and deficits, much will be learned about their cumulative and dynamic effects. These seem to be tasks worthy of our efforts.

References

Alwin, D. F., Hofer, S. M., & McCammon, R. J. (2006). Modeling the effects of time: Integrating demographic and developmental perspectives. In R. H. Binstock & L. K. George (Eds.), *Handbook of Aging and the Social Sciences* (sixth edition). (pp. 20–38). San Diego: Academic Press.

Andrews, B., Brown, G. W., & Creasey, L. (1990). Intergenerational links between psychiatric disorder in mothers and daughters: The role of parenting experiences. *Journal of Child Psychology and Psychiatry, 31*, 1115–1129.

Bifulco, A., Moran, P. M., Ball, C., Jacobs, C., Baines R., Bunn, A., & Cavagin, J. (2002). Childhood adversity, parental vulnerability, and disorder: Examining inter-generational transmission of risk. *Journal of Child Psychology and Psychiatry and Allied Disciplines, 43*, 1075–1086.

Blazer, D. G., & Hughes, D. C. (1991). Subjective social support and depressive symptoms in major depression: Separate phenomena or epiphenomena? *Journal of Psychiatric Research, 25*, 191–203.

Bosworth, H. B., Hays, J. C., George, L. K., & Steffens, D. C. (2002). Psychosocial and clinical predictors of unipolar depression outcome in older adults. *International Journal of Geriatric Psychiatry, 17*, 238–246.

Bosworth, H. B., McQuoid, D. R., George, L. K., & Steffens, D. C. (2002). Time-to-remission from geriatric depression: Psychosocial and clinical factors. *American Journal of Geriatric Psychiatry, 10*, 551–559.

Bosworth, H. B., Steffens, D. C., Kuchibhatla, M. N., Jiang, W. J., Arias, R. M. O'Connor, C. M., & Krishnan, K. R. K. (2000). The relationship of social support, social networks, and negative events with depression in patients with coronary artery disease. *Aging and Mental Health, 4*, 253–258.

Brennan, P. A., Le Brocque, R., & Hammen, C. (2003). Maternal depression, parent-child relationships, and resilient outcomes in adolescence. *Journal of the American Academy of Child and Adolescent Psychiatry, 42*, 1469–1477.

Brilman, E. L., & Ornel, J. (2001). Life events, difficulties and onset of depressive episodes in later life. *Psychological Medicine, 31*, 859–869.

Chen, Z. Y., & Kaplan, H. B. (2003). School failure in early adolescence and status attainment in middle adulthood: A longitudinal study. *Sociology of Education, 76*, 110–127.

Cherlin, A. J., Chase-Lansdale, P. L., & McRae, C. (1998). Effects of parental divorce on mental health throughout the life course. *American Sociological Review, 63*, 239–249.

Clipp, E. C., Pavalko, E. K., & Elder, G. H., Jr. (1992). Trajectories of health: In concept and empirical pattern. *Behavior, Health, and Aging, 2*, 159–179.

Cohen, S. (2004). Social relationships and health. *American Psychologist, 59*, 575–684.

Cui, X., & Vaillant, G. E. (1996). Antecedents and consequences of negative life events in adulthood: A longitudinal study. *American Journal of Psychiatry, 153*, 21–26.

Daley, S. E., Hammen, C., & Rao, U. (2000). Predictors of first onset and recurrence of major depression in young women during the 5 years following high school graduation. *Journal of Abnormal Psychology, 109*, 525–533.

Dannefer, D. (2003). Cumulative advantage/disadvantage and the life course: Cross-fertilizing age and social science theory. *Journal of Gerontology: Social Sciences, 58B*, S327–S337.

Davies, L., Avison, W. R., & McAlpine, D. D. (1997). Significant life experiences and depression among single and married mothers. *Journal of Marriage and the Family, 59*, 294–308.

Dooley, D., Prause, J., & Ham-Rowbottom, K. A. (2000). Underemployment and depression: Longitudinal relationships. *Journal of Health and Social Behavior, 41*, 421–436.

Downey, G. & Coyne, J. C. (1990). Children of depressed parents: An integrative review. *Psychological Bulletin, 108*, 50–76.

Edwards, K. J., Hershberger, P. J., Russell, R. K., & Markert, R. J. (2001). Stress, negative social exchange, and health symptoms in university students. *Journal of American College Health, 50*, 75–79.

Elder, G. H., Jr. (1974). *Children of the Great Depression.* Chicago: University of Chicago Press.

Elder, G. H., Jr. & Clipp, E. C. (1988). Wartime losses and social bonding: Influence across 40 years in men's lives. *Psychiatry, 51*, 177–198.

Elder, G. H., Jr., Johnson, M. K., & Crosnoe, R. (2003). The emergence and development of life course theory. In J. T. Mortimer & M. J. Shanahan (Eds.), *Handbook of the life course* (pp. 3–22). New York: Kluwer Academic/Plenum.

Elder, G. H. Jr., Shanahan, M. J., & Clipp, E. C. (1994). When war comes to men's lives: Life-course patterns in family, work, and health. *Psychology and Aging, 9*, 5–16.

Ellenbogen, M. A., & Hodgins, S. (2004). The impact of high neuroticism in parents on children's psychosocial functioning in a population at high risk for major affective disorder: A family-environmental pathway of intergenerational risk. *Development and Psychopathology, 16*, 113–136.

Farmer, A., Harris, T., Redman, K., Sadler, S., Mahmood, A., & McGuffin, P. (2000). Cardiff Depression Study: A sib-pair study of life events and familiarity in major depression. *British Journal of Psychiatry, 176*, 150–155.

Forthofer, M. S., Kessler, R. C., Story, A. L., & Gottlib, I. H. (1996). The effects of psychiatric disorders on the probability and timing of first marriage. *Journal of Health and Social Behavior, 37*, 121–132.

Frank, E., Tu, X. M., Anderson, B., & Reynolds, C. F. III. (1996). Effects of positive and negative life events on time to depression onset: An analysis of additivity and timing. *Psychological Medicine, 26*, 613–626.

Geddes, J. R., Carney, S. M., Davies, C., Furukawa, T. A., Kupfer, D. J., Frank, E., & Goodwin, G. M. (2003). Relapse prevention with antidepressant drug treatment in depressive disorders: A systematic review. *Lancet, 361*, 653–661.

George, L. K. (1999). Life course perspectives on mental health. In C. S. Aneshensel & J. C. Phelan (Eds.), *Handbook of the Sociology of Mental Health* (pp. 565–583). New York: Kluwer Academic/Plenum.

George, L. K. (2003). Life course research: Achievements and potential. In J. T. Mortimer & M. J. Shanahan (Eds.), *Handbook of the Life Course* (pp. 671–680). New York: Kluwer Academic/Plenum.

George, L. K., Blazer, D. G., Hughes, D. C., & Fowler, N. (1989). Social support and the outcome of major depression. *British Journal of Psychiatry, 154*, 478–485.

George, L. K. & Lynch, S. M. (2003). Race differences in depressive symptoms: A dynamic perspective on stress exposure and vulnerability. *Journal of Health and Social Behavior, 44*, 353–369.

Gilman, S. E., Kawachi, I., Fitzmaurice, G. M., & Buka, S. L. (2003). Socioeconomic status, family disruption, and residential stability in childhood: Relation to onset, recurrence, and remission of major depression. *Psychological Medicine, 33*, 1341–1355.

Goodman, S. & Gotlib, I. (1999). Risk for psychopathology in the children of depressed mothers: A developmental model for understanding mechanisms of transmission. *Psychological Bulletin, 117*, 458–490.

Gore, S., & Aseltine, R. H. (2003). Race and ethnic differences in depressed mood following the transition from high school. *Journal of Health and Social Behavior, 44*, 379–389.

Hagan, J., & Foster, H. (2003). S/he's a rebel: Toward a sequential stress theory of delinquency and gendered pathways to disadvantage in emerging adulthood. *Social Forces, 82*, 53–86.

Hallstrom, T. (1987). The relationship between childhood socioeconomic factors and early parental loss to major depression in adult life. *Acta Psyciatrica Scandinavica, 75*, 212–216.

Hammen, C., Brennan, P. A., & Shih, J. H. (2004). Family discord and stress predictors of depression and other disorders in adolescent children of depressed and non-depressed women. *Journal of the American Academy of Child and Adolescent Psychiatry, 43*, 994–1002.

Hammen, C., Henry, R., & Daley, S. E. (2000). Depression and sensitization to stressors among young women as a function of childhood adversity. *Journal of Consulting and Clinical Psychology, 68*, 782–787.

Hammen, C., Shih, J. H., & Brennan, P. A. (2004). Intergenerational transmission of depression: Test of an interpersonal stress model in a community sample. *Journal of Consulting and Clinical Psychology, 72*, 511–522.

Harris, T., Brown, G. W., & Bifulco, A. (1990). Loss of parent in childhood and adult psychiatric disorder: A tentative overall model. *Development and Psychopathology, 2*, 311–328.

Haviland, A. M. & Nagin, D. S. (2005). Causal inferences with group based trajectory models. *Psychometrika, 70*, 557–558.

Hays, J. C., Steffens, D. C., Flint, E. P., Bosworth, H. B., & George, L. K. (2001). Does social support buffer functional decline in elderly patients with unipolar depression? *American Journal of Psychiatry, 158*, 1850–1855.

Hlastala, S. A., Frank, E., Kowalski, J., Sherrill, J. T., Tu, X. M., Anderson, B., & Kupfer, D. J. (2000). Stressful life events, bipolar disorder, and the "kindling model." *Journal of Abnormal Psychology, 109*, 777–786.

Holmes-Eber, P., & Riger, S. (1990). Hospitalization and the composition of mental patients' social networks. *Schizophrenia Bulletin, 16*, 157–164.

Honkalampi, K., Hintikka, J., Haatainen, K., Kolvumaa-Honkanen, H., Tanskanen, A., & Vinamaki, H. (2005). Adverse childhood experiences, stressful life events, or demographic factors: Which are important in women's depression? A 2-year follow-up population study. *Australian and New Zealand Journal of Psychiatry, 39*, 627–632.

Horwitz, A. V., Widom, C. S., McLaughlin, J., & White, H. R. (2001). The impact of childhood abuse and neglect on adult mental health: A prospective study. *Journal of Health and Social Behavior, 42*, 184–201.

Johnson, T. P. (1991). Mental health, social relationships, and social selection: A longitudinal analysis. *Journal of Health and Social Behavior, 32*, 408–423.

Keller, M. B. Shapiro, R. W., & Lavori, P. W. (1982). Recovery in major depressive disorder: Analysis with life tables and regression models. *Archives of General Psychiatry, 39*, 905–910.

Kendler, K. S., Thornton, L. M., & Gardner, C. O. (2000). Stressful life events and previous episodes in the etiology of major depression in women: An evaluation of the "kindling" hypothesis. *American Journal of Psychiatry, 157*, 1243–1251.

Kessler, R. C. (2002). The categorical versus dimensional assessment controversy in the sociology of mental illness. *Journal of Health and Social Behavior, 43*, 125–142.

Kessler, R. C., & Magee, W. J. (1994). Childhood family violence and adult recurrent depression. *Journal of Health and Social Behavior, 35*, 13–27.

Kessler, R. C., McGonagle, K. W., Zhou, S., Nelson, C. B., Hughes, M., Eshleman, S., Wittchen, H. U., & Kendler, K. S. (1994). Lifetime and active prevalence of DSM-III psychiatric disorders in the United States: Results from the National Comorbidity Survey. *Archives of General Psychiatry, 51*, 8–19.

Kim-Cohen, J., Caspi, A., Moffitt, T. E., Harrington, H., Milne, B. J., & Poulton, R. (2003). Prior juvenile diagnoses in adults with mental disorder – Developmental follow-back of a progressive longitudinal cohort. *Archives of General Psychiatry, 60*, 709–717.

Kraaij, V., & Wilde, E. J. (2001). Negative life events and depressive symptoms in the elderly: A life span perspective. *Aging and Mental Health, 5*, 84–91.

Krause, N. & Rook, K. S. (2003). Negative interaction in late life: Issues in the stability and generalizability of conflict across relationships. *Journal of Gerontology: Psychological Sciences, 58B*, P88–P99.

Kuh, D., Hardy, B., Rodgers, B., & Wadsworth, M. E. J. (2002). Lifetime risk factors for women's psychological distress in midlife. *Social Science and Medicine, 55*, 1957–1973.

Kulka, R. A., Schlenger, W. E., Fairbank, J. A., Hough, R. L., Jordan, B. K., Marmar, C. R., & Weiss, D. S. (1990). *Trauma and the Vietnam War generation: Report of Findings from the National Vietnam Veterans Readjustment Study*. New York: Brunner/Mazel.

Landerman, R., George, L. K., & Blazer, D. G. (1991). Adult vulnerability for psychiatric disorders: Interactive effects of negative childhood experiences and recent stress. *Journal of Nervous and Mental Disease, 179*, 656–663.

Lara, M. E., Leader, J., & Klein, D. N. (1997). The association between social support and course of depression: Is it confounded with personality? *Journal of Abnormal Psychology, 106*, 478–482.

Laub, J. H., Nagin, D. S., & Sampson, R. J. (1998). Trajectories of change in criminal offending: Good marriages and the desistance process. *American Sociological Review, 63*, 225–238.

Laub, J. H., & Sampson, R. J. (2003). *Shared beginnings, divergent lives: Delinquent boys to age 70.* Cambridge, MA: Harvard University Press.

Laub, J. H., & Sampson, R. J. (2005). Coming of age in wartime: How World War II and the Korean War changed lives. In K. W. Schaie and G. H. Elder Jr., *Historical influences on lives and aging* (pp. 208–228). New York: Springer.

Lee, K. A., Vaillant, G. E., Torrey, W. C., & Elder, G. H. Jr. (1995). A 50-year prospective study of the psychological sequelae of World War II combat. *American Journal of Psychiatry, 152,* 516–522.

Lewinsohn, P. M., Allen, N. B., Seeley, J. R., & Gotlib, I. H. (1999). First onset versus recurrence of depression: Differential processes of psychosocial risk. *Journal of Abnormal Psychology, 108,* 483–489.

Long, J. V., & Vaillant, G. E. (1985). Natural history of male psychological health: XI: Escape from the underclass. *Annual Progress in Child Psychiatry and Child Development,* 159–170.

Lynch, S. M. & George, L. K. (2000). Interlocking trajectories of loss-related events and depressive symptoms among elders. *Journal of Gerontology: Social Sciences, 57B,* S117–S125.

Mazure, C. M. (1998). Life stressors as risk factors in depression. *Clinical Psychology: Science and Practice, 5,* 291–313.

McLeod, J. D. (1991). Childhood parental loss and adult depression. *Journal of Health and Social Behavior, 32,* 205–220.

McLeod, J. D., Kessler, R. C., & Landis, K. R. (1992). Speed of recovery from major depressive episode in a community sample of married men and women. *Journal of Abnormal Psychology, 101,* 277–286.

Mirowsky, J., & Ross, C. E. (1989). Psychiatric diagnosis as reified measurement. *Journal of Health and Social Behavior, 30,* 11–25.

Mirowsky, J., & Ross., C. E. (1992). Age and depression. *Journal of Health and Social Behavior, 33,* 187–205.

Monroe, S. M., & Harkness, K. L. (2005). Life stress, the "kindling" hypothesis, and the recurrence of depression: Considerations from a life stress perspective. *Psychological Review, 112,* 417–445.

Mueller, T. I., Leon, A. C., Keller, M. B., Solomon, D. A., Endicott, J., Coryell, W., Warshaw, M., & Maser, J. D. (1999). Recurrence after recovery from major depressive disorder during 15 years of observational follow-up. *American Journal of Psychiatry, 156,* 1000–1006.

Nagin, D. S., Pagani, L., Tremblay, R. E., & Vitaro, F. (2003). Life course turning points: The effect of grade retention on physical aggression. *Development and Psychopathology, 15,* 343–361.

Nasser, E. H., & Overholser, J. C. (2005). Recovery from major depression: The role of support from family, friends, and spiritual beliefs. *Acta Psychiatrica Sandinavica, 111,* 125–132.

Newsom, J. T., Rook, K S., Nishishiba, M., Sorkin, D. H., & Mahan, T. L. (2005). Understanding the relative importance of positive and negative social exchanges: Examining specific domains and appraisals. *Journal of Gerontology: Psychological Sciences, 60B,* P304–P312.

O'Connor, T. G., Thorpe, K., Dunn, J., & Golding, J. (1999). Parental divorce and adjustment in adulthood: Findings from a community sample. *Journal of Child Psychology and Psychiatry and Allied Disciplines,* 777–789.

O'Neil, M. K., Lancee, W. J., & Freeman, S. J. (1987). Loss and depression: A controversial link. *Journal of Nervous and Mental Disease, 175,* 354–357.

O'Rand, A. M. (2002). Cumulative advantage theory in life course research. *Annual Review of Gerontology and Geriatrics, 22*, 14–30.

Pevalin, D. J., & Goldberg, D. P. (2003). Social precursors to onset and recovery from episodes of common mental illness. *Psychological Medicine, 33*, 299–306.

Post, R. N. (1992). Transduction of psychosocial stress into the neurobiology of recurrent affective disorder. *American Journal of Psychiatry, 149*, 999–1010.

Roberts, R., O'Connor, T., Dunn, J., & Golding, J. (2004). The effects of child sexual abuse in later family life: Mental health, parenting, and adjustment of offspring. *Child Abuse and Neglect, 28*, 525–545.

Robins, L. N., & Regier, D. A. (Eds.) (1991). *Psychiatric Disorders in America.* New York: Free Press.

Ronka, A., Orayala, S., & Pulkkinen, L. (2003). Turning points in adults' lives: The effects of gender and the amount of choice. *Journal of Adult Development, 10*, 203–215.

Rook, K. (1984). The negative side of social interaction: Impact on psychological well-being. *Journal of Personality and Social Psychology, 46*, 1097–1108.

Ross, C. E., & Mirowsky, J. (1995). Does employment affect health? *Journal of Health and Social Behavior, 36*, 230–243.

Ross, C. E., & Mirowsky, J. (1999). Parental divorce, life course disruption, and adult depression. *Journal of Marriage and the Family, 61*, 1034–1945.

Sampson, R. J., & Laub, J. H. (1990). Crime and deviance over the life course: The salience of adult social bonds. *American Sociological Review, 55*, 609–627.

Schieman, S., Van Gundy, K., & Taylor, J. (2002). The relationship between age and depressive symptoms: A test of competing explanatory and suppression influences. *Journal of Aging and Health, 14*, 260–285.

Schulenberg, J. E., Sameroff, A. J., & Cicchetti, D. (2004). The transition to adulthood as a critical juncture in the course of psychopathology and mental health. *Development and Psychopathology, 16*, 799–806.

Scott, J., & Alwin, D. (1998). Retrospective versus prospective measurement of life histories in longitudinal research. In J. Z. Giele & G. H. Elder, Jr. (Eds.), *Methods of life course research* (pp. 98–127). Thousand Oaks, CA: Sage.

Segel, Z. V., Williams, J. M., Teasdale, J. D., & Gemar, M. (1996). A cognitive science perspective on kindling and episode sensitization in recurrent affective disorder. *Psychological Medicine, 26*, 371–380.

Seidman, E. & French, S. E. (2004). Developmental trajectories and ecological transitions: A two-step procedure to aid in the choice of prevention and promotion interventions. *Development and Psychopathology, 16*, 1141–1159.

Settersten, R. A., Jr. (2006). Aging and the life course. In R. H. Binstock & L. K. George (Eds.), *Handbook of Aging and the Social Sciences* (sixth edition) (pp. 3–19). San Diego: Academic Press.

Shaw, B. A., & Krause, N. (2002). Exposure to physical violence during childhood, aging, and health. *Journal of Aging and Health, 14*, 467–494.

Steffens, D. C., Pieper, C. F., Bosworth, H. B., MacFall, J. R., Provenzale, J. N., Payne, M. E., Carroll, B. J., George, L. K., & Krishnan, K. R. K. (2005). Biological and social predictors of long-term geriatric depression outcome. *International Psychogeriatrics, 17*, 41–56.

Turnbull, J. E., George, L. K., Landerman R., Swartz, M. S., & Blazer, D. G. (1990). Social outcomes related to age of onset among psychiatric disorders. *Journal of Consulting and Clinical Psychology, 58*, 832–839.

Turner, R. J., & Avison, W. R. (1992). Innovation in the measurement of life stress: Crisis theory and the significance of event resolution. *Journal of Health and Social Behavior, 33*, 36–50.

Turner, R. J., & Avison, W. R. (2003). Status variations in stress exposure: Implications for the interpretation of research on race, socioeconomic status, and gender. *Journal of Health and Social Behavior, 44*, 488–505.

Turner, R. J., & Lloyd, D. A. (1995). Lifetime traumas and mental health: The significance of cumulative adversity. *Journal of Health and Social Behavior, 36*, 360–376.

Turner, R. J., & Lloyd, D. A. (1999). The stress process and the social distribution of depression. *Journal of Health and Social Behavior, 40*, 374–404.

Tweed, J. L., Schoenbach, V. J., George, L. K., & Blazer, D. G. (1989). The effects of childhood parental death and divorce on six-month history of anxiety disorders. *British Journal of Psychiatry, 154*, 823–828.

Vaillant, G. E., & Vaillant, C. O. (1990). Natural history of male psychological health, XII: A 45-year study of predictors of successful aging at age 65. *American Journal of Psychiatry, 147*, 31–37.

Wade, T. J., & Pevalin, D. J. (2004). Marital transitions and mental health. *Journal of Health and Social Behavior, 45*, 155–170.

Walkup, J., & Gallagher, S. K. (1999). Schizophrenia and the life course: National findings on gender differences in disability and service use. *International Journal of Aging and Human Development, 49*, 79–105.

Wheaton, B. (1996). The domains and boundaries of stress concepts. In H. B. Kaplan (Ed.), *Psychosocial stress: Perspectives on structure, theory, life-course, and methods* (pp. 29–70). New York: Academic Press.

Wheaton, B., & Clarke, P. (2003). Space meets time: Integrating temporal and contextual influences on mental health in early adulthood. *American Sociological Review, 68*, 680–706.

Wiesner, M., Vondracek, F. W., Capaldi, D. M., & Porfeli, E. (2003). Childhood and adolescent predictors of early adult career pathways. *Journal of Vocational Behavior, 63*, 305–328.

Winfield, I., George, L. K., Swartz, M. S., & Blazer, D. G. (1990). Sexual assault and psychiatric disorders among women in a community sample. *American Journal of Psychiatry, 147*, 335–341.

Woodward, L. J., & Fergusson, D. M. (2001). Life course outcomes of young people with anxiety disorders in adolescence. *Journal of the American Academy of Child and Adolescent Psychiatry, 40*, 1086–1093.

Yama, M. F., Tovey, S. L., & Fogas, B. S. (1993). Childhood family environment and sexual abuse as predictors of anxiety and depression in adult women. *American Journal of Orthopsychiatry, 63*, 136–141.

10
Transition to Adulthood, Mental Health, and Inequality

Susan Gore, Robert H. Aseltine Jr., and Elizabeth A. Schilling

Research on the social sources of mental illness has historically given only minimal attention to specific age groups. Studies that typify sociological work, those that are concerned with social stress or with socioeconomic or gender disparities, usually involve community-residing adults of all ages and give little attention to age as a significant sociological variable. Against this background, the mental health of young adults is newly explored terrain.

Given the freshness of the topic, questions arise about the theoretical formulations that should guide research on young adults and the strategies that are needed to more explicitly incorporate attention to age and life stage. Current adult-centered formulations concerned with social inequality and social stress in mental health are a critical point of departure. Much of the current evidence on this issue confirms the importance of lifetime social stress exposure in accounting for racial/ethnic and socioeconomic differentials in mental and physical disorder (Turner & Avison, 2003; Turner, Wheaton & Lloyd, 1995). Although studies of older adults predominate, research on young adults also indicates linkages among indicators of social status, cumulative stressful adversities and both affective disorder and the onset of drug dependence during young adulthood (Gore & Aseltine, 2003; Turner, 2003). Clearly, the evidence offers compelling support for the social stress perspective as a lens for investigating processes of inequality in all age groups.

At the same time, ongoing efforts to contextualize risk processes hold special promise for research on young adult mental health. Link and Phelan (1995) have described the idea of contextualizing risk as a paradigmatic emphasis on the social conditions that shape the individual's risk exposure and that make such exposures more or less preventable. In research on the health and mental health of children and adolescents, investigators have focused on the family and neighborhood as key socialization contexts. This research retains a focus on social stress, but examines the embeddedness of these stressors in contexts over which young people have little control. In addition, measured features of context may be at a different level of analysis. Sociological research, as well as research more squarely developmental in thrust, documents the long-term effects of adverse family socioeconomic conditions into the early adult years (Wheaton & Clarke,

2003; Wickrama, Conger, Wallace, & Elder, 2003). An overview of this evidence might suggest that predictors of adaptation from early in life, both those in the realm of the family or its geographic context, and others within the person, such as delinquent behavior, tell us all we need to know about mental health processes during the transition to adulthood.

In this chapter, we specifically ask the question: Does the evidence on the importance of childhood "launching factors" (Hussong, Curran, Moffitt, Caspi, & Carrig, 2004:1031) in predicting continuity of mental disorder contradict ideas and evidence on the significance of the opportunities for change that are embedded in the transitions of this period (Schulenberg, Sameroff & Cicchetti, 2004)? This question relates to a more general debate among life course researchers regarding the degree of developmental continuity and discontinuity during the transition to adulthood. Our discussion addresses features of this general debate that are relevant to research on mental health and is guided by a central interest in young adult interpersonal and vocational contexts as social pathways into adulthood. Sociologists use the term *pathways* into adulthood to refer to a course of behavior that is relatively "laid out" as a feature of social organization, in contrast with the idea of *trajectory*, which implies a stronger role of chance and individual agency (Hogan & Astone, 1986:110). Although in most research these terms are used interchangeably, this is an important distinction in mental health studies. Echoing the debates focusing on processes of social causation and social selection, the concept of pathways directs attention to socialization environments, economic and interpersonal resources, and the constraints on and influences of behavior during the transition to adulthood. Trajectories, in contrast, reflect the more individualized decisions and choices that drive life change and are the hallmark of developmental perspectives. Life course perspectives bridge these emphases.

Research on the social demography of transition to adulthood takes a focus on pathways through descriptive attention to the social role events that mark the assumption of adult status in our society (Hogan & Astone, 1986). This population-level approach emphasizes the social nature of the pathways to adulthood through research that situates status changes involving completion of schooling, getting married, residential independence and starting a full time job in institutional conditions that vary from society to society and that are subject to historical change. Research taking a trajectories approach, as defined earlier, are likely to ask questions about developmental themes that are universal, as illustrated in Arnett's characterization of "emerging adulthood" as a distinctive developmental stage (Arnett, 2000) or they may accentuate how young people negotiate the myriad of developmental challenges. We take the contrasting pathways approach. This general disciplinary lens has figured prominently in research demonstrating that young adult transitions into stable family and work roles are linked to reductions in delinquency and problem drinking behaviors during this period (Bachman, Johnston & O'Malley, 1991; Bachman, O'Malley & Johnston, 1984; Chilcoat & Breslau, 1996; Horwitz & Raskin-White, 1991; Schulenberg, O'Malley, Bachman, & Johnston, 2000).

In the following sections we focus on additional lines of investigation that also exploit the concept of pathways to adulthood and more explicitly engage with themes of social disadvantage and the structuring of opportunity during the early adult period. We see three central foci in current investigations, all of which are sociological in character and share the "developmental stance" (Shanahan, 2000:668) that characterizes current sociological research on transition to adulthood. A first concerns the quality of *young adult transitional environments and experience* as proximal influences on mental health. Our own research on mental health in the post-secondary years examines features of vocational pathways and interpersonal relations *prior to* the assumption of the mature social roles defining adulthood, as noted above (Gore & Aseltine, 2003; Gore, Kadish, & Aseltine, 2003). A second focus emphasizes *lifetime accumulation of stress and disadvantage* and the resulting pathways into adulthood that differ in resources and well being (Dannefer, 2003; Kerckhoff, 1993; Turner & Lloyd, 1995). Finally, pathways evidencing *discontinuity or turning points in social functioning and mental health* are an important focus in mental health research due to the obvious relevance of this issue to the concept of resilience and the implications for intervention. This theme is perhaps best reflected in research that draws on life course theory (Elder, 1985; Elder, George, & Shanahan, 1996) for examining desistance of antisocial behavior among high risk youth (Laub, Nagin & Sampson, 1998).

Before we turn to a discussion of these themes, we briefly characterize the epidemiology of young adult mental health that has been so influential in stimulating research on transition to adulthood.

Epidemiology of Young Adult Mental Health

An early paper by Klerman and Weissman (1989) is perhaps the first significant report bringing to public and professional attention the high rates of depression among young adults, the increasing lifetime rates of depression in cohorts born in industrialized countries after 1940, and a decrease in the age of onset of depression with first onsets generally occurring in the late adolescent years. This report also drew attention to the increasing rate of suicide among individuals between the ages of 15 to 24, especially among white males. Recent evidence from the National Comorbidity Study (Kessler, McGonagle, Zhao, Nelson, Hughes, Eshleman, Wittchen, & Kendler, 1994), a nationally representative sample, indicates that major depression and alcohol dependence, the two most prevalent disorders among Americans, are highest in the two youngest age groups (15–24 and 25–34 years old). Specifically, depression increases from the early teens to mid-twenties, with major depression estimated as 21.2 percent for young adults between the ages of 21 and 22, which is a 45 percent increase in prevalence as individuals exit adolescence (Kessler & Walters, 1998). The NCS also finds that rates for almost all disorders are more elevated among those with lower income and education (Kessler et al., 1994; see also Newman, Moffitt, Caspi, Magdol, Silva, & Stanton, 1996). In addition, reports from the Epidemiologic Catchment Area (ECA) program indicate that about one in four individuals between the ages of 18 and 29 have experienced a mental disorder (Burke, Burke, Regier, & Rae, 1990). Miech and colleagues offer a more sobering estimate that up to 40 percent of young adults in industrialized countries meet diagnostic criteria for a major psychiatric disorder (Miech, Caspi, Moffitt, Wright & Silva, 1999).

Studies that rely on diagnostic determinations may offer fairly conservative estimates of mental health problems because they do not include the large number of individuals experiencing subclinical disorder reflected in symptoms of distress that do not meet diagnostic thresholds. A major study of clinical depression and depressed mood among college students, for example, established that those who were highly distressed as determined by a cutoff score on the CES-D inventory (Center for Epidemiologic Studies Depression) but were not designated as depressed on the basis of a clinical interview evidenced problems in social functioning at similar levels as those diagnosed with a depressive disorder (Gotlib, Lewinsohn, & Seeley, 1995). Clearly, there is a high burden of mental health problems in this age group.

For young adults who are generally well according to psychiatric standards, evidence indicates it is a time of psycho-social growth. Based on data from multiple cohorts of high school graduates, Schulenberg and associates (Schulenberg et al., 2000) have reported a consistent pattern of increments in life satisfaction, social support, self esteem and self efficacy from age 18 to 22 and, similarly, declines in loneliness, fatalism and self derogation over these years. Other research has supported this view. Young people participating in the National Longitudinal Survey of Youth (NLSY) have reported an increased perception of control during the period from age 14 to age 22 (Lewis, Ross, & Mirowsky, 1999). Finally, in one of our longitudinal studies of young adults, we contrasted change in depressive symptoms among cohorts of young people, some still in high school, and others having graduated. We found an improvement in symptom scores among the graduates that was not evidenced over the same time period among those still in school, change that was largely accounted for by improved relations with family (Aseltine & Gore, 1993).

Overall, epidemiological data establish early adulthood as an important life stage for sociological research. Depression and alcohol disorder are two highly prevalent disorders, they occur at peak rates during young adulthood, they are significantly influenced by environmental factors, and their link to gender and socioeconomic factors are all patterns that suggest needed research attention. Moreover, the evidence indicating that pathways are diverse, with many young people experiencing enhanced well being as they make normative social transitions, in contrast to others whose futures are compromised by distress and dysfunction provides compelling additional reason for accelerated research attention on young adulthood.

In the next section we further develop this theme of heterogeneity among young adults, through discussing a first focus, the importance of transitional work and educational statuses and experiences in the years after high school. As preface, we note that this is the least well developed area of research on young adult mental health, which is surprising in light of the extensive body of adult-focused work on themes related to employment, and the equally extensive body of work on adolescents concerning school transitions. As we conclude our discussion of major themes, and in our final discussion, we will link the status of research and directions for filling gaps to the central question we raised at the start of this paper, namely whether the events and circumstances of this transitional phase of life are of lesser significance to understanding mental health at this time than much earlier childhood influences. We turn now to the research on transitional environments and the school and work pathways into adulthood.

The Post-Secondary Years and Heterogeneous Pathways into Adulthood

Elder and Russell (2000) have noted that understanding change in young people's lives calls for choosing an "entry point", or developmental context, that allows us to ask questions about what happens next. The problem of choosing a point of entry is particularly thorny in research on young adulthood, a developmental period that we generally see as starting with the end of post-secondary schooling and continuing through most of the third decade of life (Arnett, 2000). The protracted end of adolescence and lengthy duration of the transition to adulthood has long been recognized and currently figures prominently in popular media attention to the new generation of "twixters," young adults in their twenties who are no longer adolescents and by society's standards not yet adults (Grossman, 2005). Inadequate employment situations and the resulting financial dependence on families are central to sociological work on the problems of these "incompletely launched" adults (Schnaiberg & Goldenberg, 1989). Furstenberg (2000), for example, has reported that by age 30, just over half of the most recent cohorts studied in the National Longitudinal Survey had worked for 2 or more years in a full time, year-around job.

This empirical portrait suggests to us constraints on the usefulness of existing research frameworks concerned with *mature* social roles, such as having continuous full time employment or being married, as an entry point for research on the link between mental health and young adult life situations during this transitional period. Large numbers of young adults have not achieved any of these stable and health-promoting adult identities and attainments. Moreover, taking a population viewpoint, young adults undertake similar activities at different times and dissimilar activities during the same time frame. A recent analysis of the National Longitudinal Survey of Youth (NLSY 79) (Mouw, 2005) indicates that in these cohorts there are sixty two distinct sequences representing the temporal relationships among leaving home, finishing school, starting work, getting married and having children.

Early efforts to grapple with this heterogeneity centered on the problem of non-normative or premature transitions to adulthood, as illustrated in research on teenage parents (Furstenberg, Brooks-Gunn & Morgan, 1987), leaving unanswered questions about the lives of the large and heterogeneous group of young people who make normative or more socially acceptable transitions. Recent approaches seek to include a broader segment of the population under the investigative lens and are approaching the issue of heterogeneity through identifying the pathways that appear conceptually important in addition to those representing significant numbers of young adults. Osgood and associates, for example, used latent class analysis to describe pathways of transition in a longitudinal sample of young adults who have been followed since early adolescence (Osgood, Ruth, Eccles, Jacobs, & Barber, 2005). Their resulting descriptive typology of pathways to adulthood includes fast starters (those having adult social roles), parents without careers, educated with partner, educated singles, working singles, and slow starters. They conclude that by age 24, most of their sample is "unsettled" in work and family roles, fitting Arnett's definition of emergent adulthood.

Having mapped some features and challenges in studying young adults in transition, we have not yet suggested how these initial descriptive efforts to gain an entry point into this developmental period can be linked to a focus on mental health. In the following sections we discuss the three themes of transitional environments, cumulative adversity and turning points as central components of current efforts to accomplish this objective.

Socioeconomic Inequality and Mental Health after the Transition from High School

Our research on a cohort of young adults making the transition from high school employs a strategy for entry into this developmental period that is linked to our interest in processes of inequality. Other researchers have also examined features of social functioning and well-being in the years immediately after high school and addressed varying concerns. For example, much of the extensive research conducted by Schulenberg and his associates (Schulenberg et al., 2005), which draws from the Monitoring the Future project (Johnston, O'Malley, & Bachman, 2003), focuses on escalations in drinking associated with off-campus residence among college students and is not prominently concerned with disadvantage and inequality.

Our emphasis on inequality led us to consider the different pathways that youth followed during the transitional period after high school. Specifically, we have been centrally interested in the heightened difficulties faced by young people who make a school-to-work transition, that is, those who seek full time employment rather than continued schooling. This large segment of the young adult population, who are necessarily omitted in mental health studies of young adults in college settings, came into public focus as the "forgotten half," in a series of reports on the career difficulties of the non-college bound (Hamilton, 1990; William T. Grant

Foundation Commission on Work, Family and Citizenship, 1988). Consistent with these aims, we selected public schools located in largely lower income urban areas, including schools serving students in two major cities in our geographic area. This resulted in a sample that was diverse in family socioeconomic background, race/ethnicity, and importantly, in post-high school educational and work pathways (Gore & Aseltine, 2003).

Although we have established that the fluidity and diversity in pathways to adulthood complicates finding a point of entry into the developmental process, our focus on a graduating cohort (and school dropouts from that cohort) and interest in vocational/educational pathways provided this point of entry for examining post-secondary life situations. The diverse composition of our sample further assisted us in contrasting the life situation and mental health of groups who had a full time college involvement, a full time work involvement, mixed involvements, and those underutilized in both spheres, when they were 2 years out of high school. In general, we found that an intra-individual or configurational approach was informative, when used in conjunction with regression methods. For example, in explaining an emergent racial/ethnic gap in depressed mood from time 1 to time 2, with Blacks and Hispanics more depressed than Whites and Asian Americans, we established that both full time school status (in a four year college) and full time work status were negatively associated with depression and important in accounting for these differentials. Descriptive data on school and work involvements indicated that Blacks and Hispanics were not very different than Whites, suggesting that the minorities should benefit from their numbers who were working at full time jobs. The distributions, however, were deceptive because they did not differentiate individuals who were designated as not working because they were in school from those who were both not working *and* not in school. Through examining different profiles of work and school involvement, we found that only 5 percent of the Whites were non-students who were not working, in contrast to 14 percent of the Blacks and 16 percent of the Hispanics.

In addition to young adults' educational/employment situations, we studied two additional features of post-secondary school experience: *the stresses* young adults were experiencing in their post-secondary situations, and the extent of *negative transition events* in their school and employment pathway over a two year period, both according to their own reports (Aseltine & Gore, 2005). Measures of these features of transitional experience draw on the dimensionality of the stress construct that is well established (Turner & Avison, 2003; Wheaton, 1994), with chronic stress in young people's work situation assessed through measures used in previous research on young people (Mortimer, Finch, Shanahan & Ryu, 1992) and adapted from the Michigan Quality of Employment Studies (Quinn & Staines, 1979). Our findings from this analysis are consistent with those obtained in our analysis of race/ethnicity, that the earlier independence that defines a post-secondary emphasis on employment can be health-promoting, but it carries with it higher stakes for stressful disruptions and failure to find developmentally suitable roles.

In framing this research study we drew heavily on the conceptualizations and research conducted by Simmons and her associates on school transitions during adolescence (Simmons & Blyth, 1987), which emphasized the importance of minimizing stressful disruptions during periods of peak individual and environment change. Within the large body of work on this issue, with much of it concerned with pubertal and cognitive change, Simmons' work stands out as significant in emphasizing the role of school structures in facilitating successful transitions. Through focusing on young people who do not transition from high school into a full time college experience, we were similarly concerned with young people at heightened risk for major stressors and mental health problems. As such, research in this vein points to the importance of educational and employment opportunity; in addition, it contextualizes the disruptions that occur within these pathways as features of stratification processes in the early adult years.

Lifetime Accumulation of Stress and Disadvantage

In conducting research on pathways into adulthood, as described in the preceding section, questions naturally arise about the prior family and personal situations to which both positive and negative young adult experiences are undoubtedly linked. For this reason, developmental frameworks that incorporate attention to environments at different points in the life course and processes of selection into and adaptation within those environments offer a compelling set of conceptual foci and methodological tools for longitudinal analysis. Within this general orientation, however, we must specify the nature of the social forces and individual actions that drive the direction of change and mental health over this period.

Our second focus concerns the study of cumulative advantage/disadvantage, which Dannefer defines as "the systematic tendency for interindividual divergence in a given characteristic (e.g., money, health, or status) with the passage of time" (Dannefer, 2003:S324). Although closely associated with the study of individual and cohort aging, an important point of departure within our field is the sociological conceptualization of the structural origins of mental health problems (Aneshensel, Rutter & Lachenbruch, 1991). This has been modeled in terms of the stresses that are embedded in the contexts of daily life, as emphasized in the Pearlin formulation of social stress theory (Pearlin, Lieberman, Menaghan, & Mullan, 1981) or through restricted access to economic, interpersonal and political resources that might alter exposure to stress and broader sociogenesis of ill health (Link & Phelan, 1995). Research in the field of social stress, for example, has addressed mental health disparities associated with socioeconomic factors and racial/ethnic group memberships and documented that cumulative stress exposure, including recent stressful events and longstanding or chronic stressors are implicated in these differentials (Turner & Avison, 2003; Turner & Lloyd, 1999). The explanatory potential of these stressors is not surprising. Stressors include significant aspects of disadvantage in work settings, threatening economic and legal stresses, problems in relationships, exposure to violence and other events that are socio-economically linked. This is important evidence that cumulative processes of disadvantage are implicated in the social stratification of mental health.

A contrasting but complementary approach that takes a life course focus seeks to understand the risks that are rooted in key developmental periods, and the unfolding of disorder as young people move from childhood to adulthood. Whereas the studies of stress we have just described examine mental health over the young adult's *lifetime*, this approach examines mental health over the young adult's *life course*. There is good reason to take this latter approach. We mentioned earlier the findings from the National Comorbidity Study concerning the high rates of disorder among young adults and the early onset nature of these disorders (Kessler et al., 1994). The research conducted by Newman and associates with a Dunedin, New Zealand sample also suggests that the prior functioning of individuals in the adolescent period may be implicated in the rates of distress and disorder evidenced among young adults. Nearly half of their sample was diagnosed with 2 or more disorders at age 21, and rates of disorder significantly increased between the ages of 13 and 15, and again between the ages of 15 and 18 (Newman et al., 1996).

Due to the importance of the adolescent period, structural perspectives on the consequences of disadvantage for the pathways into adulthood have emphasized the multiple links between family economic stress and multiple aspects of adolescent functioning. Whether disadvantage is measured at the level of the family or its neighborhood context, extensive evidence indicates that these family conditions are causally linked with child and adolescent internalizing and externalizing mental health problems and that this relationship is mediated by unsupportive and punitive socialization practices within the family environment (Conger, Conger, Elder, Lorenz, Simons, & Whitbeck, 1992; McLeod & Shanahan, 1993; Wheaton & Clarke, 2003). Importantly, this line of research illustrates the life course principle of *linked lives*, which is the embeddedness of individuals within interpersonal contexts over the life course (Elder, 1995).

In particular, studies focusing on specific types of events, such as violence exposures (Macmillan, 2001) reveal the traumatic nature of some stress exposures in the lives of the disadvantaged, and document the role of severe stress in curtailed education. Macmillan and Hagan (2004), for example, have examined the impact of an adolescent victimization on young adult socioeconomic attainment and found reductions in educational advancement that are mediated through the impact of violence on self perceptions of efficacy. In addition, experiencing victimization during adolescence is not a random event. Young people growing up in poverty have an elevated risk of experiencing violence, among other traumatic events including homelessness (McLoyd, 1998). Thus, events during adolescence which are severe and traumatic play an important role in our understanding of cumulative stress processes and the role of stratification in mental health processes linking generations.

Social Structure and the Social Embeddedness of Agency

To this point we have begun to make the case that cumulative lifetime social stress can be re-framed as a problem of cumulative life course disadvantage, a shift that serves to emphasize the underlying processes of stratification that govern the accumulation of stress and pathways into adulthood that diverge both in resources and well being (Dannefer, 2003; Kerckhoff, 1993). However, life course perspectives recognize that processes of individual action or agency are also at play, as evidenced in extensive evidence on the role of individual characteristics and behavior in selecting into environments and shaping stressful interpersonal relations (Caspi, Henry, McGee, Moffitt, & Silva, 1995; Caspi, Moffitt, Wright, & Silva, 1998; Hammen, 1991; Quinton, Pickles, Maughan & Rutter, 1993; Ronka & Pulkkinen, 1995). One such problem that can be viewed as a selection process in transition to adulthood is the role of an early onset psychiatric disorder in shaping the subsequent developmental pathways. Findings from the NCS have documented that early onset disorder predicts to failure to complete high school and/or college (Kessler, Foster, Saunders, & Stang, 1995). More extensive research has linked the escalation and exacerbation of conduct problems through adolescence and early adulthood to a childhood onset of antisocial behavior. The issue here is not the simple continuity of disorder across developmental periods but its exacerbation through multiple domains of role functioning which ultimately depletes motivation and opportunities for developing skills and forging supportive ties (Aguilar, Sroufe, Egeland, & Carlson, 2000; Moffitt, Caspi, Harrington, & Milne, 2002). Alcohol abuse, in particular, may serve to lock-in a pattern of antisocial behavior that prohibits any tendency toward reduction in conduct problems and offending that might other wise occur (Roisman, Aguilar & Egeland, 2004).

Research that establishes a strong association between prior and future disorder has not generally been of theoretical interest to sociologists because it suggests that the disease process within the individual drives social change, that is, that unwell individuals select into the environments that have fewer resources and are less optimal for development. This view would seem to be in conflict with the paradigm of structural causation that informs most sociological research and is prominently reflected more generally in developmental studies emphasizing the abilities and capacities of individuals that are generally adaptive or maladaptive. Clausen (1991) for example, has linked the idea of individual *agency*—individual effort and decision that shape one's own development—to the construct of *planful competence* or self-efficacy. He argues that the wide range of options available to young people as they exit adolescence calls for realistic goal setting and that this is likely to occur among individuals who are responsible (as opposed to rebellious), oriented toward self examination and self confident (as opposed to victimized in one's stance). Analyses emphasizing the predictive importance of these traits establish their significant impact on young adult educational and occupational attainment, marital stability and (reduced) stress exposure.

There are, however, important alternative perspectives on the role of intra-individual characteristics in cumulative stress processes. For example, the core of mental health research on the positive association between socioeconomic status and the individual's sense of control emphasizes the role of distal childhood socialization and more current life contexts in shaping individual self appraisals of this nature (Mirowsky & Ross, 2003; Wheaton, 1978). Evidence that links individual outlook and coping-related capacities to the social structure and processes of inequality is important for understanding why there is a low likelihood for change in the life situations of young people who have a history of delinquent and antisocial behavior. We have noted that one prominent explanation is that a cumulative deficit in skills and motivation ultimately functions to close doors that might have been open. However, for sociologists who are concerned with social stratification of pathways into adulthood, these models of risk accumulation overemphasize the dimension of personal responsibility (Laub & Sampson, 1993). For this reason, Shanahan and Hood (2002) have conceptualized agency as *bounded*, indicating that there are varying opportunities made available to subgroups of youth for a successful pathway into adulthood and that agency must be understood in relation to the opportunity context. A striking and well known illustration of this point is seen in Elder's research on the differences between two age cohorts in surmounting a background of family disadvantage during the Great Depression (Elder, 1974). The somewhat older men in the Oakland subsample were of age to seek employment to help support their families. In doing so, they escaped the often harsh confines of their economically stressed families and later used army service as a springboard for educational and employment opportunities made available after the war. In this way, historical events enhanced economic opportunity for the Oakland men, which was not the case for those in the younger Berkeley age cohort. Each cohort, then, embarked on the life course with different possibilities for the exercise of agency.

It is interesting to note that both Elder and Clausen conducted their analyses using the archival Oakland Growth/Berkeley Guidance data. Thus, we may conclude that interest in the limiting power of structure or the personal sense of agency is a matter of emphasis. However, more recent studies establish the choice of emphasis might best be linked to the process being investigated. We noted earlier that NLSY data indicate that for a 1990's cohort of young adults, the sense of personal control increases between the ages of 14 and 22 (Lewis et al., 1999: 1594). The investigators further established that growth in sense of control was muted for young people who dropped out of high school and that strength of control perceptions had little impact on their staying in high school. Thus, the investigators conclude that in this case the "realities of social status shape beliefs [about the self], rather than the beliefs determining the status gained."

Overall, it is safe to say that the dynamics through which the weakened bonds and continuity of disadvantage occurs involve both social structural constraints on opportunity as well as intra-individual capacities and self defeating action. Quite apart from questions about the evidence, we also think it important that investigations of young adult mental health have sparked renewed sociological interest in the concept of agency and its structural contexts. In addition, these lines of study have forged heretofore nonexistent connections between the research on criminal desistance conducted by criminologists in our field and the mental health investigations that have not been as focused on high risk young adults.

We now address the final theme that is regularly discussed in research involving young adults, namely the potential for change in life direction and its mental health impact.

Discontinuity in Pathways to Adulthood: Sources of Resilience

The idea of turning point is a life course concept that can be defined as "change in direction in the life course, with respect to a previously established trajectory, that has the long term impact of altering the probability of life destinations" (Wheaton & Gotlib, 1997:5). Wheaton and Gotlib are not distinguishing a *trajectory* from a *pathway* as we have done in emphasizing that pathways into adulthood are socially organized. They do not take a position on this issue. However, they point to the importance of turning points as altering the accumulating consequences of negative events, which we discussed in the previous section as a problem of pathways. The possibility for turning points during this transitional period is central to the fundamental question that we raised at the outset, namely, do the events and conditions of early adulthood make a difference for our understanding of mental health processes?

Turning points are often conceived as having an intervention-like quality as suggested by the idea that the direction of life can be changed. Consistent with our definition of pathways, we see turning points as coming about through environmental contingencies involving new roles and opportunities. Most discussions of this issue consider the potential for discontinuity and turning points in relation to behaviors involving the central developmental tasks of young adulthood: establishing a viable vocational pathway, and developing strong ties of intimacy outside the family of origin. Rutter's longitudinal research on the transition to adulthood among young people from the inner-city and those who were institution-reared is widely recognized as the foundation for research in this area due to its focus on the role of education in delaying marriage and preventing poor marital choices and attention to gender differences in pathways having turning point potential (Rutter, 1989).

Due to the importance of education in theories of stratification, as well as the focus on educational attainment in mental health research (Miech & Shanahan, 2000), it is not surprising that education figures prominently in research on transition to adulthood. Evidence generally indicates that the long term impact of early family adversities occurs through poor educational performance and curtailed education. However, it is also the case that schooling figures prominently in turning point potential. In their analysis of longitudinal data collected from a diverse Michigan sample, Osgood and his associates found that young people from poor families who did well in high school and evidenced high educational motivation look similar at age 24 to their more advantaged counterparts in their "upward trajectory" of employment and interest in improving themselves (Osgood et al., 2005:344). Although low family income or low parental educational attainment are not good indicators of the degree of adversity in these environments, this is an important approach in research on turning points because family social capital, or lack thereof, is so central an issue to a broad array of young people.

In general, the evidence from our work on transition from high school indicates that pathways involving postsecondary education or stable full time work contribute to improvements in functioning, as measured by reductions in depressive symptoms. We reserve use of the turning point concept for contrasts suggesting some role of education in changing an otherwise less optimal life direction among those known to be high risk. For example, to better assist in launching young people who were vocationally oriented rather than oriented toward higher education, the schools from which we recruited our sample of young adults offered a curriculum aimed to develop career-relevant skills and foster transitions to community college, keeping open the college option. This general aim follows from increasing public interest in having community schools better prepare young adults for employment, as called for by the School-to-Work Opportunities legislation (U.S. Department of Education, 1994). Programs of this nature can be conceptualized as intending to ameliorate the role of school inequality in perpetuating stratification. Taking a sociological perspective on the protective factors that drive resilient outcomes, we sought to investigate whether graduating from high school with a *career major* would boost the employment success and well being of these young people over that of their counterparts who entered the labor force in the absence of an institutional connection between the secondary school and the world of work (Gore et al., 2003). Our evidence on short term outcomes indicate that these curricular involvements promote a sense of career optimism and progress, which we interpret as features of positive mental health broadly speaking, but one that is not fully reflected in differentials involving objective features of their occupational situation.

Despite considerable research on the importance of social relationships in resilience, sociologists have not as yet fully explored the adaptive importance of young adult relationships and intimate involvements. Roisman and associates have argued that during the transition to adulthood having intimate or romantic involvements may be particularly beneficial for high risk youth as an opportunity to achieve some developmental success in an arena that differs from contexts of previous functioning that have been marked by failure (Roisman et al., 2004). Focusing on the functions of romantic ties among youth with a history of antisocial behavior, they hypothesized that although young people with early onset of disorder may be less likely to have successful intimate relationships due to the accumulation of dysfunction in their biographies, they may reap greater benefits from these ties than young people having more opportunity to develop strengths. The expectation follows from an understanding of protective factors as having potentially the greatest impact among those at heightened risk and is consistent with the idea of a conditional turning point (Wheaton & Gotlib, 1997), one that operates only for a particular subgroup. Their results support this hypothesis, though they are necessarily tentative due to concurrent measures of some variables. Specifically, for those with a longer term history of externalizing problems, having a successful romantic (and work) engagement was associated with declines in anti-social behavior by age 23, and this was not the case for those with an antisocial career that began later in adolescence. These findings are consistent with those reported by Laub and associates (Laub et al., 1998) who, on the basis of the Glueck and Glueck longitudinal data, reveal the importance of a successful marriage in a gradual process of criminal desistance.

Clearly, these intriguing lines of research on resilience should accelerate interest in the potential for turning points in young adult mental health. Specifically, they point to the powerful role of relationships in the lives of high risk young adults.

Summary and Discussion

To conclude this chapter, we return to the question we raised at the start, namely: Does the evidence on the importance of childhood "launching factors" contradict ideas and evidence on the meaningfulness of this period for mental health, includ-ing the opportunity for change? Clearly, a prominent face of research on this population is the accumulating evidence on the early childhood determinants of continuity in mental health problems from childhood to adulthood. We have suggested that this may in part be due to the challenges associated with the diversity in this age group. The heterogeneity in the timing and sequencing of educational, employment, familial and residential transitions makes it difficult to find an appropriate *point of entry* into young adults' lives. Moreover, additional variability along gender, socioeconomic and race and ethnic lines; the ambiguous length of the life stage itself; and our culture of loosened age norms for attaining adult statuses all encourage a view of individuation and personal choice in life direction during the transition to adulthood. In the absence of compelling conceptual models for rein-ing-in this variability, we are not surprised that emphases on childhood conditions and their role in processes of illness continuity have occupied center stage.

Sociologists of mental health have enthusiastically given attention to the contexts of child development and other developmental themes that reflect this prominent attention to youth. Among such themes are those emphasizing the freedoms and choices that are made and forfeited as young people negotiate change and begin to shape a life involving greater economic and socio-emotional independence from the family of origin. At the same time, we have argued that the heterogeneity in experience within this population can be conceptualized sociologically through investigations that explicitly consider pathways into adulthood as shaped by social organizational forces. Thus, ideas about individuation in the life course are balanced by concepts such as "bounded agency" (Shanahan & Hood, 2002), which underscore the social constraints that limit young people's access to opportunities and their potential to exercise agency. Taking this perspective, we see mental health (and illness) pathways as forged over time. They begin with adversity in the childhood socialization context and are maintained during adolescence through problems in mental health and social functioning and limited access to educational and employment opportunities during the early years after high school. During this latter period, the frequent job changes that economists might see as acceptable job "churning" for young people in search of a better career, are, from a mental health perspective, meaningful events and disruptions that reflect broader conditions of educational and employment opportunity.

Beyond the study of education and employment, the social relations of young adults and their connections to resources in their extended families and communities are an important and much underresearched area for investigation. Positive relationships are centrally linked to young people's ability to move in more positive life directions in the years after adolescence. The evidence we have reviewed is consistent with Coleman's (1988) understanding of the transformative potential of social capital, which is embodied in relationships. It is curious that so little research on social support has been conducted with young adults. In light of the importance of support and capital in "launching" young adults, filling this research gap is an important priority for future research.

Overall, we suggest that the dynamic nature of transition to adulthood requires more sociological attention. Themes of inequality, opportunity and the capacity for change should figure prominently in formulations that guide mental health study. This research is not diminished through attention to developmental issues and distal childhood forces. Instead, we must also find ways to more purposefully explore the mental health impact of social organizational forces during this fluid transitional period.

Acknowledgments. We greatly appreciate the help and support of the staff of the Center for Survey Research and our graduate student in the Department of Sociology, Cecilia Shiner.

References

Aguilar, B., Sroufe, L. A., Egeland, B., & Carlson, E. (2000). Distinguishing the early-onset/persistent and adolescence-limited antisocial behavior types: From birth to 16 years. *Development and Psychopathology, 12*, 109–132.

Aneshensel, C., Rutter, C. M., & Lachenbruch, P. A. (1991). Competing conceptual and analytic models: Social structure, stress and mental health. *American Sociological Review, 56*, 166–178.

Arnett, J. J. (2000). Emerging adulthood: A theory of development from late teens through the twenties. *American Psychologist, 55*, 469–480.

Aseltine, R. H., Jr., & Gore, S. (1993). Mental health and social adaptation following the transition from high school. *Journal of Research on Adolescence, 3*, 247–270.

Aseltine, R. H., Jr., & Gore, S. (2005). Work, post-secondary education and psycho-social functioning following the transition from high school. *Journal of Adolescent Research, 20*, 615–639.

Bachman, J. G., Johnston, L. D., & O'Malley, P. M. (1991). *Monitoring the Future Project after seventeen years. Design and procedures (Monitoring the Future Occasional Paper No. 33)*. Ann Arbor, Michigan: Institute for Social Research.

Bachman, J. G., O'Malley, P. M., & Johnston, L. D. (1984). Drug use among young adults: The impacts of role status and social environments. *Journal of Personality and Social Psychology, 47*, 629–645.

Burke, K. C., Burke, J. D., Regier, D. A., & Rae, D. S. (1990). Age of onset of selected mental disorders in five community populations. *Archives of General Psychiatry, 47*, 511–518.

Caspi, A., Henry, B., McGee, R., Moffitt, T., & Silva, P. (1995). Temperamental origins of child and adolescent behavioral problems: From age 3 to age 15. *Child Development, 66*, 55–68.

Caspi, A., Moffitt, T. E., Wright, B. E., & Silva, P. (1998). Early failure in the labor market: Childhood and adolescent predictors of unemployment in the transition to adulthood. *American Sociological Review, 63*, 424–451.

Chilcoat, H. D., & Breslau, N. (1996). Alcohol disorders in young adulthood: Effects of transitions into adult roles. *Journal of Health and Social Behavior, 37*, 339–349.

Clausen, J. S. (1991). Adolescent competence and the shaping of the life course. *American Journal of Sociology, 96*, 805–842.

Coleman, J. S. (1988). Social capital in the creation of human capital. *American Journal of Sociology, 94*, S95–S120.

Conger, R., Conger, K., Elder, G., Lorenz, F., Simons, R., & Whitbeck, L. (1992). A family process model of economic hardship and adjustment of early adolescent boys. *Child Development, 63*, 526–541.

Dannefer, D. (2003). Cumulative advantage/disadvantage and the life course: Cross-fertilizing age and social science theory. *Journal of Gerontology, 58*, S327–S337.

Elder, G. H., Jr. (1974). *Children of the Great Depression: Social change in life experience*. Chicago: University of Chicago Press.

Elder, G. H., Jr. (1985). Perspectives on the life course. In G. H. Elder Jr. (Ed.), *Transitions through adolescence: Interpersonal domains and context* (pp 251–284). Mahwah, NJ: Lawrence Erlbaum Associates.

Elder, G. H., Jr. (1995). The life course paradigm: Social change and individual development. In P. Moen, G. H. Elder & K. Luscher (Eds.), *Examining lives in context: Perspectives on the ecology of human development* (pp 101–139). Washington D.C.: American Psychological Association.

Elder, G. H., Jr., George, L. K., & Shanahan, M. (1996). Psychological stress over the life course. In H. B. Kaplan (Ed.), *Psychological stress: Perspective on structure, theory, life course, and methods* (pp 247–292). New York: Academic Press.

Elder, G. H., Jr., & Russell, S. T. (2000). Surmounting life's disadvantage. In L. J. Crockett & R. Silbereisen (Eds.), *Negotiating adolescence in times of social change* (pp 17–35). Cambridge, UK: Cambridge University Press.

Furstenberg, F. F. (2000). The sociology of adolescence and youth in the 1990s: A critical commentary. *Journal of Marriage and the Family, 62*, 896–910.

Furstenberg, F. F., Brooks-Gunn, J. & Morgan, S. P. (1987). *Adolescent mothers in later life*. New York: Cambridge University Press.

Gore, S., & Aseltine, R. H., Jr. (2003). Race and ethnic differences in depressed mood following the transition from high school. *Journal of Health and Social Behavior, 44*, 370–389.

Gore, S., Kadish, S., & Aseltine, R.H., Jr. (2003). Career-centered high school education and post-high school career adaptation. *American Journal of Community Psychology, 32*, 77–88.

Gotlib, I. H., Lewinsohn, P. M., & Seeley, J. R. (1995). Symptoms versus a diagnosis of depression: Differences in psychosocial functioning. *Journal of Consulting and Clinical Psychology, 63*, 90–100.

Grossman, L. (2005). Meet the twixters. *Time Magazine.* January *24*, 4–53.

Hamilton, S. (1990). *Apprenticeship for adulthood, preparing youth for the future.* New York: The Free Press.

Hammen, C. (1991). Generation of stress in the course of unipolar depression. *Journal of Abnormal Psychology, 100*, 555–561.

Hogan, D. P., & Astone, N. M. (1986). The transition to adulthood. *Annual Review of Sociology, 12*, 109–130.

Horwitz, A.V., & Raskin-White, H. (1991). Becoming married, depression, and alcohol problems among young adults. *Journal of Health and Social Behavior, 32*, 221–237.

Hussong, A. M., Curran, P. J., Moffitt, T. E., Caspi, A., & Carrig, M. M. (2004). Substance abuse hinders desistance in young adults' antisocial behavior. *Development and Psychopathology, 16*, 1029–1046.

Johnston, L. D., O'Malley, P. M., & Bachman, J. G. (2003). National Survey Results on Drug Use from the Monitoring the Future Study, (1975–2002). *Vol. I*, Secondary School Students. *Vol. 2*, College Students and Young Adults. NIH Publication No. 03–5375 and 03–5376. Bethesda, MD: National Institute on Drug Abuse.

Kerckhoff, A. C. (1993). *Diverging pathways: Social structure and career deflections.* Cambridge, UK: Cambridge University Press.

Kessler, R. C., Foster, C. L., Saunders, W. B., & Stang, P. (1995). Social consequences of psychiatric disorders I: Educational attainment. *American Journal of Psychiatry, 152*, 1026–1032.

Kessler, R. C., McGonagle, K. A., Zhao, S., Nelson, C.B., Hughes, M., Eshleman, S., Wittchen, H-U, Kendler, K. S. (1994). Lifetime and 12-month prevalence of DSM-III-R psychiatric disorders in the United States: results from the National Cormorbidity Survey. *Archives of General Psychiatry, 51*, 8–19.

Kessler, R. C., & Walters, E. E. (1998). Epidemiology of *DSM-III-R* major depression and minor depression among adolescents and young adults in the National Comorbidity Survey. *Depression and Anxiety, 7*, 3–14.

Klerman, G. L., & Weissman, M. M. (1989). Increasing rates of depression. *Journal of the American Medical Associatioin, 261*, 2229–2235.

Laub, J. H., Nagin, D. S., & Sampson, R. J. (1998). Trajectories of change in criminal offending: Good marriages and the desistance process. *American Sociological Review, 63*, 225–238.

Laub, J. H., & Sampson, R. J. (1993). Turning points in the life course: Why change matters to the study of crime. *Criminology, 31*, 301–325.

Lewis, S. K., Ross, C. E., & Mirowsky, J. (1999). Establishing a sense of personal control in the transition to adulthood. *Social Forces, 77*, 1573–1599.

Link, B. G., & Phelan, J. C. (1995). Social conditions as fundamental causes of disease. *Journal of Health and Social Behavior, 32*, 302–320.

Macmillan, R. (2001). Violence and the life course: The consequences of victimization for personal and social development. *Annual Review of Sociology, 27*, 1–22.

Macmillan, R., & Hagan, J. (2004). Violence in the transition to adulthood: Adolescent victimization, education, and socioeconomic attainment in the later life. *Journal of Research on Adolescence, 14*, 127–158.

McLeod, J., & Shanahan, M. J. (1993). Poverty, parenting, and children's mental health. *American Sociological Review, 58*, 351–366.

McLoyd, V. C. (1988). Socioeconomic disadvantage and child development. American Psychologist, 52, 185–204.

Miech, R. A., Caspi, A., Moffitt, T., Wright, B. R., & Silva, P. (1999). Low socioeconomic status and mental disorders: A longitudinal study of selection and causation during young adulthood. American Journal of Sociology, 104, 1097–1131.

Miech, R. A., & Shanahan, M. J. (2000). Socioeconomic status and depression over the life course. Journal of Health and Social Behavior, 41, 162–176.

Mirowsky, J., & Ross, C. E. (2003). Social causes of psychological distress. Second Edition. Hawthorne, NY: Aldine de Gruyter.

Moffitt, T. E., Caspi, A., Harrington, H., & Milne, B. J. (2002). Males on the life-course-persistent and adolescence-limited antisocial pathways: Follow-up at age 26 years. Developmental and Psychopathology, 14, 179–207.

Mortimer, J. T., Finch, M., Shanahan, M., & Ryu, S. (1992). Adolescent work history and behavioral adjustment. Journal of Research on Adolescence, 2, 59–80.

Mouw, T. (2005). Sequences of early adult transitions: A look at variability and consequences. In R. A. Settersten, Jr., F. F. Furstenberg, Jr., & R. G. Rumbaut (Eds.), On the frontier of adulthood (pp 256–291). Chicago, Illinois: University of Chicago Press.

Newman, D., Moffitt, T. E., Caspi, A., Magdol, L., Silva, P., & Stanton, W. (1996). Psychiatric disorder in a birth cohort of young adults: prevalence, comorbidity, clinical significance and new case incidence from ages 11–21. Journal of Consulting and Clinical Psychology, 64, 552–562.

Osgood, D. W., Ruth, G., Eccles, J. S., Jacobs, J. E., & Barber, B. (2005). Six paths to adulthood: Fast starters, parents without careers, educated partners, educated singles, working singles, and slow starters. In R. A. Settersten, Jr., F. F. Furstenberg, Jr., & R. G. Rumbaut (Eds.), On the frontier of adulthood (pp 320–355). Chicago, Illinois: University of Chicago Press.

Pearlin, L. I., Lieberman, M.A., Menaghan, E. G., & Mullan, J. T. (1981). The stress process. Journal of Health and Social Behavior, 22, 337–356.

Phelan, J. C., & Link, B. G. (1999). The labeling theory of mental disorder (I): The role of social contingencies in the application of psychiatric labels. In A.V. Horwitz & T.L. Scheid, A handbook for the study of mental health (pp 139–149). Cambridge, UK: Cambridge University Press.

Quinton, D., Pickles, A., Maughan, B., & Rutter, M. (1993). Partners, peers, and pathways: Assortative pairing and continuities in conduct disorder. Development and Psychopathology, 5, 763–783.

Quinn, R. P., & Staines, G. L. (1979). The 1977 Quality of Employment Survey. Ann Arbor: Survey Research Center, University of Michigan.

Roisman, G. I., Aguilar, B., & Egeland, B. (2004). Antisocial behavior in the transition to adulthood: The independent and interactive roles of developmental history and emerging developmental tasks. Development and Psychopathology, 16, 857–871.

Ronka, A., & Pulkkinen, Lea. (1995). Accumulation of problems in social functioning in young adulthood: A developmental approach. Journal of Personality and Social Psychology, 69, 381–391.

Rutter, M. (1989). Pathways from childhood to adult life. Journal of Child Psychology and Psychiatry, 30, 23–51.

Sampson, R. J., & Laub, J. H. (1993). Crime in the making: pathways and turning points through life. Cambridge, MA: Harvard University Press.

Schnaiberg, A., & Goldenberg, S. (1989). From empty nest to crowded nest: The dynamics of incompletely launched young adults. Social Problems, 36, 252–266.

Schulenberg, J., O'Malley, P. M., Bachman, J. G., & Johnston, L. D. (2005). Early adult transitions and their relation to well-being and substance use. In R. A. Settersten, Jr., F. F. Furstenberg, Jr., & R. G. Rumbaut (Eds.), *On the frontier of adulthood* (pp 417–453). Chicago, Illinois: University of Chicago Press.

Schulenberg, J., O'Malley, P. M., Bachman, J., & Johnston, L. (2000). Spread your wings and fly: The course of well being and substance use during the transition to young adulthood. In L. J. Crockett & R. Silbereisen (Eds.), *Negotiating adolescence in times of social change* (pp 224–255). Cambridge, UK: Cambridge University Press.

Schulenberg, J., Sameroff, A., & Cicchetti, D. (2004). The transition to adulthood as a critical juncture in the course of psychopathology and mental health. *Development and Psychopathology, 16*, 799–806.

Shanahan, M. (2000). Pathways to adulthood in changing societies: Variability and mechanisms in life course perspective. *Annual Review of Sociology, 26*, 667–692.

Shanahan, M. J., & Hood, K. (2002). Adolescents in changing social structures: bounded agency in a life course perspective. In L. J. Crockett & R. Silbereisen (Eds.), *Negotiating adolescence in times of social change* (pp 123–134). Cambridge, UK: Cambridge University Press.

Simmons, R. G. And Blyth, D. A. (1987). *Moving into adolescence*. New York: Aldine de Gruyter.

Turner, R. J. (2003). The pursuit of socially modifiable contingencies in mental health. *Journal of Health and Social Behavior, 44*, 1–17.

Turner, R. J., & Avison, W. R. (2003). Status variations in stress exposure: Implications for the interpretation of research on race, socioeconomic status and gender. *Journal of Health and Social Behavior*, 44(4), 488–505.

Turner, R. J., & Lloyd, D. A. (1995). Lifetime traumas and mental health: The significance of cumulative adversity. *Journal of Health and Social Behavior, 36*, 360–376.

Turner, R. J., & Lloyd, D. A. (1999). The stress process and the social distribution of depression. *Journal of Health and Social Behavior, 40*, 374–404.

Turner, R. J., Wheaton, B., & Lloyd, D. A. (1995). The epidemiology of social stress. *American Sociological Review, 60*, 104–125.

U. S. Department of Education. (1994). *Creating a school-to-work opportunities system.* Washington, DC.

Wheaton, B. (1978). The sociogenesis of psychological disorder: Reexamining the causal issues with longitudinal data. *American Sociological Review, 43*, 383–403.

Wheaton, B. (1994). Sampling the stress universe. In W. R. Avison & I. H. Gotlib (Eds.), *Stress and Mental Health: Contemporary Issues and Prospects for the Future* (pp 77–113). New York: Plenum.

Wheaton, B., & Clarke, P. (2003). Space meets time: Integrating temporal and contextual influences on mental health in early adulthood. *American Sociological Review, 68*, 680–706.

Wheaton, B., & Gotlib, I. H. (1997). Trajectories and turning points over the life course: Concepts and themes. In B. Wheaton & I. H. Gotlib (Eds.), *Stress and Adversity Over the Life Course: Trajectories and Turning Points* (pp 1–25). Cambridge, U.K.: Cambridge University Press.

Wickrama, K. A. S., Conger, R. D., Wallace, L. E., & Elder, G. H., Jr. (2003). Linking early social risks to impaired physical health during the transition to adulthood. *Journal of Health & Social Behavior, 44*, 61–74.

William T. Grant Commission on Work, Family, and Citizenship. (1998). The Forgotten Half: Non-college youth in America. *Youth and America's Future: The William T. Grant Commission on Work, Family, and Citizenship.*

11
Contributions of the Sociology of Mental Health for Understanding the Social Antecedents, Social Regulation, and Social Distribution of Emotion

Robin W. Simon

Introduction

While the sociology of emotion includes a number of compelling theories about the ways in which social factors influence both the experience and expression of emotion, it currently lacks a body of systematic empirical research with which to evaluate its key theories and concepts. In this chapter, I review findings from research on the sociology of mental health, which document a variety of social influences on subjectively experienced feelings and expressive behavior and which allow us to evaluate some emotion theories and concepts—particularly with respect to the social antecedents, social regulation, and social distribution of emotion in the population. However, I also discuss some ways in which theoretical developments in the sociology of emotion could enhance the sociology of mental health—especially with regard to our understanding of persistent group differences in both the experience and expression of emotional problems in the United States.

The sociology of emotion is a relatively new sub-discipline within sociology. First established as an official section of the American Sociological Association in 1986, this field of study has garnered enthusiastic interest from both micro—and macro—sociologists in a variety of substantive areas: sociologists of gender and the family, work and occupations, collective action and social movements, deviance and mental health as well as cultural, historical, medical, organizational, and political sociologists and social psychologists have all sought to enrich their understandings of their respective areas through the incorporation of emotion theories and concepts. For example, at his 2001 American Sociological Association presidential address on the evolution of human society, Doug Massey—whose own research focuses on the social demography of migration and immigration—argued that emotion is central in social life and that sociologists should turn their attention to feeling and affect (Massey, 2002). Increased sociological interest in and attention to feeling and emotion is due to a confluence of many factors, among them is the growing recognition that social life contains both rational and non-rational (i.e., emotional) forces and that individuals are both cognitive and affective beings.

However, while this relatively new field of inquiry has captured the attention of sociologists working in a variety of areas—and sociologists have increasingly recognized the centrality of feeling and emotion in a variety of aspects of social life—the sociology of emotion currently lacks a coherent body of systematic empirical work. Despite the development of a diverse and impressive set of theories about emotional experience and expression at both the micro—and macro—levels of analysis, the sociology of emotion falls short on empirical evidence with which these theories could be evaluated. The paucity of systematic empirical research in this area has been noted by both Thoits (1989) and Smith-Lovin (1995) in their excellent reviews of the field of emotion who agree that the sociology of affect is theoretically rich but limited empirically. With the exception of a handful of quantitative studies (Erickson & Ritter, 2001; Lively & Heise, 2004; Lively & Powell, 2006; Pugliesi & Shook, 1996; Ross & Van Willigen, 1996; Schieman, 1999, 2000; Simon & Nath, 2004; Sprecher, 1986; Wharton & Erickson, 1995)—many of which have based on the recent emotions module of the General Social Survey—almost all empirical work in this area has been based on small in-depth qualitative studies, which are very informative but cannot be used to adequately assess certain theoretical and substantive issues and debates.

In this chapter, I draw on findings from decades of empirical research on the sociology of mental health in order to shed light on three central but still unresolved theoretical and substantive debates in the sociology of emotion, which pertain to: (1) *the social antecedents of emotion*; (2) *the social regulation of emotion*; and (3) *the social distribution of emotion* in the United States. In particular, I review research that documents: (a) the importance of undesirable life events and chronic strains as well as other stressful social situations—such as persistent social disadvantage and inequality—in *the etiology of emotional distress*; (b) the role of *coping and social support for reducing symptoms of emotional discomfort*; and (c) the *social epidemiology of emotional disturbance* in the general population. The first part of my chapter, therefore, focuses on the contributions of the sociology of mental health for understanding the social causes, social control, and social patterning of emotion and emotional problems in the U.S.

In addition to reviewing research on mental health on the above three topics—which enhance our understanding of a myriad of social factors that influence both the experience and expression of emotion—I discuss theoretical developments in the sociology of emotion that contribute to our understanding of *persistent group differences in the manifestation (i.e., expression) of emotional problems in the U.S.*, particularly with respect to *gender, race, ethnicity, and socioeconomic status*. In the second part of the chapter, I suggest that gender, race, ethnic, and socioeconomic status variations in rates of emotional problems as well as people's emotional responses to stressful social situations may be due to important group differences in norms and beliefs about the appropriate experience and expression of emotion.

I conclude the chapter with a brief discussion of broad themes regarding the complementarity of theory and research on mental health and emotion. The sociology of mental health provides both an extensive and coherent body of empirical evidence with which several theories about emotion can be evaluated. At the same time, concepts, theories, and insights from the sociology of emotion could (and in my opinion should) be used to enrich our understanding of the social psychological mechanisms that underlie the development and persistence of mental health problems in the U.S. and group differences therein. Given their many points of overlap, it is ironic that there has been little effort to utilize theory and research from the sociology of mental health to inform theory and research on the sociology of emotion and vice-versa. *This chapter represents an attempt to integrate these separate yet highly interrelated areas of sociological inquiry.*[1] Before turning to my discussion of some overlapping and crosscutting themes in the sociologies of mental health and emotion, the following three cautionary notes are warranted.

First, while sociological theories about emotion focus on individuals' everyday feelings and expressive behavior, sociological research on mental health focuses on symptoms of emotional distress—particularly symptoms of depression and anxiety—which are considered to be *moods* or *affective states* rather than *emotions per se*. The research on mental health on which I draw, therefore, speaks more directly to the development and persistence of *emotional problems* among persons than to their immediate and short-term *feelings* and *emotions*. However, because feelings of sadness, loneliness, hopelessness, anxiety, worry, and fear are key components of both symptom scales and psychiatric diagnoses of emotional problems such as depression and anxiety, sociological research on mental health provides a window into some fundamental emotion processes that are at the center of theoretical and substantive debates about the experience and expression of everyday feelings in the general population.

It is important to mention that since symptom scales and psychiatric diagnosis of depression and anxiety are partially based on the emotions mentioned above, they actually tap into some of the same feelings that have captured the attention of emotion researchers. Indeed, it is possible, if not likely, that the experience of frequent and persistent distressing emotions underlie the development of these milder mental health problems. Although I cannot say whether these same emotions contribute to serious mental illness such as schizophrenia and personality disorders, Thoits (1985) argued that non-normative emotions and emotional displays are central in the *labeling* of serious mental illness. Her informal analysis of DSM-III diagnostic criteria revealed that "inappropriate emotional states or displays are essential defining features of 45.7% of a total of 210 disorders and are associated features of 64.8% of these disorders" (p. 224). Nevertheless, because I draw mainly on studies of milder forms of mental health problems such as depression and anxiety, keep in mind that my discussion of research on mental health and emotion does *not* apply to serious mental illness.

---

[1] This is not to say that scholars have not worked at the intersection of the sociologies of mental health and emotion. Bradburn's (1969) pioneering work and Thoits' (1984a, 1985, 1995a) later exemplary work provide excellent examples of the ways in which theory and research on mental health inform, enrich, and extend theory and research on emotion and vice versa.

Second, because most sociological research on mental health focuses on symptoms of *emotional distress* rather than on symptoms of *emotional well-being*, much of my discussion is necessarily limited to the experience and expression of *negative* feelings and emotions. I do not assume—as mental health scholars sometimes do–that the absence of negative feelings (or the absence of symptoms of emotional distress) is equivalent to the presence of positive feelings (or the presence of symptoms of emotional well-being). In his early study of the structure of psychological well-being, Bradburn (1969) found that positive and negative affect represent two separate and independent dimensions of psychological well-being. He also found that positive and negative feelings (and, by extension, positive and negative mental health) have different etiologies and are related to different things.[2] Since positive *and* negative feelings are not merely two sides of a continuum of emotional experience, unless otherwise noted, my discussion of theory and research on mental health and emotion is restricted to negative feelings and symptoms of emotional distress.

Finally, while the empirical findings on the social antecedents, regulation, and distribution of emotion that I discuss may apply to persons residing in other industrialized (and possibly non-industrialized) societies, the literature I draw on is based largely on studies conducted in the U.S. and, therefore, cannot be generalized to the emotions of and emotion processes among persons residing in other cultural contexts. Cross-cultural work on emotion and mental health finds considerable cultural variability in both the experience and expression of emotion and psychiatric illness (see Kleinman [1986] for a comparative psychiatric study in China; Scherer, Wallbott, & Summerfield [1986] for a cross-cultural study of emotional experience across several European countries, and Kleinman & Good [1985]). Evidence from anthropological and historical studies of emotion and mental health also strongly suggests that there is cultural variation in the social situations individuals perceive as stressful and which are emotionally distressing; for example, while the death of a loved one in the contemporary U.S. is stressful

---

[2] Interestingly, Bradburn (1969) found that interpersonal and role-related problems are related to negative affect, whereas social participation and affiliation are associated with positive affect. These findings differ somewhat from the predictions of Kemper's social interactional theory of emotion (1978, 1990) that I will elaborate on later, which claims that persons with relatively low status and power in social relationships experience more negative feelings, while those with comparatively high status and power in interpersonal relationships experience more positive feelings. It is, however, possible that interpersonal and role-related problems are associated with negative emotions because they represent declines in individuals' relative status and power in role-relationships; conversely, unproblematic social participation may be associated with positive emotions because it enhances individuals' perceptions of their relative status and power. Given these rich theoretical and empirical insights about negative and positive feelings, it is unfortunate that sociological research on mental health focuses only on symptoms of emotional distress rather than on symptoms of both emotional well-being and emotional distress as Bradburn did over three decades ago. For a rare example of recent research on mental health that focuses on negative *and* positive well-being, see Keyes (2002).

and emotionally distressing (and is associated with negative feelings such as sadness and grief), this does not appear to be the case in high mortality societies where death is a frequent occurrence and common feature of social life (Aries, 1981; Lofland, 1985). A pivotal question for future research on both emotion and mental health is whether the social factors that are closely associated with negative emotions and emotional distress (and positive emotions and emotional well-being) in the U.S. are the same or different in other, particularly non-western, societies.

Contributions of the Sociology of Mental Health for Understanding Emotion

The Social Antecedents of Emotion

Along with their social science colleagues in anthropology, history, and psychology (e.g., Brody, 1999; Corrigan, 2002; Kleinman, 1986; Kleinman & Good, 1985; Lazarus & Folkman, 1984; Lutz, 1988; Lutz & White, 1986; McMahon, 2006; Rosaldo, 1980, 1984; Schachter & Singer, 1962; Scherer, et al., 1986; Seligman, 2004; Shields, 2002; Stearns & Stearns, 1986), emotions scholars in sociology argue that there is a strong social basis of emotion, and that social situations influence people's feelings and expressive behavior (e.g., Gordon, 1981; Hochschild, 1975, 1979, 1983; Lively & Heise, 2004; Shott, 1979; Simon & Nath, 2004; Smith-Lovin, 1995; Thoits 1985, 1989). Most, if not all, sociological theories about the social antecedents of emotion assert that social situations are *crucial* for individuals to have an emotional experience and influence whether they experience positive or negative feelings. As a case in point, Kemper's (1978, 1990) social interactional theory about emotion argues that decrements in individuals' status and power in social relationships produce negative emotions, while increments in their relationship status and power contribute to positive feelings. In contrast, Heise's (1979) affect control theory posits that social situations that disconfirm people's social identities result in negative feelings, whereas social situations that confirm their social identities lead to positive emotions (also see Smith-Lovin, 1990; Smith-Lovin & Heise, 1988).

The importance of social situations for shaping individuals' feelings and emotions is nowhere more evident than in current definitions of emotion. While there are numerous definitions of emotion with some important differences between them, most current ones in sociology emphasize four distinct but interrelated elements—among them the social situation. Contemporary emotions theorists generally agree that emotions involve complex combinations of: (1) physiological (i.e., bodily) sensations; (2) cognitive appraisals of social situations; (3) expressive gestures or emotional behaviors; and/or (4) cultural meanings, definitions, and labels.[3]

---

[3] See Thoits (1985, 1989) for this particular formulation of emotion and Schachter and Singer (1962) for an earlier two-factor theory of emotion, which also emphasizes the importance of social situations for feelings and emotions.

However, while they assume that social situations influence whether or not people experience an emotion and shape the type of emotion they experience (as well as contribute to both the intensity and duration of the emotion), sociologists of emotion have ironically not specified *which* situations are most likely to elicit emotional responses from persons (for exceptions, see Heise [1979] and Smith-Lovin [1987]). With the exception of a handful of in-depth qualitative studies of specific emotions such as anger (e.g., Stearns & Stearns, 1986; Tavris, 1982;), love (e.g., Cancian, 1987; Simon, Eder, & Evans, 1992; Swidler, 1980, 2001), gratitude (Hochschild, 1989), sadness (e.g., Karp, 1996; Kleinman, 1986; Kleinman & Good, 1985), sympathy (Clark, 1987, 1997), grief (Lofland, 1985), and shame (Scheff, 1990), there has unfortunately been little research that has systematically assessed individuals' negative (or for that matter positive) emotional reactions to various social situations.[4]

Decades of research on the sociology of mental health—particularly on the etiology (or causes) of emotional problems—have identified several critical emotion eliciting situations. In fact, most, if not all, research on mental health conducted from a stress process theoretical paradigm has focused on specifying those social situations that individuals perceive as stressful and are emotionally distressing. Dozens of studies document that undesirable life events, chronic strains, and other stressful social situations are associated with elevated levels of emotional distress and contribute to the onset and persistence of emotional disturbance among persons. This research also finds that socially disadvantaged persons—such as those with low levels of education and income, the unmarried, women, and racial and ethnic minorities—report greater exposure to undesirable events and chronic strains than their socially advantaged peers.

Life Events

A considerable body of work in this area has focused on the impact of life events on both symptoms of emotional distress and psychiatric disorders, particularly depression and anxiety, in the general population of adults and more recently adolescents (e.g., Aneshensel, 1992; Aneshensel, Rutter, & Lachenbruch, 1991; Avison & McAlpine, 1992; Brown & Harris, 1978, 1989; Dohrenwend & Dohrenwend, 1974; Gore, Aseltine, & Colten, 1992; Thoits, 1995b). In an effort to sample the "universe of stressors" (Aneshensel, 1992; Turner & Lloyd, 1999;

---

[4] Similar to their mental health colleagues, emotions researchers in sociology tend to study negative rather than positive emotions. With the exception of research on love noted above and some limited work on happiness (e.g., Bradburn & Caplovitz, 1965), most sociological studies of specific emotions have examined negative feelings such as anger, sadness, grief, and shame. The almost exclusive scholarly focus on negative affect may reflect an underlying cultural preoccupation with negative rather than positive feelings. Consistent with this idea, Easterbrook (2003) who is an economist recently argued that despite tremendous progress in a variety of aspects of social (including economic) life, there has been a steady decline in happiness in the U.S. over the past 50 years. Also, see McMahon (2006) for an interesting description and analysis of the history of happiness in western thought and society.

Turner, Wheaton, & Lloyd, 1995; Wheaton, 1994, 1999), life events research now includes a large number and wide range of events that people experience over the life course. Although researchers find that the magnitude of the association between exposure to eventful stress and emotional disturbance is relatively modest (see Aneshensel [1992] and Thoits [1995b] but also Turner et al., [1995]), it is clear that certain types of events—especially undesirable, uncontrollable, and unpredictable (or non-normative) ones—are perceived as highly stressful and are emotionally distressing (Aneshensel, 1992; Thoits, 1995b). Among the most problematic of these events for depression and anxiety are those involving loss such as the loss of a job, divorce, and death of a loved one (e.g., Kessler, Turner, & House, 1989; Menaghan & Lieberman, 1986; Simon, 2002; Thoits, 1983; Umberson, 2003; Wortman, & Kessler, 1992; Wheaton, 1990).

Some of these events (e.g., a job loss or divorce) may be emotionally harmful because they accompany decrements in people's status and power in social relationships as Kemper's social interactional theory about emotion argues. Alternatively, loss and other types of undesirable events may be emotionally damaging because they disconfirm person's social identities as Heise's affect control theory posits. It is, of course, equally possible that these undesirable life events are emotionally distressing simply because they threaten individuals' sense of emotional and material (i.e., financial) security. In any case, findings from this research strongly suggest that people respond to undesirable life events with an array of negative feelings such as sadness, loneliness, hopelessness, anxiety, worry, fear, and possibly anger, frustration, insecurity, embarrassment, humiliation, and shame. Extending these insights, this research also suggests that people may respond to desirable life events—especially controllable and predictable (or normative) ones such as marriage, the birth of a child, a graduation, promotion, or new job—with a variety of positive feelings including happiness, satisfaction, contentment, security, joy, excitement, and pride as well as symptoms of emotional well-being. It would be useful for future research on life events to investigate these possibilities—particularly the degree to which desirable events contribute to the development and persistence of emotional well-being.

Chronic Strains

In addition to identifying life events that are associated with elevated levels of emotional distress and the onset of psychiatric disturbance, mental health researchers have examined the role and significance of chronic strains for the development and persistence of emotional problems, particularly depression and anxiety, in the general population. In contrast to eventful stressors, which are discrete social situations that often involve a role or status change or transition, chronic stressors refer to situations that are part of routine social life and are ongoing and recurrent (Pearlin, 1989; Pearlin & Lieberman, 1987; Pearlin, Menaghan, Lieberman, & Mullan, 1981). Since they are rooted in everyday social life, chronic strains encompass a wide range of social situations and circumstances that individuals perceive as stressful—including conflicts in (and between) work and family roles and relationships, financial difficulties, health problems or disability, challenges associated with providing on-going care to dependent or ill family members, prejudice and discrimination, as well as social inequality and disadvantage. An accumulation of studies now document that persistent and recurrent stressors are major precursors of emotional disturbance (e.g., Aneshensel, 1992; House, Landis, & Umberson, 1988; Liem & Liem, 1978; Ross & Huber, 1985; Ross & Mirowsky, 1989; Thoits, 1995b; Wheaton, 1990, 1994). Research further shows that exposure to chronic strains is more strongly associated with emotional distress than exposure to eventful stressors (Aneshensel, 1992; Avison & Turner, 1988; Turner et al., 1995). Several scholars have noted that a reason why undesirable life events are causally related to emotional problems is because they usher in a host of chronic challenges and difficulties for persons (e.g., Aneshensel, 1992; Mirowsky & Ross, 2003; Pearlin, 1989; Thoits, 1995b; Wheaton, 1983, 1990).

Here again, it is possible that chronic strains are emotionally distressing because they decrease individuals' perceptions of status and power in social relationships or disconfirm their social identities as Kemper and Heise argue, respectively. There is actually some support for the idea that certain situations (e.g., having an employed wife) are emotionally disturbing because they reduce individuals' perceptions of power and control in social relationships (Rosenfield, 1989; Ross, Mirowsky, & Huber, 1983). There is also some evidence that chronic strains in valued role domains are highly stressful and distressing because they threaten role-identities that are salient to persons (see Simon [1992] but also Thoits [1995c] who does not find support for the identity-salience hypotheses with respect to life events). Whatever the exact underlying theoretical mechanism is, findings from this research strongly suggest that people respond to chronic strains with an assortment of negative emotions including sadness, loneliness, hopelessness, anxiety, worry, and fear, and possibly anger, frustration, insecurity, embarrassment, humiliation, and shame. This research also suggests that individuals may respond to on-going social situations that either bolster their perception of status and power, confirm their social identities, or simply increase their sense of emotional and material security with a host of positive emotions such as happiness, satisfaction, contentment, security, excitement, joy, and pride. It would be helpful for research on chronic strains to examine these possibilities, especially the extent to which on-going positive social situations contribute to positive feelings and the development of long-term emotional well-being.

Taken together, research on the etiology of emotional distress has identified a large number and wide range of social situations that influence the development and persistence of emotional problems and which undoubtedly precipitate a sequelae of negative feelings among people. Indeed, this research demonstrates that exposure to stressful life events and chronic strains explain some of the variance in emotional distress in the population (e.g., Aneshensel et al., 1991; Dohrenwend & Dohrenwend, 1976; Kessler, 1979; Mirowsky & Ross, 2003; Turner et al., 1995). Simply stated, sociodemographic and social status differences in the prevalence of emotional problems and psychiatric disorders in the U.S. are partially due to sociodcmographic and social status differences in exposure to stressful social situations. Emotions scholars should draw on this useful typology of undesirable life events and chronic strains in order to pinpoint the social situations that underlie decrements in individuals' power and status in social relationships and that disconfirm their social identities—which have both been hypothesized to increase negative feelings and emotions.

However, at the same time that the sociology of mental health contributes to our understanding of the social antecedents of emotion, theory and research in this area would benefit from the addition of a broader range of life events and on-going social situations (including life-affirming desirable events and on-going positive situations) as well as a broader range of emotional outcomes—particularly measures of emotional well-being. Consistent with Aneshensel and colleagues' (1991, 1992, 1996) argument about the need for research to consider multiple sources and outcomes of stress, the inclusion of measures of emotional well-being would allow mental health researchers to more fully capture the ways in which social experiences affect the emotions and health of individuals in the population. This would also permit them to directly assess whether the absence of symptoms of emotional distress is different from the presence of symptoms of emotional well-being as Bradburn (1969) argued and found some time ago.

The Social Regulation of Emotion

In addition to developing innovative theories about the social antecedents of emotion, sociologists of emotion have developed provocative theories about the *social regulation of emotion*. Most notable among these is Hochschild's (1975, 1979, 1982, 1988) seminal theoretical work on emotion management. In this cultural theory about emotion, Hochschild argues that societies contain cultural beliefs about emotion, which give rise to social norms about appropriate emotional experience and expression. She claims that cultural beliefs about emotion influence individuals' emotions vis-à-vis feeling and expression norms, which specify the emotions they should and should not feel and express both in general and in specific settings. Feeling rules are social norms that specify the appropriate type, intensity, duration, and target of subjectively experienced feelings. Expression rules are social norms that regulate the type, intensity, duration, and target of emotional behavior or affective displays. According to Hochschild, feeling and expression rules are standards by which we judge our own and other people's emotions; when our feelings and expressions depart from emotion norms, we often engage in emotion management, expression management, or both in order to create a more appropriate response. She emphasizes that individuals learn social norms about emotion through the same processes and in the same contexts in which they learn other normative information, which is in everyday social interaction with parents, siblings, teachers, and peers. That is, people acquire cultural knowledge about socially permissible and unacceptable feelings and affective behavior from childhood throughout adulthood vis-à-vis emotional socialization.

As the most influential of the sociological theories about emotion (Smith-Lovin, 2003), there is now a significant body of work that has elucidated the processes through which individuals manage their own and other people's emotions (e.g., Erickson & Ritter, 2001; Erickson & Wharton, 1997; Frude & Goss, 1981; Gatta, 2002; Harlow, 2003; Hochschild, 1983, 1988; Leavitt & Power, 1989; Leidner, 1993; Lively, 2000, 2002; Lois, 2003; Pierce, 1995; Pollak & Thoits, 1989; Simon et al., 1992; Smith & Kleinman, 1988; Thoits, 1995a). This research has also identified the content of feeling and expression norms and documented emotional socialization in a variety of social contexts.[5] However, while these studies shed light on emotion management (as well as emotion norms and emotion socialization) in various social settings, they provide little insight into the social regulation of emotion in the general population.

For instance, we still do not know the extent to which individuals manage their non-normative (or "deviant") emotions and whether there are sociodemographic and social status variations in the use (and effectiveness) of emotion management. Once again, decades of research on the sociology of mental health—particularly on *coping and social support*—demonstrate that people regulate (i.e., manage) their own and other's negative emotions through a variety of coping and social support resources and strategies. This research also shows that coping and social support are not randomly distributed in the population; certain groups of people—including those with lower levels of education and income, the unmarried, racial and ethnic minorities, and (depending on the specific type of resource and strategy) women— have fewer coping and social support resources and use less effective coping strategies than others with which to manage their negative feelings.

Coping Resources & Strategies

Because emotional distress and psychiatric disturbance are not inevitable consequences of exposure to undesirable life events and chronic strains, researchers have sought to identify social factors that intervene between stressful social situations and people's emotional reactions to them. To date, researchers have identified a number of coping and social support resources and strategies that mediate and

---

[5] Following Hochschild's (1983) seminal work on flight attendants, most sociological research on emotion management has been conducted at the workplace (Erickson & Wharton, 1997; Erickson & Ritter, 2001; Gatta, 2002; Hochschild, 1983; Leidner, 1993; Lively, 2000, 2002; Pierce, 1995), although there has been some work in the family (Frude & Goss, 1981; Hochschild, 1989; Wharton & Erickson, 1995). There is also some research on emotion norms, emotion socialization, and emotion management in educational institutions such as professional school (Cahill, 1999; Smith & Kleinman, 1989), college (Harlow, 2003), middle-school (Simon et al., 1992), and preschool (Leavitt & Powell, 1989; Pollak & Thoits, 1989) as well as among "deviant" subgroups including sexual minorities (Schrock, Holden, & Reid, 2004) and the disabled (Cahill & Eggleston, 1994). Potentially fruitful are- nas for this genre of work are psychiatric and other types of hospitals as well as athletic, political, and military organizations. See Lois (2003) for an interesting investigation of the emotion culture of a search and rescue organization.

moderate the relationship between stress exposure and emotional disturbance (Pearlin & Schooler, 1978). For example, studies show that *coping resources*—which refer to individuals' personal characteristics such as their sense of control or mastery and self-esteem—directly reduce symptoms of emotional distress as well as buffer the deleterious effects of stress exposure (Mirowsky & Ross, 1990; Turner & Noh, 1983; Turner & Roszell, 1994). Similarly, studies find that *coping strategies*—which refer to peoples' actual behavior such as problem-focused and emotion-focused coping efforts—have both direct and indirect effects on emotional problems that are associated with eventful and chronic stressors (Menaghan, 1983). Men and women turn to these coping strategies in order to deal with demands of stressful social situations themselves as well as their emotional reactions to them. Not surprisingly, studies indicate that problem-focused coping is most efficacious for dealing with the demands themselves, while emotion-focused coping is most efficacious for dealing with one's emotional reactions to difficult life events, situations, and circumstances (Thoits, 1991a, 1995b).[6] For these and other reasons, coping researchers have concluded that people often use multiple strategies when coping with acute and chronic stressors.[7]

Since coping resources and strategies reduce symptoms of emotional distress and buffer the harmful emotional effects of life stress, it is likely that they also affect individuals' immediate and short-term negative emotional reactions to social situations more generally. For example, people who believe that they have control over life outcomes, who have high self-esteem, and who have an active coping style (i.e., who regularly use coping behaviors) may be less likely to experience negative feelings than those who lack coping resources and have a passive coping orientation. When faced with a demand, these persons may also experience negative emotions with less intensity and for a shorter duration than those who lack resources. Moreover, the negative feelings they experience may not as readily develop into chronic feelings of emotional distress and emotional problems.

However, while all coping resources and strategies are likely to be important for reducing negative feelings, emotion-focused coping efforts may be particularly significant. In her highly innovative work on this topic, Thoits (1984a, 1985) argued that emotion-focused coping operates in much the same way as emotion management (also see Folkman & Lazarus, 1985 and Lazarus & Folkman, 1984).

---

[6] It is important to emphasize that coping *resources* such as a sense of control and self-esteem are *intra*-individual characteristics of persons that inadvertently protect them from the negative emotional effects of stress. In contrast, coping *strategies* such as problem-focused and emotion-focused coping refer to individual's actual *efforts* to manage specific situational demands, which they appraise as taxing (Lazarus & Folkman, 1984; Thoits, 1995a).

[7] Studies further indicate that people use a greater number of coping strategies when they appraise the situation as severe (Cronkite & Moos 1984; Folkman & Lazarus, 1980) and that problem-focused coping is more likely when stressors are appraised as controllable, while emotion-focused coping is more likely when they are appraised as uncontrollable (Coyne, Aldwin, & Lazarus, 1981; Folkman, 1984; Folkman & Lazarus, 1980, 1985; Stone & Neal, 1984; Thoits, 1991a).

Utilizing concepts from the sociology of emotion, she showed that people cope with persistent and recurring negative emotions—especially *non*-normative and *distressing* feelings—in a number of different social contexts through emotion management by suppressing the negative feelings they have and replacing them with more appropriate or pleasant (i.e., positive) emotions. These findings suggest that individuals routinely *transform* their emotions so that they are more consistent with cultural emotion norms. Coping researchers should pay greater attention to both the use and effectiveness of emotion management for reducing feelings of emotional distress as well as for increasing feelings of emotional well-being among persons in the population.

Social Support

An additional psychosocial resource that sociologists of mental health frequently study is social support, which includes both functional and structural support. Unlike the coping resources and strategies discussed above—which consist of individuals' *own* response to managing stressful situations and their emotional reactions to them—functional support refers to "functions performed for the individual by significant others such as family members, friends, and coworkers" (Thoits, 1995b: 64). Three types of functional support have been identified in the literature; significant others provide instrumental, informational, and emotional support (House & Kahn, 1985).[8] Moreover, functional support may be received or perceived; people may actually receive these various forms of assistance from others or simply perceive that such assistance is available if needed. One of the most interesting findings of this research is that perceived emotional support is associated with fewer symptoms of emotional distress than received social support (Wethington & Kessler, 1986).[9] Similar to research on coping resources discussed above, studies show that perceived emotional support directly reduces emotional disturbance as well as buffers the damaging emotional effects of undesirable life events and chronic strains. Studies further indicate that the most efficacious type of social support in the face of life stress is simply having an intimate confiding relationship (Cohen & Wills, 1985).

In contrast to functional support, structural support refers to the social networks in which people are embedded and the characteristics of these networks—such as the number of social relationships they have and the frequency with which they have contact with these persons; structural support is the degree to which

---

[8] As the terms imply, instrumental support refers to concrete services or resources that others provide to individuals who are dealing with stress, including such things as childcare, meals, transportation, housing, and money. Similarly, informational support refers to information that others provide, while emotional support refers to the understanding and sympathy (i.e., the emotional assistance) they give.

[9] Paralleling the ideas in Kemper's social interactional theory of emotion, Wethington and Kessler (1983) claim that a reason why the receipt of social support is not as effective for reducing symptoms of emotional distress as the perception of social support is because it results in declines in power and status in the social relationship.

individuals are socially integrated. Although structural support (including the size of the social network) is associated with fewer symptoms of emotional distress, research indicates that it does not buffer the negative emotional impact of stressors on persons (Cohen & Wills, 1985; House et al., 1988).

Since social support mediates (and sometimes moderates) the relationship between stress exposure and emotional disturbance, it may also affect individuals' immediate and short-term negative emotional responses to stressful social situations. It is possible, if not likely, that social support—especially *emotional* support—operates in much the same way as do coping resources and strategies with respect to the social regulation of negative emotions. For example, people with supportive social networks may experience less frequent negative emotions to begin with. Additionally, either the perception or receipt of all forms of assistance—including instrumental, informational, and particularly emotional support—may reduce negative feelings that tend to arise in stressful social situations. Emotional support from a partner, close friend, relative, and/or coworker may also be directly involved in emotion management; persons who have emotional support may be better able to manage their own negative feelings when dealing with stressors and supportive others may help them manage their emotions, their affective displays, or both.

In her seminal work in this area, Thoits (1984a, 1985, 1986a) identified several techniques of interpersonal coping assistance—many of which involve emotion-focused coping. It appears that supportive others help individuals manage their distressing emotions by: (1) reinterpreting situations so they are less negative or threatening; (2) distracting them so they do not dwell on the stressful situation or the unpleasant emotions; (3) helping them alter their physiological sensations with substances, prayer, meditation, and physical exercise; as well as (4) encouraging them to actually transform their current feelings by suppressing the unpleasant emotions they are experiencing and invoking more positive emotions. Inspired by Thoits' pioneering work on this topic, several in-depth qualitative studies of emotion management, especially interpersonal and reciprocal emotion management, have elucidated the content of emotion-focused social support in a variety of social settings, contexts, and relationships (Francis, 1997; Lively, 2000; Schrock, Holden, & Reid, 2004; Staske, 1996; Thoits, 1995a). Social support researchers should examine the various ways in which supportive members of people's social networks help them reduce their negative emotions and perhaps increase their positive feelings vis-à-vis emotion management.

Taken as a whole, research on the sociology of mental health has identified a variety of coping and social support resources and strategies through which individuals regulate their own (and other people's) distressing emotions. Since they directly reduce feelings of emotional discomfort as well as buffer the emotional impact of stressors, it is likely that coping and social support also help persons regulate their immediate and short-term negative emotional responses to a plethora of stressful social situations. Emotion-focused coping and emotional support may be particularly important for the management of negative feelings. Not surprisingly, with the exception of the availability of supportive emotional relationships—which women report the same as or more of than men—stress theory predicts and mental health research generally finds that the epidemiology of coping and social support closely corresponds to the epidemiology of emotional distress and psychiatric disorder in the population (e.g., Mirowsky & Ross, 2003; Pearlin & Schooler, 1978; Pearlin, 1985; Thoits, 1987, 1995b; Turner & Marino, 1994; Turner & Noh, 1983). That is, socially disadvantaged persons—including those with lower levels of education and income, the unmarried, women, and racial and ethnic minorities— have fewer coping resources and use less effective coping strategies than their socially advantaged peers. Interestingly, the observation that women are more likely than men to both perceive that they have emotional support and use emotion-focused coping strategies (Simon & Nath, 2004; Thoits, 1991b) contradicts stress theories' explanation of women's higher rates of emotional distress but provides support for Hochschild's (1983) assertion that emotion management is more common among women than among men. Emotions scholars would be wise to draw on this exhaustive inventory of coping and social support resources and strategies in order to broaden their knowledge about the multitude of ways in which individuals manage their own (and others') negative feelings.

Nevertheless, at the same time that research on coping and social support contributes to our understanding of the social regulation of emotion in the general population, it would be enhanced by following Thoits' lead and more explicitly examining the degree to which people manage their own and others' negative (and possibly positive) emotions. By doing so, mental health scholars could begin to identify social norms that underlie individuals' understandings of and beliefs about appropriate and inappropriate feelings and expressive behavior.

The Social Distribution of Emotion

In addition to theorizing about the social antecedents and social regulation of emotion, emotions scholars have theorized about the *social distribution of emotion*. Indeed, a core insight of the sociology of emotion is that feelings are *socially patterned* and are, therefore, *not* randomly distributed in the population. For instance, Kemper's (1990) and Hochschild's (1979) influential structural theories about emotion posit that individuals' social location influences both their subjectively experienced feelings and their affective behavior. Kemper argues that people with high status and power in society (i.e., those with high levels of education and income, the married, men, and white persons) experience more frequent positive emotions, whereas people with low status and power in society (i.e., those with low levels of education and income, the unmarried, women, and racial and ethnic minorities) experience more frequent negative feelings. Hochschild further claims that individuals who are employed in low status occupations not only experience more frequent negative and less frequent positive emotions, but are also the targets of other people's negative feelings.

Despite these rich theoretical insights, with the exception of a handful of recent quantitative studies (Lively & Heise, 2004; Ross & Van Willigen, 1996; Schieman, 1999, 2000; Simon & Nath, 2004; Sprecher, 1986), data limitations have prevented emotion researchers from assessing the social distribution of emotion in the population. The few studies that exist provide support for structural theories about emotion. As a case in point, based on analyses of data from the 1996 emotions module of the General Social Survey, Nath and I (Simon & Nath, 2004) found that people with lower levels of education and household income, the unmarried, women, and ethnic minorities report negative feelings more often than those with higher levels of education and income, the married, men, and white persons. In contrast, individuals with higher levels of education and men report positive emotions more often than those with lower levels of education and women. Not surprisingly, our research also reveals sociodemographic and social status differences in the frequency with which people experience specific emotions; individuals with higher levels of education and men report more frequent feelings of calm and excitement, whereas those with lower levels of education and household income and women report more frequent feelings of anxiety and sadness. However, in contrast to the predictions of structural theories about emotion, we also found that there are no sociodemographic or social status differences in self-reports of feelings of anger and shame.[10]

Because symptom scales and psychiatric diagnoses of depression and anxiety include negative emotions such as sadness, loneliness, hopelessness, worry, anxiety, and fear, it should come as no surprise that the findings from Nath's and my recent research and other quantitative studies of the social structuring of emotion closely parallel findings from research on mental health with respect to the social epidemiology (i.e., the social patterning) of emotional distress and psychiatric disturbance in the general population. Dozens of studies based on both community and national samples of adults and more recently adolescents document that persons with disadvantaged social statuses—including those with low socioeconomic status, the unmarried, females, and some ethnic groups—have higher rates of certain types of emotional problems than their more advantaged peers. In fact, the search for the underlying causes of sociodemographic and social status differences in mental health problems in the U.S. is responsible for the abundance of sociological

---

[10] Although Nath and I did not find gender differences in the frequency with which people report angry feelings, Ross and Van Willigen (1996) found that women report angry emotions more often than men. Differences between the findings of these two studies may be due to differences in the measurement of anger in these different studies, which Nath and I discuss in our paper. However, although they do not report more frequent feelings of anger than men, our study revealed that women report that their anger is both more intense and of longer duration than men's and that men and women differ in the ways in which they cope with (i.e., manage) their angry feelings. Consistent with Thoits' study (1991b), we found that women cope with their angry feelings by talking with others and praying to God, whereas men cope with their anger by using substances, including having a drink or taking a pill. Using these same data (i.e., the GSS emotions module), Lively and I (Simon & Lively, 2005) are currently investigating whether women's more intense and longer lasting anger play a role in their more frequent feelings of emotional distress relative to men. Our analyses indicate that these two dimensions of anger are involved in women's more frequent feelings of both sadness and anxiety and that angry feelings are associated with emotional distress.

research on both the social etiology of emotional distress and the role of coping and social support for reducing emotional discomfort that I discussed earlier.

Socioeconomic Status

Consistent with sociologists' long-term preoccupation with the ways in which social class affects individuals, groups, and societies, sociologists of mental health have documented social class differences in emotional distress. Epidemiological studies in the U.S. dating as far back as the 1930's (Faris & Dunham, 1939) consistently indicate a close association between socioeconomic status and mental health problems in the general population of adults and that all types of emotional problems (ranging from the mildest forms of emotional discomfort to the most severe forms of mental illness) are more common among persons with lower levels of education and family income and lower status occupations (e.g., Dohrenwend & Dohrenwend, 1969; Hollingshead & Redlich, 1958; Kessler, 1979; Kessler & Cleary, 1980; Link, Lennon, & Dohrenwend, 1993; Yu & Williams, 1999).

However, while the association between socioeconomic status and mental health is irrefutable, the underlying social factors that are responsible for this relationship are more elusive and continue to be the subject of debate. For example, some studies show that social causation processes are of greater significance than social selection processes for understanding socioeconomic status differences in mental health, while others find that both social causation and social selection contribute to the social class-emotional distress relationship (Dohrenwend, Levan, Shrout, Schwartz, Naveh, Link, Skodal, & Stueve, 1992; McLeod & Kaiser, 2004). Moreover, although some scholars maintain that lower class persons experience greater emotional distress because they are more exposed to acute and chronic stressors (e.g., Turner et al., 1995), others claim that deficits in coping and social support resources among the lower class (which render them more vulnerable to the harmful emotional effects of stress) are responsible (e.g., Kessler & McLeod, 1990; Pearlin & Schooler, 1978; Thoits, 1984b, 1995b). No matter which of these arguments they embrace, mental health researchers have interpreted the available evidence to mean that individuals' location in the stratification system and other structural factors influence their emotional well-being.

The fact that persons with limited educations, occupations, and financial resources report higher levels of emotional distress and are more likely to have certain types of psychiatric problems than their more advantaged counterparts closely corresponds to findings from Nath's and my study of the social distribution of emotion in the U.S. discussed above. It is worth noting that although research on mental health typically does not examine the social distribution of emotional well-being in the population, an early study showed that happiness is associated with socioeconomic status and is more frequently experienced by members of advantaged social classes (Bradburn & Caplovitz, 1965). These earlier findings are also consistent with Nath's and my recent research on emotion. In short, decades of research in the sociology of mental health provide support—albeit indirect support—for Kemper's and Hochschild's structural theories about emotion. At the same time, findings from Nath's and my recent work and Bradburn and Caplovitz's early study illustrate that research on the relationship between socioeconomic status and mental health would benefit from the inclusion of measures of emotional well-being since it would allow researchers in this area to directly assess whether social advantaged persons actually report better mental health than their disadvantaged peers.

Marital Status

In addition to socioeconomic status, sociologists of mental health have long been interested in the relationship between marital status and emotional distress. First documented by Gove over a quarter of a century ago (Gove, 1972; Gove & Tudor, 1973), dozens of studies since then have demonstrated that unmarried persons—including both never and previously married persons such as the widowed and divorced—report more emotional problems (ranging from the mildest forms of emotional discomfort to more severe forms of mental illness) than their married peers (e.g., Barrett, 2000; Kessler & McRae, 1984; Menaghan, 1989; Menaghan & Lieberman, 1986; Pearlin & Johnson, 1977; Simon, 1998, 2002; Thoits, 1986b; Umberson, Chen, House, Hopkins, & Slaten, 1992; Williams, 2003; Williams, Takeuchi, & Adair, 1992). It is worth noting that the marital status difference in emotional well-being is one of the most oft cited findings from the sociology of mental health. In fact, the greater emotional discomfort experienced by unmarried compared to married people was initially observed over one hundred years ago in Durkheim's (1951) classic study of the social basis of suicide.[11]

However, here again, while the association between marital status and mental health is indisputable, scholars debate about the underlying social factors that are responsible for this relationship. Although numerous studies show that social causation processes are of greater importance than social selection processes for understanding marital status differences in emotional distress (Marks & Lambert, 1998; Menaghan, 1989; Menaghan & Lieberman, 1986; Simon, 2002; Thoits, 1986b), other studies find that social selection processes also contribute to this relationship (Mastekaasa, 1992; Menaghan, 1985; Simon, 2002). For example, longitudinal research shows that depressed persons are more likely to become divorced than non-depressed persons. Moreover, as

---

[11] Although much less studied than marital status, sociological research on mental health also documents employment status differences in emotional disturbance (Lennon, 1999); not surprisingly, unemployed persons report more mental health problems than their employed peers. However, while married and employed persons report fewer symptoms of emotional distress, studies also show that parenthood does *not* confer a mental health advantage for individuals. Based on a nationally representative sample of adults, Evenson and I (Evenson & Simon, 2005) found that recently found that there is no type of parent who reports less depression than non-parents. We do, however, find considerable variation in depression among parents and that certain types of parenthood are associated with more depressive symptoms than others.

in the case of socioeconomic status differences in mental health, some researchers argue that unmarried persons report greater emotional distress because they are more exposed to acute and chronic stressors (Pearlin & Johnson, 1977; Thoits, 1986), whereas others claim that deficits in coping and social support resources among the unmarried (which render them more vulnerable to the harmful emotional effects of stress) are responsible for their comparatively poorer mental health (Kessler & Essex, 1982; Thoits, 1984b, 1995b). Whichever explanation they embrace, mental health scholars agree that marital status represents a structural location in systems of inequality in the U.S. that influences people's emotional well-being. As such, epidemiological findings on marital status—which dovetail findings from Nath's and my research on the social distribution of emotion in the U.S.—also support Kemper's and Hochshild's structural theories about emotion. Although our study revealed that married people do *not* report more frequent positive emotions than their unmarried peers, future research on the relationship between marital status and mental health should nonetheless examine symptoms of emotional well-being as well as symptoms of emotional distress in order to assess whether the married actually experience better mental health than unmarried persons.

Before leaving the topic of marital status differences in emotional distress, one additional point is in order; in his influential sex-role theory of mental illness, Gove (1972; Gove & Tudor, 1973) argued that the emotional advantages of marriage are only available to men and that marriage is emotionally *dis*advantageous for women. Gove attributed married women's relatively higher rates of emotional distress in modern industrial societies to their social roles in the family, which he claimed were unrewarding and highly stressful. While these ideas are provocative, in a recent empirical test of Gove's theory I found that the emotional benefits of marriage apply to men *and* women when male and female types of mental health problems are *both* considered (Simon, 2002). This finding reflects the more general finding from epidemiological research that men and women manifest (i.e., *express*) emotional distress in gender-specific ways (Dohrenwend & Dohrenwend, 1976)—a finding to which I now turn.

Gender

Motivated in large part by Gove's sex-role theory of mental illness, mental health researchers have also focused on the relationship between gender and emotional disturbance. Because most studies on this topic are based on symptoms of generalized distress, depression, and anxiety (which are more common among women), and do *not* include symptoms of distress that are more common among men (such as antisocial personality disorders and substance problems), scholars have long assumed that women have higher rates of mental health problems than men. To explain women's elevated levels of emotional distress, researchers emphasize their greater exposure to role-related stress (e.g., Aneshensel et al., 1991; Gore & Mangione, 1983; Kessler & McRae, 1984; Menaghan, 1989; Mirowsky & Ross, 2003; Ross & Huber, 1985; Simon, 1992, 1995; Thoits, 1986b) as well as their greater vulnerability to stress due to their lack of coping and social support resources (e.g., Kessler, 1979; Rosenfield, 1989; Thoits, 1984a).

However, while these explanations are compelling and have advanced our understanding of the relationship between gender and mental health in the U.S., epidemiological studies of life-time and recent prevalence rates of mental disorders among adults document that men and women experience *different types* of emotional problems; while women have higher rates of affective and anxiety disorders (and their psychological corollaries of non-specific emotional distress, depression, and anxiety), men have higher rates of antisocial personality and substance abuse disorders (and their psychological corollaries of antisocial behavior and substance problems) (Aneshensel et al., 1991; Dohrenwend & Dohrenwend, 1976; Kessler, McGonagle, Schwartz, Blazer, & Nelson, 1993; Meyers, Weissman, Tischler, Holzer, Leaf, Orvaschel, Anthony, Boyd, Burke, Kramer, & Stoltzman, 1984; Robins, Helzer, Weissman, Orvaschel, Burke, & Rieger, 1984). Moreover, studies show that gender differences in these types of emotional problems are evident in early adolescence (Avison & McAlpine, 1992; Gore et al., 1992; Rosenfield, Lennon, & White 2005; Rosenfield, Vertefuille, & McAlpine, 2000). Based on these findings, scholars have concluded that men and women *manifest* distress with different *types* of emotional problems. In fact, epidemiologists assert that when male and female types of psychiatric disorders and mental health problems are *both* considered there are *no* gender differences in overall rates of mental illness among adults and adolescents in the U.S.

That males and females manifest emotional distress with different types of emotional problems and respond to stress with gender-typical emotional disorders strongly suggest that they also differ in the frequency with which they experience everyday negative (and positive) emotions more generally. There is some evidence of this in Nath's and my study of gender and emotion discussed above; although we found that women are not more emotional than men, women report negative feelings more often than men, whereas men report positive feelings more often than women. We also found gender differences in self-reports of specific emotions; while there are no gender differences in feelings of anger and shame, men report more frequent feelings of calm and excitement, whereas women report more frequent feelings of sadness and anxiety. Interestingly, our analyses further revealed that gender differences in the frequency of some negative feelings (as well as some positive emotions) disappear once sociodemographic and social status variables (i.e., structural factors) are held constant.

To the extent that women are structurally disadvantaged in the U.S.—and there is strong evidence indicating that they are—Nath's and my findings provide support for Kemper's and Hochschild's structural theories about emotion. However, at the same time, by documenting that males and females express emotional discomfort with different *types* of mental health problems, epidemiological studies reveal a more complex set of patterns, which provide support for *both* structural *and* cultural theories about emotion. Regardless of which theory is more accurate, it is clear from this research that future work on the relationship between gender and mental health should include a variety of measures of emotional distress (and emotional well-being) in order to capture the ways in which males and females express emotional distress.

Race and Ethnicity

A much less studied and subsequently less understood source of variation in mental health in the U.S. is race. In general, studies that assess the mental health of minorities report few differences between blacks and whites. Both community and national epidemiological studies indicate that rates of anxiety and depressive disorders are lower for blacks than whites (Kessler, McGonagle, Zhao, Nelson, Hughes, Eshelman, Wittchen, & Kendler, 1994; Turner & Gil, 2002 Williams & Harris-Reid, 1999) and that African Americans report the same (or fewer) symptoms of emotional distress than their white peers when statistical controls for socioeconomic status are included in analyses (Kessler & Neighbors, 1986). These findings have led to the conclusion that race does not have an independent effect on mental health.[12]

Paradoxically, while African Americans do *not* have higher rates of *mental* health problems than whites, they *do* have higher rates of *physical* health problems. Even less well understood are ethnic variations in mental health; although there is too little information about Asians and Native Americans to draw meaningful conclusions at this time, rates of emotional problems are higher for Hispanics than for whites (Williams & Harris-Reid, 1999). Interestingly, the only difference in self-reports of feelings between blacks and whites that Nath and I found in our study were for anxiety. However, and paralleling epidemiological findings on race, African Americans report anxious feelings *less* rather than more often than their white peers. Research on the relationship between race and mental health, therefore, provides only limited support for structural theories about emotion. Here again, future work on this relationship should include measures of emotional well-being as well as measures of emotional distress in order to determine whether African American's actually enjoy better mental health than white persons.

Overall, sociologists of mental health have made important contributions to our understanding of the social distribution of emotion in the U.S. Epidemiological studies document that socially disadvantaged persons—including those with lower socioeconomic status and the unmarried—are more distressed than their more advantaged peers. Gender differences in mental health are more complex and depend on the type of emotional problem considered; while women have higher rates of *internalizing* emotional problems such as depression and anxiety, men have higher rates of *externalizing* emotional problems such as substance abuse. Moreover, despite their social disadvantage, African Americans do *not* report

---

[12] The one exception to this observation is the race difference in emotional distress among socially disadvantaged persons; African Americans with low socioeconomic status report higher levels of distress than their low socioeconomic status white counterparts (Kessler & Neighbors, 1986).

more emotional problems than white persons. Sociological research on mental health, therefore, provides some though not complete support for Kemper's and Hochschild's structural theories about emotion. Emotions researchers should make use of this extraordinary body of work to test, refine, and expand their theories about sociodemographic and social status differences in the experience of negative emotions in the general population of adolescents and adults.

However, at the same time that epidemiological research provides a window into the social distribution of negative emotions in the U.S., it would be greatly enriched by including measures of emotional well-being as well as measures of emotional distress so that mental health researchers could directly assess whether those social groups who report less distress also report greater well-being. Nath's and my recent work on the social distribution of both negative and positive "everyday" emotions in the general population of adults strongly suggest that this would be a worthwhile addition to sociological theory and research on mental health.

Contributions of the Sociology of Emotion for Understanding Group Differences in the Manifestation of Emotional Problems

Emotion Cultures, Emotion Norms, and Emotional Socialization

At the same time that sociological research on mental health sheds light on theoretical debates in the sociology of emotion regarding the social causes, social control, and social patterning of emotion, theoretical insights from the sociology of emotion enhance our understanding of persistent group differences in rates of emotional problems—particularly with respect to gender, race, ethnicity, and socioeconomic status. Although epidemiological studies document gender differences in the prevalence of certain types of mental health problems, with the exception of only a few scholars (Rosenfield, 1999; Rosenfield et al., 2000, 2006; Simon, 2000, 2002; Simon & Nath, 2004), there has been little theoretical work specifying *why* men and women *express* distress with gender-typical emotional problems. There has also been little theoretical work specifying *why* blacks report fewer emotional but more physical health problems than white persons (see Brown, Sellers, Brown, & Jackson [1999] and Williams & Harris-Reid [1999] for exceptions). Moreover, while studies show that socioeconomic status differences in exposure and vulnerability to stress help explain socioeconomic status differences in emotional disturbance, other factors may also contribute to this relationship. Theoretical developments in the sociology of emotion—especially cultural theories about emotion, which highlight the importance of emotion cultures, emotion norms, and emotional socialization—provide a conceptual framework with which to interpret group differences in the experience and expression of emotional problems in the U.S. as well as a useful direction for future research on these issues.

Recall that Hochschild's (1975, 1979, 1982) cultural theory about emotion asserts that societies contain ideological beliefs about feelings, which include cultural norms about their proper experience and expression; social norms about emotion (i.e., feeling and expression rules) specify the emotions individuals should and should not feel and express in general and in particular social settings. According to Hochschild and others (e.g., Gordon, 1981; Smith-Lovin, 1995; Thoits, 1985), feeling and expression rules provide standards by which people judge their own and others' emotions; when people's feelings and expressions depart from emotion norms, they often engage in emotion management, expression management, or both in order to create a more appropriate response. As noted earlier, a central tenet of cultural theories about emotion is that individuals learn the feeling and expression norms of their respective cultures and subcultures in social interaction with others and acquire knowledge about socially permissible and unacceptable feelings and expressive behavior throughout the life course vis-à-vis emotional socialization. In my opinion, Hochschild's compelling cultural theory about emotion can be used to understand persistent group differences in emotional distress and psychiatric disturbance in the population. Simply stated, gender, race, ethnic, and socioeconomic status differences in rates of emotional problems in the U.S. may be a function of group differences in *cultural norms* and *beliefs* about the appropriate experience and expression of emotion.

Gender

Drawing on these and other theoretical developments in the sociology of emotion, I have argued elsewhere (Simon, 2000, 2002; Simon & Nath, 2004) and maintain that U.S. emotion culture includes beliefs about the "proper" emotional styles of males and females as well as gendered feeling and expression rules, which specify the appropriate experience and expression of emotion for males and females. In addition to deeply held cultural beliefs that females are more emotional than males, the experience and expression of sadness is not only accepted but is expected for females, though it is considered inappropriate for males. In contrast, the experience and expression of anger is culturally appropriate for males but not for females. A consequence of gender-linked emotional socialization is that females learn to express emotional upset with internalizing emotional problems such as depression and anxiety, whereas males learn to express emotional discomfort with externalizing problems such as substance abuse and antisocial behavior. Another consequence of gendered emotional socialization is that males and females learn to manage (i.e., inhibit, suppress, and/or transform) their "deviant" feelings and expressions when they depart from culturally based emotion norms. In short, gender differences in rates of internalizing and externalizing emotional problems in the U.S. may be micro— level reflections of our larger (i.e., macro— level) emotion culture.

Indirect support for this hypothesis is evident in Nath's and my study of gender and emotion, which shows that women report sadness more often than men even when sociodemographic and status differences between men and women are held constant (Simon & Nath, 2004). In another study, I found that men and women respond to the stress of marital loss (i.e., including both divorce and widowhood) with gender-typical emotional problems (Simon, 2002). Indirect support for these ideas is evident in other research as well (see Aneshensel et al. [1991]; Rosenfield et al. [2000; 2006]; and Umberson et al. [1992] but not Umberson et al. [1996]). However, while this theoretical framework is promising for understanding *why* men and women express emotional distress in different ways, future research on this topic should directly assess men's and women's *beliefs* about culturally appropriate emotional experience and expression for males and females as well as the degree to which they manage their "deviant" feelings and expressions.

It is important to point out that the theoretical perspective about gendered-responses to stress advanced above compliments Rosenfield's (1999; Rosenfield et al., 2000, 2006) important work on this topic. Rosenfield posits that gender differences in the manifestation of emotional disorders reflect gender-differentiated self-structures, which are a by-product of gender role socialization. Drawing on prior theoretical work on gender differences in personality and the social self (Chodorow, 1978), she argues and finds that females have other-focused self-structures, which predispose them to manifest distress vis-à-vis internalizing emotional problems such as depression. In contrast, males have ego-focused self-structures, which predispose them to manifest distress vis-à-vis externalizing problems such as antisocial behavior and substance abuse. A potentially fruitful and exciting area for future work on this topic is the *interrelationships* among culture, gender, the self, and emotion.[13]

Race and Ethnicity

These same theoretical ideas about the role and significance of emotion cultures, emotion norms, and emotional socialization for understanding gender differences in the manifestation of emotional problems can also be used to shed light on a paradoxical finding in the literature on health disparities in the U.S. (briefly touched on earlier) that has long puzzled health scholars. That is, while African Americans are less likely to have psychiatric disorders and report the same (or lower) levels of emotional distress than their white counterparts, they experience more (and more severe) physical disorders and health problems than their white peers (Brown et al., 1999; Dohrenwend & Dohrenwend, 1969; Dresser & Badger,1985; George & Lynch, 2003; Jackson, Williams, Torres, Sellers, & Brown, 1996; Kessler et al., 1994; Schulz, Israel, Williams, Parker, Becker, & James, 2000; Smaje, 2000; Turner & Gil, 2002; Williams & Collins, 1997; Williams & Harris-Reid, 1999, Williams & Collins, 1997; Williams & Harris-Reid, 1999). Scholars suggest that the lower rates of emotional problems among blacks are due to highly supportive extended families and social networks in the black community, which buffer the deleterious emotional effects of stress. Health researchers also argue that the higher rates of physical health problems among

---

[13] See Rosaldo (1980, 1984), Kleinman (1986, Kleinman & Good 1985), Lutz (1988), Lutz and White (1986), Kondo (1990), Mageo (1998), and Milton and Svasek (2005) as well as Marcus and Kitayama (1991) and Kitayama and Marcus (1994) for fascinating discussions of the implications of cultural differences in the social self (e.g., the implications of ego versus other-focused self-structures) for the experience, expression, and meaning of emotion.

blacks are a by-product of racism, discrimination, and social disadvantage, which affect their health directly as well as restrict their access to health care.

However, it is conceivable that black-white differences in rates of mental and physical health problems also reflect deeply embedded sub-cultural norms and beliefs about appropriate feelings and expressive behavior. For example, the experience and expression of negative emotions such as sadness, loneliness, hopelessness, anxiety, worry, fear, and possibly anger may be viewed as inappropriate in African American culture. To the extent that this is the case—and there is some reason to believe that it may be—black individuals may learn from childhood on through emotional socialization to avoid, suppress, and transform (i.e., manage) these non-normative negative feelings and expressions. Some indirect support for this notion is evident in Nath's and my study of emotion; for example, we found that blacks report negative emotions in general—and feelings of sadness, anxiety, and anger in particular—*less* frequently than whites even after sociodemographic and social status variables are held constant. Together, these patterns strongly suggest that the stressors to which black persons are exposed take their toll on their *physiological* rather than on their *emotional* health and well-being.

To the extent that African Americans respond to stressful social situations with physical rather than emotional problems, it is crucial that research on racial inequalities in stress and mental health also examine physical health problems. Future research on racial disparities in health should also directly assess individuals' beliefs about culturally appropriate and inappropriate emotional experiences and expressions as well as the extent to which they manage their "deviant" feelings and affective behavior when they depart from social norms. Research on ethnic (i.e., Hispanic, Asian, & Native American) variations in mental (and physical) health should be particularly sensitive to these possibilities as well.

Note that these empirical observations for both gender and race differences in mental health in the U.S. provide unequivocal support for Aneshensel's (1992; Aneshensel et al., 1991) proposition that the effects of stress are highly specific and depend on the social characteristics of the person, the type of stressor involved, and the particular health problem examined (also see Barrett [2003] and Simon [1998, 2002]). That men and women as well as black and white individuals manifest emotional upset with distinctly different types of health problems also highlights the need for stress researchers to sample the "universe of stress outcomes" and include multiple health (i.e., multiple mental *and* physical health) outcomes in research on social group differences in the consequences of social stress, as Aneshensel (1999) argued several years ago.

Socioeconomic Status

Finally, although research demonstrates that socioeconomic status differences in symptoms of emotional distress and psychiatric disorders in the U.S. are partially explained by socioeconomic status differences in exposure and vulnerability to acute and chronic stressors (Turner et al., 1995), social class differences in emotion culture, emotion norms, and emotional socialization may also contribute to this relationship. I mentioned earlier that studies have long shown that all types of emotional problems (ranging from the mildest forms of emotional discomfort to the most severe forms of mental illness) are more common among persons with lower levels of education and family income and lower status occupations than those with higher levels of education and family income and higher status occupations (Dohrenwend & Dohrenwend, 1969; Faris & Dunham, 1939; Hollingshead & Redlich, 1958; Kessler, 1979; Kessler & Cleary, 1980; Link et al., 1993; Yu & Williams, 1999). However, while there is little doubt that members of disadvantaged social classes are more exposed to stressful situations and lack coping and social support resources with which to buffer the negative emotional impact of stressors (Pearlin & Schooler, 1978), it is reasonable to posit that they are also less likely to manage their emotions by suppressing their negative feelings and invoking more positive ones.

Although there has been no empirical research on this topic to my knowledge, Hochschild (1979, 1983, 1990) claims that there are social class differences in emotion cultures, emotion norms, and emotional socialization, which ultimately result in class differences in the use of emotion management. Extrapolating from Kohn's (1969) classic work on class differences in parental values and childhood socialization, Hochschild argues that persons with higher status occupations routinely manage their emotions in order to satisfy occupational requirements. Consequentially, parents with these occupations value and put a greater emphasis than those with lower status occupations on emotional introspection and control and socialize their children to both attend to and manage their negative and non-normative feelings and expressions. To the extent that this argument is correct, long observed socioeconomic status differences in mental health may also reflect socioeconomic status differences in the *management* of negative emotions. While studies document class differences in coping resources such as mastery and self-esteem (Mirowsky & Ross, 2003; Pearlin & Schooler, 1978; Thoits, 1995b; Turner & Roszell, 1994), future research should examine socioeconomic status differences in the use of coping strategies—especially emotion-focused coping behaviors—in order to assess the accuracy of Hochschild's provocative ideas.[14]

---

[14] In addition to gender, race, ethnic, and socioeconomic differences in emotional disturbance, epidemiological studies of mental health in the U.S. find that younger adults report higher levels of emotional distress including depression and anxiety than older persons (e.g., Mirowsky & Ross, 2003). Closely paralleling these findings, research on the social distribution of everyday emotions in the U.S. finds that younger adults report negative feelings such as sadness, anxiety, and anger more frequently than older adults (Schieman, 1999; Simon & Nath, 2004). Scholars attribute age differences in emotion and mental health to structural factors that are associated with the early adult life course—a stage of life when individuals are establishing themselves in jobs and marriage and raising children. However, it is equally possible that observed age differences in emotion and emotional distress reflect age-related norms about appropriate feeling and expressive behavior. Because the experience and expression of negative emotions may be less accepted for older than for younger persons in American culture, future research should examine whether age-based emotion norms exist and if there are age and/or cohort differences in individuals' beliefs about appropriate feeling and expressive behavior. Future research should also investigate whether older persons are more likely than younger people to manage their negative feelings and expressions.

In sum, theoretical developments in the sociology of emotion enhance our understanding of persistent group differences in mental health problems in the U.S. As such, insights, concepts, and theories about emotion open up promising new directions for future research on these important issues. In my opinion, a logical next step for research on gender, race, ethnic, and socioeconomic status variations in mental health is to elucidate the many complex linkages among cultural (and subcultural) norms and beliefs about appropriate feelings and expressions, the content of emotional socialization, the use of emotion management (by self and others) to regulate non-normative feelings, and the types of emotional (as well as physical) health problems members of different social groups typically experience and express. The integration of theory and research from the sociologies of mental health and emotion would go far towards broadening and deepening our collective knowledge about social group differences in mental and physical health problems as well as group differences in affective responses to a range of social situations.

Conclusions: The Complementarity of the Sociologies of Mental Health & Emotion

In the first part of this chapter, I drew on findings from decades of research on the sociology of mental health in order to shed light on unresolved theoretical issues and debates in the sociology of emotion regarding the social antecedents, social regulation, and social distribution of emotion. However, in discussing these findings, I also took the opportunity to suggest some ways in which insights from the sociology of emotion could enhance research on the etiology of emotional distress, the role of coping and social support for reducing emotional problems, and the social epidemiology of emotional disturbance in the population. In the second part of the chapter, I turned my attention to theoretical developments in the sociology of emotion that can contribute to theory and research in the sociology of mental health with respect to our understanding of persistent group differences in the experience and expression of emotional (and physical) health problems. There are undoubtedly other points of overlap between the sociologies of mental health and emotion that would benefit from this type of integration and cross-fertilization. I conclude the chapter by briefly highlighting some broad themes I touched on regarding the complementarity of theory and research on mental health and emotion and point to some topics that would profit from greater integration of these separate, yet highly interrelated, areas of sociological inquiry.

Since symptoms scales that are employed in research on mental health include some of the same feelings that are of interest to emotions researchers, sociologists of emotion can use findings from this body of work to evaluate as well as refine and expand theories and concepts about feeling and emotion.

With respect to the *social antecedents of emotion*, sociologists of mental health have developed an elaborate typology of social situations that are responsible for the development and persistence of emotional problems among individuals in the general population. Emotions scholars should draw on this useful typology in order to assess whether everyday negative feelings can be traced to undesirable life events and on-going strains, and if so, whether these events and social situations are stressful because they decrease people's status in social relationships or disconfirm their social identities as Kemper and Heise argue, respectively. At the same time, sociologists of mental health should make greater use of these and other theories about emotion in order to elaborate the *social psychological mechanisms* that underlie people's emotional reactions to acute and chronic stressors. This would enhance their understanding of *why* these social experiences are emotionally distressing.

With regard to the *social regulation of emotion*, sociologists of mental health have developed an exhaustive inventory of coping and social support resources and strategies that individuals use to control their own and others' distressing emotions. Emotions researchers should draw on this rich source of data in order to broaden their knowledge about the multitude of ways in which people manage their own and other people's negative feelings. By the same token, coping and social support researchers should follow Thoits' lead by utilizing theoretical insights from the sociology of emotion and examining group differences in the use of emotion management in the population. Mental health researchers should also make use of Hochschild's cultural theory about emotion and investigate both cultural and sub-cultural norms variations in norms and beliefs about appropriate and inappropriate feelings and expressive behavior.

Finally, in terms of the *social distribution of emotion*, sociologists of mental health have provided a wealth of information about sociodemographic and social status variations in emotional distress in the U.S. Emotions researchers should utilize this extraordinary body of work in order to evaluate a number of different theories, including both structural and cultural theories about emotion. On the other hand, epidemiologists should draw on these theories about emotion and examine a broader range of emotional outcomes—particularly symptoms of emotional well-being—so that they could determine whether the absence of symptoms of distress is equivalent to presence of symptoms of well-being as Bradburn claimed and found several decades ago. Sociologists of mental health should also make use of rich theoretical insights from the sociology of emotion—especially theories that highlight the importance of emotion cultures, emotion norms, and emotional socialization for influencing individuals' perceptions about appropriate and inappropriate feelings and expressive behavior—in order to better understand persistent group differences in the manifestation of emotional problems in the population.

Thus, at the same time that emotions researchers should draw on research from the sociology of mental health in order to evaluate, refine, and expand their concepts and theories, mental health researchers should take advantage of concepts, theories, and insights from the sociology of emotion in order to explicate the mechanisms that underlie the development of mental health problems in the U.S. and persistent group differences therein. In addition to including a broader range of health outcomes (including emotional well-being as well as physical health problems and physical well-being), mental health research should include a broader range of social situations that people experience—particularly life affirming desirable events and on-going positive social situations. The inclusion of positive *and* negative social experiences as well as measures of emotional and physical health problems *and* well-being in their work would allow mental health and emotions researchers to more fully capture the multitude of ways in which social life and social experience affect the emotional lives and health of individuals.

Acknowledgments. I gratefully acknowledge Kathryn Lively as well as Bill Avison, Jane McLeod, and Bernice Pescoscolido for their helpful comments and suggestions on an earlier version of this chapter.

References

Aneshensel, C. S. (1992). Social stress: Theory and research. *Annual Review of Sociology, 18*, 15–38.

Aneshensel, C. S. (1996). Consequences of psychosocial stress: The universe of stress outcomes. In H. B. Kaplan (Ed.), *Psychosocial stress: Perspectives on structure, theory, life-course, and methods* (pp. 111–136). New York: Academic.

Aneshensel, C. S. (1999). Outcomes of the stress process. In A. V. Horwitz & T. L. Scheid (Eds.), *A handbook for the study of mental health: Social contexts, theories, and systems* (pp.211–227). New York: Cambridge.

Aneshensel, C. S., Rutter, C. S. & Lachenbruch, P. (1991). Social structure, stress, and mental health: Competing conceptual models. *American Sociological Review, 56*, 166–178.

Aries, P. (1981). *The hour of death.* New York: Oxford University.

Avison, W. R., & McAlpine, D. (1992). Gender differences in symptoms of depression among adolescents. *Journal of Health and Social Behavior, 33*, 77–96.

Avison, W. R., & Turner, R. J. (1988). Stressful life events and depressive symptoms: Disaggregating the effects of acute stressors and chronic strains. *Journal of Health and Social Behavior, 29*, 253–264.

Barrett, A. E. (2000). Marital trajectories and mental health. *Journal of Health and Social Behavior, 41*, 451–464.

Barrett, A. E. (2003). Race differences in the mental health effects of divorce. *Journal of Family Issues, 24*, 995–1019.

Berkman, L. F. (1984). Assessing the physical health effects of social networks and social support. *Annual Review of Public Health, 5*, 413–432.

Bradburn, N. M. (1969). *The structure of psychological well-being.* Chicago: Aldine.

Bradburn, N. M., & Caplovitz, D. (1965). *Reports on happiness.* Chicago: Aldine.

Brody, L. (1999). *Gender, emotion, and the family.* Cambridge: Harvard University.

Brown, G. W., & Harris, T. O. (1978). *The social origins of depression: A study of psychiatric disorder in women.* New York: Free Press.

Brown, T. N., Sellers, S. L., Brown, K. T., & Jackson, J. (1999). Race, ethnicity, and culture in the sociology of mental health. In C. S. Aneshensel & J. C. Phelan (Eds.), *The handbook of the sociology of mental health* (pp. 67–182). New York: Plenum.

Cahill, S. E. (1999). Emotional capital and professional socialization: The case of mortuary science students (and me). *Social Psychology Quarterly, 62*, 101–116.

Cahill, S. E., & Eggleston, R. (1994). Managing emotions in public: The case of wheel-chair users. *Social Psychology Quarterly, 57*, 300–312.

Cancian, F. M. (1987). *Love in America: Gender and self development.* New York: Cambridge University.

Chodorow, N. (1978). *The reproduction of mothering.* Berkeley: University of California.

Clark, C. (1987). Sympathy biography and sympathy margin. *American Journal of Sociology, 93*, 290–321.

Clark, C. (1997). *Misery and company: Sympathy in everyday life.* Chicago: University of Chicago.

Cohen, S., & Wills, T. A. (1985). Stress, social support, and the buffering hypothesis. *Psychological Bulletin, 98*, 310–357.

Corrigan, J. (2002). *Business of the heart: Religion and emotion in the nineteenth century.* Berkeley: University of California.

Coyne, J., Aldwin, C. & Lazarus, R. S. (1984). Depression and coping in stressful episodes. *Journal of Abnormal Psychology, 90*, 439–447.

Cronkite, R. C., & Moos, R. H. (1984). The role of predisposing and moderating factors in the stress-illness relationship. *Journal of Health and Social Behavior, 25*, 372–393.

Dohrenwend, B. P., & Dohrenwend, B. S. (1969). *Social status and psychiatric disorders: A causal inquiry.* New York: Wiley.

Dohrenwend, B. P., & Dohrenwend, B. S. (1976). Sex differences in psychiatric disorders. *American Journal of Sociology, 81*, 1447–1454.

Dohrenwend, B. P., Levan, I., Shrout, P. E., Schwartz, S. Naveh, G., Link, B. G. Skodal, A. E., & Stueve, A. (1992). Socioeconomic status and psychiatric disorders: The causation-selection issue. *Science, 255*, 946–952.

Dresser, W., & Badger, L. (1985). Epidemiology of depressive symptoms in black communities: A comparative analysis. *Journal of Nervous and Mental Disease, 173*, 212–230.

Durkheim, E. (1951). *Suicide: A study in sociology.* New York: Free Press.

Easterbrook, G. (2003). *The progress paradox: How life gets better while people feel worse.* New York: Random House.

Erickson, R., & Ritter, C. (2001). Emotional labor, burnout, and inauthenticity: Does gender matter? *Social Psychology Quarterly, 64*, 146–163.

Erickson, R., & Wharton, A. S. (1997). Inauthenticity and depression: Assessing the consequences of interactive service work. *Work and Occupations, 24*, 188–213.

Evenson, R. J., & Simon, R. W. (2005). Clarifying the relationship between parenthood and depression. *Journal of health and Social Behavior, 46*, 341–358.

Faris, R. E. L., & Dunham, H. W. (1939). *Mental disorders in urban areas.* New York: Hafner.

Folkman, S. (1984). Personal control and stress and coping processes: A theoretical analysis. *Journal of Personality and Social Psychology, 46*, 839–852.

Folkman, S., & Lazarus, R. S. (1980). An analysis of coping in a middle-aged community sample. *Journal of Health and Social Behavior, 21*, 219–239.

Folkman, S., & Lazarus, R. S. (1985). If it changes, it must be a process: Study of emotion and coping during three stages of a college examination. *Journal of Personality and Social Psychology, 48*, 150–170.

Francis, L. (1997). Ideology and interpersonal emotion management: Redefining identity in support groups. *Social Psychology Quarterly, 60*, 153–171.

Frude, N., & Goss, A. (1981). Maternal anger and the young child. In N. Frude (Ed.), *Psychological approaches to child abuse* (pp. 52–63). Totowa, N.J.: Rowman & Littlefield.

Gatta, M. L. (2002). *Juggling food and feelings: Emotional balance in the workplace.* New York: Lexington Books.

George, L. K., & Lynch, S. M. (2003). Race differences in depressive symptoms: A dynamic perspective on stress exposure and vulnerability. *Journal of Health and Social Behavior, 44,* 353–369.

Gordon, S. L. (1981). The sociology of sentiment and affect. In M. Rosenberg & R. H. Turner (Eds.), *Social psychology: Sociological perspectives* (pp. 562–592). New York: Basic Books.

Gore, S., Aseltine, R. H. Jr., & Colten, M. E. (1992). Social structure, life stress, and depressive symptoms in a high school-age population. *Journal of Health and Social Behavior, 33,* 97–113.

Gore, S., & Mangione, T. (1983). Social roles, sex roles, and psychological distress: Additive and interactive models. *Journal of Health and Social Behavior, 24,* 300–312.

Gove, W. R. (1972). The relationship between sex roles, marital status, and mental illness. *Social Forces, 51,* 34–44.

Gove, W. R., & Tudor, J. F. (1973). Adult sex roles and mental illness. *American Journal of Sociology, 78,* 50–73.

Harlow, R. (2003). Race doesn't matter, but. . .: The effect of race on professors' experiences of emotion management in the undergraduate classroom. *Social Psychology Quarterly, 66,* 348–363.

Heise, D. R. (1979). *Understanding events: Affect and the construction of social action.* New York: Cambridge University Press.

Hochschild, A. R. (1975). The sociology of feeling and emotion: Selected possibilities. In M. Millman & R. M. Kantor (Eds.) *Another voice: Feminist perspectives on social life and social science* (pp. 208–307). New York: Anchor.

Hochschild, A. R. (1979). Emotion work, feeling rules, and social structure. *American Journal of Sociology, 85,* 551–575.

Hochschild, A. R. (1983). *The managed heart: Notes on the commercialization of human feeling.* Berkeley: University of California.

Hochschild, A. R. (1989). *The second shift.* Berkeley: University of California Press.

Hochschild, A. R. (1990). Ideology and emotion management: A perspective and path for future research. In T. D. Kemper (Ed.), *Research agendas in the sociology of emotions* (pp. 17–144). Albany, N.Y.: State University of New York.

Hollingshead, A. B., & Redlich, F. C. (1958). *Social class and mental illness: A community study.* New York: Wiley.

House, J. S., & Kahn, R. L. (1985). Measures and concepts of social support. In S. Cohen & S. L. Syme (eds.), *Social support and health* (pp. 83–108). Orlando, FL: Academic Press.

House, J. S., Landis, K. R., & Umberson, D. (1988). Social relationships and health. *Science, 241,* 540–545.

Jackson, J. S., Williams, D. R., Torres, M., Sellers, S., & Brown, K. (1996). Racism and the physical and mental health of African Americans: A thirteen year national panel study. *Ethnicity and Disease, 6,* 132–147.

Karp, D. A. (1996). *Speaking of sadness: Depression, disconnection, and the meanings of illness.* New York: Oxford.

Kemper, T. D. (1978). *A social interactional theory of emotions.* New York: Wiley.

Kemper, T. D. (1990). Social relations and emotions: A structural approach. In T. D. Kemper (Ed.), *Research agendas in the sociology of emotions* (pp. 207–237). Albany, New York: State University of New York.

Kessler, R. C. (1979). Stress, social status, and psychological distress. *Journal of Health and Social Behavior, 20,* 259–272.

Kessler, R. C., & Cleary, P. D. (1980). Social class and psychological distress. *American Sociological Review, 49,* 620–631.

Kessler, R. C., & Essex, M. (1982). Marital status and depression: The importance of coping resources. *Social Forces, 61,* 484–507.

Kessler, R. C., McGonagle, K. A., Schwartz, M., Blazer, D. G., & Nelson, C. B. (1993). Sex and depression in the national co-morbidity survey I: Lifetime prevalence, chronicity, and recurrence. *Journal of Affective Disorders, 25,* 85–96.

Kessler, R. C., McGonagle, K. A., Zhao, S., Nelson, C. B., Hughes, M., Eshelman, S., Wittchen, H-U., & Kendler, K. S. (1994). Lifetime and 12-month prevalence of DSM-III-R psychiatric disorders in the United States. *Archives of General Psychiatry, 51,* 8–19.

Kessler, R. C., & McLeod, J. D. (1990). Socioeconomic status differences in vulnerability to undesirable life events. *Journal of Health and Social Behavior, 31,*162–172.

Kessler, R. C., & McRae, J. A. (1984). Trends in the relationship between sex and psychological distress: 1957–1976. *American Sociological Review, 46,* 443–452.

Kessler, R. C., & Neighbors, H. W. (1986). A new perspective on the relationships among race, social class, and psychological distress. *Journal of Health and Social Behavior, 27,* 107–115.

Kessler, R. C., Turner, B., & House, J. (1989). Unemployment, reemployment, and emotional functioning in a community sample. *American Sociological Review, 54,* 648–657.

Keyes, C. L. (2002). The mental health continuum: From languishing to flourishing in life. *Journal of Health and Social Behavior, 43,* 207–222.

Kitayama, S., & H. Marcus. (1994). *Emotion and culture: Empirical studies of mutual influence.* New York: American Psychological Association.

Kleinman, A. (1986). *Social origins of distress and disease: Depression, neurasthenia, and pain in modern China.* New Haven: Yale University.

Kleinman, A., & Good, B. (1985). Culture and depression: Studies in the anthropology and cross-cultural psychiatry of affect and disorder. Berkeley: University of California.

Kohn, M. (1969). *Class and conformity: A study in values.* Homewood, IL: Dorsey Press.

Kondo, D. K. (1990). *Crafting selves: Power, gender, and discourses of identity in a Japanese workplace.* Chicago: University of Chicago Press.

Lazarus, R. S., & Folkman, S. (1984). *Stress, appraisal, and coping.* New York: Springer.

Leavitt, R. L., & Power, M. B. (1989). Emotional socialization in the postmodern era: Children in day care. *Social Psychology Quarterly, 52,* 35–43.

Leidner, R. (1993). *Fast food, fast talk: Service work and the routinization of everyday life.* Berkeley: University of California.

Lennon, M. C. (1999). Work and unemployment as stressors. In A. V. Horwitz & T. Scheid (Eds.), *A handbook for the study of mental health: Social contexts, theories, and systems* (pp. 284–294). New York: Cambridge.

Liem, R., & Liem, J. (1978). Social class and mental illness reconsidered: The role of economic stress and social support. *Journal of Health and Social Behavior, 19,* 139–156.

Link, B. G., Lennon, M. C., & Dohrenwend, B. P. 1993. Socioeconomic status and depression: The role of occupations involving direction, control, and planning. *American Journal of Sociology, 98,* 1351–1387.

Lively, K. J. (2000). Reciprocal emotion management: Working together to maintain stratification in private law firms. *Work and Occupations, 27,* 32–63.

Lively, K. J. (2002). Client contact and emotional labor: Upping the balance and evening the field. *Work and Occupations, 29*, 198–225.

Lively, K. J., & Heise, D. (2004) Sociological realms of emotional experience. *American Journal of Sociology, 109*, 1109–1136.

Lively, K. J., & Powell, B. (In press). Emotional expression at work and at home: Domain, status, or individual characteristics? *Social Psychology Quarterly*.

Lofland, L. H. (1985). The social shaping of emotion: Grief in historical perspective. *Symbolic Interaction, 8*, 171–190.

Lois, J. (2003). *Heroic efforts: The emotional culture of search and rescue volunteers.* New York: New York University.

Lutz, C. A. (1988). *Unnatural emotions: Everyday sentiments on a Micronesian atoll and their challenge to western theory.* Chicago: University of Chicago.

Lutz, C. A., & White, G. M. (1986). The anthropology of emotions. *Annual Review of Anthropology, 15*, 405–436.

Mageo, J. M. (1998). *Theorizing self in Samoa: Emotions, genders, and sexualities.* Ann Arbor, Michigan: University of Michigan Press.

Marcus, H. R., & Kitayama, S. (1991). Culture and the self: Implications for cognition, emotion, and motivation. *Psychological Review, 98*, 224–253.

Marks, N. F., & Lambert. J. D. (1998). Marital status continuity and change among young and midlife adults: Longitudinal effects on psychological well-being. *Journal of Family Issues, 19*, 652–686.

Massey, D. S. (2002). A brief history of human society: The origin and role of emotion in social life. *American Sociological Review, 67*, 1–29.

McLeod, J. D., & Kaiser, K. (2004). Childhood emotional and behavioral problems. *American Sociological Review, 69*, 636–658.

McMahon, D. H. (2006). *Happiness: A history.* New York: Atlantic Monthly Press.

Menaghan, E. G. (1983). Individual coping efforts: Moderators of the relationship between life stress and mental health outcomes. In H.B. Kaplan (Ed.), *Psychosocial stress: Trends in theory and research* (pp. 157–191). New York: Academic.

Menaghan, E. G. (1985). Depressive affect and subsequent divorce. *Journal of Family Issues, 6*, 296–306.

Menaghan, E. G. (1989). Role changes and psychological well-being: Variations in effects by gender a role repertoire. *Social Forces, 68*, 296–306.

Menaghan, E. G., & Lieberman, M. A. (1986). Changes in depression following divorce: A panel study. *Journal of Marriage and the Family, 48*, 319–328.

Meyers, J. K., Weissman, M. M., Tischler, G. L., Holzer, C. E., Leaf, P. J., Orvaschel, H., Anthony, J. C., Boyd, J. H., Burke, J. D. Jr., Kramer, M., & Stoltzman, R. (1984). Six month prevalence of psychiatric disorders in three communities. *Archives of General Psychiatry, 41*, 959–967.

Milton, K., & Svasek, M. (2005). *Mixed emotions: Anthropological studies of feeling.* New York: Berg.

Mirowsky, J., & Ross, C. E. (1990). Control or defense? Depression and the sense of control over good and bad outcomes. *Journal of Health and Social Behavior, 31*, 71–86.

Mirowsky, J., & Ross, C. E. (2003). *Social causes of psychological distress* (2nd Ed). New York: Aldine de Gruyter.

Pearlin, L. I. (1985). Social structure and processes of social support. In S. Cohen & S.L. Syme (Eds.), *Social support and health* (pp. 43–60). Orlando, FL: Academic Press.

Pearlin, L. I. (1989). The sociological study of stress. *Journal of Health and Social Behavior, 30*, 241–256.

Pearlin, L. I., & Johnson, J. S. (1977). Marital status, life strains, and depression. *American Sociological Review, 42*, 704–715.

Pearlin, L. I., & Lieberman, M. A. (1987). Social sources of emotional distress. In R Simmons (Ed.), *Research and community mental health*, Volume 1 (pp. 217–248). Greenwich: JAI Press.

Pearlin, L. I., Menaghan, E. G., Lieberman, M. A. & Mullan, J. T. (1981). The stress process. *Journal of Health and Social Behavior, 22*, 337–356.

Pearlin, L. I., & Schooler, C. (1978). The structure of coping. *Journal of Health and Social Behavior, 19*, 2–21.

Pierce, J. I. (1995). *Gender trials: Emotional lives in contemporary law firms*. Berkeley: University of California.

Pollak, L. H., & Thoits, P. A. (1989). Processes in emotional socialization. *Social Psychology Quarterly, 52*, 22–34.

Pugliesi, K., & Shook, S. L., (1997). Gender, jobs, and emotional labor in a complex organization. *Social Perspectives on Emotion, 4*, 283–316.

Robins, L. N., Helzer, J. E., Weissman, M. M., Orvaschel, E. G., Burke, J. D., & Regier, D. A., (1984). Lifetime prevalence of specific psychiatric disorders in three sites. *Archives of General Psychiatry, 41*, 949–958.

Rosaldo, M. Z. (1980). *Knowledge and passion*. New York: Cambridge University.

Rosaldo, M. Z. (1984). Toward an anthropology of self and feeling. In R. Shweder & R. Levine (Eds.), *Culture theory: Essays on mind, self, and society* (pp. 137–157). New York: Cambridge University.

Rosenfield, S. (1989). The effects of women's employment: Personal control and sex differences in mental health. *Journal of Health and Social Behavior, 30*, 77–91.

Rosenfield, S. (1999). Splitting the difference: Gender, the self, and mental health. In C. S. Aneshensel & J. C. Phelan (Eds.), *Handbook of the sociology of mental health* (pp. 209–224). New York: Kluwer Academic/Plenum.

Rosenfield, S., Lennon, M. C., & White, H. R. (2006). The self and mental health: Self-salience and the emergence of internalizing and externalizing problems. *Journal of Health and Social Behavior, 46*, 323–340.

Rosenfield, S., Vertefuille, J. & McAlpine, D. (2000). Gender stratification and mental health: Dimensions of the self. *Social Psychology Quarterly, 63*, 208–223.

Ross, C. E., & Huber, J. (1985). Hardship and depression. *Journal of Health and Social Behavior, 26*, 312–327.

Ross, C. E., & Mirowsky, J. (1989). Explaining the social patterns of depression: Control and problem solving–or support and talking? *Journal of Health and Social Behavior, 30*, 206–219.

Ross, C. E., Mirowsky, J., & Huber, J. (1983). Dividing work, sharing work, and in-between: Marital patterns and depression. *American Sociological Review, 48*, 809–823.

Ross, C. E., & Van Willigen, M. (1996). Gender, parenthood, and anger. *Journal of Marriage and the Family, 58*, 572–584.

Schachter, S., & Singer, J. E. (1962). Cognitive, social, and physiological determinants of emotional state. *Psychological Review, 69*, 379–399.

Scheff, T. J. (1990). Socialization of emotions: Pride and shame as causal agents. In T. D. Kemper (Ed.), *Research agendas in the sociology of emotions* (pp. 281–304). Albany, N.Y.: State University of New State University of New York Press.

Scherer, K. R., Wallbott, H. G., & Summerfield, A. B. (Eds.). (1986). *Experiencing emotion: A cross-cultural study*. Cambridge, UK: Cambridge University.

Schieman, S. (1999). Age and anger. *Journal of Health and Social Behavior, 40*, 273–289.

Schieman, S. (2000). Education and the activation, course, and management of anger. *Journal of Health and Social Behavior, 41*, 20–39.

Schrock, D. Holden, D., & Reid, L. (2004). Creating emotional resonance: Interpersonal emotion work and emotional framing. *Social Problems, 51*, 61–81.

Schulz, A. Israel, B., Williams, D., Parker, E., Becker, A., & James, S. (2000). Social inequalities, stressors, and self-reported health status among African American and white women in the Detriot metropolitan area. *Social Science and Medicine, 51*, 1639–1653.

Seligman, M. (2004). *Authentic happiness: Using the new positive psychology to realize your potential for lasting fulfillment.* New York: Free Press.

Shields, S. A. (2002). *Speaking from the heart: Gender and the social meaning of emotion.* New York: Cambridge University.

Shott, S. (1979). Emotion and social life: A symbolic interactionist perspective. *American Journal of Sociology, 84*, 1317–1334.

Simon, R. W. (1992). Parental role strains, salience of parental identity, and gender differences in psychological distress. *Journal of Health and Social Behavior, 33*, 25–35.

Simon, R. W. (1995). Gender, multiple roles, role meaning, and mental health. *Journal of Health and Social Behavior, 36*, 182–194.

Simon, R. W. (1998). Assessing sex differences in vulnerability among employed parents: The importance of marital status. *Journal of Health and Social Behavior, 39*, 38–54.

Simon, R. W. (2000). The importance of culture in sociological theory and research on stress and mental health: A missing link? In C. E. Bird, P. Conrad, & A.M. Fremont (Eds.), *Handbook of medical sociology* (pp. 68–78). New York: Prentice Hall.

Simon, R. W. (2002). Revisiting the relationships among gender, marital status, and mental health. *American Journal of Sociology, 107*, 1065–1096.

Simon, R.W., Eder, D., & Evans, C. (1992). The development of feeling rules underlying romantic love among female adolescents. *Social Psychology Quarterly, 55*, 29–46.

Simon, R. W., & Lively, K. J. (2005). Gender differences in dimensions of anger and their implications for distressing emotions. Paper presented at the annual meetings of the American Sociological Association, Philadelpia, PA.

Simon, R. W., & Nath, L. K (2004). Gender and emotion in the United States: Do men and women differ in self-reports of feelings and expressive behavior? *American Journal of Sociology, 109*, 1137–1176.

Smaje, C. (2000). Race, ethnicity, and health. In C. E. Bird, P. Conrad, & A. M. Fremont (Eds.), *Handbook of medical sociology* (pp. 114–128). New Jersey: Prentice-Hall.

Smith, A. C., III, & Kleinman, S. (1989). Managing emotions in medical school: Students' contacts with the living and the dead. *Social Psychology Quarterly, 52*, 56–69.

Smith-Lovin, L. (1987). Impressions from events. *Journal of Mathematical Sociology, 13*, 35–70.

Smith-Lovin, L. (1990). Emotion as the confirmation or disconfirmation of identity: An affect control model. In T. D. Kemper (Ed.), *Research agendas in the sociology of emotions* (pp. 238–270). Albany, N.Y.: State University of New York.

Smith-Lovin, L. (1995). The sociology of affect and emotion. In K. Cook, G. A. Fine, & J. S. House (Eds.), *Sociological perspectives on social psychology* (pp. 118–48). New York: Allyn & Bacon.

Smith-Lovin, L. (2003). They got the feeling, but they missed the Marx: Twenty years of the managed heart. Paper presented at the annual meetings of the American Sociological Association, Atlanta GA.

Smith-Lovin, L., & Heise, D. R. (1988). *Analyzing social interaction: Advances in affect control theory.* New York: Gordon & Break.

Sprecher, S. (1986). The relationship between inequity and emotions in close relationships. *Social Psychology Quarterly, 49*, 309–321.

Staske, S. A. (1996). Talking feelings: The collaborative construction of emotion in talk between close relational partners. *Symbolic Interaction, 19*, 111–142.

Stearns, C. Z., & Stearns, P. N. (1986). *Anger: The struggle for emotional control in America's history*. Chicago: University of Chicago Press.

Stone, A. A., & Neale, J. M. (1984). New measure of daily coping: Development and preliminary results. *Journal of Personality and Social Psychology, 46*, 892–906.

Swidler, A. (1980). Love and adulthood in American culture. In N. J. Smelser & E. H. Erickson (Eds.), *Themes of work and love in American culture*, (pp. 120–147). Cambridge, Mass.: Harvard University Press.

Swidler, A. (2001). *Talk of love: How culture matters*. Chicago: University of Chicago Press.

Tavris. C. (1982). *Anger: The misunderstood emotion*. New York: Touchstone.

Thoits, P. A. (1983). Dimensions of life events that influence psychological distress: An evaluation and synthesis of the literature. In H. B. Kaplan (Ed.), *Psychological stress: Trends in theory and research* (pp.33–103). New York: Academic.

Thoits, P. A. (1985). Self-labeling processes in mental illness: The role of emotional deviance. *American Journal of Sociology, 92*, 221–249

Thoits, P. A. (1986a). Social support as coping assistance. *Journal of Consulting and Clinical Psychology, 54*, 416–423.

Thoits, P. A. (1986b). Multiple identities: Examining gender and marital status differences in psychological distress. *American Sociological Review, 51*, 259–272.

Thoits, P. A. (1987). Gender and marital status differences in control and distress: Common stress versus unique stress explanations. *Journal of Health and Social Behavior, 28*, 7–22.

Thoits, P. A. (1989). The sociology of emotions. *Annual Review of Sociology, 61*, 837–857.

Thoits, P. A. (1990). Emotional deviance: Research agendas. In T. D. Kemper (Ed.), *Research agendas in the sociology of emotions* (pp. 180–206). Albany, N.Y.: State University of New York Press.

Thoits, P. A. (1991a). Patterns of coping with controllable and uncontrollable events. In E. M. Cummings, A. L. Greene, & K. H. Karraker (Eds.), *Life-span developmental psychology: Perspectives on stress and coping* (pp. 235–258). Hillsdale, N.J.: Lawrence Earlbaum.

Thoits, P. A. (1991b). Gender differences in coping with emotional distress. In J. Eckenrode (Ed.), *The social context of coping* (pp. 107–138). New York: Plenum.

Thoits, P. A. (1995a). Managing the emotions of others. *Symbolic Interaction, 19*, 85–109.

Thoits, P. A. (1995b). Stress, coping, and social support: Where are we? what next? *Journal of Health and Social Behavior, 35*, 53–79.

Thoits, P. A. (1995c). Identity relevant events and psychological symptoms: A cautionary tale. *Journal of Health and Social Behavior,36*, 72–83.

Turner, R. J., & Gil, A. G. (2002). Psychiatric and substance use disorders in South Florida. *Archives of General Psychiatry, 59*, 43–50.

Turner, R. J., & Lloyd, D. A. (1999). The stress process and the social distribution of depression. *Journal of Health and Social Behavior, 40*, 374–404.

Turner, R. J., & Marino, F. (1994). Social support and social structure: A descriptive epidemiology. *Journal of Health and Social Behavior, 35*, 193–212.

Turner, R. J., & Noh, S. (1983). Class and psychological vulnerability: The significance of social support and personal control. *Journal of Health and Social Behavior 24*, 2–15.

Turner, R. J., & Roszell, P. (1994). Psychosocial resources and the stress process. In W. R. Avison & I. H. Gottlib (Eds.), *Stress and mental health: Contemporary issues and prospects for the future* (pp. 179–210). New York: Plenum.

Turner, R. J., Wheaton, B., & Lloyd, D. A. (1995). The epidemiology of social stress. *American Sociological Review, 60,* 104–25.

Umberson, D. (2003). *Death of a parent: Transition to a new adult identity.* New York: Cambridge University Press.

Umberson, D., Chen, M. D., House, J. S. Hopkins, K., & Slaten, E. (1996). The effects of social relationships on psychological well-being: Are men and women really so different? *American Sociological Review, 61,* 837–857.

Umberson, D., Williams, K., & Anderson, K. (2002). Violent behavior: A measure of emotional upset? *Journal of Health and Social Behavior, 43,* 189–206.

Umberson, D., Wortman, C. B., & Kessler, R. C. (1992). Widowhood and depression: Explaining long-term gender differences in vulnerability. *Journal of Health and Social Behavior, 33,* 10–24.

Wethington, E., & Kessler, R. C. (1986). Perceived social support, received social support, and adjustment to stressful life events. *Journal of Health and Social Behavior,27,* 78–89.

Wharton, A. S., & Erickson, R. J. (1995). The consequences of caring: Exploring the links between women's job and family emotion work. *Sociological Quarterly, 36,* 301–324.

Wheaton, B. (1990). Life transitions, role histories, and mental health. *American Sociological Review, 55,* 209–223.

Wheaton, B. (1994). Sampling the stress universe. In W. R. Avison & I. H. Gotlib (Eds.), *Stress and mental health: Contemporary issues and prospects for future research* (pp. 77–114). New York: Plenum.

Wheaton, B. (1999). Social stress. In C. S. Aneshensel & J. C. Phelan (Eds.), *Handbook of the sociology of mental health* (pp. 277–300). New York: Kluwer.

Williams, D. R., & Collins, C. (1997). Socioeconomic status and racial differences in health: Patterns and explanations. *Annual Review of Sociology, 21,* 349–386.

Williams, D. R., & Harris-Reid, M. (1999). Race and mental health: Emerging patterns and promising approaches. In A.V. Horwitz & T. Scheid (Eds.), *Handbook for the study of mental health: Social contexts, theories, and systems* (pp. 295–327). New York: Cambridge.

Williams, D. R., Takeuchi, D., & Adair, R. K. (1992). Marital status and psychiatric disorders among blacks and whites. *Journal of Health and Social Behavior,33,* 140–157.

Williams, K. (2003). Has the future of marriage arrived? A contemporary examination of gender, marital status, and psychological well-being. *Journal of Health and Social Behavior, 44,* 470–487.

Yu, Y., & Williams, D. R. (1999). Socioeconommic status and mental health. In C. S. Aneshensel & J. C. Phelan (Eds.), *Handbook for the sociology of mental health* (pp. 151–166). New York: Kluwer/Plenum.

12
Social Psychology and Stress Research

Jane D. McLeod and Kathryn J. Lively

The stress process is a microcosm of the society-individual interface, where structural and cultural constraints are manifest in human thought and action. Macro-level constraints become visible in population patterns of stress exposures as well as in the strategies that individuals use to avoid and respond to potentially stressful circumstances. Proximal social interactions that are embedded in this broader set of constraints serve as the sites at which the meanings of stressful life experiences are constructed, thereby acting as conduits for macro-level influences. The selves that engage stressful experiences participate in, and are shaped by, this process of meaning construction, closing the circle between society and individual. If we accept all this to be true, research on the stress process must invoke the full range of sociological theories regarding the nature of the society-individual interface. In turn, stress research has potential to inform the development of those theories by applying their insights to analyses of specific life transitions and challenges.

We advance these two claims through a critical examination of the current status of stress research within sociology. Stress research is an interdisciplinary field with important contributions from sociology, psychology, and allied mental health disciplines. Sociological stress researchers distinguish themselves by their explicit attention to the macro-foundations of the stress process. Pearlin's influential statement that sociologists are uniquely positioned "to observe how deeply well-being is affected by the structured arrangements of people's lives and by the repeated experiences that stem from these arrangements" (Pearlin, 1989, p. 241) has been embraced by sociological stress researchers, leading to important insights into the nature of social stratification and its implications for individual lives. Complementary statements followed on the heels of Pearlin's, calling for greater recognition of the links between stratification research and stress research (Aneshensel, 1992), for integration of diverse outcomes into stress research (Aneshensel, Rutter, & Lachenbruch, 1991), and for attention to population-based health processes (Schwartz, 2002). Together, these commentators asserted a unique sociological contribution grounded in the "social facts" about which Durkheim wrote (Schwartz, 2002).

While not disagreeing with the importance of analyzing the macro-foundations of individual stressful circumstances, we contend that the "social" in social stress is not confined to the macro-world but can be found also in the world of interpersonal relations and self, central concerns of sociological social psychology. If stress research can connect with the concerns of mainstream sociology through an emphasis on the macro-world, it can also do so through an emphasis on meso- and micro-interactions.

In this chapter, we identify new opportunities for stress research that emerge from deeper integration of social psychological principles, especially the tenets of symbolic interactionism. Specifically, we propose a vision for stress research which complements consideration of the macro-foundations of the stress process with equal emphasis on meaning construction as its central dynamic.[1] Inasmuch as meaning construction is an inherently social process, our vision for stress research reveals another layer of social influence in the stress process, both in the construction itself and as the process of construction is shaped by macro- and meso-structural constraints. Our vision encourages greater attention to the interactional basis of stressful experiences and to the centrality of self in the stress process. We illustrate our points by considering traditional and contemporary conceptualizations of social roles in stress research.

A Brief History of Social Stress Research

Social stress research traces its origins to the foundational works of W.B. Cannon, Adolf Meyer, and Hans Selye. Cannon (1929), a neurologist and physiologist, reviewed laboratory research on animals and case studies of medical patients to argue that emotionally provocative experiences (e.g., fear, pain) produce increases in levels of physiological activity that help animals cope with the experience (e.g., heightened adrenal gland activity). While often adaptive, these increases may promote disease if not relieved. Meyer, a psychiatrist, extended Cannon's work by asserting that normative changes, such as graduating from school or the birth of a child, also have the potential to affect physical and mental health. Selye (1956), a physician and endocrinologist, conducted extensive animal experiments which demonstrated that a variety of physical stressors (e.g., cold, pain) elicited that same syndrome of physiological reactions, which he called the General Adaptation Syndrome. The syndrome is characterized by stages of alarm, resistance, and exhaustion, the last of which follows only if the stressors overwhelm the animal's adaptive capacity.

These foundational works have been elaborated in a sustained program of research concerned with the consequences of life stress for humans. The basic tenet of this program is that stress affects health by overwhelming adaptive capacities.

---

[1] Our comments are not intended to deny the existence of obdurate realities (see Fine, 1992). Poverty, oppression, hunger, technology are all tangible features of the social system that have real implications for the lives of individuals. We contend, however, that an exclusive focus on those material realities diverts our attention from much of the "social" in social stress.

Studies by sociologists, psychologists, and allied social and behavioral scientists estimate the physical and mental health effects of diverse stressors—including major life events, chronic strains, daily hassles, and major lifetime traumas—and the determinants of variation in stress responses. As a group, these studies reveal both the vulnerability and resilience of humans, the essential importance of meaningful social relations to human health, and the creativity of human thought and action in the face of threat.

Since the early 1980s, sociological research on stress has followed Pearlin's stress process framework (Pearlin, Lieberman, Menaghan, & Mullan, 1981). This framework sees the outcomes of stress as a function of the primary stressors to which persons are exposed (such as job loss), the secondary stressors that follow from them (such as marital tensions), and the resources that mediate or moderate their effects on mental health. The resources that have received the most attention from sociologists are mastery, social support, and coping strategies. Consistent with the stress process framework, much research in the late 1970s and 1980s investigated the role of social support and coping in ameliorating the effects of stressors on mental health. It is in this context that Pearlin published his influential 1989 article in which he urged sociologists to remember that the components of the stress process are not randomly distributed but, rather, "can be traced back to surrounding social structures and people's locations within them (p. 242)."

Two types of studies deriving from this framework currently dominate sociological stress research.[2] The first type of study evaluates social status differences in the components of the stress process framework as a means to document inequitable societal arrangements. Studies of this type collect information on the variety of stressors to which members of general population samples are exposed, and use comparisons of stress exposure across population subgroups to document the individual-level implications of macro-structural conditions. For example, Turner and his colleagues (1995) observed that chronic stressors and life events occurring to self were more commonly experienced by persons with low occupational statuses than by those with high occupational statuses, and that these differences in stress exposure explained approximately 33% of observed differences in depression across occupational groups. Based on that evidence, the authors concluded that systemic stressors importantly contribute to the distribution of depression in the general population. Studies such as this are faithful to the current vision of stress research in that they link concepts from the stress process model to macro-structural phenomena and to individual-level psychological states.

The second type of study uses the stress process framework to understand the implications of specific social conditions or statuses for individual mental health. For example, Aneshensel and her colleagues (1993) used the stress process framework to conceptualize the experiences of family members caring for a person with Alzheimer's disease. Their use of the stress process model led them to

---

[2] Within psychology, studies of coping currently dominate the field, with a recent search finding 13,744 published articles concerned with "coping behaviors" between 1967 and 1999 (Somerfield & McCrae, 2000).

ask questions about perceptions of stress among caregivers, the distribution of material and social resources across caregivers, and the implications of those resources for caregivers' abilities to maintain their own emotional health. The goal of studies such as this is to understand socially-patterned variations in the meanings that challenging circumstances come to have for individuals, in responses to those circumstances, and in mental health outcomes. Although studies of specific life events (e.g., divorce) have fallen out of favor among sociological stress researchers, they have similar potential to offer insight into the social origins of stress responses.

Theoretical Origins of Sociological Stress Research

While stress researchers take an eclectic approach to theory, both current traditions within sociological stress research draw primary inspiration from the social structure and personality tradition in sociological social psychology. The social structure and personality (SSP) tradition is concerned with the relationship between macro-social systems or processes and individual feelings, attitudes, and behaviors.[3] The SSP perspective conceives of the world as a series of embedded circles with the individual at the core surrounded by progressively larger and more complex social groupings, including dyads, small groups, communities, organizations and institutions, and the larger social system. In much the same way that one can peel away the layers of an onion to reveal the inner core, SSP researchers attempt to trace the processes through which components of the social system influence individuals and, less often, through which individuals affect social systems (House, 1981; McLeod & Lively, 2003).

This tradition of research is distinguished from the general macro-micro project of sociology by its adherence to three analytic principles: the components principle, the proximity principle, and the psychological principle. The components principle stipulates that researchers identify the specific components of the social system that are most relevant to understanding the phenomenon of interest. The proximity principle directs our attention to the proximate social experiences through which macro-social structures impinge on individual lives, in particular, micro-interactions and small group processes. The psychological principle involves an examination of the psychological mechanisms through which proximal structures and processes affect individual attitudes, feelings, and behaviors. The application of this framework to sociological stress research is straightforward, with macro-social structures such as socioeconomic hierarchies influencing experiences within proximal social environments that, in turn, affect mental health.

---

[3] Among SSP researchers, social structure is defined as "a *persisting* and bounded *pattern* of social relationships (or pattern of behavioral intention) among the units (persons or positions) in a social system" (House 1981, p. 542, emphasis in original).

By attending to these principles, stress research has made important contributions to sociological research on the nature of stratification hierarchies, their implications for daily life, and their effects on individual health and well-being. With respect to the components principle, stress researchers have disaggregated the dimensions of stratification that are linked with stress through analyses that estimate the associations of gender, race, income, education, and occupational status with stress exposure and coping resources (e.g., Kessler & Neighbors, 1986; McLeod & Kessler, 1990; Pearlin & Schooler, 1978; Turner & Avison, 2003; Turner, Wheaton, & Lloyd, 1995). These analyses reveal that the different components of socioeconomic stratification are related to stressful experiences in different ways. For example, income predicts the risk of marital separation/divorce but education does not, whereas education is a stronger predictor of negative events in one's social network (McLeod & Kessler, 1990). Women report more chronic stress and more negative network events than men, but do not report more events occurring to themselves (Turner et al., 1995). Similarly, stress research highlights the complexity of race as a system of stratification that is enacted within multiple levels of social life by documenting the mental health implications of both obvious and insidious forms of discrimination (Williams & Williams-Morris, 2000; Brown, 2003). In sum, stress research has contributed to general conceptual understandings of contemporary stratification systems by affirming their complex, multidimensional character (Mirowsky, Ross, & Reynolds, 2000).

Stress research has also contributed to many sub-disciplines of sociology through its systematic investigations of the proximal environments through which stratification affects health and well-being. Stressors are defined with reference to the geographic, organizational, and interpersonal contexts in which people live their lives, including the family, work, and neighborhoods (Aneshensel & Sucoff, 1996; Conger, Conger, Elder, Lorenz, Simons, & Whitbeck, 1992; Kohn & Schooler, 1983; Hill, Ross, & Angel, 2005). The resources with which people anticipate, avoid, and respond to stress are also attached to these contexts and are enacted within them. By defining and measuring major status-based experiences (e.g., financial deprivation), role strains and role conflicts (e.g., marital problems), and contextual stressors (e.g., neighborhood violence), stress researchers have taken from, and given back to, other sub-disciplines by developing tools with which to analyze the structure and content of major social organizations and institutions. For example, research on the stressful aspects of work environments has yielded a highly differentiated conceptualization of those environments that has informed research on work and occupations (Fenwick & Tausig, this volume).

Finally, stress researchers have given careful attention to the nature of psychological experience as well as to the processes through which proximal stressors affect mental health. With respect to the former, sociologists have questioned dominant psychiatric conceptualizations of mental health and asserted the relevance of more generic forms of distress and of positive mental health (e.g., Horwitz, 2002; Keyes, 2002). By so doing, sociologists aim to broaden the realm of psychological experiences worthy of research attention.

With respect to the latter, stress research illustrates the relevance of self-constructs as mediators in the association between stressful experiences and mental health (Pearlin et al., 1981; Williams & Williams-Morris, 2000), and the importance of identity to definitions and responses to stress (Thoits, 1992, 1995; Burke, 1991). In their early analysis of the stress process, Pearlin and colleagues (1981) demonstrated that stressors have implications for mental health, in part, because they are associated with declines in self-esteem and mastery. Similarly, Williams and Williams-Morris's (2000) review highlighted the centrality of internalized racism to the processes through which racism affects mental health (see also Brown, Sellers, & Gomez, 2002). Thoits (1992) and Burke (1991) applied different versions of identity theory to the stress process but came to similar predictions: stressors that challenge valued identities have the most profound implications for distress. Research on self and identity in the stress process complements basic social psychological research by providing further evidence that the self is both social product and social force (Rosenberg, 1979) and by specifying the processes through which the self responds to threats.

In sum, stress research demonstrates the profound implications of stratification hierarchies for individuals. These hierarchies have effects that move beyond their narrow domains (e.g., status attainment processes) into the most personal aspects of people's lives. These contributions conform to social stress research's goal "to identify elements of social life that have dysfunctional consequences" (Pearlin, 1999, p. 410) as well as to social structure and personality's traditional emphasis on the macro-determinants of individual feelings, attitudes, and behaviors (House, 1981).

As impressive as these contributions are, they nevertheless yield a surprisingly sterile portrait of the stress process. SSP-oriented research has yielded thorough definitions and descriptions of the components of the stress process, but little understanding of how the process itself works—of the underlying interpersonal and self processes through which stressors come to have meaning for individuals and, thereby, influence their physical and emotional well-being. We believe that integrating the tenets of symbolic interactionism, the other major theoretical tradition within sociological social psychology (House, 1977; Stryker, 1977), into stress research would yield a richer understanding of the social origins of the stress process.

The social structure and personality framework and symbolic interactionism offer complementary insights into the nature of macro-micro relations. Social structure and personality research encourages careful identification of the macro- and meso-structures that are implicated in individual outcomes as well as precise estimation of the relative contributions of these structures to explaining variance in those outcomes. Perhaps by necessity, its tenets bias models of the stress process towards unidirectional causal influences that begin with macro-social conditions and end with the individual (Thoits, 1994). In contrast to the social structure and personality tradition's "top-down" view of macro-micro relations, symbolic interactionism emphasizes meaning construction and creativity in human action—the interpersonal and self processes through which people make sense of their worlds and act towards them.

Following from these basic claims, we offer a complementary, but distinct, vision for stress research which emphasizes the centrality of meaning negotiation to the stress process. More explicitly, we contend that, although the stress process is importantly shaped by broad structural and cultural imperatives, its social origins cannot be revealed by consideration of those imperatives alone. Rather, what makes the stress process "social" is that it is constructed and enacted in interpersonal interactions—in dyads, small groups, organizations, and social institutions—the proximal environments of the social structure and personality tradition. These meso-level interactions—where society meets the self—have received surprisingly little attention from sociological stress researchers. They are important both because they are the sites in which structural and cultural imperatives become most directly visible, but also because they form the basis of meaning construction. Our vision suggests new directions for research that would enhance our understanding of how people respond when confronted with potentially stressful events, and that would contribute to important theoretical debates within sociology.

We begin our argument by introducing three foundational tenets of symbolic interactionism: the centrality of meaning to human life, the interactional basis of meaning construction, and the self. We then turn to a description of how meaning, interaction, and self have been conceptualized by stress researchers in the past and of new opportunities that would arise from taking the insights of symbolic interactionists seriously. Our arguments build on the work of previous scholars (see, for example, Thoits, 1995b; Pearlin, 1999), to present a more general theoretical argument for the integration of diverse theoretical frameworks within sociological social psychology.

Symbolic Interactionism

Symbolic interactionism assumes that meaning is central to human life.[4] This central tenet asserts that meaning shapes not only how individuals interpret particular events, but also how they interpret others, their environments, and, perhaps, most importantly, themselves (Heise, 2002; Smith-Lovin & Heise, 1988). These interpretations, in turn, color how individuals respond to events and situations, regardless of the objective reality of the event itself (Charmaz, 1980; 1991).

One of the more enduring insights of symbolic interaction is that meaning is not static. Instead, meaning is expected to change over time as individuals

---

[4] There are many different versions of symbolic interactionist thought, which vary with respect to the degree of fluidity they attribute to meaning (Blumer, 1989; Heise, 1977; Mead, 1934; Stryker, 1988). Whereas early articulations of the theory that sought to distinguish symbolic interaction from other forms of sociological social psychology emphasized the negotiated nature of meaning and self, later versions (Stryker, 1980) reintroduced the constraining, albeit not determining influence of structure. Stryker, for one, explained the relative consistency of social life by attaching meaning to the self. The self, from this perspective is comprised not only of individuals' social positions but also by corresponding roles that are maintained vis-à-vis interaction with stable and enduring social relations.

develop new understandings of their situations (Blumer, 1969; Orbuch, 1997). New understandings may result from the changing nature of the situation itself or from self-reflection but may also arise out of social interactions with real and imagined others. The interactionist view of meaning as dynamic and negotiated contrasts sharply with more traditional conceptualizations of meaning which treat concepts such as culture and beliefs as obdurate and therefore resistant to individual influences.

Social comparisons play an important role in the process of meaning construction. Symbolic interactionists contend that we routinely gauge our own reactions to particular events against how we believe we *should* react or how we believe others would react in a similar circumstance. Individuals who come to see their reaction as exceeding (or otherwise not adhering to) valued social norms may attempt to change their reaction, either by altering their interpretation of the event (e.g. reinterpreting the event as an opportunity rather than a disaster), or by changing their views of themselves.

In contrast to the static, trait-like conceptualizations of self that characterize social structure and personality research (represented by, for example, measures of self-esteem or mastery), symbolic interactionists conceptualize self as both precursor and product of action and meaning. Whether viewed as a collection of salient social roles that individuals actively pursue and support (Stryker, 1980) or as a cybernetic system of situated identities that individuals are motivated to maintain (Heise, 1977; Burke, 1991), definitions of the self (and its related cognitions and behaviors) are dependent upon the presence, the acceptance, and, oftentimes, the support of others (Stryker & Burke, 2000). As a central meaning system, the self is subject to reinterpretation and reconstruction over time.

Together, these tenets of symbolic interactionism assume an agentic model of human action (Charmaz, 1991; Heise, 1977; Hochschild, 1983; Mead, 1934; Stryker, 1994) which contrasts with the more deterministic image of social structure within the social structure and personality tradition (McLeod & Lively, 2003).[5] If we accept the tenet that meaning is constructed by such social processes as making comparisons and seeking and receiving support, it follows that the stress process is, at its heart, interactional. It is here, at the level of face-to-face interactions, that people come to construct and to reconstruct meaning not only about the events in their lives, but also about themselves.

By proposing that stress researchers be more attentive to the insights of symbolic interactionism we are, in effect, proposing a paradigmatic reorientation. Our proposed approach requires a significant shift from stress researchers' over-reliance on an intrapsychic view of self to one that is inherently more social. To

---

[5] The notion of human agency found new expression in the structure-agency debate which dominated sociological writings in the 1980s, and remains central to contemporary social theory (Alexander, 1982, 1984; Bourdieu, 1977; Emirbayer & Mische, 1998; Giddens, 1976, 1984; Sewell, 1992).

make this shift, stress researchers would have to be willing to expand the view of the self as a protective, yet passive, set of predetermined characteristics or roles and adopt a more fluid conceptualization of self as negotiated interpersonally and dependent upon social interaction. By examining how the self and consequent meanings and behaviors are influenced by others, a more interactive approach has the potential to shed light into why some people construct particular life events and situations as stressful and others do not. It would also provide greater insight into how the meanings of identities and life events are constructed and the effects of these negotiations on psychological and emotional outcomes. As we hope our argument demonstrates, stress research and sociological social psychology have much to gain from such a shift.

Meaning in the Stress Process

Stress researchers agree that the effects of stressors on mental health depend on their meanings to the individual (Brown & Harris, 1978; Pearlin, 1983; Pearlin, 1989; Simon, 1995; Thiots, 1991, 1992; Wortman, Silver, & Kessler, 1993; see Simon's (1997) excellent review for more details). Traditional approaches to the measurement of meaning depend on the assumptions that the meanings of stressors can be determined objectively, and that better measures of meaning will yield more powerful associations between stress exposures and mental health.

Psychologists have traditionally favored measures of stress appraisals that are based on subjective ratings of threat, controllability, change, and the like (see for example Cohen et al., 1983; Peacock and Wong, 1990). Sociologists (and some psychologists) reject these measures out of hand based on the reasonable criticism that they confound reactions to events with their appraisals (see Monroe & Kelley, 1995 for a review). It comes as no surprise, critics claim, to find that events rated as more stressful or threatening by respondents have stronger associations with psychological well-being than less stressful or threatening events because ratings of stress appraisals depend on the outcome of the event.

In response to these concerns, some researchers have developed elaborate coding systems designed to yield objective ratings of event characteristics. For example, Brown and Harris's (1978) Life Events and Difficulties Schedule elicits a narrative about each reported event or difficulty which is then evaluated by a panel that rates the event for its long-term contextual threat, severity, as well as several other characteristics (see Wethington, Brown, & Kessler, 1995 for a review). Event/difficulty ratings are made without reference to the respondent's subjective reactions or emotional responses to ensure that the ratings are independent of the effects of the stressors on mental health outcomes. Dohrenwend and colleagues (1993) developed the Standardized Event Rating system which follows a similar format, but which deletes all information pertaining to social vulnerability from the narratives in order to permit analysis of how social vulnerabilities modify the effects of stressful circumstances.

Other researchers have inferred meaning from the context in which events occur. For example, Wheaton (1991) demonstrated that the effect of events vary with the sequence of life-course experiences in which they are embedded, thereby inferring variation in meaning from variation in effects (see also Thoits, 1995b). Similarly, Umberson and her colleagues (1992) observed stronger effects of widowhood on depression among women who experienced subsequent financial and household strain. In each case, the context of the event is used to define its meaning for the respondent.

Finally, most in keeping with symbolic interactionist principles, another group of researchers has argued for an approach to meaning that more directly considers identity, beliefs, and values (Pearlin, 1989; Simon, 2000; Thoits, 1992). Thoits (1992) proposed that the meanings of stressors depend on the importance of the identity domain in which they occur. Pearlin (1989) asserted that social values shape the meaning of stressors. Extending that point, Simon (1995, 2000) directed attention to "gender-linked cultural norms, values, expectations, and beliefs (2000, p. 73)" as they influence men's and women's subjective interpretations of potentially stressful role-based experiences. She found, for example, that working women were more distressed by work-family conflict than were working men because women perceived their roles as workers as in conflict with their roles as caregivers whereas men did not.

As these examples illustrate, most analyses of meaning in the stress process have been oriented towards developing better estimates of the effects of stressful experiences on individual outcomes rather than towards the study of meaning itself. As a result, these analyses fail to provide even basic descriptive information about the meanings that people give to stressful circumstances and about their origins in macro- and meso-level experiences. In particular, we know little about whether men and women view the "same" circumstances similarly or differently (with Simon's (1995) research an important exception) or whether meanings vary systematically by race/ethnicity, socioeconomic status, or other important status characteristics. We also know little about how meanings change as the stress process unfolds.

Following from traditional conceptualizations of meaning, a social structure and personality approach would encourage studies of the associations of SES, gender, race, and other important social and cultural indicators with self-reported stress appraisals. Studies of this type would allow us to determine whether the "same" event is viewed differently depending on one's social location. For example, we would be able to determine whether persons with lower levels of income rate a significantly greater number of events as "very stressful" than persons with higher levels of income. Analyses of this type would complement prior analyses of the social distribution of stress exposure (e.g., McLeod & Kessler, 1990; Turner et al., 1995) by showing how social location shapes the interpretation of stressors at a particular moment in time.

Such traditional analyses rest on the assumption that appraisals are resistant to change. Integrating the interactionist assumption that appraisals are fluid and dynamic would require that we take a different approach to the study of meaning, more in line with research on accounts (Orbuch, 1997).[6] Research on accounts analyzes the spontaneous or solicited stories that people present to explain and interpret stressful (or potentially stressful) experiences. The goals of the analyses are diverse, including understanding the content of the account (their temporal form, attributional statements, embedded affect), the conditions under which different types of accounts are given and by whom, and the conditions under which other people accept or reject accounts. Beyond Weiss's (1975) research on divorce, stress researchers have paid little attention to extant research on accounts, perhaps because it is often focused on specific life traumas (e.g., Orbuch's research on sexual abuse (Orbuch, Harvey, David, & Merbach, 1994), Silver's research on incest (Silver, Boon, & Stones, 1983)).

Analyses of accounts of specific stressful experiences offer several advantages to stress researchers. When abstracted across stressful experiences, they provide answers to general questions about how people make sense of, and impose order on, those experiences. What common forms and themes appear across accounts of different types of experiences? What causal attributions appear and what do they tell us about how the respondent conceptualizes her or his relationship with the world? How are accounts influenced by position in the life course and by important social locations? Answers to these questions address general concerns in research on meaning construction, the self, and social stratification.

In addition, by their very nature, accounts constitute coping strategies. By telling the story of their experience, people are explaining and interpreting the experience in a way that helps them make sense of what happened for themselves and others. Accounts may include descriptions of coping efforts, but are also forms of coping themselves and, thereby, relevant to stress research. As Orbuch (1997) notes, the process of confiding implicit in the construction of an account has physical and mental health benefits (Harvey, Orbuch, Chwalisz, & Garwood, 1991; Orbuch et al., 1994). Thus, accounts can inform our understanding of how people cope with problems in their lives. Because accounts often elicit information about the responses and actions of others, they also offer insight into how people use, maintain, and repair interpersonal relations during times of stress.

Finally, accounts are dynamic. They change over time in response to the individual's changing understanding of the experience as well as based on the feedback of others and collective understandings (Harvey, Orbuch, & Weber, 1990; Orbuch, Harvey, Davis, & Merbach, 1993; Orbuch, Veroff, & Holmberg, 1994). Analyses of changes in accounts over time have the potential to reveal macro- and meso-influences on meaning that are more subtle than those gleaned from traditional survey-based approaches as well as individual acceptance or resistance to those influences. Such analyses straddle the traditional concerns of

---

[6] Although the terms "account" and "narrative" are often used interchangeably, Orbuch (1997) offers a useful distinction. The term narrative usually refers to an individual's story as told to someone else; an account may be presented publicly, but may also be represented in private activities such as diary-writing. Accounts also involve causal attributions that are intended to make sense of a troubling situation.

social structure and personality research and symbolic interactionism. In sum, although accounts cannot be used to develop precise estimates of the effects of stressful experiences on mental health, they can be used to understand the *process* through which people construct the meaning of those experiences.

Orbuch (1997) notes one important limitation in extant research on accounts: research has not yet evaluated whether and how accounts are related to subsequent behavior. Stress research is ideally suited for this task inasmuch as it can evaluate the implications of current accounts for subsequent efforts to avoid and cope with stressors.

The Interactional Basis of the Stress Process

Our discussion of meaning asserted that meaning is fluid and constructed, a result not only of individual perceptions but also of social feedback. In this section, we consider the interactional basis of the stress process in greater depth.

Sociological stress researchers acknowledge social interactions in the stress process through analyses of social networks and social support. Social network conceptualizations emphasize the structural connections—the presence or absence of links—among individuals or groups (see Lin & Peek, 1999 for a review). Common network concepts such as density (the degree of overlap among the links within a given domain), reciprocity (whether exchanges occur in both directions across a link), and multiplexity (whether a given link involves an exchange of more than one function or activity) further specify the nature of the connections among groups of individuals and the possible pathways for the exchange of information and resources. Social network characteristics have inconsistent associations with mental health and are only occasionally found to buffer the effects of stressors on mental health, perhaps, as Lin and Peek (1999) speculate, because their associations with social support have not been fully specified.[7]

The concept of social support highlights the content of social networks and their provision of caring and instrumental assistance (House, Umberson, & Landis, 1988; Turner & Turner, 1999). As several other chapters in this volume review, the perception that one is loved and cared for, and the availability of an emotional confidant, buffer the effects of stressful experiences on mental health (Kessler & McLeod, 1985). While the concepts of social networks and social support are distinct, several researchers have studied their interconnections, for example, how the size and density of networks relates to their capacity to provide emotional and instrument support (e.g., Acock & Hurlbert, 1993; Lin, 1982; Wellman & Wortley, 1989).

Studies of social networks and social support in the stress process have contributed importantly to our understanding of interpersonal resources as moderators of stress

---

[7] Or, perhaps social networks not only define the support to which people have access but also influence how effective that support is, a point raised by Bernice Pescosolido.

effects. However, they take us only partway towards appreciating the interactional basis of the stress process because they are embedded in a conceptual paradigm that places the individual actor at the center of the inquiry. When thinking about how people experience stress, stress researchers tend to envision isolated individuals who encounter potentially stressful experiences, appraise and interpret those experiences, make decisions about how to respond to them, and then either become distressed or not depending on the effectiveness of their responses. This conceptualization aligns with dominant rational actor models of human behavior, but is not true to how people understand and respond to complex problems (see Pescosolido, 1992).

In addition, although studies of social networks and social support ably demonstrate the many health-related benefits of receiving information, assistance, and emotional support, they fail to acknowledge that interpersonal interactions also serve as the basis for meaning construction. In other words, supportive (and non-supportive) interactions transmit more than practice and emotional assistance. What we argue for here, then, are the benefits of conceptualizing stress as a cybernetic, interactionally-based process, consistent with Pescosolido's (1992) reconceptualization of help-seeking.

A cybernetic, interactionally-based process refers to a process in which the form and content of communication places limits on the meanings that can be constructed by actors within any given interaction Applied to the case of stress, it implies a process in which individual understandings of stressful experiences are subject to the scrutiny and evaluation of others (real or imagined), and change in response. The scrutiny and evaluation of others may occur through subtle, and even unrecognized, social comparisons or through direct confrontation and conflict.

Symbolic interactionist theory offers insight into both types of processes. Beginning with the more subtle, the meanings that other people hold are invoked when individuals check their own reactions against those of the "generalized other"—the whole of a society's shared values and norms (Mead, 1934). Although this process of construction does not involve direct contact with other people, it is nonetheless social. When individuals compare their own reactions against those of the generalized other, they see themselves as they believe others would see them and gauge their reactions to a particular event against how they believe they *should* react or how they believe other people would react in a similar circumstance (Hochschild, 1983; Thoits, 1984, 1985).

The ways in which individuals use (and, even, determine the content of) the generalized other in stressful times inform our understanding of how and why people make comparisons more generally. For example, while some individuals may come to define the nebulous "they" as compassionate and kind, others may hold a much harsher or unforgiving view of society's norms. Because stress researchers tend to look at large aggregates of people, and study a broad range of potentially stressful events, they would be advantageously positioned to investigate the circumstances under which individuals adopt or construct different norms by which to judge their behaviors, identities, and or reactions (Smith-Lovin & Douglass, 1992. Thomassen, 2002). Moreover, inasmuch as such views of what constitutes society's values are products of socialization, life experiences, and interpersonal interactions, the study of social comparisons represents another point of convergence for social structure and personality research and symbolic interactionism.

While the generalized other serves as one point of reference, people also engage in more strategic comparisons with both real and imagined others to preserve their sense of self (Rosenberg, 1979). For example, some people make upward comparisons in order to feel better about their futures whereas others make downward comparisons in order to feel better about their present situations (Major, Testa, & Bylsma, 1991; Pearlin & Skaff, 1996; Wills, 1991; Wood & Taylor, 1991). People may also look to specific others in order to seek examples of either appropriate ("I'd like to be able to handle this like her") or inappropriate ("please don't let me act like that") responses and then model their actions accordingly. The comparisons that people choose to make are a function not only of how they see themselves in the present, but also of how they would like to see themselves in the future. Social comparisons convey the values and beliefs of both broad (i.e., macro) and local (e.g., meso) cultures *and* serve as primary means for pursuing self-motives such as self-verification (Swann, 1983) and self-enhancement (Tesser, 1986). Stressful experiences threaten the self and trigger social comparisons, making the stress process an ideal site in which to analyze how culture becomes relevant to meaning as well as how social comparisons are invoked to achieve self-motives. Despite impressive research on the cultural foundations of psychological experience (Heine, Lehman, Peng, & Greenholz, 2002; Kitayama, Markus, Matsumoto, & Norasakkunkit, 1997), much remains to be known about the use of general and specific comparisons to enhance or maintain the self in different structural and cultural contexts.[8]

Complementing the extant literature on the link between perceived inequity in the household division of labor and distress (Glass & Fujimoto, 1994; Lennon & Rosenfield, 1994), Hochschild's (1989) qualitative work on the "second shift" demonstrated that husbands and wives managed their anger and resentment over what they each perceived as an unequal division in the division of household labor by making strategic comparisons that simultaneously protected the self and obscured blatant disparities in the division of household tasks. Wives who were committed to having an egalitarian marriage made comparisons with other women who had greater household responsibilities, rather than comparing the work they did against that performed by their husbands. Husbands, too, chose their comparisons carefully, oftentimes comparing their contributions around the house to those of other men that they knew or to their fathers (also see Bylsma & Major, 1994).

---

[8] A full discussion of the role of culture is outside of the scope of this review. Here, we note simply that, although stress research focuses most of its attention on the structural origins of stress, stressors also arise from contradictions among and between cultural ideals and material realities (e.g. the conflict between dominant attitudes against mothers seeking employment and high rates of employment among mothers of preschool children; Treas & Widmer, 2000). Culture also shapes the meaning and emotional significance of stressors and defines the range of coping responses that seem possible (see Simon, 2000).

These strategic comparisons allowed couples not only to better manage their feelings of distress (or unfairness) regarding domestic schedules, but also to construct and maintain a meaning system that supported their idealized views of themselves (as, for example, feminist/egalitarian), their spouses (e.g., egalitarian male/primary caretaker), and their marriages. Hochschild's observations of how comparisons are used to avoid potential conflict within the household have implications for research on stress avoidance as well as for theories of culture, emotions, and self-verification.

Shifting to more direct forms of meaning negotiation, other people become involved when individuals seek or are offered support from friends, family members, or—in some cases—professionals. While social support can be viewed as strictly instrumental, the advice and assistance we receive from others also communicates the social and cultural meaning of our life experiences—whether they are seen as desirable, important, devastating. Thinking about social support as a form of meaning construction offers new ways to understand established findings. For example, research on social support suggests that similar others may be the best source of interpersonal coping (Thoits, 1986). The benefits of support from similar others may reflect their greater ability to offer salutary interpretations of the experience. Similar others may also be better able to neutralize residual feelings, such as embarrassment, shame, or guilt, that exacerbate stress (Lively, 2000; Thoits, 1985; also see Lazarus and Folkman, 1984) by reinterpreting those feelings as normal and understandable.

In sum, reframing the study of stress in terms of interactionally-based meaning construction helps us to ask new questions about how the meanings of life circumstances are created in interaction—which important others (real and imagined) are invoked in definitional processes, in what settings those processes occur, and how their character varies depending on both. It directs us to the flows of interpretation as well as information and resources to and from the individual over time—another component of the "social" in social stress. Perhaps more fundamentally, what it suggests is that the concept of social support, while useful for delimiting an important component of the stress process, is a proxy for much more complex interpersonal processes that are only partially reflected in its narrow and static conceptualization. Interpersonal interactions are a central focus of the symbolic interactionist framework, emphasizing the importance of that framework in the study of stress.

A Social Self

The linchpin of our argument is that sociological stress research relies on an overly static, individualistic, and (ironically) psychological conceptualization of self. General theories of self acknowledge that self is a social product, created in interpersonal interaction rather than existing as a purely psychological phenomenon (Cooley, 1902; Mead, 1934; Stryker, 1980). By implication, self and identity are fluid and negotiated, changing across time and space in response to others' actions and to situational imperatives. Although stress researchers recognize that stressful experiences have implications for self-conceptions (e.g., Krause, 1991; Pearlin et al., 1981), they have been slow to incorporate a fully realized conceptualization of self into their models. Social psychological theories of identity hold considerable promise for this purpose.

Identity theory as proposed by Sheldon Stryker (1980) posits that the self is made up of multiple role identities that are organized in a salience hierarchy; identities at the top of the salience hierarchy are more likely to be enacted in given social situations than identities at the bottom. According to identity theory, identity salience is a function of commitment (ties to other social actors) and will decrease under conditions in which identity claims are not supported interactionally. An individual for whom teacher is a salient identity, for example, may be forced to rearrange his or her salience hierarchy (of identities) if he or she is unable to relate to or with students. Likewise, a man who loses custody of his children may reduce the salience of "father". Losses of, or challenges to, highly salient identities are predicted to cause greater levels of distress than losses of or challenges to less salient identities (see also Burke, 1991; Large & Marcussen, 2000).

Empirical evidence for these predictions is mixed. Thoits' community-based studies (1992, 1994, 1995) find little support for the hypothesis that events occurring in salient life domains have stronger effects on mental health than other events. In contrast, Hammen (Hammen et al., 1985; Hammen & Goodman-Brown, 1990) finds that events that threaten dominant self-schema are associated with higher levels of depression. Simon (1992) observed stronger effects of child problems on parental distress among fathers who were highly committed to the parental role than among fathers who were not, but no difference in effects among mothers. Possible explanations for the different results include the use of different outcomes and different measures of identity salience. As plausibly, people may change their identity salience hierarchies in response to stressors (e.g., Pearlin & Skaff, 1996; Thoits, 1995a) attenuating the association of those rankings with distress. Far from discouraging further research on identity and stress, these results encourage those efforts by pointing to the need for more precise and dynamic measurement of identity in studies of stress (see also Stryker (1980)).

Affect control theory (ACT; Heise, 1977, 2002; MacKinnon, 1994; Smith-Lovin & Heise, 1988) is another theory of role-based identities that has potentially profound implications for our understanding of stress processes. More than most theories within sociological social psychology, ACT integrates elements of social cognition, social structure, culture, and affect to address the question of how meaning influences individual behavior, and attributions about self, others, behaviors (or actions) and settings. It acknowledges the importance of situationally/role-based interaction and culturally shared norms (or sentiments) in meaning negotiation and allows for feedback between actors and objects as they collectively re-shape meaning, behavior, attributions, and emotion. It has the potential to inform our general understanding of the social origins of meaning in the stress process, and of the processes through which meaning can be renegotiated in interaction.

In brief, affect control theory specifies that individuals hold culturally shared sentiments regarding the degree to which social identities (both as actors and objects), behaviors, and settings are good or bad, powerful or powerless, and active or inactive (Heise, 1977; Smith-Lovin & Heise, 1988).[9] Situational events create transient meanings that are juxtaposed against these fundamental sentiments. The difference in meaning produced by a particular event is known as deflection and is experienced as a sense of likelihood: the more unlikely an event is perceived to be in that situation, the more deflection is likely to occur. For example, the event "mother hits child" creates a large deflection because the behavior is inconsistent with fundamental cultural sentiments regarding mothers' behaviors towards their children. Because individuals are motivated to reduce deflection in their own interactions (as well as when witnessing the interactions of others) actors are motivated to either change their own behavior or their definitions of one or more elements of the situation (e.g. change their definition of the event to "mother *disciplines* child").

Although there have been few empirical examinations of the relationship between deflection and stress, Francis's (1997) research on support groups for divorcees and widowers demonstrates that individuals' definitions of situations and resultant deflections have real consequences for emotional well-being. Most ACT research focuses on the ways in which individuals redefine situations (also see Hochschild, 1983). Francis illustrates that some definitional changes are, in fact, motivated by interpersonal interactions (also see Thoits, 1995a). In her analysis, support group members worked together to reduce deflection and its concomitant emotional responses by changing the meanings of their spousal losses through the reconfiguration of actor-behavior-object relations. Specifically, widows and widowers who viewed themselves as being "bad, weak, and inactive," and their deceased spouse as "good, weak, and inactive," were often encouraged to view themselves as "good, weak, and inactive," and their spouses as "bad, strong, and active." In other words, individuals who came into the group believing that they had failed their spouse were encouraged to redefine the event as their spouse abandoning them. Once the survivor saw him or herself in a more positive light (as someone who was guiltless, as opposed to someone who was guilty), the group leader could then encourage the formation of a "survivor" identity, which is characterized as being not only good, but also strong and active. Lively and Heise (2004) have shown, using survey data, that individuals who routinely occupy good, strong, and active identities are more likely to also report experiencing good, positive, and active emotions (e.g., happiness) and less likely to experience bad, weak and inactive emotions (e.g., distress).

These analyses, taken together, ably illustrate the potential of ACT-informed studies to advance research agendas tied specifically to stress research. They

---

[9] The social identity "mother", for example, is viewed as being very good, slightly powerful, and somewhat active, whereas a "child" is viewed as exceptionally good, very powerless, and very active.

reveal that social support can work by encouraging identity transformation and that identity transformations may result in reduced feelings of sadness or distress. Following from this example, studies of stress have the potential to contribute to more general theoretical development in sociology regarding how meaning is constructed in social interaction. An important extension of this work would be to evaluate whether individuals who occupy different social locations or have access to different forms of individual and or interpersonal resources define or redefine elements of situations (e.g., themselves, others, behaviors, or settings) using dif-ferent strategies and in ways that more or less successfully reduce deflection and or feelings of distress.

Social Roles in the Stress Process

The potential benefits of integrating symbolic interactionist principles into stress research are evident in the revitalization of role theory since the 1980s. Social roles have historically been, and continue to be, one of the primary ways in which stress researchers have defined domains of stress exposure and conceptualized meaning (Pearlin, 1983). Social roles are also a central concept associated with social structure and personality research (House, 1981) and with structural symbolic interactionism (Stryker, 1980). Social roles reflect the broad social structure but they are also sources of meaning for individuals. Our review of the revitalization of the concept demonstrates the added value to be gained from drawing on both conceptualizations, particularly as they are related to meaning construction, in stress research.

Traditional conceptualizations of social roles define them as behavioral expectations that are associated with, and emerge from, identifiable positions in social structure (e.g., Merton, 1957). In this view, social roles exist prior to social interactions and serve as constraints on behavior. They are predetermined positions that we enter and exit in patterned ways over the life course (George, 1993).

This conceptualization of social roles has motivated stress research on structurally-based variation in role occupancy and role expectations as determinants of individual functioning, an area of research to which stress research has made significant contributions. Drawing on traditional sociological interests in the fit (or lack thereof) between structural requirements and individual personality, researchers have also studied the implications of role incongruity, role conflict, and role overload for physical and mental health and for deviant behavior (Meton, 1957; Thoits, 1983). There is also a well-established literature on multiple role occupancy and well-being that tests the competing hypotheses that multiple roles offer greater potential for self-actualization (Linville, 1987) and that multiple roles create tension and stress (Thoits, 1983). Sequences of role exits and entries matter for mental health, in different ways for different groups (Jackson, 2002), a finding that bridges role theory and the life course. More generally, role-based stressors serve as a central mechanism through which macro-structures come to have relevance for individual lives (Pearlin, 1983, 1999).

These applications of role theory to stress research can be usefully extended through consideration of more general theoretical developments within role theory. Specifically, traditional role theory has been repeatedly criticized for its lack of attention to individual agency. In response, several attempts have been made to revitalize our understanding of role and, therefore, role theory through the introduction of interactionist principles. The first of these theoretical innovations shifted the conceptualization of role-based human behavior from role-playing to role-making (Stryker & Statham, 1985; Turner, 1962). The concept of role-making emphasizes situational dynamics, meaning construction, bargaining, and personal control in role-based behavior. In essence, the interactionist conceptualization views individuals as creative negotiators of role expectations within specific interactions.

The concept of role-making identifies one strategy through which individuals avoid and respond to stress: renegotiating the meaning of the role. For example, men and women who feel conflict between their roles as workers and as parents can attempt to redefine what those roles mean in order to reduce the conflict, an attempt to "modify the situation" in Pearlin and Schooler's (1978) terms. What is particularly interesting (and uniquely social) about role-making may not be captured by a pure coping conceptualization, however. Role-making represents another point at which macro-social and interpersonal influences on meaning construction can be made visible by the stress process. Role-making is structurally and situationally bound; cultural and structural constraints limit the perceived desirability of role redefinition (e.g., men may feel less motivated than women to redefine the worker role) and draw boundaries around possible role redefinitions (e.g., the definition of the worker role cannot be extended beyond relations involving some exchange of skills for resources). Moreover, not everyone has the same power to assert redefinitions, implying that status-based characteristics enter into interpersonal negotiations regarding the meaning and importance of role-based experiences. In sum, the natural link between the concept of role-making and current conceptualizations of coping responses affirms that the stress process is fluid, flexible, and interactionally-based. It also suggests an alternative way to view coping processes that may yield new information about stress responses and about constraints on role-making processes.

Callero (1994) recently extended the concept of role-making by introducing the notion of "role-using" which begins from the premise that roles are not just bundles of rights and obligations but are also cultural objects that serve as resources in interaction. In addition to their situationally-based realities, roles also have independent symbolic and cognitive realities, named variously "typifications" (Hewitt, 1991; Schutz, 1970) or "gestalts" (Turner, 1978), that transcend specific pragmatic applications. These symbolic realities involve generalized images of what it means to hold specific role positions that can be used by individuals as identity claims (as when a woman asserts her identity as a mother) but also to claim resources (e.g. assistance with child rearing) and to understand behaviors or feelings (e.g., men can invoke the role of mother to explain their nurturing behaviors even if they cannot claim the role).

We use the example of work-family conflict to illustrate the utility of integrating contemporary conceptualizations of social roles into stress research. Several studies document that combining work and family roles can be stressful, particularly for women (Menaghan, 1989; Thoits, 1986). Simon's (1995) research usefully builds upon this work by demonstrating that the *meaning* of the combination of work and family roles varies by sex due to different normative expectations regarding men's and women's roles within the family. Integrating the more interactionally based processes of role-making and role-using into this line of research could add further richness to our understanding the meaning of family-related stress. For example, despite a general tendency for women in Simon's study to be more distressed by work-family conflict than men, some women perceived work and family roles as interdependent and, thereby, avoided distress. Drawing on our understanding of role-making, we might analyze how these women were able to construct their role within the family as a provider, as well as a caregiver, and whether and how members of their social networks supported (or rejected) their constructions (see Hochschild, 1989).

Role-using offers additional insight into the process of meaning construction, one that is particularly attentive to macro-level constraints and which is, therefore, consistent with stress researchers' traditional interests in inequality. Analyses of role-using would direct our attention to individuals' abilities to assert role-based identity claims in order to cope with potentially stressful circumstances. To continue our substantive example, we could analyze the ability of men and women in different structural locations to assert their identities as parents or workers in order to manage the stress of conflicting work-family roles. Consider, for instance, the contrast between welfare mothers' inabilities to collectively assert the priority of their roles as mothers over their roles as workers as compared to middle and upper-class women's abilities to collectively negotiate flexibility in work contracts to allow for maternal leave, flexible hours, and even stopped tenure clocks. In sum, identity claims are resources that individuals and collectives can invoke in their efforts to create a less stressful life, but their success is contingent on culturally and structurally-bound processes of negotiation. Analyses of these processes have the potential to reveal additional pathways through which macro-structures influence the stress process.

A Call to Action

Over the past fifty years, stress research has evolved from a model concerned with physiological processes of alarm, resistance, and exhaustion (Selye, 1956) into a model that can be applied to understanding the fabric of social life and the consequences of social inequalities for individual well-being (Pearlin, 1989). We have seen a shift from studies that equated stress with the experience of major life events (Holmes & Rahe, 1967) to studies that recognize the diversity of potentially stressful experiences through the life course and across life domains (see Wheaton,

1999 for a review). The stress process model has been applied to many different substantive topics, including the transition to adulthood (Gore & Aseltine, 2003), labor force conditions (Fenwick & Tausig, 1994), caregiving for persons with Alzheimer's disease and HIV (Aneshensel, Botticello, & Yamamoto-Mitani, 2004; Pearlin, Aneshensel, & LeBlanc, 1997), immigration (Mossakowski, 2003; Noh & Avison, 1996), and teen parenting (Turner, Sorenson, & Turner, 2000), among others, yielding insights into how people maintain equilibrium in the face of potentially disruptive life circumstances.

Given that progress, how do we justify a paradigmatic shift in stress research? Why should we broaden our image of the social in social stress? What is to be gained from redefining the stress process as meaning construction, from incorporating interactionist models of human action, and from giving serious attention to the social dimensions of self?

There are at least four reasons to consider alternative approaches to stress research. First, from a purely political perspective, sociological stress researchers' disinterest in the determinants of meaning cedes too much to the discipline of psychology by implying that the meanings of stressors are purely intrapsychic constructions. We contend, in contrast, that the meanings of stressors are inherently social and, therefore, amenable to sociological analysis. Research concerned with meaning construction has potential implications that go far beyond our understanding of the stress process to inform core social psychological theories pertaining to the construction of meaning, self as a motive, and power, control, and bargaining in interpersonal interactions.

Second, stress research cannot answer the questions it wants to answer without broadening the scope of its inquiries. As articulated in several recent publications (Aneshensel & Phelan, 1999; Pearlin, 1999), stress researchers are concerned with the consequences of social structures for mental health because those consequences illuminate the dysfunctions inherent in social systems. While one can question the utility of that goal (Schwartz, 2002), assuming that it is reasonable, we miss critical evidence for those dysfunctions if we focus exclusively on the beginning and endpoint of the process. Our common mediators and moderators—social support, coping, and intrapsychic resources—are proxies for much more complex social processes that beg attention as instantiations of the macro-micro nexus. In-depth analyses of these processes have the potential to reveal additional effects of structural conditions that are not evident in simple measures of stress exposures and responses.

Even our more pragmatic goals related to stress intervention cannot be achieved unless we acknowledge the socially constructed nature of stress. The weak observed associations between stressors and mental health have stimulated considerable research on the factors that distinguish those individuals who fare well in the face of stressful life experiences from those who do not, with attention given primarily to social support and coping. Yet, despite over "(t)wo decades of concentrated research," studies of coping and support "have yielded relatively little of either clinical or theoretical value (Somerfield & McCrae,

2000, p. 620)". A recent series of commentaries in the *American Psychologist* locates the problem in an overemphasis on between-person, cross-sectional designs to the neglect of within-person, process-oriented studies, in the failure to acknowledge unconscious processes in stress responses, and in our lack of attention to the needs and goals of individuals (Tennen, Affleck, Armeli, & Carney, 2000; Cramer, 2000; Coyne & Racioppo, 2000). Each of these critiques orients us towards a deeper analysis of the role of meaning in stress responses, a reorientation that is consistent with the documented successes of cognitively-based stress interventions (e.g., Wolchik et al., 2002, although see Coyne & Racioppo, 2000 for cautions). Sociologists' unique contribution to this endeavor is the recognition that meanings are social products rather than intrapsychic constructions. They cannot arise or be maintained without support from others.

Finally, the future of stress research within sociology depends on asserting its relevance to the questions that dominate current sociological and social psychological theory. These questions challenge the dominant model of stress by invoking a less deterministic image of social structure, by placing social interaction at the center of efforts to understand macro-structural effects, and by taking the self seriously. Whereas we could imagine other interpretations of these challenges, we focus here on their relevance as potential points of expansion for stress research, reaching out into new directions that elaborate the social underpinnings of the stress process. Stress research has contributed importantly to illustrating the dysfunctions inherent in social systems but its analyses are incomplete. Social systems shape not only who is exposed to stress and the resources to which they have access, but also whose situational definitions dominate, how stressors are perceived, and how those perceptions affect emotions. More generally, we cannot adequately describe the nature of our society, now and into the future, without attending to the nature and content of interpersonal interactions and their implications for individual psychological processes (Pescosolido & Rubin, 2000). By orienting itself to this more general disciplinary concern, stress research has the potential to become central, rather than peripheral, to our sociological mission.

Acknowledgments. An earlier version of this paper was presented at the 52nd annual meeting of the Society for the Study of Social Problems, August, 2002, Chicago, IL and, subsequently, at the University of Akron and at the seminar for the Indiana University Program in Identity, Self, Role, and Mental Health. Peggy Thoits' comments as SSSP discussant, and the comments of the Akron and Indiana participants strongly influenced the direction this paper took. Special thanks are due Sheldon Stryker for his thoughtful reading of the paper, and to Bernice Pescosolido and Bill Avison for their comments. Partial support for this work was provided by NIMH training grant T32 MH 14588 and NICHD grant R01 HD 050288 (McLeod, PI) and by the Norman Rockefeller Center for Public Policy at Dartmouth College (Lively).

References

Acock, A. C., & Hurlbert, J. S. (1993). Social networks, marital status, and well-being. *Social Networks, 15*, 309–334.

Alexander, J. C. (1982). *Theoretical logic in sociology: Positivism, presuppositions, and current controversies*. Berkeley: University of California Press.

Alexander, J. C. (1984). Social-structural analysis: Some notes on its history and prospects. *Sociological Quarterly, 25*, 5–26.

Aneshensel, C. S. (1992). Social stress: Theory and research. *Annual Review of Sociology, 18*, 15–38.

Aneshensel, C. S. (1993). Stress, role captivity, and the cessation of caregiving. *Journal of Health and Social Behavior, 34*, 54–70.

Aneshensel, C. S., Botticelli, A. L., & Yamamoto-Mitani, N. (2004). When caregiving ends: The course of depressive symptoms after bereavement. *Journal of Health and Social Behavior, 45*, 422–440.

Aneshensel, C. S., & Phelan, J. C. (1999). *Handbook of the sociology of mental health*. New York: Kluwer Academic/Plenum Press.

Aneshensel, C. S., Rutter, C. M., & Lachenbruch, P. A. (1991). Competing conceptual and analytic models: Social structure, stress, and mental health. *American Sociological Review, 56*, 166–178.

Aneshensel, C. S., & Sucoff, C. A. (1996). The neighborhood context of adolescent mental health. *Journal of Health and Social Behavior, 37*, 293–311.

Blumer, H. (1969). *Symbolic interactionism: Perspective and method*. Englewood Cliffs, NJ: Prentice-Hall.

Bourdieu, P. (1977). *Outline of a theory of practice*. Cambridge, UK: Cambridge University Press.

Brown, G. W., & Harris, T. O. (1978). *Social origins of depression: A study of psychaigtric disorder in women*. New York: Free Press.

Brown, T. N. (2003). Critical race theory speaks to the sociology of mental health: Mental health problems produced by racial stratification. *Journal of Health and Social Behavior, 44*, 292–301.

Brown, T. N., Sellers, S. L., & Gomez, J. P. (2002). The relationship between internalization and self-esteem among black adults. *Sociological Focus, 35*, 55–71.

Burke P. J. (1991). Identity processes and social stress. *American Sociological Review, 56*, 836–49.

Bylsma, W. H., & Major, B. (1994). Social comparisons and contentment: Exploring the psychological costs of the gender wage gap. *Psychology of Women Quarterly, 18*, 241–249.

Callero, P. L. (1994). From role-playing to role-using: Understanding role as resource. *Social Psychology Quarterly, 5*, 228–243.

Cannon, W. B. (1929). *Bodily changes in pain, hunger, fear, and rage*. New York: Appleton.

Charmaz, K. (1980). The social construction of self-pity in the chronically ill. In N. K. Denzin (Ed.) *Studies of symbolic interaction* (Vol. 3, pp. 123–146). Greenwich, CT: JAI Press.

Charmaz, K. (1991). *Good days, bad days: The self in chronic illness and time*. New Brunswick, NJ: Rutgers University Press.

Cohen, S., Kamarck, T., & Mermelstein, R. (1983). A global measure of perceived stress. *Journal of Health and Social Behavior, 24*, 385–396.

Conger, R. D., Conger, K. J., Elder, G. H., Jr., Lorenz, F. O., Simons, R. L., & Whitbeck, L. B. (1992). A family process model of economic hardship and adjustment of early adolescent boys. *Child Development, 63*, 526–541.

Cooley, C. H. (1902). *Human nature and the social order*. New York: Scribner's Sons.

Coyne, J. C., & Racioppo, M. W. (2000). Never the twain shall meet?: Closing the gap between coping research and clinical intervention research. *American Psychologist, 55*, 655–664.

Cramer, P. (2000). Defense mechanisms in psychology today: Further processes for adaptation. *American Psychologist, 55*, 637–645.

Dohrenwend, B. P. Raphael, K. G., Schwartz, S., Stueve, A., & Skodol, A. (1993). The structured event probe and narrative rating method for measuring stressful life events. In L. Goldberger & S. Breznotz (Eds.) *Handbook of stress* (pp. 174–199). New York: Free Press.

Emirbayer, M., & Mische, A. (1998). What is agency? *American Journal of Sociology, 103*, 962–1023.

Fenwick, R., & Tausig, M. (1994). The macroeconomic context of job stress. *Journal of Health and Social Behavior, 35*, 266–282.

Fine, G. A. (1991). On the macrofoundations of microsociology: Constraint and the exterior reality of structure. *The Sociology Quarterly, 32*, 161–177.

Francis, L (1997). Ideology and interpersonal emotion management: Redefining identity in two support groups. *Social Psychology Quarterly, 60*, 153–171.

George, L. (1993). Sociological perspectives on life transitions. *Annual Review of Sociology, 19*, 353–373.

Giddens, A. (1976). *The new rules of sociological method*. New York: Basic Books.

Giddens, A. (1984). *The constitution of society: Outline of the theory of structuration*. Berkeley, CA: University of California Press.

Glass, J. &, Fujimoto, T. (1994). Housework, paid work, and depression among husbands and wives. *Journal of Health and Social Behavior, 3*, 179–91.

Gore, S., & Aseltine, R. H., Jr. (2003). Race and ethnic differences in depressed mood following the transition from high school. *Journal of Health and Social Behavior, 44*, 370–389.

Hammen, C., & Goodman-Brown, T. (1990). Self-schemas and vulnerability to specific life stress in children at risk for depression. *Cognitive Research and Therapy, 14*, 215–227.

Hammen, C., Marks, T., Mayol, A., & deMayo, R. (1985). Depressive self-schemas, life stress, and vulnerability to depression. *Journal of Abnormal Psychology, 94*, 308–319.

Harvey, J. H., Orbuch, T. L., Chwalisz, K. D., & Garwood, G. (1991). Coping with sexual assault: The roles of account-making and confiding. *Journal of Traumatic Stress, 4*, 515–531.

Harvey, J. H., Orbuch, T. L., & Weber, A. L. (1990). A social psychological model of account-making in response to severe stress. *Journal of Language and Social Psychology, 9*, 191–207.

Heine, S. J., Lehman, D. R., Peng, K., & Greenholtz, J. (2002). What's wrong with cross-cultural comparisons of subjective Likert scales?: The reference-group effect. *Journal of Personality and Social Psychology, 82*, 903–918.

Heise, D. R. (1977). Social action as the control of affect. *Behavioral Sciences, 22*, 163–177.

Heise, D. R. (2002). Understanding social interaction with affect control theory. In J. Berger and M. Zelditch (Eds.), *New directions in contemporary sociological theory* (pp. 17–40). Boulder CO: Rowman and Littlefield.

Hewitt, J. P. (1991). *Self and society* (5th ed). Boston: Allyn and Bacon.

Hill, T. D., Ross, C. E., & Angel, R. J. (2005). Neighborhood disorder, psychophysiological distress, and health. *Journal of Health and Social Behavior*, *46*, 170–186.

Hochschild, A. R. (1983). *The managed heart: The commercialization of feeling*. Berkeley: University of California Press.

Hochschild, A. R. (with A. Manchung). (1989). *The second shift: Working parents and the revolution at home*. New York: Avon Books.

Holmes, T. H., & Rahe, R. H. (1967). The social readjustment rating scale. *Journal of Psychosomatic Research*, *11*, 213–218.

Horwitz, A. V. (2002). Outcomes in the sociology of mental health and illness: Where have we been and where are we going? *Journal of Health and Social Behavior*, *43*, 143–151.

House, J. S. (1977). The three faces of social psychology. *Sociometry, 40*, 161–177.

House J. S. (1981). Social structure and personality. In M. Rosenberg & R. H. Turner (Eds.) *Social psychology: Sociological perspectives* (pp. 525–61). New York: Basic Books.

House, J. S., Umberson, D., & Landis, K. (1988). Structures and processes of social support. *Annual Review of Sociology*, *14*, 293–318.

Jackson, P. B., & Finney, M. (2002). Negative life events and psychological distress among young adults. *Social Psychology Quarterly*, *65*, 186–201.

Kessler, R. C., & McLeod, J. D. (1985). Social support and mental health in community samples. In S. Cohen & S. L. Syme (Eds.), *Social support and health* (pp. 219–240). New York: Academic.

Kessler, R. C., & Neighbors, H. W. (1986). A new perspective on the relationships among race, social class, and psychological distress. *Journal of Health and Social Behavior*, *27*, 107–115.

Keyes, C. L. M. (2002). The mental health continuum: From languishing to flourishing in life. *Journal of Health and Social Behavior*, *43*, 207–222.

Kitayama, S., Markus, H. R., Matsumoto, H., & Norasakkunkit, V. (1997). Individual and collective processes in the construction of the self: Self-enhancement in the United States and self-criticism in Japan. *Journal of Personality and Social Psychology*, *72*, 1245–1267.

Kohn, M. L., & Schooler, C. (1983). *Work and Personality: An inquiry into the impact of social stratification*. Norwood, NJ: Ablex Publishing Corporation.

Krause, N. (1991). Financial strain and psychological well-being among the American and Japanese elderly. *Psychology and Aging, 6*, 170–181.

Large, M. D., & Marcussen, K. (2000). Extending identity theory to predict differential forms and degrees of psychological distress. *Social Psychology Quarterly*, *63*, 49–59.

Lazarus, R. S. and S. Folkman. (1984). *Stress appraisals and coping*. New York: Springer.

Lennon, M. C., & Rosenfield, S. (1994). Relative fairness and division of housework: The importance of options. *American Journal of Sociology, 100*, 506–31.

Lin, N. (1982). Social resources and instrumental action. In P. W. Marsden & N. Lin (Eds.) *Social structure and network analysis* (pp. 131–145). Beverly Hills, CA: Sage.

Lin, N., & Peek, M. K. (1999). Social networks and mental health. In A. V. Horwitz & T. L. Scheid (Eds.) *A handbook for the study of mental health* (pp. 241–258). New York: Cambridge University Press.

Linville, P. W. (1987). Self-complexity as a cognitive buffer against stress-related illness and depression. *Journal of Personality and Social Psychology*, *58*, 1040–1047.

Lively, K. J. (2000). Reciprocal emotion management. *Work and Occupations, 27*, 32–63.

Lively, K. J., & Heise, D. R. (2004). Sociological realms of emotional experience. *American Journal of Sociology, 109*, 1109–36.

MacKinnon, N. J. (1994). *Symbolic interactionism as affect control*. Albany: State University of New York Press.

Major, B., Testa. M., & Bylsma, W. H. (1991). Responses to upward and downward social comparison: The impact of esteem-relevance and perceived control. In J. Suls & T. A. Wills (Eds.) *Social comparison: Contemporary theory and research* (pp. 237–60). Hillsdale, NJ: Lawrence Erlbaum Associates.

McLeod J. D., & Kessler R. C. (1990). Socioeconomic status differences in vulnerability to undesirable life events. *Journal of Health and Social Behavior, 31*, 162–72.

McLeod J. D., & Lively, K. J. (2003). Social structure and personality. In J. D. Delamater (Ed.) *Handbook of social psychology* (pp. 77–102). New York: Kluwer/Plenum.

Mead, G. H. (1934). *Mind, self, and society*. Chicago: University of Chicago Press.

Menaghan, E. G. (1989). Role changes and psychological well-being: Variations in effects by gender and role repertoire. *Social Forces, 67*, 693–714.

Merton, R. K. (1957). The role-set: Problems in sociological theory. *British Journal of Sociology, 8*, 106–120.

Mirowsky, J., Ross, C. E., & Reynolds, J. (2000). Links between social status and health status. In C. E. Bird, P. Conrad, & A. M. Fremont (Eds.) *Handbook of medical sociology* (Fifth edition; pp. 47–67). Upper Saddle River, NJ: Prentice-Hall.

Monroe, S. M., & Kellery, J. M. (1995). Measurement of stress appraisal. In S. Cohen, R. C. Kessler, & L. U. Gordon (Eds.) *Measuring stress: A guide for health and social scientists* (pp. 122–147). New York: Oxford University Press.

Mossakowski, K. N. (2003). Coping with perceived discrimination: Does ethnic identity protect mental health? *Journal of Health and Social Behavior, 44*, 318–31.

Noh, S., & Avison, W. R. (1996). Asian immigrants and the stress process: A study of Koreans in Canada. *Journal of Health and Social Behavior, 37*, 192–206.

Orbuch, T. L. (1997). People's accounts count: The sociology of accounts. *Annual Review of Sociology, 23*, 455–478.

Orbuch, T. L., Harvey, J., David, S., & Merbach, N. (1994). Account-making and confiding as acts of meaning in response to sexual assault. *Journal of Family Violence, 9*, 249–264.

Orbuch, T. L., Veroff, J., & Holmberg, D. (1993). Becoming a married couple: The emergence of meaning in the first years of marriage. *Journal of Marriage and the Family, 55*, 815–26.

Peacock, E. J., & Wong. P. T. P. (1990). The Stress Appraisal Measure (SAM): A multidimensional approach to cognitive appraisal. *Stress Medicine, 6*, 227–236.

Pearlin, L. I. (1983). Role strains and personal stress. In H. B. Kaplan (Ed.) *Psychosocial stress: Trends in theory and research* (pp. 3–32). New York: Academic Press.

Pearlin, L. I. (1989). The sociological study of stress. *Journal of Health and Social Behavior, 30*, 241–256.

Pearlin, L. I. (1999). The stress concept revisited. In C. A. Aneshensel and J. C. Phelan (Eds.) *Handbook of the sociology of mental health* (pp. 395–415). New York: Kluwer Academic/ Plenum.

Pearlin, L. I., Aneshensel, C. A., & LeBlanc, A. J. (1997). The forms and mechanisms of stress proliferation: The case of AIDS caregivers. *Journal of Health and Social Behavior, 38*, 223–236.

Pearlin, L. I., Lieberman, M. A., Menaghan, E. G., & Mullan, J. T. (1981). The stress process. *Journal of Health and Social Behavior, 22*, 337–356.

Pearlin, L. I., & Schooler, C. (1978). The structure of coping. *Journal of Health and Social Behavior, 19*, 2–21.

Pearlin, L. I., & Skaff, M. M. (1996). Stress and the life course: A paradigmatic alliance. *The Gerontologist, 36*, 239–247.

Pescosolido, B. A. (1992). Beyond rational choice: The social dynamics of how people seek help. *American Journal of Sociology, 97*, 1096–1138.

Pescosolido, B. A., & Rubin. B. A. (2000). The web of group affiliations revisited: Social life, postmodernism, and sociology. *American Sociological Review, 65*, 52–76.

Rosenberg, M. (1979). *Conceiving the self.* New York: Basic Books.

Schutz, A. (1970). *On phenomenology and social relations.* Chicago: University of Chicago Press.

Schwartz, S. (2002). Outcomes for the sociology of mental health: Are we meeting our goals? *Journal of Health and Social Behavior, 43*, 223–235.

Selye, H. (1956.) *The stress of life.* New York: McGraw-Hill.

Sewell, W. H., Jr. (1992). A theory of structure: Duality, agency, and transformation. *American Journal of Sociology, 98*, 1–29.

Silver, R. L., Boon, C., & Stones, M. H. (1983). Searching for meaning in misfortune: Making sense of incest. *Journal of Social Issues, 39*, 81–101.

Simon, R. W. (1992). Parental role strains, salience of parental identity and gender differences in psychological distress. *Journal of Health and Social Behavior, 33*, 25–35.

Simon, R. W. (1995). Gender, multiple roles, role meaning, and mental health. *Journal of Health and Social Behavior, 36*, 182–194.

Simon, R. W. (1997). The meanings individuals attach to role-identities and their implications for mental health. *Journal of Health and Social Behavior, 38*, 256–274.

Simon, R. W. (2000). The importance of culture in sociological theory and research on stress and mental health: A missing link? In C. E. Bird, P. Conrad, & A. M. Fremont (Eds.) *Handbook of medical sociology* (Fifth edition; pp. 68–78). Upper Saddle River, NJ: Prentice-Hall.

Smith-Lovin, L., Douglass, W. (1992). An affect control analysis of two religious subcultures. In V. Gecas & D. Franks (Eds.), *Social Perspectives on Emotion, 1*, (pp. 217–48). Greenwich, CT: JAI Press.

Smith-Lovin, L., & Heise, D. R. (1988). *Analyzing social interaction: Advances in affect control theory.* New York: Gordon and Breach Science Publishers. (Reprint of a special issue of the *Journal of Mathematical Sociology*, Vol. 13.).

Somerfield, M. R., & McCrae, R. R. (2000). Stress and coping research: Methodological challenges, theoretical advances, and clinical applications. *American Psychologist, 55*, 620–625.

Stryker, S. (1977). Developments in "two social psychologies": Toward an appreciation of mutual relevance. *Sociometry, 40*, 145–160.

Stryker, S. (1980). *Symbolic interactionism: A social structural version.* Menlo Park, CA: Benjamin/Cummings.

Stryker, S. (1994). Freedom and constraint in social and personal life: Toward resolving the paradox of self. In G. M. Platt & C. Gordon (Eds.) *Self, collective behavior and society: Essays honoring the contributions of Ralph H. Turner* (pp. 119–138). Greenwich, CT: JAI Press.

Stryker, S., & Burke, P.J. (2000). The past, present, and future of an identity theory. *Social Psychology Quarterly, 63*, 284–297.

Stryker, S., & Statham A. (1985). Symbolic interaction and role theory. In G. Lindzey & E. Aronson (Eds.) *Handbook of social psychology, 1*, (pp. 311–78). New York: Random House.

Swann, W. B., Jr. (1983). Self-verification: Bringing social reality into harmony with the self. In J. M. Suls & A. G. Greenwald (Eds.) *Social psychological perspectives on the self* (Vol. 2) (pp. 33–66). Hillsdale, NJ: Lawrence Erlbaum.

Tennen, H., Affleck, G., Armeli, S., & Carney, M. A. (2000). A daily process approach to coping: Linking theory, research, and practice. *American Psychologist, 55*, 626–636.

Tesser, A. (1986). Some effects of self-evaluation maintenance on cognition and action. In R. M. Sorrentino & E. T. Higgins (Eds.) *Handbook of motivation and cognition: Foundations of social behavior* (pp. 435–464). New York: Guilford Press.

Thoits, P. A. (1985). Self-labeling processes in mental illness: The role of emotional deviance. *American Journal of Sociology, 91*, 221–249.

Thoits, P. A. (1986). Multiple identities: Examining gender and marital status differences in distress. *American Sociological Review, 51*, 259–272.

Thoits, P. A. (1991). On merging identity theory and stress research. *Social Psychology Quarterly, 54*, 101–112.

Thoits, P. A. (1992). Identity structures and psychological well-being: Gender and marital status comparisons. *Social Psychology Quarterly, 55*, 236–256.

Thoits, P. A. (1994). Stressors and problem-solving: The individual as psychological activist. *Journal of Health and Social Behavior, 35*, 143–159.

Thoits, P. A. (1995a). Identity-relevant events and psychological symptoms: A cautionary tale. *Journal of Health and Social Behavior, 36*, 72–82.

Thoits, P.A. (1995b). Stress, coping, and social support processes: Where are we? What next? *Journal of Health and Social Behavior, Special Issue*, 53–79.

Thoits, P. A. (2005). Personal agency in the stress process. Leonard I. Pearlin Award for Distinguished Contributions to the Sociological Study of Mental Health address, Annual Meeting of the American Sociological Association, August, 2005.

Thomassen, L. (2002). An alcoholic is good and sober: sentiment change in AA. *Deviant Behavior: An Interdisciplinary Journal, 23*, 177–200.

Treas, J., & Widmer, E. D. Married women's employment over the life course: Attitudes in cross-national perspective. *Social Forces, 78*, 1409–1436.

Turner, R. H. (1962). Role-taking, role standpoint, and reference group behavior. In A.M. Rose (Ed.), *Human behavior and social processes* (pp. 20–40). Boston: Houghton Mifflin.

Turner, R. H. (1978). Role and the person. *American Journal of Sociology, 84*, 1–23.

Turner, R. J., & Avison, W. R. (2003). Status variations in stress exposure: Implications for the interpretation of research on race, socioeconomic status, and gender. *Journal of Health and Social Behavior, 44*, 488–505.

Turner, R. J., Sorenson, A. J., & Turner, J. B. (2000). Social contingencies in mental health: A seven-year follow-up study of teenage mothers. *Journal of Marriage and the Family, 62*, 777–791.

Turner, R. J., & Turner, J. B. (1999). Social integration and support. In C. S. Aneshensei & J. C. Phelan (Eds.) *Handbook of the sociology of mental health* (pp. 301–320). New York: Kluwer/Plenum.

Turner, R. J., Wheaton, B., & Lloyd, D. (1995). The epidemiology of social stress. *American Sociological Review, 60*, 104–125.

Umberson, D., Wortman, C. B., & Kessler, R. C. (1992). Widowhood and depression: Explaining long-term gender differences in vulnerability. *Journal of Health and Social Behavior, 33*, 10–24.

Weiss, R. S. (1975). *Marital separation.* New York: Basic Books.

Wellman, B., & Wortley, S. (1989). Brother's keepers: Situating kin relations in broader networks of social support. *Sociological Perspectives, 32*, 273–306.

Wheaton, B. (1990). Life transitions, role histories, and mental health. *American Sociological Review, 55*, 209–223.

Wheaton, B. (1999). The nature of stressors. In A. V. Horwitz & T. L. Scheid (Eds.) *A handbook for the study of mental health: Social contexts, theories, and systems* (pp. 176–197). New York: Cambridge University Press.

Williams D. R., & Williams-Morris, R. (2000). Racism and mental health: the African American experience. *Ethnicity and, Health, 5*, 243–68.

Wills, T. A. (1991). Similarity and comparison. In J. Suls and T, A. Wills (Eds.) *Social comparison: Contemporary theory and research* (pp. 51–78). Hillsdale, NJ: Lawrence Erlbaum Associates.

Wolchik, S. A., Sandler, I. N., Milsap, R. E., Plummer, B. A., Greene, S. M., Anderson, E. R., Dawson-McClure, S. R., Hipke, K., & Haine, R. A. (2002). Six year follow-up of preventive interventions for children of divorce: A randomized controlled trial. *Journal of the American Medical Association, 288,* 1874–1881.

Wood, J. V., & Taylor, K. L. (1991). Serving goals through social comparison. In J. Suls and T, A. Wills (Eds.) *Social comparison: Contemporary theory and research* (pp. 24–50). Hillsdale, NJ: Lawrence Erlbaum Associates.

Wortman, C. B., Silver, R. C., & Kessler, R. C. (1993). The meaning of loss and adjustment to bereavement. In M. S. Stroebe & R. O. Hansson (Eds.) *Handbook of bereavement: Theory and research intervention* (pp. 349–366). New York: Cambridge University Press.

Part IV
Social Responses to Mental Illness

13
Stigma and the Sociological Enterprise

Bernice A. Pescosolido and Jack K. Martin

Introduction

Stigma is an attribute that, according to prevailing social norms, is deeply discrediting, marks a person as tainted and allows the target to be denigrated (Goffman, 1963). The targeted person, whose identity and belonging are called into question, is devalued, compromised, and considered less than fully human (Crandall, 2000; Crocker, Major, & Steele, 1998). As a result, stigma deprives the target of his or her dignity, limits opportunities, challenges humanity, and interferes with full participation in society (Dovidio, Major, & Crocker, 2000). Even those associated with stigmatized persons are often affected, experiencing a "courtesy" stigma.

Not surprisingly, the concept of stigma occupies a central place in the sociology of mental health, focusing on the impact of mental illness on individuals, families, treatment systems and societies. The stigma of mental illness has been blamed for low service utilization, poor individual medical and social outcomes surrounding mental illness, inadequate funding of research and treatment infrastructures, and hindered policy attention (Estroff, 1981; Markowitz, 2001; Okazaki, 2000; Wahl, 1999). Despite perceptions among some providers and researchers in the medical arena that the stigma associated with mental illness has dissipated in the face of deinstitutionalization, prejudice and discrimination toward persons with mental health problems persist (Baxter, 1994; Dain, 1994; Hyman, 2000; Pang, 1985; Rose, 1988; Swan, 1999). Indeed, sociological research continues to demonstrate that high levels of prejudice and discrimination are common (e.g., Link, Phelan, Bresnahan, Stueve, & Pescosolido, 1999; Martin, Pescosolido, & Tuch, 2000; Pescosolido, Monahan, Link, Stueve, & Kikuzawa, 1999; Phelan, Link, Stueve, & Pescosolido, 2000; see also Keusch, Wilentz, & Kleinman, 2006).

There would appear to be no question about the continued importance of stigma in the sociology of mental health. The question we ask here directly addresses the charge of reflection, rather than relevance. In particular, we are concerned with the interplay between general sociological theory and relevant concepts which surround the social consequences of mental illness. This task does not simply telescope backward to past contributions and building blocks, but, more importantly, trains the analytical lens forward to consider the future interplay between the sociology of mental health and the discipline of sociology.

To this end, we trace the various theoretical traditions that have either addressed or contributed to the sociological perspective on the stigma of mental illness. We first lay out the contemporary state of affairs, focusing on both the reliance on general sociological theory and on arguments over time that produced the current state of theoretical and empirical research. We end with a reconsideration of the untapped potential in original formulations and recent developments, examining how new directions can enhance contributions to the current resurgence in stigma research and the general stock of sociological knowledge.

Sociological Traditions and the Development of the Sociology of Stigma

Goffman's (1963) *Stigma: Notes on the Management of Spoiled Identity* is often held up as the beginning of serious sociological attention to stigma. In fact, the study of the stigma attached to mental illness drew its foundational inspirations from at least two additional lines of basic research—the societal reaction perspective to deviance and the study of racial prejudice and discrimination. We briefly describe the three traditions below.

The Continuing Prominence of Goffman

While a classic statement that highlighted a key moment in the sociology of mental health, the scope of Goffman's book was broad, covering a range of substantive areas that produced a general perspective on the social conse-quences of difference. He considered the situation of being an orphan, facing hearing impairment or a wide spectrum of disabilities, engaging in criminal behavior, and holding identities from prostitute to revolutionary, in addition to having a mental illness.

Basic to the insights in *Stigma* are the four key ingredients relative to the social consequences of devalued attributes. First, individuals who face stigma are disqualified from full social citizenship. Stigma is a mark that separates and isolates. Second, while stigma can be seen as an attribute that is somehow known to others, its effects materialize only in and through social interaction. Social relationships, rather than attributes, are central to the conceptualization and language of stigma. Third, Goffman distinguished different types of stigma: abominations of the body (e.g., physical deformities), blemishes of individual character (e.g., mental illness), and tribal stigma (e.g., race, religion, national identities). Fourth, Goffman suggests that stigma is not static over the moral career. Individuals may go from a stigmatized identity to a "normal" one, as in the case of orphans who grow up. Others may start out within range of societal norms for acceptance and move to a stigmatized iden-tity through illness or behavioral transgressions. While the fundamental base and continued reference point for stigma (Keusch et al., 2006), Goffman's contributions have been complemented by other lines of research, most prominently, labeling theory, and sociological research into the bases of racial prejudice and discrimination.

The Social Construction of Deviance: Labeling Theory and Stigma

As Link and Phelan (1999, p. 482) point out, theory and research on stigma has been closely intertwined with the debates over the labeling perspective in sociology. This realization is perhaps best detailed in *Being Mentally Ill: A Sociological Theory* (Scheff, 1966). In this work, Scheff begins by mapping the lines of agreement and disagreement with other theoretical models (e.g., psychoanalytic, medical, Marxist, biocultural, psychological) of mental illness. Unlike Goffman, however, who ultimately rejects much of the sociological use of the term "deviance" (1963, Chapter 5), Scheff finds a critical start there, particularly as articulated in the work of Howard Becker (1963) and Edward Lemert (1951; 2000). Deviance, from the standpoint of this alternate perspective, is less usefully seen as an inherent quality or characteristic of any act. Rather, deviance lies in people's reaction to any act or behavior. Thus, Scheff takes as central the distinction between rule-breaking and deviance; that is, the difference between violations of social norms and the subset that becomes officially labeled as norm violations.

Basic to Scheff's labeling theory of mental illness is a solid description of the underlying social process that leads to chronic mental illness, combined with a detailed accounting of the contingencies that shape societal reactions. As depicted in Figure 13.1, the process begins with norm violations or "offensive acts" in the context of a particular social setting. Many norm violation acts have readily available categories into which they may be classified; for example, crime, perversion, or bad manners. The potential for being labeled with a mental illness comes when behavior or appearance does not fit existing categories, becoming "residual rule breaking" or "residual deviance."

Here Scheff outlines three basic propositions: rule-breaking is 1) diverse in origin – psychological conditions, defiance or resistance, and biological changes, for example; 2) very prevalent compared to treated rates of mental illness; and 3) most often unnoticed, rationalized away, or denied. Further, whether or not the residual rule-breaking is noticed depends on a complex interplay of contingencies that shape the reaction of others to individual behavior. The severity, visibility and frequency of the rule-breaking all push toward a more severe reaction, as do the existence of cultural biases and stereotypes that predispose a judgment of mental illness (e.g., the depressed housewife). However, rule-breakers who have social power are likely to be protected from negative responses by taking an alternative role or label for behavior (e.g., the eccentric millionaire). Finally, the social distance between the rule-breaker and those observing the behavior matter: When the target person occupies the lower

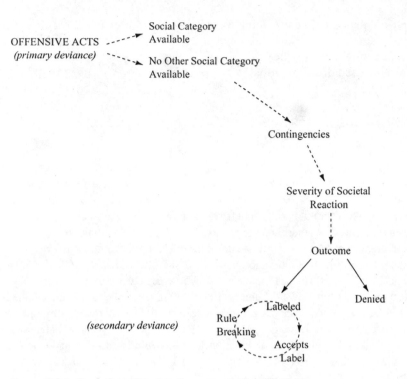

FIGURE 13.1. Depiction of the labeling process (Scheff, 1966).

social status and is observed in transgressions by those with greater social power, the probability of a negative societal reaction is increased. In the end, the constellation of contingencies surrounding a behavior or appearance results in a societal reaction.

Much residual rule-breaking is ignored at this point, having only transitory import. However, if the outcome of the interactional process is a severe societal reaction, then the individual is labeled "mentally ill" and enters into a positive feedback loop. That is, because culture holds images in language and media of what "appropriate" behaviors are for persons with mental illness, the labeled individuals begin to act in conformity with that label, engaging in more residual rule-breaking (secondary deviance), solidifying the societal reaction and the "just" application of the label. Since labels define for others and for the targeted individuals what persons with mental illness are "like," labels become potent influences. Stigma is one price to be paid for mental illness.

Not surprisingly, the reaction to labeling theory was anything but quiet. In fact, as discussed in the "Introduction" to this volume, much of the attention in the main-stream sociological journals that addressed the sociology of mental health revolved around the debates about the power of labels. Prominent among those who opposed the idea that mental illness and the subsequent reaction are socially constructed was Walter Gove. In a series of articles, Gove and his associates argued that the societal reaction perspective is largely a theoretical exercise accompanied by very little empirical data. Further, Gove found that existing empirical data that could address the power of labeling theory also called the perspective into question. He contended that individuals who are hospitalized, indeed, have a "serious disturbance." In addition, the idea that a label sets in motion a self-fulfilling prophecy that shapes future behavior or an individual's fate, he argued, was at best over-blown (Gove, 1970). In fact, Gove and Tudor (1973) concluded that their data show that when biases suggested in labeling theory are taken into account (e.g., greater likelihood of women to offer socially desirable responses), the difference in rates of mental illness between men and women actually increase (see also Gove & Howell, 1974). In support, Dunham (1971) argued that labeling theorists "turned their backs on two centuries of clinical data collected by psychiatrists" (1971, p. 313) and failed to understand "the consequences of hospitalization, especially in the new climate of hospital treatment for mental illness" (1971, p. 313). Thus, opponents of labeling theory rejected what they considered to be an extreme social constructivist view, even as they disagreed about the effects of the aftermath of hospitalization on individuals' futures.

This critique was also contested. A number of individuals saw Gove as misinterpreting their research (Mechanic, 1971) or misunderstanding the theory itself (Scheff, 1974). As Link and Phelan (1999) point out, stigma was a central point of disagreement in these debates. Those opposing labeling theory argued that stigma was "relatively inconsequential" (1999, p. 483), while others continued to find negative attitudinal responses to mental illness and effects on unemployment. In the end, Link and his colleagues (1989) offered modified labeling theory (MLT) that argued that while labeling does not always produce an acceptance of the diagnosis and automaton-like behavior in line with cultural stereotypes, it certainly has important consequences, including stigma (see also Pescosolido, McLeod, & Alegria, 2000, pp. 418–420). According to MLT, cultural stereotypes of mental illness create powerful expectations of devaluation and discrimination in people with mental illness, and these expectations have important consequences for self-esteem, treatment seeking, and social functioning. Studies of consumer populations continue to show that while treatment may have positive effects on individuals' quality of life, stigma continues to produce adverse effects (Link, Struening, Rahav, Phelan, & Nuttbrick, 1997; Rosenfield, 1997).

The labeling tradition continues to shape how sociologists see the effects of mental illness, though its influence on research has focused almost entirely away from its role in shaping diagnosis. As a useful perspective on stigma, labeling theory suggests that devaluation of individuals is fundamentally attached to the acquisition of a diagnosis, even if the presence of "strange" behaviors plays a clear role in conferring and disclosing the "mark" (Martin et al., 2000). The attitudes and behavior of others towards the stigmatized person comprise the prejudice and discrimination that persons with mental illness face. However, the impetus for understanding the role of cultural climate has always had a tie to the study of public attitudes, most notably, sociological attention to race and race relations.

Theories of Prejudice and Discrimination

The prominence of theories of prejudice and discrimination in the development of the sociological enterprise is well-established. Indeed, perhaps the most enduring focus in the study of Americans' attitudes can be found in national surveys of attitudes dealing with issues of racial/ethnic prejudice and preferences for social distance from devalued racial/ethnic groups (Bobo, Kluegel, & Smith, 1997). While the extent to which inquiry into the roots and prevalence of stigmatizing attitudes toward mental illness has been influenced by the race literature is not certain, what is clear is that these parallel lines of inquiry have emphasized two common substantive themes and have embraced a common methodological approach. These are: 1) the role of interpersonal contact, 2) the role of causal attributions, and 3) the reliance on nationally representative survey data to estimate the levels and correlates of intolerance.

The Role of Interpersonal Contact

Early on, social science theories focused on the "binding power of common experiences" (Calavita & Serron, 1992, p. 766). Particularly in the area of race relations, social psychologists (Allport, 1954) and sociologists (Williams, 1947) focused on interpersonal interaction as key to reducing discrimination and prejudice. Indeed, as Biernat and Dovidio (2000, p. 110) point out, intergroup contact has long been psychology and sociology's prescription for changing attitudes and stereotypes. Indeed, in early studies in workplaces, neighborhoods, and schools, there was wide support for the notion that increasing interaction between those "marked" and "unmarked" increased sentiments of "liking" (Caplow, 1964; Homans, 1951).

Several studies have demonstrated that interpersonal contact lessens negative racial attitudes (Desforges, Lord, Ramsey, Mason, VanLeeuwen, West, & Lepper, 1991; Ellison & Powers, 1994; Jackman & Crane, 1986; Jones, Farina, Hastorf, Markus, Miller, & Scott, 1984; Sigelman & Welch, 1993). These findings are also reflected in a number of studies of contact with persons with mental health problems. For example, individuals who have experiences with persons with mental health problems have been found to have fewer negative reactions, display fewer discriminatory behaviors, and endorse more tolerant attitudes (Adams & Partee, 1998; Jones et al., 1984; Penn, Guynan, Daily, Spaulding, & Sullivan, 1994). In fact, much of the recent effort to reduce the stigma attached to mental illness has taken these findings as the starting point for new policies and programs (Corrigan, 2000).

The Role of Causal Attributions

The inquiry into the roots and consequences of both racial prejudice and mental illness stigma also came to emphasize the potentially liberalizing impact of the endorsement of extra-individual causal attributions on levels of prejudice and stigma. As Phelan (2005, p. 308) points out, the beliefs that individuals hold about causes of stigmatized behaviors presumed to be attributable to flaws of individual character as with mental illness, and by extension, about the bases of racial inferiority and disadvantage will impact affect, expectations, and behavioral responses to the stigmatized behavior or group.

Attention to the role of causal attributions in the race relations literature can be traced back to the 1970s and 1980's when sociologists of race searched for models that might explain the persistent decline (since the 1940s and 1950s) in Americans' expressions of what has been termed traditional or 'Jim Crow' racism. While explanations for this trend vary widely, according to some, the decline of a traditional, biologically-based racist ideology was partially the result of the adoption of a structural stratification ideology, particularly among younger and better-educated whites. This ideology holds that disadvantage among blacks is at least partly the result of environmental factors that limit achievement opportunities (i.e., discriminatory practices in employment and education), not in innate and/or biological causes (Hughes & Tuch, 2000; Tuch & Hughes, 1996). Simply stated, the acceptance of socioeconomic attributions, as indexed by the endorsement of the notion of social responsibility for black disadvantage, has been found to be an important correlate of the *rejection* of traditional racial stereotypes (Bobo et al., 1997; Martin & Tuch, 1997).

Sociological inquiry into the role of causal attributions relative to the stigmatization of mental health problems has, for the most part, followed a parallel line of reasoning. Based largely on the literature on the 'medicalization' of deviance (see, for example, Conrad, 2000; Conrad & Schneider, 1992), and the efforts of advocacy groups (e.g., the National Alliance for the Mentally Ill), sociological studies of the stigma of mental illness and stigmatization processes have also focused on cognitions relative to individual versus social structural and/or medical-genetic causes of mental health problems. There is, however, a notable divergence between these parallel lines of inquiry. Specifically, much like the race literature, research into the role of attributions for the causes of mental illness has found that contemporary Americans are much less likely to endorse individual-level attributions for mental health problems (i.e., bad or weak individual character), and are significantly more likely to endorse medical, genetic, or structural (i.e., stress) causes (Martin et al., 2000; Martin, Pescosolido, Olafsdottir, & McLeod, 2007; Pescosolido, Martin, Link, Kikuzawa, Burgos, & Swindle, 2000; Phelan & Link, 2002). Unlike patterns evidenced in the race literature, however, the endorsement of these extra-individual attributions for mental illness have not *consistently* been found to reduce levels of prejudicial attitudes (i.e., perceptions of dangerousness) or the willingness to discriminate against persons with mental health problems (i.e., social distance preferences, Martin et al., 2007; Phelan, 2005). Forthcoming; Phelan, 2005).

Reliance on Survey Data

As noted above, perhaps the most enduring focus in the study of Americans' attitudes can be found in national surveys dealing with issues of racial/ethnic prejudice and preferences. Applied to the case of mental illness, however, survey-based studies of public attitudes began somewhat later, with the pioneering work conducted in the 1950s (Star, 1952; 1955; see also Cumming & Cumming, 1957; Woodward, 1951). Much like the early literature on levels of racial intolerance, where non-rational and 'Jim Crow' sentiments were found to be predominant, early surveys of attitudes toward mental illness documented a generalized ignorance of mental illness; negative attitudes surrounding the issues of cause, treatment and outcomes; and a high level of public sentiment that favored the social rejection of persons with mental illness. Subsequent survey work in the 1970s and 1980s did not dispute these earlier findings (Armstrong, 1976; Rabkin, 1974; Roman & Floyd, 1981; Townsend, 1975). Moreover, levels of stigma reported among the general population continued to be distressingly high into the 1990s. Indeed, in 1996, over two-thirds of individuals reported fear and a desire to avoid persons with mental illness (Martin et al., 2000; Pescosolido et al., 1999). Further, at least in Western nations, findings from recent representative regional and national studies are remarkably consistent with these earlier patterns (Crisp, Gelder, Rix, Meltzer, & Rowlands, 2000; Stuart & Arboleda-Florez, 2000).

However, much like the survey data that point to a liberalization of Americans' attitudes toward race, the recent data relative to public attitudes toward mental illness also indicate that the public has become much more sophisticated in their knowledge and understanding of the range of mental health problems, and in their acceptance of scientific advances suggesting biological and genetic causes. In addition, these studies show a differentiation in the public mind regarding the challenges posed by diverse mental health problems and the utility of the range of treatments (Crisp et al., 2000; McKeon & Carrick, 1991; Stuart & Arboleda-Florez, 2000). Yet, as much progress as these recent surveys reveal, studies continue to suggest a deep concern about the dangerousness of people with mental health problems; the belief that genetic causes underlie dangerousness and the desire to reject family members of those with mental health problems as marital partners; the willingness to use the legal system to coerce people with mental health problems into treatment; and high levels of rejection of persons with mental health problems in workplace and intimate relationships (Crisp et al., 2000; Link et al., 1999; Martin et al., 2000; Pescosolido et al., 1999; Phelan, 2005; Phelan et al., 2000).

In sum, sociologists of mental health have fruitfully borrowed from complementary lines of sociological research and theory. However, there is little, if any, evidence that sociological research on race relations has ever taken notice of efforts in the sociology of mental health, even the potential relevance of Goffman's work. These realizations notwithstanding, two questions remain in addressing the power of the reflective interplay between the mainstream of the discipline and the subfield of mental health: Has the sociological study of stigma continued to draw from relevant developments in sociology and other relevant fields? And, how can new directions pursued in the sociological study of complementary fields offer additional insights into social processes? We now turn to the sociology of mental health's ability to reflect the cutting edge of the discipline and to reflect back to the general stock of sociological knowledge.

The Current State of Affairs: Resurgence and the Need for Rethinking

The last decade has witnessed an increase in research and policy attention to stigma. Across the social and socio-medical sciences, special issues have appeared in journals (e.g., *Schizophrenia Bulletin, The Lancet, Psychiatric Services*), national data collections have been mounted (e.g., the General Social Survey modules in 1996, 1998, 2002, and 2006), conferences have been organized (e.g., 2001 Conference, "Stigma and Global Health: Developing a Research Agenda;" see Keusch et al., 2006), and targeted grant initiatives have become available (see Michels, Hofman, Keusch, & Hrynkow, 2006). Moreover, for the first time in U.S. history, the Surgeon General focused attention on mental illness, beginning with a review of recent evidence on stigma and concluding that stigma constitutes the "foremost barrier to treatment and recovery" (U.S. Department of Health and Human Services, 1999, p. 3). This report was followed, four years later, by the President's New Freedom Commission on Mental Health Report, *Achieving the Promise: Transforming Mental Health Care in America* (U.S. Department of Health & Human Services, 2003) which outlined a set of recommendations necessary to address problems identified in the Surgeon General's *Report*. First among these recommendations was a call for a national campaign to eradicate stigma, an effort currently headed by the Substance Abuse and Mental Health Administration in concert with the National Ad Council. Other major initiatives have included the development of a series of anti-stigma campaigns (e.g., *"Real Men, Real Depression," "Eliminating the Barriers Initiative"*), and an information clearinghouse which catalogues campaigns, research, and other resources, and offers training and technical assistance (SAMHSA's Resource Center to Address Discrimination and Stigma (ADS Center); see websites for complete listing: *www.adscenter.org; www.adcouncil.org/default.aspx?id=303*). Further, this resurgence in stigma research, intervention and policy efforts extends beyond national borders. Under the *"Open the Doors"* initiative spearheaded by Norman Sartorius and the World Psychiatric Association (e.g., see Sartorius, 1997; Sartorius & Schulze, 2005), a number of national and regional studies have been mounted and almost two dozen countries have launched hundreds of interventions to decrease stigma.

While these reports and initiatives suggest that research priorities must now target interventions and change, we contend that without additional basic research on the underlying roots of stigma, the results of efforts toward change may be underwhelming. Below, we suggest some areas that would continue to elaborate the understanding of stigma, and in the process, address central issues in sociological theory and offer a more promising foundation for interventions.

Moving Toward Synthesis

Link and Phelan (1999) argue that the either-or view that characterized the debate over labeling theory is fruitless. We agree. On that particular count, our own research, based on the 1996 General Social Survey, suggests that both the particular behaviors associated with mental health problems *and* the application of the label of being "mentally ill" affect the public's stigmatizing responses in terms of perceptions of dangerousness and social rejection (Link et al., 1999; Martin et al., 2000; Pescosolido et al., 1999). As such, this research points to a need to recalibrate empirical efforts around a synthesis of what is known from a variety of perspectives.

While addressing medical sociology more broadly and not specifically the sociology of mental health, Sol Levine's (1995) call for "creative integration" addresses the benefits and costs of the impressive growth of sociological research trained on health, illness and healing. Levine contrasts the "rich and abundant benefits of our growing diversity and specialization" with "a form of intellectual parochialism that splinters . . . and impedes productive discourse. . ." (1995, p. 1). Aside from the labeling theory debates of the 1970s, the study of stigma has not been beset by an explicit or fractious line of division. But Levine's (1995) analysis signals a greater challenge: Have our efforts in understanding stigma drawn creatively from our own discipline and from the other disciplines that have addressed prejudice and discrimination?

There is much work to be done here, including a simple synthesis of all of the - factors best considered in an overall model. By now, there is no shortage of efforts to identify the critical ingredients that exacerbate or moderate stigmatizing reactions and their effects on persons with mental illness. For the most part, however, these efforts have focused on one issue or another; for example, an "attribution model" (Corrigan, 2000; Corrigan, Markowitz, Watson, Rowan, & Kubiak, 2003) or the "contact hypothesis" (Kolodziej & Johnson, 1996). In an attempt to move

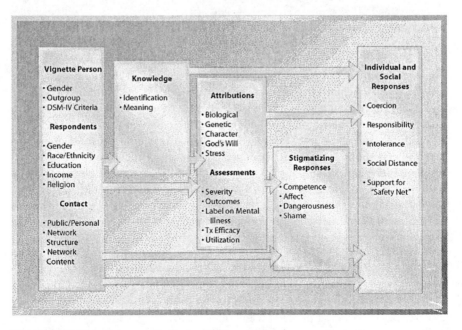

FIGURE 13.2. The etiology and effects of stigma model.

beyond these piece-meal approaches, we offer the Etiology and Effects of Stigma (EES) Model (Figure 2a; for a child adaptation see Martin et al., 2007).

The EES attempts to organize existing concepts and known relationships into a comprehensive system. It brings together a set of concerns as they shape the prejudice and discrimination associated with mental illness; specifically the race, gender, and SES characteristics of the person with mental health problems (i.e., the target person or "receiver," as often called in stigma research) and the person in a position to stigmatize (i.e., the respondent or "sender"); the nature of their relationship (i.e., personal/impersonal, positive or negative); and knowledge, attributions, and assessments of mental illness. Evidence in the recent GSS studies suggests that some social characteristics of the respondent (i.e., education) matter in public reactions to mental illness; overall, however, findings suggest that these characteristics are not as powerful as suggested by past research (see Schnittker, 2000, for example, on how gender shapes perceptions of dangerousness). As a result, we bring in social network ideas to develop a more elaborated and precise set of hypotheses on how the influence of contact with persons with mental illness depends on the structure of the relationship and the effects of the mental illness on the relationship. For example, having a close relationship and seeing it grow stronger as a result of the mental illness will likely shape stigmatizing responses differently from relationships which ended as a consequence of the mental illness.

The combination of socio-demographic characteristics and social networks influences public knowledge (e.g., recognition of mental illness), attributions (e.g., chemical imbalance, genes, stress, home life) and assessments (e.g., severity, the label of mental illness or other status). Together, these factors, in turn, influence stigmatizing beliefs and discrimination against people with mental health problems in the workplace or family.

This type of framework allows us to suggest, as we noted earlier, that both Gove's (1970) and Scheff's (1966) ideas operate to shape stigma. That is, the nature of the problem behaviors described or exhibited do matter; however, independently, individuals who label such variant behaviors as characteristic of "mental illness" are also more likely to report prejudicial attitudes towards persons with mental health problems. The label, itself, may shape discrimination because "mental illness" is associated in the public's mind with danger (Pescosolido et al., 1999). In this way, the EES incorporates Link and Phelan's (1999) admonition to integrate, rather than adjudicate among, ideas from different sociological theories and begins the effort to bring recent theoretical developments from the mainstream into the study of stigma.

Insights Ignored from and by Sociology: Reflection Reconsidered

The EES Model represents only a first step. Sociologists have never been alone in their concern with stigma, as much of the research and theory reported above indicates. A deeper synthesis would begin to bring in relevant research from sociology, psychology, cognitive science, and telecommunications to understand how personality, social position, social networks, media, and the manifestations of disorders shape the processes and structures underlying stigma. For example, have we integrated fully the "lessons" from psychological social psychology or even our own sociological social psychology into understanding the interactions in which the effects of stigma are delivered or experienced? Remember, Allport (1954) argued that "contact" only "breeds liking" under a restricted set of conditions—i.e., equal status, a high degree of collaboration, repeated contact, personal rather than formal interaction, and institutional support. This configuration of interactional requisites occurs very infrequently in day-to-day life or in interventions. Below, we focus on two issues—"contact" viewed from recent developments in network theory, and a consideration of how affect, noted in the race literature and coming to prominence as a research focus over the last two decades in sociology, may hold promise to "get underneath" stigma.

Network Elaborations

Have we employed all of the theoretical and empirical developments in social network theory that might provide a richer elaboration of the contact hypothesis (see, for example, Carrington, Scott, & Wasserman, 2005)? Along this line, network theory has shown that it is not just a particular interaction or relationship that matters, but an individual's stock of social network ties and experiences that shape attitudes and behaviors. This includes the number and density of ties, the structure of the set of ties that surrounds the individual, the valence of those ties, and the cultural beliefs that are held in those ties (Wellman, Wong, Tindall, & Nazer, 1996). Most markedly, in contemporary times, network theory maintains that cultural opportunities for social interaction are less bounded by traditional cleavages such as race, age, or gender. In earlier times, these opportunities were circumscribed effectively and narrowly by sociodemographic characteristics because they imposed strict restrictions on social interactions.

Recent studies on stigma using the General Social Survey have, indeed, shown a remarkable lack of socio-demographic influence. This is the case for both the "target" (e.g., the gender, race, education, age of the vignette person) and the "respondent" (e.g., the gender, race, age, education of the interviewee). Understanding whether this lack of socio-demographic effects is real or an artifact has implications, not only for stigma research, but also for anti-stigma efforts and for the discipline of sociology. This absence of sociodemographic differences may represent problems of inadequate statistical power, the difference between ideal and real response, and/or the result of some other methodological factor (i.e., the method of administration of the "case"). But in continuing to pursue this question, our findings with regard to stigma will support or refute the classic and more recent claims of social network theorists that socio-demographics have lost explanatory power in marking cultural cleavages (Pescosolido & Rubin, 2000; Simmel, 1955; White, Boorman, & Brieger, 1976).

If the research indeed turns out to support network theory, then mapping social interactions, rather than listing sociodemographics, must be considered more directly in stigma research designs. We would need to enumerate the frequency, nature, duration, and outcomes of network ties with persons with mental health problems. Further, we would need to ask about and understand the knowledge, beliefs, and meanings held in an individual's social circle. Finally, interventions would need to target networks, not individuals.

Elaborations from the Sociology of Race and Race Relations

Do we understand, and have we incorporated, recent developments from the study of race relations (see, for example, Forman, 2004; Pettigrew, 1997)? For example, the potential of apathetic concern noted in the race literature could be, but has not yet been, applied to questions regarding responses to those with mental illness. That is, some researchers suggest that racial issues no longer represent a significant social cleavage for the U.S. public (Forman, 2004). This conclusion is based on two sets of findings. First, Bobo, Kluegel and Smith (1997, p. 29), among others, contend that the source of a liberalizing trend in tolerance toward racial out-groups lies in key beliefs about individual-level differences that have "suffered a direct cultural assault and quickly eroded." Second, however, Americans' support for policy initiatives to ameliorate racial disadvantage also receive low levels of support. Faced with this apparent contradiction between Americans' rejection of racist ideology and their continued unwillingness to support policies designed to ameliorate race-based disadvantage, recent commentators (e.g., Forman, 2004; Sniderman & Carmines, 1997) have argued that Americans have become apathetic or disinterested in racial issues, assuming that race no longer 'matters.' Only when their own opportunities may be restricted in order to reduce disadvantage for others do individuals take notice.

It may be the case that Americans' assessments of persons with mental health problems have traveled a parallel course. Specifically, following the movement to "deinstitutionalize" mental health treatment, the specter of "the mental hospital patient" has largely vanished from the contemporary scene. Coupled with Americans' overwhelming faith in the effectiveness of psychiatric medications for treating mental health problems (see Martin & Pescosolido, 2005), the problem of mental illness and persons with mental health problems may be "off the radar" of the majority of Americans. What remains unclear, however, is whether this hypothesized disinterest in mental health-related problems translates into new or changing attitudes that stigmatize mental illness. Will it be only in response to policies to support "recovery" that the public responds with a generalized opposition to targeted programs and resources?

Elaborations from the Sociology of Emotions

An additional shortcoming of both the race-based and mental illness stigma literatures is found in the absence of concern with affect, that is, the emotional response to members of other racial/ethnic groups or persons with mental illness. Simply stated, inconsistent support for the "contact hypothesis" might best be understood with reference to an absence of concern for the role of emotion in interaction. This gap has been noted in the race literature by both Pettigrew (1997) and Welch et al. (2001). Specifically, these theorists argue that the public's reports of the emotions experienced during interactions with members of out-groups have a direct impact on prejudicial attitudes toward members of that group. That is, interpersonal contact that eventuates in feelings of "closeness" or "friendship" reduces the endorsement of prejudice and the willingness to discriminate. Similar concerns have been only infrequently discussed, however, by researchers examining the impact of interpersonal contact on stigmatizing responses to mental illness. We have argued elsewhere that the major emotion driving stigmatizing responses is the fear associated with mental illness. How individuals evaluate the "dangerousness" of individuals attenuates, and nearly eliminates, the influence of the label and the "disturbing" behaviors (see, for example, Martin et al., 2000). While Thoits (1985; 2005) has considered the role of emotions in the process of self-labeling, we have yet to consider which emotions, other than fear, may be at work in shaping prejudice and discrimination toward persons with mental illness. For example, how does empathy, sympathy or disgust influence the willingness to interact with individuals with mental illness or even support the provision of social services or policies to assist in recovery?

Summary

Creative integration requires a rethinking of how the best ideas and evidence within and across disciplines, may produce insights on the cultural climate of stigma and offer a way to restart stalled lines of basic research. For example, the sociology of culture has taken on a prominence in recent years, bridging cognition, meaning-making and network structures (Swidler, 2001). However, what it has abandoned is the direct study of cultural "products" in favor of a focus on the production of culture. This leaves stigma researchers turning to the relatively new discipline of telecommunications for theoretical and empirical insights. Their recent research indicates that production features matter: emotional, vivid or distinct content are more readily available (i.e., capable of being recalled) and accessible (i.e., more easily or quickly recalled; Busselle, 2001; Busselle & Greenberg, 2000; Lang, 2000). Further, Gerbner's work has documented that "heavy" T.V. viewers are more likely affected by media images, and that they are more likely to hold negative images of less powerful groups (Gerbner, Gross, Signorielli, Morgan, & Jackson-Beeck, 1979; Gerbner, Gross, Morgan, & Signorielli, 1980; Gerbner & Signorielli, 1979). Yet, the meaning and impact of these images are "sifted through" personal experiences.

Thus, how social network structures and cultures operate together to affect attitudes and behaviors is central. Telecommunication's emphasis on production features (e.g., pacing) and the way they are processed by individuals could be combined with the features of individuals' social networks to consider how contact can counter, filter, or reinforce the stereotypes, information, and images that media offer. Overall, this suggests that both sets of researchers, working in relative isolation from one another, is not the most productive strategy to advance the understanding of stigma or more general social processes. The critical questions that face the study of stigma require synthesizing insights from social networks, culture, media, intergroup relations, and emotions into a comprehensive theoretical system. Resulting research would provide answers that would greatly enhance the stock of sociological knowledge, as well as uncover the roots of stigma.

Conclusion: Drawing from and Reflecting Back to the Social Science Core of Theory and Research

Despite the variety of theoretical debates and policy priorities outlined above, a number of conclusions about stigma would seem to be clear-cut. *First*, stigma continues to surround mental illness, and its existence is widely acknowledged. Correspondingly, individuals with mental health problems, their families, providers, and policymakers report deep, wide and continuous experiences of stigma and discrimination. In other words, stigma-based criticism and rejection are commonplace in communities, families, churches, workplaces and treatment systems (Chernomas, Clarke, & Chisholm, 2000; Hinshaw & Cicchetti, 2000; Pescosolido et al., 2000; Wahl, 2000).

Second, recent studies show progress in an increased public understanding of the genesis of both mental illness problems and their effective medical treatments as compared to sentiments expressed in earlier decades. However, these studies continue to reveal distressingly high levels of rejection, fear and punitive social reactions toward persons with mental health problems (Crisp et al., 2000; Fabrega, 1991; Phelan et al., 2000).

Third, and encouragingly, there has been widening scholarly interest in stigma and its consequences across countries, adding the potential to understand larger cultural and structural influences on stigma (Keusch et al., 2006; Sartorius & Schulze, 2005). This has been accompanied by a parallel resurgence in interest from consumers and providers, and from policymakers and funders.

Fourth, whatever changes in stigma that may have occurred in recent years, mental illness continues to exert a heavy toll on individuals, caretakers, and policies targeting mental illness. Individual-level research on persons' experiences of stigma and its effects continues to present a clear, consistent, and distressing picture. Numerous studies document profound effects, including a lower quality of life, education selection effects (Link et al., 1997; McLeod & Kaiser, 2004; Mechanic, McAlpine, Rosenfield, & Davis, 1994), persistent social stress (Wright, Gronfein, & Owens, 2000), lower self-esteem (Penn & Martin, 1998), interference with the process of recovery (Markowitz, 1998; Wahl, 2000) and even a shortened life span (Ben Noun, 1996; Farnham, Zipple, Tyrell, & Chittinanda, 1999; Fuller, Edwards, Procter, & Moss, 2000; Rost, Smith, & Taylor, 1993). In fact, vulnerability to stigma is greater for mental illness than for coronary heart disease, tuberculosis or cancer

(Lai, Hong, & Chee, 2001; Ohaeri, 2001) and includes institutional as well as personal concerns such as the loss of legal rights (Burton, 1999), and discrimination in intensive care (Bailey, 1998; Failer, 2002; Scholsberg, 1993).

All of these conclusions call for a more integrative and creative effort, an assessment of the current state of research, and a reconsideration of theory and methods. While the manifest function of a reconsidered research agenda on stigma would target the sociology of mental health, it would also hold great potential to strengthen our contributions to the larger discipline. Sociology, as a discipline, has experienced the same positive growth and fractures of specialization to which Levine (1995) alludes. In the development of theoretical lines, it has veered toward some issues and away from others.

In the preface of *Reducing the Stigma of Mental Illness*, Norman Sartorius, one of the preeminent psychiatrists of his generation, elaborates on the importance of taking up such challenges. He notes that,

"The level of our ignorance is such that it is safe to predict that much more time is necessary before we learn enough about schizophrenia to be able to prevent it. . . .[however] . . . We know what obstacles stand in the way of recovery and rehabilitation. Among these obstacles undoubtedly the most serious and the most difficult is the stigmatization of mental illness and of all those in contact with it – the sufferers, their families, the medications used for treatment, the institutions in which treatment is provided, staff in mental health institutions and even the sites on which they are located" (Sartorius & Schulze, 2005).

As Goffman reminded us early on, stigma is fundamentally a social phenomenon rooted in social relationships and shaped by the culture and structure of society (Goffman, 1963). We hope our current consideration of the study of stigma has shown us that understanding the stigma attached to mental illness shines a harsh light on the social fault lines of a society, illuminating the diminished life chances of some of the most vulnerable individuals. If, as Keusch et al. (2006) contend, too little research has been done of late and that a new science of stigma is needed, then our review and Sartorius' claim suggests that the sociology of mental health, the discipline of sociology, and all of the social sciences need to be front and center in the creative integration of stigma research.

Note

1. Curiously, as we have discussed above, a similar liberalizing trend is not yet evidenced in recent surveys of Americans' views toward those with mental illness. Despite the apparently effective efforts of advocate groups to convince the American public that mental health problems are actually medical problems, the majority of Americans continue to endorse sentiments that stigmatize persons with mental health problems. Interestingly, efforts of groups like the National Alliance for the Mentally Ill (NAMI) have been opposite those of race-based struggles—their explanation toward, rather than away from, support for biological attributions. The implications of these diverse arguments for acceptance may be usefully examined.

Acknowledgments. Support was provided by grants R01 TW006374, R01 MH065950, R01 MH074985 (from the Fogarty International Center, the National Institute of Mental Health, and the Office of Behavioral and Social Science Research), the College of Arts and Sciences, and the Indiana Consortium for Mental Health Services Research. Thanks to Steven Tuch, Jane McLeod and Bill Avison for comments and to Alex Capshew and Mary Hannah for administrative assistance.

References

Adams, S. M., & Partee, D. J. (1998). Integrating psychosocial rehabilitation in a community-based faculty nursing practice. *Journal of Psychosocial Nursing and Mental Health Services, 36*, 24–28.

Allport, G. E. (1954). *The nature of prejudice.* Garden City, NY: Doubleday.

Armstrong, B. (1976). Preparing the community for the patient's return. *Hospital and Community Psychiatry, 27*, 349–356.

Bailey, S. R. (1998). An exploration of critical care nurses' and doctors' attitudes towards psychiatric patients. *Australian Journal of Advanced Nursing, 15*, 8–14.

Baxter, W. E. (1994). American psychiatry celebrates 150 years of caring. *Psychiatric Clin North America, 17*, 683–693.

Becker, H. S. (1963). *Outsiders: Studies in the sociology of deviance.* New York: The Free Press.

Ben Noun, L. (1996). Characterization of patients refusing professional psychiatric treatment in a primary care clinic. *Israel Journal of Psychiatry, 33*, 167–174.

Biernat, M., & Dovidio, J. F. (2000). Stigma and stereotypes. In T. F. Heatherton, R. E. Kleck, M. R. Hebl & J. G. Hull (Eds.), *The social psychology of stigma* (pp. 88–125). New York, NY: The Guilford Press.

Bobo, L., Kluegel, J. R., & Smith, R. A. (1997). Laissez faire racism: The crystallization of a "Kinder, gentler" Anti-black ideology. In S. A. Tuch & J. K. Martin (Eds.), *Racial attitudes in the 1990s: Continuity and change* (pp. 15–44). Greenwood, CT: Praeger.

Burton, V. S. J. (1999). The consequences of official labels: A research note on rights lost by the mentally ill, mentally incompetent, and convicted felons. *Community Mental Health Journal, 26*, 267–276.

Busselle, R. W. (2001). Television exposure, perceived realism, and exemplar accessibility in the social judgment process. *Media Psychology, 3*, 43–67.

Busselle, R. W., & Greenberg, B. S. (2000). The nature of television realism judgments: A re-evaluation of their conceptualization and measurement. *Mass Communication & Society, 3*, 249–268.

Calavita, K., & Serron, C. (1992). Postmodernism and protest: Recovering the sociological imagination. *Law and Society Review, 26*, 765–771.

Caplow, T. (1964). *Principles of organization.* New York: Harcourt, Brace and World.

Carrington, P. J., Scott, J., & Wasserman, S. (2005). *Models and methods in social network analysis.* Cambridge and New York: Cambridge University Press.

Chernomas, W. M., Clarke, D. E., & Chisholm, F. A. (2000). Perspectives of women living with schizophrenia. *Psychiatric Services, 51*, 1517–1521.

Conrad, P. (2000). Medicalization, genetics and human problems. In C. E. Bird, P. Conrad & A. M. Fremont (Eds.), *Handbook of medical sociology* (pp. 322–333). Upper Saddle River, NJ: Prentice Hall.

Conrad, P., & Schneider, J. W. (1992). *Deviance and medicalization: From badness to sickness*. Philadelphia, PA: Temple University Press.

Corrigan, P. W. (2000). Mental health stigma as social attribution: Implications for research methods and attitude change. *Clinical Psychology: Science and Practice, 7,* 48–67.

Corrigan, P. W., Markowitz, F. E., Watson, A. C., Rowan, D., & Kubiak, M. A. (2003). An attribution model of public discrimination towards persons with mental illness. *Journal of Health & Social Behavior, 44,* 162–179.

Crandall, C. S. (2000). Idiology and lay theories of stigma: The justification of stigmatization. In T. F. Heatherton, R. E. Kleck, M. R. Hebl & J. G. Hull (Eds.), *The social psychology of stigma* (pp. 126–152). New York, NY: The Guilford Press.

Crisp, A. H., Gelder, M. G., Rix, S., Meltzer, H. I., & Rowlands, O. J. (2000). Stigmatization of people with mental illness. *British Journal of Psychiatry, 177,* 4–7.

Crocker, J., Major, B., & Steele, C. M. (1998). Social stigma. In D. Gilbert, S. T. Fiske & G. Lindzey (Eds.), *The handbook of social psychology* (pp. 504–553). New York: McGraw-Hill.

Cumming, E., & Cumming, J. (1957). *Closed ranks: An experiment in mental health education*. Cambridge, MA: Harvard University Press.

Dain, N. (1994). Reflections on antipsychiatry and stigma in the history of american psychiatry. *Hospital and Community Psychiatry, 45,* 1010–1014.

Desforges, D. M., Lord, C. G., Ramsey, S. L., Mason, J. A., VanLeeuwen, M. D., West, S. C., & Lepper, M. P. (1991). Effects of structured cooperative contact on changing negative attitudes toward stigmatized social groups. *Journal of Personality and Social Psychology, 60,* 531–544.

Dovidio, J. F., Major, B., & Crocker, J. (2000). *The social psychology of stigma*. New York, NY: The Guilford Press.

Dunham, H. W. (1971). Comment on gove's evaluation of societal reaction theory as an explanation for mental illness. *American Sociological Review, 36,* 313–314.

Ellison, C. G., & Powers, D. A. (1994). The contact hypothesis and racial attitudes among black americans. *Social Science Quarterly, 75,* 385–400.

Estroff, S. E. (1981). *Making it crazy: An ethnography of psychiatric clients in an american community*. Berkeley, CA: University of California Press.

Fabrega, H. J. (1991). The culture and history of psychiatric stigma in early modern and modern western societies: A review of recent literature. *Comprehensive Psychiatry, 32,* 97–119.

Failer, J. L. (2002). *Who qualifies for rights? Homelessness, mental illness, and civil commitment*. Ithaca, NY: Cornell University Press.

Farnham, C. R., Zipple, A. M., Tyrell, W., & Chittinanda, P. (1999). Health status risk factors of people with severe and persistent mental illness. *Journal of Psychosocial Nursing and Mental Health Services, 37,* 16–21.

Forman, T. A. (2004). Color-blind racism and racial indifference: The role of racial apathy in facilitating enduring inequalities. In M. Krysan & A. E. Lewis (Eds.), *The changing terrain of race and ethnicity* (pp. 43–66). New York: Russell Sage Foundation.

Fuller, J., Edwards, J., Procter, N., & Moss, J. (2000). How definition of mental health problems can influence help-seeking in rural and remote communities. *Australian Journal of Rural Health, 8,* 148–153.

Gerbner, G., Gross, L., Morgan, M., & Signorielli, N. (1980). Violence profile no. 11: Trends in network television trauma and viewer conceptions of social reality, 1967–1979. Philadelphia: Annenberg School of Communications, University of Pennsylvania.

Gerbner, G., Gross, L., Signorielli, N., Morgan, M., & Jackson-Beeck, M. (1979). The demonstration of power, violence profile no. 10. *Journal of Communication, 27*, 177–196.

Gerbner, G., & Signorielli, N. (1979). Women and minorities in television drama 1969–1978. Philadelphia: Annenberg School of Communications, University of Pennsylvania.

Goffman, E. (1963). *Stigma: Notes on the management of spoiled identity.* Englewood Cliffs, NJ: Prentice-Hall.

Gove, W. R. (1970). Societal reaction as an explanation of mental illness: An evaluation. *American Sociological Review*, 873–884.

Gove, W. R., & Howell, P. (1974). Individual resources and mental hospitalization: A comparison and evaluation of the societal reaction and psychiatric perspectives. *American Sociological Review, 39*, 86–100.

Gove, W. R., & Tudor, J. F. (1973). Adult sex roles and mental illness. *American Journal of Sociology, 78*, 812–835.

Hinshaw, S. P., & Cicchetti, D. (2000). Stigma and mental disorder: Conceptions of illness, public attitudes, personal disclosure and social policy. *Development and Psychopathology, 12*, 555–598.

Homans, G. (1951). *The human group.* London: Routledge and K. Paul.

Hughes, M., & Tuch, S. A. (2000). How beliefs about poverty influence racial policy attitudes: A study of whites, african-americans, hispanics, and asians in the U.S. In D. O. Sears, J. Sidanius & L. Babo (Eds.), *Racialized politics: Values, ideology and prejudice in american public opinion* (pp. 165–190). Chicago: University of Chicago Press.

Hyman, S. E. (2000). The millennium of mind, brain and behavior. *Archives of General Psychiatry, 57*, 88–89.

Jackman, M. R., & Crane, M. (1986). Some of my best friends are black. . .: Interracial friendship and whites' racial attitudes. *Public Opinion Quarterly, 50*, 459–486.

Jones, E., Farina, A., Hastorf, A., Markus, H., Miller, D. T., & Scott, R. (1984). *Social stigma: The psychology of marked relationships.* New York, NY: Freeman.

Keusch, G. T., Wilentz, J., & Kleinman, A. (2006). Stigma and global health: Developing a research agenda. *The Lancet, 367*, 525–527.

Kolodziej, M. E., & Johnson, B. T. (1996). Interpersonal contact and acceptance of persons with psychiatric disorders: A research synthesis. *Journal of Consulting and Clinical Psychology, 64*, 1387–1396.

Lai, Y. M., Hong, C., & Chee, C. Y. (2001). Stigma and mental illness. *Singapore Medical Journal, 42*, 111–114.

Lang, A. (2000). The information processing of mediated messages: A framework for communication research. *Journal of Communication, 50*, 46–70.

Lemert, E. M. (1951). *Social pathology.* New York: McGraw-Hill.

Lemert, E. M. (2000). *Crime and deviance: Essays and innovations of edwin m. Lemert.* Lanham, MD: Rowman & Littlefield.

Levine, S. (1995). Time for creative integration in medical sociology. *Journal of Health and Social Behavior, 35*, 1–4.

Link, B. G., Cullen, F. T., Struening, E. L., Shrout, P. E., & Dohrenwend, B. P. (1989). A modified labeling theory approach to mental disorders: An empirical assessment. *American Sociological Review, 54*, 400–423.

Link, B. G., & Phelan, J. C. (1999). The labeling theory of mental disorder (i): The role of social contingencies in the application of psychiatric labels. In A. V. Horwitz & T. L. Scheid (Eds.), *A handbook for the study of mental health* (pp. 139–150). Cambridge: Cambridge University Press.

Link, B. G., Phelan, J. C., Bresnahan, M., Stueve, A., & Pescosolido, B. A. (1999). Public conceptions of mental illness: Labels, causes, dangerousness and social distance. *American Journal of Public Health, 89,* 1328–1333.

Link, B. G., Struening, E. L., Rahav, M., Phelan, J. C., & Nuttbrick, L. (1997). On stigma and its consequences: Evidence from a longitudinal study of men with dual diagnoses of mental illness and substance abuse. *Journal of Health and Social Behavior, 38,* 177–190.

Markowitz, F. E. (1998). The effects of stigma on the psychological well-being and life satisfaction of persons with mental illness. *Journal of Health and Social Behavior, 39,* 335–347.

Markowitz, F. E. (2001). Modeling processes in recovery from mental illness: Relationships between symptoms, life satisfaction, and self-concept. *Journal of Health and Social Behavior, 42,* 64–79.

Martin, J. K., & Tuch, S. A. (1997). *Racial attitudes in the 1990s. Continuity and change.* Westport, CT: Praeger.

Martin, J. K., & Pescosolido, B. A. (2005). *Public views of psychiatric medications in light of health and health care.* Bloomington, IN: Indiana Consortium for Mental Health Services Research.

Martin, J. K., Pescosolido, B. A., Olafsdottir, S., & McLeod, J. D. (2007). The construction of fear: Modeling Americans' preferences for social distance from children and adolescents with mental health problems. *Journal of Health and Social Behavior, 48,* (in press).

Martin, J. K., Pescosolido, B. A., & Tuch, S. A. (2000). Of fear and loathing: The role of disturbing behavior, labels and causal attributions in shaping public attitudes toward persons with mental illness. *Journal of Health and Social Behavior, 41,* 208–233.

McKeon, P., & Carrick, S. (1991). Public attitudes to depression: A national survey. *Irish Journal of Psychological Medicine, 8,* 116–121.

McLeod, J. D., & Kaiser, K. (2004). Childhood emotional and behavioral problems in educational attainment. *American Sociological Review, 69,* 636–658.

Mechanic, D. (1971). Comment on "Mental illness". *American Sociological Review, 36,* 314.

Mechanic, D., McAlpine, D., Rosenfield, S., & Davis, D. (1994). Effects of illness attribution and depression on the quality of life among persons with serious mental illness. *Social Science and Medicine, 39,* 155–164.

Michels, K. M., Hofman, K. J., Keusch, G. T., & Hrynkow, S. H. (2006). Stigma and global health: Looking forward. *The Lancet, 367,* 538–539.

Ohaeri, J. U. (2001). Caregiver burden and psychotic patients' perception of social support in a nigerian setting. *Social Psychiatry & Psychiatric Epidemiology, 36,* 86–93.

Okazaki, S. (2000). Treatment delay among asian-american patients with severe mental illness. *American Journal of Orthopsychiatry, 70,* 58–64.

Pang, J. J. (1985). Partial hospitalization: An alternative to inpatient care. *Psychiatric Clin North America, 8,* 587–593.

Penn, D. L., Guynan, K., Daily, T., Spaulding, W. D., & Sullivan, M. (1994). Dispelling the stigma of schizophrenia: What sort of information is best? *Schizophrenia Bulletin, 20,* 567–577.

Penn, D. L., & Martin, J. K. (1998). The stigma of severe mental illness: Some potential solutions for a recalcitrant problem. *Psychiatric Quarterly, 69,* 235–247.

Pescosolido, B. A., Martin, J. K., Link, B. G., Kikuzawa, S., Burgos, G., & Swindle, R. (2000). *Americans' views of mental illness and health at century's end: Continuity and change. Public report on the MacArthur mental health module, 1996 General*

Social Survey. Bloomington, IN: Indiana Consortium for Mental Health Services Research.

Pescosolido, B. A., McLeod, J. D., & Alegria, M. (2000). Confronting the second social contract: The place of medical sociology in research and policy for the twenty-first century. In C. E. Bird, P. Conrad & A. M. Fremont (Eds.), *Handbook of medical sociology* (pp. 399–426). Upper Saddle River, NJ: Prentice-Hall.

Pescosolido, B. A., Monahan, J., Link, B. G., Stueve, A., & Kikuzawa, S. (1999). The public's view of the competence, dangerousness, and need for legal coercion of persons with mental health problems. *American Journal of Public Health, 89*, 1339–1345.

Pescosolido, B. A., & Rubin, B. A. (2000). The web of group affiliations revisited: Social life, postmodernism, and sociology. *American Sociological Review, 65*, 52–76.

Pettigrew, T. (1997). The affective component of prejudice: Empirical support for the new view. In S. A. Tuch & J. K. Martin (Eds.), *Racial attitudes in the 1990s: Continuity and change* (pp. Westport, CT: Praeger.

Phelan, J. C. (2005). Geneticization of deviant behavior and consequences for stigma: The case of mental illness. *Journal of Health and Social Behavior, 46*, 307–322.

Phelan, J. C., & Link, B. G. (2002). Public perceptions that people with mental illness are dangerous: The role of impersonal public contact. International Stigma Conference, Leipzig.

Phelan, J. C., Link, B. G., Stueve, A., & Pescosolido, B. A. (2000). Public conceptions of mental illness in 1950 and 1996: What is mental illness and is it to be feared? *Journal of Health and Social Behavior, 41*, 188–207.

Rabkin, J. (1974). Public attitudes toward mental illness: A review of the literature. *Schizophrenia Bulletin, 10*, 9–33.

Roman, P. M., & Floyd, H. H. (1981). Social acceptance of psychiatric illness and psychiatric treatment. *Social Psychiatry, 16*, 21–29.

Rose, R. (1988). Schizophrenia, civil liberties and the law. *Schizophrenia Bulletin, 14*, 1–15.

Rosenfield, S. (1997). Labeling mental illness: The effects of received services and perceived stigma on life satisfaction. *American Sociological Review, 62*, 660–672.

Rost, K., Smith, G. R., & Taylor, J. L. (1993). Rural-urban differences in stigma and the use of care for depressive disorders. *Journal of Rural Health, 9*, 57–62.

Sartorius, N. (1997). Fighting schizophrenia and its stigma. A new world psychiatric association educational programme. *British Journal of Psychiatry, 170*, 297.

Sartorius, N., & Schulze, H. (2005). *Reducing the stigma of mental illness: A report from a global association.* New York: Cambridge University Press.

Scheff, T. J. (1966). *Being mentally ill: A sociological theory.* Chicago, IL: Aldine.

Scheff, T. J. (1974). The labeling theory of mental illness. *American Sociological Review, 39*, 444–452.

Schnittker, J. (2000). Gender and reactions to psychological problems: An examination of social tolerance and perceived dangerousness. *Journal of Health & Social Behavior, 41*, 224–240.

Scholsberg, A. (1993). Psychiatric stigma and mental health professionals (stigmatizers and destigmatizers). *Medicine and Law, 12*, 409–416.

Sigelman, L., & Welch, S. (1993). The contact hypothesis revisited: Black-white interaction and positive racial attitudes. *Social Forces, 71*, 781–795.

Simmel, G. (1955). *Conflict and the web of group affiliations.* New York: Free Press.

Sniderman, P. M., & Carmines, E. G. (1997). *Reaching beyond race.* Cambridge, MA: Harvard University Press.

Star, S. A. (1952). What the public thinks about mental health and mental illness. National Association for Mental Health, Annual Meeting.

Star, S. A. (1955). The public's ideas about mental illness. Chicago: National Opinion Research Center.

Stuart, H., & Arboleda-Florez, J. (2000). Community attitudes toward persons with schizophrenia. *Canadian Journal of Psychiatry, 46,* 245–252.

Swan, J. (1999). Wearing two hats. Consumer and provider. *Journal of Psychosocial Nursing and Mental Health Services, 37,* 20–24.

Swidler, A. (2001). *Talk of love: How culture matters.* Chicago, IL: University of Chicago Press.

Thoits, P. A. (1985). Self-labeling processes in mental illness: The role of emotional deviance. *American Journal of Sociology, 91,* 221–249.

Thoits, P. A. (2005). Differential labeling of mental illness by social status: A new look at an old problem. *Journal of Health and Social Behavior, 46,* 102–119.

Townsend, J. M. (1975). Cultural conceptions, mental disorders, and social roles: A comparison of Germany and America. *American Sociological Review, 40,* 739–752.

Tuch, S. A., & Hughes, M. (1996). Whites' racial policy attitudes. *Social Science Quarterly, 77,* 1048–1060.

U.S. Department of Health & Human Services (2003). *Achieving the promise: Transforming mental health care in America. The President's new freedom commission on mental health report.* Bethesda, MD: U.S. Department of Health & Human Services.

U.S. Department of Health and Human Services (1999). *Mental health: A report of the Surgeon General.* Rockville, MD: U.S. Department of Health and Human Services.

Wahl, O. F. (1999). Mental health consumers' experience of stigma. *Schizophrenia Bulletin, 25,* 467–478.

Wahl, O. F. (2000). *Telling is risky business.* New Brunswick, NJ: Rutgers University Press.

Welch, S., Sigelman, L., Bledsoe, T., & Combs, M. (2001). *Race and place: Race relations in an american city.* New York: Cambridge University Press.

Wellman, B., Wong, R., Tindall, D., & Nazer, N. (1996). A decade of network change: Turnover, persistence and stability in personal communities. *Social Networks, 19,* 27–50.

White, H. C., Boorman, S. A., & Brieger, R. L. (1976). Social structure from multiple networks. I. Blockmodels of roles and positions. *American Journal of Sociology, 88,* 135–160.

Williams, R. M. (1947). *The reduction of intergroup tensions.* New York: Social Science Research Council.

Woodward, J. L. (1951). Changing ideas on mental illness and its treatment. *American Sociological Review, 16,* 443–454.

Wright, E. R., Gronfein, W. P., & Owens, T. J. (2000). Deinstitutionalization, social rejection, and the self-esteem of former mental patients. *Journal of Health and Social Behavior, 41,* 68–90.

14
Social Integration: A Conceptual Overview and Two Case Studies

Stephanie W. Hartwell and Paul R. Benson

Introduction

The study of social integration and its effects on health and well-being has been at the center of theory and research in sociology since its inception. Broadly defined as the extent to which individuals are socially linked to one another, social integration has consistently been shown to exert positive effects on a diverse array of physical and mental health problems, including cancer, myocardial infarction, depression, and even the common cold (see reviews by Cohen, Gottlieb, & Underwood, 2000; House, Landis, & Umberson, 1988; Turner & Turner, 2000). The concept has also been utilized in research related to a variety of other important social concerns, including, among others, crime (Gibson, Jihong, Nicholas, & Gaffney, 2002; Sampson, 2003; Sampson & Laub, 2003), political participation (Putnam, 1993a; 1995; Verba, Lehman-Scholzman, & Brady, 1995), and community care of "deviant" populations, such as those with mental illness and other disabilities (Hughes & Gove, 1989; Meyer, Christen, Graf, Ruesch, & Hell, 2002; Segal, Baumohl, & Moyles, 1980).

This chapter clarifies the concept of social integration by (1) providing a brief history of the key theoretical perspectives underlining the study of social integration; (2) organizing a framework to integrate these perspectives; (3) illustrating the framework using two of our on-going studies; and (4) highlighting limitations and directions for future research.

Classical and Contemporary Approaches

The seminal contribution of French sociologist, Emile Durkheim, to the study of social integration lies in his examination of suicide rates across societies and social groups. In *Suicide*, Durkheim (1951) concluded that there were four basic forms of suicide. The first, *egoistic suicide*, stems from the individual's lack of social ties to society. The second, *anomic suicide*, is most likely to occur when society's ability to regulate its members is weakened or destroyed due to rapid social change or major social upheavals. According to Durkheim, the third and fourth types, *altruistic* and *fatalistic suicide*, are most likely to occur when society's grasp on the individual is excessive (for example, when Hindu religious tradition demands that a widow climb onto her husband's funeral pyre). Thus, either too much or too little social integration can be harmful.

In addition to his work on suicide, Durkheim (1933) also discussed the importance of social integration in his earlier work, *The Division of Labor in Society*. In *The Division of Labor*, Durkheim noted that simple societies function primarily through "mechanical solidarity" where informal networks and controls predominate, while more complex societies function through "organic solidarity," a process involving more formal social bonds and forms of social control. In this way, Durkheim demonstrated how social integration is related to historical and social structural context. For instance, in more complex societies, the ties between individuals and large-scale social institutions, such as schools, the government, and the criminal justice system, are likely to be particularly critical.

The importance of social integration is also reflected in the work of early American sociologists. Social disorganization theorists, such as Park, Burgess and McKenzie (1925) and Shaw and McKay (1942) for example, found that urban areas with less social cohesion and stability had higher rates of crime and delinquency. Similarly, Faris and Dunham's (1939) work on isolation and schizophrenia also emphasized the role played by social instability and disorganization in the genesis of mental disorder. Like Durkheim, these early American sociologists viewed community ties as requisite for both normal development and for the maintenance of appropriate social behavior. This emphasis on the role of macrosocial community characteristics in fostering beneficial social relations is echoed in the recent work of "social capital" theorists and researchers (Kawachi & Berkman, 2000).

The Need for an Integrating Framework

As noted earlier, it is now widely acknowledged that social relationships and affiliations have powerful effects on a host of health and mental outcomes. However, as Berkman and her colleagues (2000) have noted: "When investigators write about the impact of social relationships on health, many terms are used loosely and interchangeably, including social networks, social support, social ties, and social integration" (p. 844). The lack of clarity has caused confusion and slowed progress in the field. Thus, we present a framework we found useful in articulating the social integration concept. This framework (see Figure 14.1) suggests that social integration is most clearly viewed as a "meta-construct" composed of distinct, but interrelated, concepts – in this case, social networks, social support, social engagement, and social capital. Each of these concepts emphasizes a different way of thinking about social ties (between individuals, between individuals and groups, and between groups) and their effects on individual and group outcomes. While our framework emphasizes that there are many different ways of thinking about social integration and its effects, in our rendition, social integration is fundamentally anchored by *social networks*. Linked to the social networks in

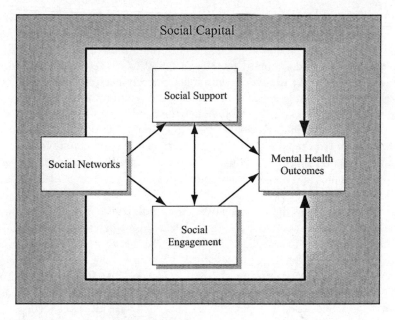

FIGURE 14.1. Conceptual framework.

which individuals and groups are embedded are *social support* (the emotional and instrumental resources flowing between individuals and groups within networks) and *social engagement* (the extent to which individuals participate in a broad array of social roles, relationships, and activities). Each of these elements of social integration potentially affects one another as well as a variety of outcomes of interest, including adjustment, health and emotional well-being. Additionally, each is influenced by *social capital* (the extent to which a community, neighborhood, or social group provide its members with the opportunities needed to increase their personal and family resources). Each of these four aspects of social integration is briefly outlined below.

Social Networks

In formal network theory, the term *network* refers to the ties that connect a specific set of actors (Burt & Minor, 1983; Marsden, 1990). Although network research typically has studied ties between individuals, the approach can also be used to investigate the linkages between other social entities including families, corporations, prisons, and social service agencies (Brissette, Cohen, & Seeman, 2000; Pescosolido, 1992, 2005). Using network analysis, investigators have examined a variety of network characteristics, including size, density, composition, and range, and their relationship to health and mental health outcomes (Acock & Hurlbert, 1993; Bowling & Browne, 1991; Burt & Minor, 1987; Lin & Ensel, 1989; Lin & Peek 1999). Importantly, researchers have also investigated the relationship between social network characteristics and the provision and receipt of social support. This work has indicated that different types of networks are better at allocating different kinds of support. For example, access to informal support have been found to be associated with dense, homophilous networks (networks with many interconnections between socially similar members), while access to formal support is more likely to be linked to wide-ranging networks made up of socially dissimilar members (Fischer, 1982; Haines & Hurlbert, 1992; Hurlbert, Haines, & Beggs, 2000; Suitor, Pillemer, & Keeton, 1995; Wellman & Wortley, 1990). Low-density networks have also been found to be particularly valuable during difficult life transitions including divorce, unemployment, and geographic relocation (Granovetter, 1973; Hirsch, 1980; Wilcox, 1981).

A major strength of the social network approach rests on its assumption that human behavior and experience is largely structured by the web of social relations in which individuals are embedded. Thus, the emphasis of social networks is eminently sociological – focusing on the effects (positive and negative) of social interaction within society (Pescosolido, 2005; Pescosolido & Rubin, 2000). Social networks, in short, provide the relational structure within which social resources, social support, and social engagement, are generated, provided, and received.

Social Support

Over the past twenty-five years there have been hundreds of studies on social support and its effects on health and mental health (Cohen & Wills, 1985; Cohen et al., 2000; House et al., 1988). However, as Turner and Turner (2000) observed, what exactly is meant by "social support" is not always clear, with the concept often being used by different investigators to refer to many different kinds of social, social psychological, and psychological processes. Thus, similar to social integration, social support is best viewed as a multidimensional construct "composed of several legitimate and distinguishable theoretical constructs" (Vaux, 1988, p. 28).

There are several different conceptualizations of social support common in the literature. One important distinction is between *perceived support* (support that is perceived to be available if needed) and *received support* (support that is reported to have been recently provided by others). While both types of support have been studied extensively, two decades of research indicates that it is the primarily the subjective appraisal of support (that is, perceived support) that is responsible for social support's positive impact on adjustment, health, and well-being (Turner & Turner, 2000). Evidence, in fact, suggests that the benefits of "objective" social support indicators, such as receipt of supportive behaviors and network ties, may be primarily mediated through the subjective perception of being supported and cared for by others (House, 1981; Wethington & Kessler, 1986). Research also indicates that measures of perceived and received support are not interchangeable and that the processes tapped by these two types of support are not identical (Willis & Shinar, 2000).

The multidimensional nature of the social support concept is also evident when considering the different functions potentially provided through social relationships, including *emotional support, instrumental support, informational support, companionship*, and *social validation* (Argyle, 1992; House, 1981). Different forms of social support can also be distinguished based on who provides the support – *informal support* provided by family, friends, coworkers, and neighbors or *formal support* provided by bureaucratic organizations and professional help-givers. Each of these different dimensions of support are likely to be more useful in dealing with particular kinds of problems than with others – for example, one would hypothesize that emotional support would be particularly useful in buffering individuals against interpersonal stress, while informational support would be less helpful in this regard. Similarly, one would expect different types of social support to be related to adjustment through differing mechanisms such as altering appraisal of the stressful event, enhancing mastery and self-esteem, improving problem-solving ability, and facilitating behavior change (Turner & Turner, 2000; Vaux, 1988; Willis & Shinar, 2000; Umberson, 1987). Finally, it should be emphasized that not all forms of social support have positive consequences. Indeed, research has clearly demonstrated that social relationships can also engender conflict and stress, leading to increased distress and decreased emotional well-being (Goode, 1960; Rook, 1984; Rook & Pietromonaco, 1987).

Social Engagement

Social engagement can be defined as the extent to which an individual participates in a broad range of social roles and relationships. Like social networks and social support, increased social participation has been found to have beneficial effects on health and well-being (Berkman & Syme, 1979; Burton, 1998; Greenfield, Rehm, & Rogers, 2000). Social engagement has also been linked to favorable social and behavioral outcomes in areas such as family functioning (Dunst, Trivette, & Jodry, 1996), child and adolescent development and behavior (Cochran, Larner, Riley, Gunnarsson, & Henderson, 1990; Cotterell, 1996), and crime (Gibson et al., 2002; Sampson, 2003; Sampson & Laub, 2003). The benefits of performing multiple social roles have also been noted by a number of researchers (Cohen, 1988; Marks, 1977; Sieber, 1974). Thoits (1983), for example, has suggested that social roles provide people with meaningful social identities and purpose in life. Thus, as individuals accumulate valued social roles (for example, spouse, parent, worker, and friend), the sense that life has meaning and purpose increases, leading to improved well-being. In a similar vein, it has been suggested that increased social involvement positively affects health and well-being through a variety of social and informational influences, for example, by encouraging health-promoting behaviors and discouraging unhealthy ones (Berkman et al., 2000; Rook, 1990; Umberson, 1987). While its benefits are clear, social engagement can also have adverse effects, for example, participation in a delinquent gang may encourage illegal drug use and other forms of deviant or criminal behavior. Similarly, multiple roles can also be detrimental, particularly when role expectations are conflicting, discrepant, or overwhelming (Coser, 1974; Goode, 1960; Simon, 1995).

Social Capital

The notion of social capital offers a different perspective on the concept of social integration by refocusing analytic attention on the broader social contexts in which support is embedded. Based on the writings of Bourdieu (1986) and Coleman (1990), among others, social capital has been be defined as "those features of social structures—such as levels of interpersonal trust and norms of reciprocity and mutual aid—which act as resources for individuals and facilitate collective action" (Kawachi & Berkman, 2000, p. 175). As such, social capital is conceptualized as a macro-social feature of neighborhoods, communities, and societies. From this perspective, collectives possessing high levels of social capital are marked by strong levels of interpersonal trust and mutual obligation as well as by the existence of what Coleman (1990) has termed "appropriate" social organizations, that is, voluntary groups, such as resident's associations and civic organizations, whose purpose is to facilitate beneficial interactions among members and to improve the quality of life of the wider community.

The positive effects of social capital have been examined in a variety of areas, including education (Coleman & Hoffer, 1987), political science (Putnam, 1993a; 1995; Verba, et al., 1995), criminology (Samson, Raudenbush, & Earls, 1997), and public health (Kawachi, Kennedy, & Lochner, 1997). In criminology, for example, Sampson and his colleagues (1997) found that neighborhoods where the residents reported higher levels of social cohesion and mutual trust (what they termed "collective efficacy") had lower rates of violent crime compared to neighborhoods where residents reported lower levels of trust and cooperation. Similarly, Kawachi et al. (1999) conducted a multilevel study of the relationship between state-level social capital and health. In that investigation, they found aggregate measures of trust and reciprocity to be significantly correlated with self-reported health, even after controlling for potentially confounding individual-level variables such as income, education, and health insurance coverage.

Like other forms of capital, access to social capital is unequally distributed across social groupings. Minorities and the poor, in particular, are less likely than others to reside in communities possessing high levels of social capital. In addition, because social capital requires social stability, social disruption and instability can be highly damaging to the creation and maintenance of this social resource (Kawachi & Berkman, 2000). In socially disorganized communities, low levels of trust and cooperation among residents are likely to constrain the ability of the community as a whole to garner needed economic and social resources, thus leading to further deterioration and loss of social capital (Putnam, 1993b; Wilson, 1987; Woolcock, 1998).

As our overview has shown, the concept of social integration is multidimensional, encompassing the social structure in which individuals are embedded as well as the content of their interpersonal and institutional interactions. The concepts we highlighted as influential in integration outcomes—social networks, social support, social engagement, and social capital—are interrelated and occur both within and across collectives (formal and informal social institutions) and individuals (social ties). In addition, as our discussion hopefully makes clear, the effects of each facet of social integration on outcomes are also multifaceted, potentially encompassing both positive and negative consequences.

Case Studies: Social Integration Applied to Mental Health

In the next two sections of this chapter, we examine social integration using two studies that reflect the expanse of concept and the utility of separating out its components. The first is a longitudinal study of children with autism and their families, and the second is a research program on criminal offenders with mental illness released from prison into the community.

Social Integration and Family Adaptation to Childhood Disability: The Family-School Autism Project

Sam was a full-term baby who appeared normal and healthy at birth. According to his mother, aside from a little colic, Sam's first year of life was uneventful. By age 18 months, however, Sam's family became concerned over his increasing lack of social responsiveness, poor eye contact, and failure to acquire any meaningful speech. When brought to the attention of the family pediatrician, the parents were told "not to worry" since "all children develop differently." By age 2, however, Sam's parents become increasingly alarmed by his continued language delays, as well as by his frequent tantrums, lack of play skills, and strange behaviors (for example, staring at lights and waving his fingers in front of his eyes). Family life was further disrupted by Sam's chronic sleep problems, extreme mood fluctuations, and refusal to eat most foods. Finally, at their wit's end, Sam's parents brought him for an evaluation at a nearby children's hospital. After several days of testing, they were informed that Sam had autism. While in one sense relieved that they at last had a label for their son's puzzling and disturbing behaviors, Sam's parents also experienced a range of conflicting emotions, including depression, guilt, anger, and frustration. "What is autism and what will it mean for Sam and our family?"

The extent to which parents of children with autism are socially integrated, that is, are able to access key network ties in order to receive and utilize informal and formal support is currently being studied as part of the Family-School Autism Project, an ongoing longitudinal study of children with autism and their families (Benson, in press; Benson & Karlof, 2003a, 2003b; Benson, Karlof, & Siperstein, In submission; Benson, Siperstein, Karlof, & Widaman, 2004). Social integration has been shown to be crucial to their ability to successfully cope with the demands and stresses associated with their child's disorder (Albanese, San Miguel, & Koegel, 1996; Beresford, 1994; Boyd, 2002; Bristol, 1987; Konstantareas & Homatidis, 1991). However, for many families, the intense and unremitting demands of caring for a child with autism may come to ellipse other family priorities, in some cases, severely compromising the ability of family members to develop and sustain critical social connections, both within and outside the home (Domingue, Cutler, & McTarnaghan, 2000; Gray, 1998; Moes, 1995; Norton & Drew, 1994). Integrative family activities, such as dinners together, weekend outings, and summer vacations, are often severely limited or curtailed (Fox, Vaughn, Wyatte, & Dunlap, 2002; Gray, 1998; Turnbull & Ruef, 1996), while marital discord may result as parents disagree on how to manage the cacophony of difficulties emanating from their child's pervasive developmental disorder (Fisman, Wolf, & Noh, 1989; Marcus, Kunce, & Schopler, 1997; Rodrigue, Morgan, & Geffken, 1990).

Family members of children with autism may restrict their social activities and relationships outside the home. Siblings, for example, may avoid inviting friends over for fear that their autistic brother or sister may have a tantrum or behave strangely (Bagenholm & Gilberg, 1991; Fisman et al., 1989; Harris, 1994), while parents may come to increasingly isolate themselves from extended family, friends and other, potential sources of social support (Fox et al., 2002; Koegel, Schreibman, Britten, Burke, & O'Neil, 1982; Marcus et al., 1997; Moes, 1995). Similarly, parents (particularly mothers) may curtail or end employment outside the home in order to provide care for their autistic child (Freeman, Litchfield, & Warfield, 1995; Shearn & Todd, 2000). Thus, in a variety of ways and for various reasons, the social integration of families with autistic children often becomes increasingly constricted as family members are overwhelmed by the stresses and strains of caring for their severely disabled relative.

As the family's social networks decline, social engagement decreases, and social support from others becomes less available. At the same time, overwhelmed family members may also find it increasingly difficult to effectively seek out and make use of what supports they have (Benson, in press). Evidence regarding the adverse impact of caretaking stress and burden on the social integration of families of children with autism is consistent with the stress process framework (Pearlin, 1999) and with research on caregiver stress associated with other disabling conditions such as mental illness, HIV/AIDS and Alzheimer's Disease (Fisher, Benson, & Tessler, 1990; Pearlin, Aneshensel, & LeBlanc, 1997; Pearlin, Mullan, Semple, & Skaff, 1990; Zarit, Orr, & Zarit, 1985).

When asked to estimate the extent to which their child's autism limited their relationships and activities in a variety of life areas, a large percentage of participating parents reported *severe* restrictions in areas such as family activities (41%), social activities outside the home (43%), participation in community groups or organizations (40%), and work (31%), as well as their relationships with friends (21%), extended family members (19%), their spouse (19%), and their children (18%). The multifaceted impact of autism on truncated family networks and engagement is illustrated by the comments of one parent, who noted:

There is really no area (of life) that it autism doesn't affect. . .I spend nearly all of my time looking after "Alex" (her five year-old child with autism). . .Everything else suffers. You eat in shifts so someone can keep on eye on Alex. . .You don't go out, either as a couple or a family . . . I quit my job to be with Alex after school. . .You end up drained and isolated. . .

Not surprisingly, significant positive correlations were found between restricted parent social engagement and parents' report of child symptom severity, with the parents of more severely impaired children reporting greater restrictions in their family and social life. Further, while parental mental health is directly affected by child autism severity, some of autism's impact on parent depression is also indirect, with higher levels of child symptom severity (e.g., social unresponsiveness, aggression, repetitive, self-stimulatory behaviors) resulting in reduced parent social ties and engagement, which, in turn, results to poorer parent adjustment and well-being.

Findings flowing from the first year of the project also show marked variation in the perceived availability and helpfulness of different sources of social support. The sources of informal support rated as most helpful by respondents were spouses and parents, while school personnel and child's primary physician were rated as the most helpful sources of formal support (with 54% rating school staff as being either "very" or "extremely helpful").

Despite the perceived helpfulness of some sources of informal and formal support, what is perhaps most striking about these data, however, is the high percentage of parents reporting a potential source of support was either "unavailable" or "not at all helpful" to them in coping with their child's disorder. Among those potential sources of support viewed as least available or supportive were clergy (80%), coworkers (77%), private and public agencies (64%), and extended family members (43%). These data suggest that many parents of children with autism perceive themselves as being bereft of supportive social ties, both to potential informal sources of assistance and to existing formal support services provided by public and private agencies. In addition, they suggest, at least in some cases, that sources of social "support" may, in fact, be unsupportive, potentially resulting in negative interactions, increased family stress, and an increased likelihood of poor mental health outcomes for parents and other family members (Rook, 1984; Rook & Pietromonaco, 1987).

Institutional Connections: School and Capital

Although preliminary, results from Family-School Autism Project suggest that parents play a pivotal role in the development of their autistic children (Benson et al., 2005). However, higher SES parents and the parents of less severely disabled children are significantly more involved than their peers. This supports prior research on school participation by the parents of nondisabled children indicating that parents with greater cultural and social capital tend to be more actively involved in their children's education than are those with fewer socioeconomic resources (Coleman & Hoffer, 1987; Lareau, 1989; McNeal, 2000).

Based on preliminary findings, there appears to be several avenues through which SES either promotes or hinders parents' educational involvement. In a few cases, lower-SES parents in sample were so preoccupied with securing basic family needs, such as food and housing, that they were simply unable to invest much time or effort in their child's education. In other cases, poorer and less well-educated parents appeared uncertain about how best to engage their child educationally, while in still other cases, these parents appeared to view home and school as largely separate spheres of activity, with teachers and school personnel being primarily responsible for their child's education rather than parents.

Analyses also indicate that the level of support and assistance provided to parents by their child's school is a highly significant predictor of the extent to which parents are educationally involved with their autistic child, with different forms of school support facilitating different forms of parent involvement. Evidence indicates, for example, that parents are most likely to participate in school-based activities when the school provides parents with an open and welcoming environment as well as a variety of specific opportunities for them to participate in their child's education through classroom visits, volunteer work, and participation in school-related groups and organizations. On the other hand, active parent educational involvement in the home was found to be most likely to occur when the school provided the family with direct training, consultation, and other home-based services. Not surprisingly, families with children residing in more affluent communities were significantly more likely to receive home-based school supports compared to families living in communities with fewer economic and social resources.

In sum, the foregoing discussion of parent educational involvement illustrates a number of issues related to the study of social integration. As noted earlier, the extent to which individuals are connected to others, including key groups, organizations, and institutions, has been shown to affect a variety of social and behavioral outcomes, including parent and child adjustment. One particularly important institution affecting the lives of children (and indirectly, families) is the school. In addition, consistent with the findings of the current study, the extent to which parents are able to effectively participate in their child's education has been shown to be influenced by a variety of factors, including the cultural and social capital that socially-resourced families have at their disposal. Similarly, the availability of supportive social networks and other community resources also been linked, more generally, to adaptive parenting practices and to improved child outcomes in a variety of studies of families of both disabled and nondisabled children (Burchinal, Follmer, & Bryant, 1996; Cochran et al., 1990; Hauser-Cram, Warfield, Shonkoff, & Krauss, 2001).

Finally, despite positive societal changes and legal requirements, the relationship between parents and schools is clearly not always positive. While strained relations between parents and schools is not uncommon in regular education (Chrispeels & Rivero, 2001; Fine, 1993; Lareau, 1989; Lareau & Horvat, 1999), home-school conflict in special education is particularly pronounced, with litigation against school systems by parents of children with autism becoming increasingly frequent (Lake & Billingsley, 2000; Stoner, Bock, Thompson, Angell, Barbara, Heyl, & Crowley, 2005; Yell & Drasgow, 2000). In this regard, it is noteworthy that several features specific to autism have contributed to this increased conflict between parents and schools, chief among them the "epidemic" rise in new cases of autism since the early 1990s coupled with the very high cost of providing educational services to these children (in many cases, exceeding $40,000 a year per child).

Under such circumstances, it is almost inevitable that the interests of families and schools will at times collide, leading, at least in some instances, to weakened home-school bonds, increased family stress, and more problematic child outcomes.

Social Integration and Offenders with Mental Illness: Massachusetts FTT Community Re-entry Studies

Victoria is a 28-year-old black female with schizophrenia who has been incarcerated for shoplifting, armed robbery, and assault and battery. According to Victoria she has been "doing time" most of her life. As a youth she spent time in juvenile detention for stealing cars and running away from home. She attributes her criminality to "wanting money, knowing how to shoplift / hustle, drug and liquor use and hanging around with the wrong people," in particular, "the wrong men." Victoria can be violent, and has been homeless with a drug problem, but has never prostituted, "my mom taught me that my cooch is my pride and my joy. I will never give that up for money, but I will stick somebody up with a face mask on." She grew up with one sister and 2 brothers in "the projects" and was first incarcerated as an adult for shoplifting, "I like money and fly clothes." She was released with 2 years probation, violated her probation and returned to prison for 2 more years. Upon release this time, she went, "buck wild," back to drinking and getting high. She had a job at McDonalds, but was arrested and incarcerated for trying to rob a store with a baseball bat. Subsequently, she spent 3 more years in prison. "This is when I turned my life around. I participated in all these programs." However, when she was released, "nothing was stable, going back and forth between people's houses. I felt homeless. I stayed at shelters for a week at a time, but mostly hotels." She had entitlements, an intake appointment at a local mental health clinic, and a case manager who wanted to help her with housing, but, "I never met him because I started using heroin. He was trying to get me my own place, but I was off my meds and using heroin." She began shoplifting, "I was actually taking orders. I had fences. One lady might want 20 pairs of jeans from the GAP and if you insulate a duffle bag with duct tape the beepers don't go off, or you carry in a huge Bed, Bath and Beyond bag and a pair of wire cutters, you're all set . . . they have so many clothes don't notice them missing." She was arrested again, "I was getting greedy and sloppy." Victoria describes living in the community as difficult, "sometimes it is difficult for me, it's hard. I don't like being without money and my attitude is I am going to do what I have to for money."

A large number of studies have examined the ability of individuals with mental illness to reside in the community and their potential for social integration (Bachrach & Lamb, 1989; Grob 1991; Rice & Harris, 1997). However, these studies focus primarily on individuals released from psychiatric hospitals (Hiday, 1996; Perlick, Rosenheck, Clarkin, Sirey, & Raue, 1999; Satsumi, Inada, & Yamauchi, 1998; Swanson, Borum, & Swartz, 1996). For instance, Steadman and colleagues (1998) studied community re-entry of people discharged from acute psychiatric facilities and found that the co-occurrence of a substance abuse disorder is a major factor contributing to community violence. Additionally, a large body of research on specialized case management, such as assertive community treatment, concludes that intensive case management can reduce the risk of violence and re-hospitalization and improve community tenure for individuals discharged from the hospital (Dvoskin & Steadman, 1994; Mueser, Bond, Drake, & Resnick, 1998; Phillips, Burns, Edgar, Mueser, Linkins, Rosenheck, Drake, & Herr, 2001). Thus, for recently released hospitalized individuals, approaches to integration focus on personal characteristics and community or social service resources (networks and capital).

We are only now beginning to address what happens to people with a mental illness who are released from correctional facilities. Recent research on individuals with mental illness released from correctional custody suggests that specialized services are also needed to help integrate this population in the community (Hartwell, Friedman, & Orr, 2001c; Hartwell & Orr, 1999). However, existing service models and the justice system's post release oversight mechanisms do not necessarily take into account the unique experience of ex-inmates returning to the community with mental illness. To begin, criminal justice research on the community reintegration of released inmates rarely distinguishes persons with psychiatric disabilities from the general population of offenders (Gendreau, Goggin, & Cullen, 1999; Vose, 1990), and models predicting recidivism emphasize criminal history variables (Bonta, Law, & Hanson, 1998; Kempf, 1989; Loeber & LeBlanc, 1990).

There is, however, a growing body of literature that examines the impact of specialized or intensive case management programming (formal mechanisms of social networks, support and engagement) for individuals with mental illness involved with the criminal justice system (Draine & Solomon, 1994; Roskes, Feldman, Arrington, & Leisher, 1999; Solomon & Draine, 1995; Wilson, Tien, & Eaves, 1995; Wolff, Diamond, & Helminiak, 1997; Ventura, Cassel, Jacoby, & Huang, 1998). Wolff and colleagues (1997) found that clients receiving the most intensive mental health services also had the most law enforcement contacts. Conversely, Wilson and colleagues (1995) found that intensive case management programs improved the chances of community tenure for offenders with mental illness by providing them a network to rely on at times of crisis, suggesting the buffering feature of support. The most definitive program of research to date, however, indicates that closer surveillance of offenders with mental illness can have an iatrogenic effect and lead to more frequent contact with the criminal justice system (Draine & Solomon, 1994; Solomon & Draine, 1995, 1999; Solomon, Draine, & Marcus, 2002; Solomon et al., 1994;).

During the past several years, a series of studies have been underway in Massachusetts that continue to examine the social integration of offenders with mental illness as they attempt to traverse the divide from correctional custody to the community (see Hartwell, 2001a, b, c, 2003a, b, 2004a, b, 2005). This research consists of ongoing data collection, analysis of a large secondary data set, and qualitative interviews with ex-inmates with psychiatric disabilities. The secondary data originate from the Massachusetts' Department of Mental Health (DMH) Forensic Transition Team (FTT) program. The goal of the FTT program is to help address the needs of individuals with mental illness being released from correctional custody.

In Massachusetts, study data indicate that gender and substance abuse are major factors influencing offender integration due to the influence personal characteristics on configurations of social support, engagement, and networks. For instance, female offenders with mental illness tend to be younger and have less education than their male counterparts. They are more likely to be substance abusers, mood disordered, and have a mental health service history indicating that prior to incarceration they had linkages to community mental health resources or formal supports in the community (Hartwell, 2001b). Still, difficulties in finding meaningful employment post incarceration, a history of service need and reliance, and the shorter sentences they receive for public order and property crimes cycle female offenders through the criminal justice system at a faster rate. This cycling ultimately inhibits their ability to network or make meaningful connections in the community (Hartwell, 2001b). Instead, women are more likely to remain in the community under the supervision of the criminal justice system on probation. Again, individuals with mental illness often fare poorly with mandated formal supports in the community such as probation because they violate their conditions of release, enmeshing themselves further with the criminal justice system (Solomon & Drain, 1999). Rather than returning to the community, they become further entrenched in the justice system network that may provide community and institutional engagement at a formal level, but offers few informal social network ties.

Women also emphasize the importance of engagement in social roles in families (such as mother, daughter, sister) and other networks of informal supports for affirmation. While the benefits of these relationships seem clear, they can also have adverse effects. To begin, most females anticipate returning to their families post incarceration. However, family ties are often attenuated due to serving sentences in an institution far from home, providing an example of environmental or contextual constraints affecting social supports. Additionally, previous social relationships based on deviant behaviors such as drug dealing and use may encourage subsequent forms of deviant or criminal behavior upon release from correctional custody. Essentially, for these females, their engagement with the criminal justice system shapes the nature and configuration of their social engagement after release.

Ex-offenders who are mentally ill and substance abusers have social networks in the community. However, they are misfits in the mental health and substance abuse service systems, and their presence in the criminal justice system is indicative of their disenfranchisement. The high rates of substance abuse including the common use of multiple illicit substances among individuals with mental illness (rates that increase as they age) might provide some measure of the quality of their social ties (Hartwell, 2004a). Substance abuse increases the community integration degree of difficulty for individuals with mental illness (Albercht, Walker, & Levy, 1982; Drake, Bartels, Teague, Noordsy, & Clark, 1993; Solomon & Draine, 1999). For ex-offenders who are also mentally ill substance abusers, these difficulties are compounded. They are older and generally have more services needs. They are more likely to serve misdemeanor sentences in correctional custody and be lost to follow-up by service systems post release (Hartwell, 2004b).

Nearly 70% offenders with mental illness released from correctional custody in Massachusetts are dually diagnosed with mental illness and substance abuse problems (Hartwell, 2004a, b). The dually diagnosed serve sentences related to their substance use (public order offenses, property crimes, and drug dealing offenses). They are also more likely to be female, homeless, and are more likely to violate probation and recidivate to correctional custody after release (Hartwell, 2004a, b). The economic and ecological context and the biological necessity of drug addiction can propel the dually diagnosed ex-offenders into criminal activity as a survival strategy and, in turn, increase the potential for re-arrest. Still, drug use is a social activity creating social networks and resources. However, the characteristics of these networks and quality of their resources (drugs, drug using associates) are negligible and indicative that certain social factors and personal characteristics, including age and gender, impede integration of drug users (Albrecht et al., 1982).

While substance abuse decreases social integration potential, taking prescribed medications in the community enhances individuals' social networks and community reintegration success by helping individuals address their illness and manage symptomatology (Hartwell, 2005). To keep their prescription filled, individuals must be in contact with clinicians and social service providers that offer resources and work to galvanize connections to the community. Most ex-offenders with mental illness understand that taking their medications helps to manage their mental illness and improves their functioning in the community (Hartwell, 2005). Nevertheless, many complain that they have to take "too much medication," and that medications produce socially unacceptable side effects ("they make me drool sometimes"). Many individuals resent having to adhere to strict medication regimens because they remind them of being "sick." Finally, when street drugs enter the picture, prescribed medication is usually abandoned. For many, using street drugs becomes a priority shifting attention from other aspects of their lives and health including medication and symptom management and, consequently, pro-social ties (Hartwell, 2005).

Institutional Connections, Housing, and Social Capital

In Massachusetts as elsewhere, finding a safe place to live after incarceration is difficult. Research has shown that psychiatric symptoms and criminal history are more likely to result in decreased family bonds (Tessler, Gamache, Rossi, Lehman, & Goldman, 1992). For instance, Victoria describes having family, but is bouncing from place to place and describes, "feeling homeless." Essentially, her mental illness and substance abuse make her difficult to live with, and she is "expendable" to the current household because she has little to offer and disrupts its organization. When individuals are released from correctional custody into environments that lack resources or capital to support them, they have a difficult time making strides toward pro-social connections and activities including work, school, and treatment. This emphasis on the role of contextual characteristics of communities and their ability to ameliorate or perpetuate social problems highlights the importance of social integration and its relationship to social capital at both micro-social and macro-social levels.

Communities with little social capital have truncated networks resulting in problems such as limited housing options. In this scenario, nearly a third of ex-offenders with mental illness are homeless at release from correctional custody, but when asked about their housing preferences ex-offenders with mental illness say they would like to live "on their own." In reality, living on their own can prove isolating and lonely due to their limited social supports. Supportive housing is the next favored option, but supportive housing is not always available for ex-inmates and for individuals with psychiatric disabilities, and living amongst others with similar disabilities, and living amongst challenging. Nonetheless, in the short-term, individuals that remain in the community for the longest time post release often live in supportive housing arrangements or with their families (Hartwell, 2003a; 2005). In both these scenarios ex-offenders are living amongst other people, engaged as a part of a larger network, sharing resources and supports. Whether with family or in supportive housing, social networks are a requisite for both housing resources and the maintenance of appropriate social supports necessary for community engagement post incarceration.

Still, the characteristics of the neighborhoods and communities where ex-offenders reside offer important dimensions to understand the complexities of integration. For example, many ex-offenders return to communities with institutional resources and supports in place to ease their transitions. Although institutional resources and supports are a facet of social capital, they are not usually the features that facilitate collective action and cohesion. Poor, disorganized communities have institutional supports in place because they tend to lack formal social supports and networks. Conversely, ex-offenders are not welcome in communities with informal supports and rich social networks of engaged individuals. These more cohesive communities are essentially socially integrated and have the collective efficacy to keep crime and criminals away (Sampson et al., 1997; Gibson, 2002), while areas lacking social cohesion or collective efficacy are more prone to crime and other types of deviance. Thus, although social integration appears to be a goal during community re-entry, integrated communities can also be an ecological/contextual barrier for psychiatrically disabled ex-offenders returning to the community. In many scenarios, psychiatrically disabled ex-offenders ultimately drift to disorganized communities where they can be integrated into more formal service systems in lieu of developing more informal community networks.

Findings from the Massachusetts FTT research program also support the thesis that the experience of offenders with mental illness released from correctional custody is largely shaped by their criminal history and formal entanglements with institutions (courts, social services). Most recent criminal charge and length of incarceration affect their return to the community (Hartwell, 2003 a, b). The challenge of release from a penal institution and the stigma inevitably encountered in the community includes both public perception/acceptance and the response of the social service system. For instance, high profile offenders with mental illness (sex offenders, individuals who have committed homicide) are more often "stepped-down" from prisons directly to locked hospitals. That is, individuals with certain personal characteristics are generally kept from the community and are rather moved through a system reliant on formal supports and institutions.

In sum, individuals with mental illness are released from correctional custody to the community where their personal characteristics and social linkages, both formal and informal, influence the systems charged in their control and treatment, and, in turn, ascribe their social location upon release (Horwitz, 1990; Kitsuse, 1962; Scheff, 1966). Social distance theory asserts that individuals that are considered deviant negotiate a separate or distant social reality (Horwitz, 1990; McCall & Simmons, 1966). They are outsiders, isolated, and set furthest away from normative social interaction (Horwitz, 1990; McCall & Simmons, 1966). Link and colleagues (1999) noted that when the mentally ill are perceived as dangerous, that they have limited social interaction with others who desire social distance from them. The salience of social integration in this distant social reality where social controls include segregated institutions such as prisons and hospitals is negligible until individuals attempt to traverse the distance from these institutions to the community.

The Limitations of Social Integration as a Meta-Concept

While our two research programs differ in their substantive focus, they nevertheless share certain commonalities, which tie them to the study of social integration generally and the sociology of mental health specifically. Both studies, for example, clearly illustrate the critical importance of social integration to successful social adaptation. For the families of autistic children, the availability and use of supportive social ties both reduces stress and promotes child learning and development, while for mentally ill offenders, successful community integration is clearly contingent upon supportive pro-social connections with family members, service providers and even institutions. At the same time, both studies underscore how social networks can erode due to macro and micro social processes. Finally, both studies also point to the ways that supportive social relationships are embedded in the wider social structure in which they occur.

Understanding social integration through a framework that includes social networks, social support, levels of social engagement, and social capital enables us to better understand the sociology of mental health and the importance of social structure. However, there needs to be much more work on identifying the specific causal mechanisms and empirically delineating the relationships among all the potential components of the social integration construct. For example, while our conceptual framework (see Figure 1) posits a bi-directional relationship between social networks and social engagement, no research examining this relationship currently exists. Similarly, evidence concerning the relationship between social support and social engagement is equivocal, with research generally suggesting that the correlation between social engagement and perceived support is only modest (Cohen, 1988; Cohen & Wills, 1985). Research indicates that different elements of social support (for example, perceived and received support) are, themselves, often only weakly related.

Measures of social integration are not interchangeable and thus investigators should think carefully about what aspects of social integration they believe are most pertinent to assess in their research. It is also advisable, where possible, to employ multiple integration measures (including community-level measures of social capital) in the same study. This would allow investigators to examine the relationships among measures and to assess their individual and combined effects on outcomes of interest. As this chapter elucidates, social integration can mean different things to different groups. There are clear variations in human capital and social structure that alter the ways in which investigators should measure and understand social integration. For instance, what does it mean to be integrated to families with a child with a disability or individuals with multiple stigmas? Are the "preferred" outcomes informal rather than reliance on formal networks and supports (institutions). Finally, in some ways, although social integration can be understood at individual and aggregate levels, it seems to operate most fluidly at the aggregate level.

The appeal of social integration as a sociological construct is that it shifts attention from individual characteristics and behaviors to the environment or context and allows us to address questions about the availability of resources, macro-level dynamics that shape environments, and behavior/adaptation in relation to resources. Social integration is both a feature and consequence of social conditions and social arrangements influencing the lives of individuals and aggregates. Focusing on interpersonal interaction in social structural context, social integration permits researchers to examine social participation both based on and resulting in social arrangements and well-being. Thus, while mental health research continues to make a contribution to key theoretical and empirical debates regarding social integration, social integration remains mainstream concept used in sociology to provide insights into the experience of mental health and illness.

Acknowledgments. Preparation of this chapter was partially supported by U.S. Department of Education Grants H324C010125 and H324C040092.

References

Acock, A. C., & Hurlbert, J. S. (1993). Social networks, marital status, and well-being. *Social Networks, 15*, 309–334.

Albanese, L. A., San Miguel, S. K., & Koegel, R. L. (1995). Social support for families. In R. L. Koegel & L. K. Koegel (Eds.), *Teaching Children with Autism* (pp. 95–104). Baltimore: Brookes.

Albrecht, G. L., Walker, V. G., and Levy, J. A. (1982). Social distance from the stigmatized: A test of two theories. *Social Science and Medicine, 16*, 1319–1327.

Argyle, M. (1992). Benefits produced by supportive social relationships. In H. O. F. Veisel & U. Baumann (Eds.), *The Meaning and Measurement of Social Support*. New York: Hemisphere.

Bachrach, L., &. Lamb, H. R. (1989). What we have learned from deinstitutionalization. *Psychiatric Annuals, 19*, 12–21.

Bägenholm, A., & Gillberg, C. (1991). Psychosocial effects on siblings of children with autism and mental retardation: A population-based study. *Journal of Mental Deficiency Research, 35*, 291–307.

Benson, P. R. (in press). The impact of child symptom severity on depressed mood among parents of children with autism spectrum disorders: The mediating role of stress proliferation. *Journal of Autism and Developmental Disorders*.

Benson, P. R., & Karlof, K. L. (2003a). *The role of the family in the education of children with autism*. Presentation given at the Second Annual Conference on the Shared Implementation of IDEA. Arlington, VA (April).

Benson, P. R., & Karlof, K. L. (2003b). *Parent involvement in the education of young children with autism*. Presentation given at the Annual Meetings of the Association of the Severely Handicapped. Chicago (December).

Benson, P. R., Karlof, K. L., & Siperstein, G. N. (In submission). Parent involvement in the education of young children with ASD.

Benson, P. R., Siperstein, G. N., Karlof, K. L., & Widaman, K. F. (2004). Preliminary findings from a longitudinal study of children with autism and their families. Presentation given at the Office of Special Education Programs Project Directors' Meetings, Washington, D.C. (July).

Beresford, B. A. (1994). Resources and strategies: How parents cope with the care of a disabled child. *Journal of Child Psychology and Psychiatry, 35*, 171.

Berkman, L. F., & Glass, T. (2000). Social integration, social networks, social support and health. In L. F. Berkman & I. Kawachi (Eds.), *Social Epidemiology* (pp. 137–173). Oxford: Oxford University Press.

Berkman, L. F., Glass, T., Brissett, I., & Seeman, T. E. (2000). From social integration to health: Durkheim and the new millennium. *Social Science and Medicine, 51*, 843–857.

Berkman, L. F., & Syme, S. L. (1979). Social networks, host resistance and mortality: A nine-year follow-up study of Alameda County residents. *American Journal of Epidemiology, 109*, 186–204.

Bonta, J., Law, M., & Hanson, K. (1998). The prediction of criminal and violent recidivism among mentally disordered offenders: A meta-analysis. *Psychological Bulletin, 123*, 123–142.

Bourdieu, P. (1986). The forms of capital. In J. G. Richardson (Ed.), *A Handbook of Theory: Research for the Sociology of Education* (pp. 241–58). New York: Greenwood Press.

Bowling, A., & Browne, P. D. (1991). Social networks, health, and emotional well-being among the oldest old in London. *Journal of Gerontology, 46*, 20–32.

Boyd, B. A. (2002). Examining the relationship between stress and lack of social support in mothers of children with autism. *Focus on Autism and Other Developmental Disabilities, 17*, 208–215.

Brissette, I., Cohen, S., & Seeman, T. E. (2000). Measuring social integration and social networks. In S. Cohen, I. G. Underwood, and B. H. Gottlieb (Eds.), *Social Support Measurement and Intervention: A Guide for Health and Social Scientists* (pp. 53–85). New York: Oxford University Press.

Bristol, M. M. (1987). Mothers of children with autism or communication disorders: Successful adaptation and the Double ABCX Model. *Journal of Autism and Developmental Disorders, 17*, 469–486.

Burchinal, M. R., Follmer, A., & Bryant, D. M. (1996). The relations of maternal social support and family structure with maternal responsiveness and child outcomes among African-American families. *Developmental Psychology, 32*, 1073–83.

Burt, R. S., & Minor, M. (Eds.) (1987). *Applied network analysis.* Beverly Hills, CA: Sage.

Burton, R. P. D. (1998). Global integrative meaning as a mediating factor in the relationship between social roles and psychological distress. *Journal of Health and Social Behavior, 39*, 201–215.

Chrispeels, J. H., & Rivero, E. (2001). Engaging Latino families for student success: How parent education can reshape parents' sense of place in the education of their children. *Peabody Journal of Education, 76*, 119–169.

Cochran, M., Larner, M., Riley, D., Gunnarsson, L., & Henderson, C. (Eds.) (1990). *Extending families: The social networks of parents and their children.* New York: Cambridge University Press.

Cohen, S. (1988). Psychosocial models of the role of social support in the etiology of physical disease. *Health Psychology, 7*, 269–297.

Cohen, S. (2001). Social relationships and health. *Advances in Mind-Body Medicine 17*, 5–7.

Cohen, S., Gottlieb, B., & Underwood, I.G. (2000). Social relationships and health: Challenges for measurement and intervention. In S. Cohen, L. G. Underwood, & B. H. Gottlieb (Eds.), *Social support measurement and intervention: A guide for health and social scientists* (pp. 3–28). New York: Oxford University Press.

Cohen, S., & Wills, T. A. (1985). Stress, social support, and the buffering hypothesis. *Psychological Bulletin, 98*, 310–357.

Coleman, J. S. (1990). *Foundations of social theory.* Cambridge, MA: Harvard University Press.

Coleman, J. S., & Hoffer, T. (1987). *Public and private high schools: The impact of communities.* New York: Basic Books.

Coser, R. (1974). *Greedy institutions.* New York: Free Press.

Cotterell, J. (1996). *Social networks and social influences in adolescence.* London: Routledge.

Dominigue, B., Cutler, B., & McTarnaghan, J. (2000). The experience of autism in the lives of families. In A. M. Wetherby and B. M. Prizant (Eds.), *Autism Spectrum Disorders: A Transactional Developmental Perspective* (pp. 269–284). Baltimore, MD: Brookes.

Draine, J., & Solomon, P. (1994). Jail recidivism and the intensity of case management services among homeless persons with mental illness leaving jail. *Journal of Psychiatry and Law 22*, 245–261.

Drake, R. E., Bartels, S. J., Teague, G. B., Noordsy, D. L., & Clark, R. E. (1993). Treatment of substance abuse in severely mentally ill patients. *The Journal of Nervous and Mental Disease, 181*, 606–611.

Dunst, C. J., Trivette, C. M., & Jodry, W. (1997). Influences of social support on children with disabilities and their families. In M. Guralnick (Ed.), *The effectiveness of early intervention* (pp. 499–522). Baltimore: P.H. Brookes.

Durkheim, E. (1933). *The division of labor in society.* New York: The Free Press.

Durkheim, E. (1951). *Suicide.* New York: The Free Press.

Dvoskin, J. A., & Steadman, H. J. (1994). Using intensive case management to reduce violence by mentally ill persons in the community. *Hospital & Community Psychiatry, 45*, 679–684.

Faris, E. L., & Dunham, H. W. (1939). *Mental disorder in urban areas: An ecological study of schizophrenia and other psychoses*. Chicago: University of Chicago Press.

Fine, M. (1993). [Ap]parent involvement: Reflections on parents, power, and urban public schools. *Teachers College Record, 94*, 682–710.

Fischer, C. S. (1982). *To dwell among friends: Personal networks in town and city*. Chicago: University of Chicago Press.

Fisher, G. A., Benson, P. R., & Tessler, R. (1990). Family response to mental illness: Developments since deinstitutionalization. In J. Greenley (Ed.), *Research in Community and Mental Health* (vol. 6, pp.203–36). Greenwich, CT: JAI Press.

Fisman, S. N., Wolf, L. C., & Noh, S. (1989). Marital intimacy in parents of exceptional children. *Canadian Journal of Psychiatry, 34*, 519–525.

Fox, L., Vaughn, B. J., Wyatte, M.L., & Dunlap, G. (2002). "We can't expect other people to understand": Parent perspectives on problem behavior. *Exceptional Children, 68*, 437–450.

Freeman, R., Litchfield, L., & Warfield, M. E. (1995). Balancing work and family responsibilities: Perspectives of parents of children with developmemtal disabilities. *Families in Society: The Journal of Contemporary Human Services, 76*, 506–514.

Gendreau, P., Goggin, C., & Cullen, F. (1999). The effects of prison sentences on recidivism. *The Department of the Solicitor General Canada*. User Report, No. 24.

Gibson, C. L., Jihong, Z., Nicholas, L. P., & Gaffney, M. J. (2002). Social integration, individual perceptions of collective efficacy, and fear of crime in three cities. *Justice Quarterly, 19*, 538–563.

Goode, W. J. (1960). A theory of role strain. *American Sociological Review, 25*, 483–96.

Granovetter, M. (1973). The strength of weak ties. *American Journal of Sociology, 25*, 1360–1380.

Gray, D. E. (1998). *Autism and the family: Problems, prospects, and coping with the disorder*. Springfield, IL: Charles C. Thomas.

Greenfield, T. K., Rehm, J., & Rogers, J. D. (2001). Effects of depression and social integration on the relationship between alcohol consumption and all-cause mortality. *Addiction, 97*, 29–38.

Grob, G. N. (1991). *From asylum to community: Mental health policy in America*. Princeton, NJ: Princeton University Press.

Haines, V. A., & Hurlbert, J. S. (1992). Network range and health. *Journal of Health and Social Behavior, 33*, 254–268.

Harris, S. L. (1994). *Siblings of children with autism: A guide for families*. Bethesda, MD: Woodbine House.

Hartwell, S. W. (2001a). An examination of racial differences among mentally ill offenders in Massachusetts. *Psychiatric Services, 52*, 234–236.

Hartwell, S. W. (2001b). Female mentally ill offenders and their community reintegration needs. An initial examination. *International Journal of Law and Psychiatry, 24*, 1–11.

Hartwell, S. W. (2003a). Short-term outcomes for offenders with mental illness released from incarceration. *International Journal of Offender Therapy and Comparative Criminology, 47*, 145–158.

Hartwell, S. W. (2003b). Prison, hospital or community: Community re-entry and mentally ill offenders. *Research in Community and Mental Health, 12*, 199–220.

Hartwell, S. W. (2004a). Triple stigma: persons with mental illness and substance abuse problems in the criminal justice system. *Criminal Justice Policy Review, 15*, 89–99.

Hartwell, S. W. (2004b). Comparisons of offenders with mental illness only and offenders with dual diagnoses. *Psychiatric Services*, *55*, 145–149.

Hartwell, S. W. (2005). The organizational response to community re-entry. In S.W. Hartwell (Ed.), *The organizational response to persons with mental illness involved with the criminal justice system.* Research in Social Problems and Public Policy Series, Volume 12 (pp. 197–217). Elsevier Science.

Hartwell, S. W., Friedman, D., & Orr, K. (2001). From correctional custody to community: The Massachusetts Forensic Transition Team. *New England Journal of Public Policy*, *19*, 73–82.

Hartwell, S. W., & Orr, K. (1999). The Massachusetts Forensic Transition Program for mentally ill offenders re-entering the community. *Psychiatric Services*, *50*, 1220–1222.

Hauser-Cram, P., Warfield, M. E., Shonkoff, J. P., & Krauss, M. W. (2001). Children with disabilities: A longitudinal study of child development and parent well-being. *Monographs of the Society for Research in Child Development*, *66*, 1–131.

Hiday, V. A. (1996). Outpatient commitment: Official coercion in the community. *Coercion and Aggressive Community Treatment: A New Frontier in Mental Health Law.* New York, NY: Plenum Press.

Hirsch, B. J. (1980). Natural support systems and coping with major life events. *American Journal of Community Psychology*, *8*, 159–172.

Horwitz, A. V. (1990). The logic of social control. New York: Plenum Press.

House, J. S. (1981). Work, stress, and social support. Reading, MA: Addison-Wesley.

House, J. S., Landis, K. R., & Umberson, D. (1988). Social relationships and health. *Science*, *241*, 540–545.

Hughes, M., & Gove, W. R. (1989). Explaining the negative relationship between social integration and mental health: The case of living alone. *American Sociological Association, Sociological Abstracts*.

Hurlbert, J. S., Haines, V. A., & Beggs, J. J. (2000). Core networks and tie activation: What kind of routine networks allocate resources in nonroutine situation? *American Sociological Review*, *65*, 598–618.

Kawachi, I., & Berkman, L. (2000). Social cohesion, social capital, and health. In L. F. Berkman & I. Kawachi (Eds.), *Social Epidemiology* (pp. 174–190). New York: Oxford University Press.

Kawachi, I., Kennedy, B. P., & Glass, R. (1999). Social capital and self-rated health: A contextual analysis. *American Journal of Public Health*, *89*, 1187–1193.

Kawachi, I., Kennedy, B. P., & Lochner, K. (1997). Long live community: Social capital as public health. *American Prospect*, *35*, 56–59.

Kempf, K. (1989). Delinquency: Do the dropouts drop back in? *Youth and Society*, *20*, 269–289.

Kessler R. C., McGonagle, K. A. Zhao S., Nelson C. B., Hughes M., Eshleman S., Wittchen, H. U., & Kendler K. S. (1994) Lifetime and 12-month prevalence of DSM-III-R psychiatric disorders in the United States. Results from the National Comorbidity Survey. *Archives of General Psychiatry, 51, 8-19.*

Kituse, J. (1962). Social reaction to deviant behavior: problems in theory and method. *Social Problems*, *9*, 247–256.

Koegel, R. L., Schreibman, L., Britten, K., Burke, J. C., & O'Neil, R. E. (1982). A comparison of parent training to direct clinic treatment. In R. Koegel, A. Rinover, & A. L. Engle (Eds.), *Educating and understanding autistic children* (pp.260–279). San Diego: College Hill Press.

Konstantareas, M. K., & Homatidis, S. (1991). Effects of developmental disorder on parents: Theoretical and applied considerations. *The Psychiatric Clinics of North America, 14,* 183–198.

Lake, J., & Billingsley, B. (2000). An analysis of factors that contribute to parent-school conflict in special education. *Remedial and Special Education, 21,* 240–252.

Lareau, A. (1989). *Home advantage: Social class and parental intervention in elementary education.* Philadelphia: Falmer.

Lareau, A., & Horvat, E. M. (1999). Moments of social inclusion and exclusion: Race, class, and cultural capital in family-school relationships. *Sociology of Education, 72,* 37–53.

Lin, N., & Ensel, W. M. (1989). Life stress and health: Stressors and resources. *American Sociological Review, 54,* 382–99.

Lin, N., & Peek, K. (1999). Social networks and mental health. In A. V. Horwitz & T. L Schneid (Eds.), *Handbook for the study of mental health: Social contexts, theories, and systems* (pp. 239–283). Cambridge University Press.

Link, B. G., Phelan, J. C., Bresnahan, M., Stueve, A., & Pescosolido, B. A. (1999). Public conceptions of mental illness: Labels, causes, dangerousness, and social distance. *American Journal of Public Health, 89,* 1328–1333.

Loeber, R., & LeBlanc, M. (1990). Towards a developmental criminology. In M. Tonry & N. Morris (Eds.), *Crime and justice Vol. 12* (pp. 375–473). Chicago: University of Chicago Press.

Marcus, L. M., Kunce, L. J., & Schopler, E. (1997). Working with families. In D. R. Cohen & F. R. Volkmar (Eds.), *Handbook of autism and pervasive developmental disorders.* New York: Wiley.

Marsden, P. V. (1990). Network data and analysis. *Annual Review of Sociology, 18,* 435–463.

Marks, S. (1977). Multiple roles and role strain: Some notes on human energy, time, and commitment. *American Sociological Review, 42,* 921–936.

McCall, G. J., & Simmons, J.L. (1966). *Identities and interactions.* New York: The Free Press.

McNeal, R. B. (2000). Differential effects of parent involvement on cognitive and behavioral outcomes by sociodemographic status. *Journal of Socio-Economics, 30,* 171–179.

Meyer, P. C., Christen, S., Graf, J., Ruesch, P., & Hell, D. (2002). Determinants of quality of life of mentally ill persons. *Osterreichische Zeitschrift Fur Soziologie, 27,* 63–79.

Moes, D. (1995). Parent education and parent stress. In R. L. Koegel, & L. K. Koegel (Eds.), *Teaching Children with Autism* (pp.79–94). Baltimore: Brookes.

Mueser, K. T., Bond, G. R., Drake, R. E., & Resnick, S. G. (1998). Models of community care for severe mental illness: A review of research on case management. *Schizophrenia Bulletin, 24,* 37–74.

Norton, P., & Drew, R. (1994). Autism and potential family stressors. *American Journal of Family Therapy, 22,* 67–76.

Park, R. E., Burgess, E. W., & McKenzie, R. D. (1925). *The city.* Chicago: University of Chicago Press.

Pearlin, L. I. (1999). The stress process revisited: Reflections on concepts and their interrelationship. In C. S. Aneshensel, & J. C. Phelan (Eds.), *Handbook for the study of mental health: Social contexts, theories, and systems* (pp. 395–415). New York: Cambridge University Press.

Pearlin, L. I., Aneschensel, C. A., & LeBlanc, A..J. (1997). The forms and mechanisms of stress proliferation: The case of AIDS caregivers. *Journal of Health and Social Behavior, 38,* 223–236.

Pearlin, L. I., Mullan, J. T., Semple, S. J., & Skaff, M. M. (1990). Caregiving and the stress process: An overview of concepts and measures. *Journal of Gernotology, 30,* 583–94.

Perlick, D. A., Rosenheck, R. A., Clarkin, J. F., Sirey, J., & Raue, P. (1999). Symptoms predicting inpatient service use among patients with bipolar affective disorder. *Psychiatric Services, 50,* 806–812.

Pescosolido, B. A. (1992). Beyond rational choice: The social dynamics of how people seek help. *American Journal of Sociology, 97,* 1096–1138.

Pescosolido, B. A. (2005). Social Networks. In G. Albrecht (Ed.) *Encyclopedia of disability.* Thousand Oaks, CA: Sage Publications.

Pescosolido, B. A., & Rubin, B. (2000). The web of group affiliations revisited: Social life, postmodernism, and sociology. *American Sociological Review, 65,* 52–76.

Phillips, S., Burns, B., Edgar, E., Mueser, K., Linkins, K., Rosenheck, R., Drake, R., & Herr, E. (2001). Moving assertive community treatment into standard practice. *Psychiatric Services, 52,* 771–779.

Putnam, R. D. (1993a). *Making democracy work: Civic traditions in modern Italy.* Princeton, N.J.: Princeton University Press.

Putnam, R. D. (1993b). The prosperous community: Social capital and public life. *American Prospect, 13,* 35–42.

Putnam, R. D. (1995). Bowling alone: America's declining social capital. *Journal of Democracy, 6,* 65–78.

Radloff, L. S. (1977). The CES-D scale: A self-report depression scale for research in the general population. *Journal of Consulting and Clinical Psychology, 56,* 893–897.

Regier, D. A., Narrow, W. E., Rae, D. S., Manderscheid, R. W., Locke, B. Z., & Goodwin, F. K. (1993). The de facto US mental and addictive disorders service system: Epidemiologic catchment area retrospective 1-year prevalence rates of disorders and services. *Archives of General Psychiatry, 50,* 85–94.

Rice, M. E., & Harris, G. T. (1997). The treatment of mentally disordered offenders. *Psychology, Public Policy, and the Law, 3,* 126–183.

Rodrigue, J. R., Morgan, S. B., & Geffken, G. R. (1990). Families of autistic children: Psychosocial functioning of mothers. *Journal of Clinical Child Psychology, 19,* 371–379.

Rook, K. S. (1984). The negative side of social interaction. *Journal of Personality and Social Psychology, 46,* 1097–1108.

Rook, K. S. (1990). Social networks as a source of social control in older adults' lives. In H. Giles, N. Coupland, & J. Wiemann (Eds.). *Communities, health, and the elderly* (pp. 45–63). Manchester: University of Manchester Press.

Rook, K. S., & Pietromonaco, P. (1987). Close relationships: Ties that heal or ties that bind? *Advances in Personal Relationships, 1,* 1–33.

Roskes, E., Feldman, R., Arrington, S., & Leisher, M. (1999). A model program for the treatment of mentally ill offenders in the community. *Community Mental Health Journal, 35,* 461–475.

Sampson, R. J. (2003). The neighborhood context of well-being. *Perspectives in Biology and Medicine, 46,* S53–64.

Sampson, R. J., & Laub, J.H. (2003). Desistance from crime over the life course. In J. T. Mortimer, & M. Shanahan (Eds.), *Handbook of the life course* (pp. 295–310). New York: Kluwer Academic/Plenum.

Sampson, R. J., Raudenbush, S. W., & Earls, F. (1997). Neighborhoods and violent crime: A multilevel study of collective efficacy. *Science, 277*, 918–924.

Satsumi, Y., Inada, T., & Yamauch, T. (1998). Criminal offenses among discharged mentally ill individuals: Determinants of the duration of discharge and absence of diagnostic specificity. *International Journal of Law and Psychiatry, 21*, 197–207.

Scheff, T. J. (1966). *Being mentally ill*. Chicago: Aldine Publishing Company.

Segal, S. P., Baumohl, J., Moyles, E. W. (1980). Neighborhood types and community reaction to the mentally ill: A paradox of intensity. *Journal of Health and Social Behavior, 21*, 345–359.

Shaw, C. R., & McKay, H. D. (1942). *Juvenile delinquency in urban areas*. Chicago: University of Chicago Press.

Shearn, J., & Todd, S. (2000). Maternal employment and family responsibilities: The perspectives of mothers of children with intellectual disabilities. *Journal of Applied Research in Intellectual Disabilities, 13*, 109–131.

Sieber, S. (1974). Toward a theory of role accumulation. *American Sociological Review, 39*, 567–578.

Simon, R. W. (1995). Gender, multiple roles, role meaning, and mental health. *Journal of Health and Social Behavior, 36*, 182–94.

Solomon, P., & Draine, J. (1995). Jail recidivism in a forensic case management program. *Health & Social Work, 20*, 167–173.

Solomon, P., & Draine, 0. (1999). Explaining lifetime criminal arrests among clients of a psychiatric probation and parole service. *Journal of the American Academy of Psychiatry and Law, 27*, 239–251.

Solomon, P., Draine, J., & Marcus, S.C. (2002). Predicting incarceration of clients of a psychiatric probation and parole service. *Psychiatric Services, 53*, 50–56.

Solomon, P., Draine, J., & Meyerson, A. (1994). Jail recidivism and receipt of community mental health services. *Hospital & Community Psychiatry, 45*, 793–797.

Steadman, H. J., Mulvey, E. P., Monahan, J., Robbins, P. C., Appelbaum, P. S., Grisso, T., Roth, L. H., & Silver, E. (1998). Violence by people discharged from acute psychiatric inpatient facilities and by others in the same neighborhoods. *Archives of General Psychiatry, 55*, 393–401.

Stoner, J. B., Bock, S. J., Thompson, J. R., Angell, M., Barbara, E., Heyl, S., & Crowley, E. P. (2005). Welcome to our world: Parent perceptions of interactions between parents of young children with ASD and education professionals. *Focus on Autism and Other Developmental Disabilities, 20*, 39–51.

Suitor, J. J., Pillimer, K., & Keeton, S. (1995). When experience counts: The effects of experiential and structural similarity on patterns of support and interpersonal stress. *Social Forces, 73*, 1573–1588.

Swanson, J., Borum, R., Swartz, M. (1996). Psychotic symptoms and disorders and the risk of violent behavior in the community. *Criminal Behavior and Mental Health, 6*, 317–338.

Tessler, R. C., Gamache, G., Rossi, P., Lehman, A., & Goldman, H. (1992). The kindred bonds of mentally ill homeless persons. In P. O'Malley (Ed.), *Homelessness: New England and beyond* (pp. 265–280). Amherst, MA: University of Massachusetts Press.

Thoits, P. A. (1983). Multiple identities and psychological well-being: A reformulation and test of the social isolation hypothesis. *American Sociological Review, 48*, 174–187.

Thoits, P. A. (1999). Sociological approaches to mental illness. In A. V. Horwitz & T. L. Scheid (Eds.), *A handbook for the study of mental health* (pp. 121–138). New York: Cambridge University Press.

Turnull, A., & Ruef, M. (1996). Family perspectives on problem behavior. *Mental Retardation, 34,* 280–294.

Turner, R. J., & Turner, J. B. (2000). Social integration and support. In C. S. Aneshensel, & J. C. Phelan (Eds.), *Handbook of the sociology of mental health* (pp. 301–319). New York: Plenum.

Umberson, D. (1987). Family status and health behaviors: Social control as a dimension of social intergration. *Journal of Health and Social Behavior, 28,* 306–319.

Vaux, A. (1988). *Social support: Theory, research, and intervention.* New York: Praeger.

Verba, S., Lehman-Schlolzman, K., & Brady, H. E. (1995). *Voice and equality: Civic volunteerism and American politics.* Cambridge, MA: Harvard University Press.

Ventura, L. A., Cassel, C. A., Jacoby, J. E., & Huang, B. (1998). Case management and recidivism of mentally Ill persons released from jail. *Psychiatric Services, 49,* 1330–1337.

Vose, G. (1990). The effect of community reintergration on rates of recidivism: A statistical overview of data for the years 1971 through 1987. Massachusetts Department of Correction. July, 16, 389–421.

Wellman, B., & Wortley, S. (1990). Different strokes from different folks: Community ties and social support. *American Journal of Sociology, 96,* 558–588.

Wethington, E., & Kessler, R. C. (1986). Perceived support. received support, and adjustment to stressful life events. *Journal of Health and Social Behavior, 27,* 78–90.

Wilcox, B. L. (1981). Social networks in adjusting to marital separation. In B. H. Gottlieb (Ed.), *Social networks and social support* (pp. 97–115). Beverly Hills, CA: Sage.

Wilson, D., Tien, G., & Eaves, D. (1995). Increasing the community tenure of mentally disordered offenders: An assertive case management program. *International Journal of Law and Psychiatry, 18,* 61–69.

Wilson, W. J. (1987). *The truly disadvantaged.* Chicago: University of Chicago Press.

Wolff, N., Diamond, R. J., & Helminiak, T. W. (1997). A new look at an old issue: People with mental illness and the law enforcement system. *The Journal of Mental Health Administration, 24,* 152–165.

Woolcock, M. (1998). Social capital and economic development: Toward a theoretical synthesis and policy framework. *Theory and Society, 27,* 151–208.

Yell, M. L. & Drasgow, E. (2000). Litigating a free appropriate public education: The Lovaas hearings and cases. *The Journal of Special Education, 33,* 205–214.

Zarit, S. H., Orr, N., & Zarit, J. M. (1985). *The hidden victims of Alzheimer's Disease: Families under stress.* New York: New York University Press.

15
Sociological Traditions in the Study of Mental Health Services Utilization

Donna D. McAlpine and Carol A. Boyer

Sociological accounts of the utilization of mental health services echo the conceptual frameworks and language that have long been the domain of the discipline. There is a rich tradition of research describing individuals who use care and their interactions with health care professionals and the institutions that define the mental health care system. This body of research demonstrates that pervasive social influences that go beyond the characteristics of the illness or its symptoms shape individuals' help-seeking behavior and treatment experiences. In the earliest work that incorporated sociological theory, Talcott Parsons (1951) defined help-seeking in terms of the social roles of the sick and their physicians; social norms and expectations exerted powerful influences on decision-making when ill and on the structure and organization of care. Although Parsons' concept of the sick role fit less well with mental illnesses, his conceptualization of the doctor-patient relationship as essentially socially defined, informed research on utilization for all health problems. Similarly when closely tied to disciplinary interests, mental health utilization research offers a platform for studying larger sociological concepts of attribution, social inequalities, countervailing power relationships, social organization, and socialization. Mental health utilization research likewise informs the broader discipline about the social context of individual, group and organizational behavior.

The search for how and why individuals seek and use mental health services is fundamentally rooted in the process of social selection (Greenley & Mechanic, 1976; Mechanic, 1978), a dominating concept in much of social science research. Studies with both treated and community samples document large variation in treatment patterns for persons with mental health problems and have reinforced the need to examine the social processes by which persons are selected into care. Models of help-seeking that give sole or primary emphasis to either physiological distress, symptoms or "need" (medical models) or to rational decision making processes (economic models) overlook critical social processes that facilitate, delay, or impede persons getting into treatment. Fully understanding variations in treatment patterns for mental health problems, therefore, is essentially a sociological enterprise.

In this chapter, we provide an overview of research that has contributed to the understanding of social selection into mental health treatment. We locate findings from this research in the broader sociological tradition that gives preeminence to the social context of people's lives, and their relationships with other individuals and institutions. A coherent approach for advancing knowledge about mental health services utilization would benefit from using theoretical models that organize existing research findings and guide future research. Three broad perspectives meet this challenge: 1) societal reaction theories; 2) theories of illness behavior; and 3) social network theories. The contributions of each of these perspectives for understanding variation in help-seeking are reviewed. Moreover, we highlight the potential for these sociological perspectives to contribute to unanswered questions about the gaps and variation in treatment rates for persons with mental health problems. Finally, we critically examine theories of seeking and using mental health services to identify the concepts that link them to the wider discipline of sociology.

Social Selection as the Core of Sociological Inquiry

In most or all sub-fields of sociology, social selection has been a central concept challenging the equally essential presumption in sociology that social conditions are causally related to outcomes. Understanding selection processes matters, whether one's interests concern health, occupation, education, marriage, deviance or a myriad of other statuses (Mechanic, 1978). The principles underlying how individuals or groups are sorted into various social roles – married or unmarried, employed or unemployed, educated in what schools and colleges, treated or not treated, sentenced to jail terms or not – represent powerful processes in understanding social life. For instance, to understand whether marriage offers social, psychological or economic advantages, the question of whether persons with these advantages are more likely to be selected into marriage must be resolved.

Individuals are selected into various positions or groups based on a wide variety of factors: genetics and biology, temperament or innate intelligence may all be the basis of selection. The observation that persons with serious mental illness may be selected into lower socioeconomic statuses is an example of the importance of health selection, which has received wide attention in the literature. The contribution of sociologists is their attention to social selection—or the social characteristics that account for "the sorting and resorting that continuously go on among social groups" (Mechanic, 1975, p. 394).

The social characteristics of individuals partially determine those who do (and do not) enter various positions. Likewise organizations exert selective processes that facilitate, delay or deny entry based on social criteria. The mental health system has an array of public and private facilities that selectively admit inpatients based not on the severity of their illness alone, but on social class (Minkin, Stoline, & Sharfstein, 1994).

What makes social selection especially vexing to sociologists is their having to discount its influence when studying the impact of social characteristics, interventions or treatments on various outcomes (Mechanic, 1975). Whether a new motivational approach to treatment adherence, a promising social policy initiative or innovative educational program, the effects of these strategies must be separated from the individuals who were recruited, selected or drawn into these interventions. Unmeasured or unknown personal motivations, interests and efforts and other social characteristics can have a strong and confounding influence on the results attributed to the interventions. Randomization can minimize selection effects although they are difficult to use with many social experiments. A myriad of statistical techniques are able to handle potential selection biases (Winship & Mare, 1992), but are not always able to eliminate their influence. Given the prominence of social selection in so many areas of study and its insidiousness in interpreting results, it is surprising why "so few sociologists take selection itself as the object of their theory and inquiry" (Mechanic, 1975, p. 394).

Just as individuals enter various social roles, so they are selected into treatment. A tradition of research in mental health services utilization has taken social selection seriously. The earliest studies of treated cases of mental illness showed that individuals were not randomly entering treatment or entering based solely on a mental health problem, need or psychiatric illness. Individuals with psychiatric symptoms and illnesses sought and avoided entering care selectively. Some choices were likely made intentionally, others under coercion or unintentionally. Within the mental health treatment system, insurance policies, the social processes of interactions among clinicians and patients and the organizations in which they practice have differentially favored some groups over others. Individuals have selected themselves into care as providers selected who would be treated, the types of treatment and where treatment occurred.

When examining the selective flow of individuals into mental health treatment, social factors also need to be distinguished from the social causes associated with the mental health problem or psychiatric illness. Clinicians as well as policymakers need to be aware and clear about the differences between the social causes of psychiatric illnesses and the social factors influencing the course of illness and help-seeking behaviors (Mechanic, 1980). Some of the same social factors can affect both the illness and actions taken in response to the symptom, and support exists for both social causation and social selection arguments (Wheaton, 1978). However, the implications for treatment, care, and policy would be vastly different depending on whether the factors were associated with social causation of the illness or social selection in help-seeking.

In the remainder of this chapter, we examine sociological contributions to our understanding of selection into mental health treatment. We review influential studies of treated populations to highlight the importance of selection that could then only be fully investigated with studies of community samples. We discuss the main social factors, social class, gender, age, and race and ethnicity, that have been shown to be the most consistent predictors of entering mental health treatment. While a variety of studies have documented these and other social correlates of the use of mental health services, we focus on three traditions of research that use and elaborate the concepts and language of sociology to understand mental health services utilization. We offer reflections on how these bodies of work (societal reaction, illness behavior, and social networks theories) contribute to our understanding of variation in help seeking and treatment, as well as how they contribute to our understanding of broader sociological concerns with processes of social selection.

Early Work with Treated Populations

Prior to the 1950s, most studies that examined the utilization of services for persons with mental health problems used samples of persons who were already in treatment. Two early studies that were immensely influential illustrate the nature of this research. In a study in Chicago conducted in the early 1930s, Faris and Dunham (1960) undertook a complete census of patients receiving care in public and private mental hospitals and examined the correlation between treatment rates and patients' area of residence. They concluded that schizophrenia was associated with living in socially disorganized areas, although they failed to find such a pattern for bipolar disorder.

A second example of early influential work from the 1950s was conducted by Hollingshead and Redlich (1958). The researchers completed a census of persons in the New Haven region who were treated by psychiatrists in private offices, clinics or mental hospitals and compared the social characteristics of these patients to a random community sample. One of the central hypotheses of this research was that social class was associated with differences in thresholds for identifying mental illnesses and entry into treatment. Among other conclusions, the researchers found that "a distinct inverse relationship does exist between social class and mental illness" (Hollingshead & Redlich, 1958, p. 217).

The authors of both of these studies acknowledged that unobserved selection processes might account for their findings. In interpreting their findings that the rates of mental disorder were concentrated in specific areas of the city, Faris and Dunham (1960) wrote: ". . .the patterns of rates distribution [may] represent only a concentration of cases of mental disorder which have been institutionalized because of poverty" (p. 161). They went on to dismiss this possibility, arguing that including both private and public hospitals minimized this potential selection bias.

These studies generated a substantial body of research about the social characteristics that produce or "cause" mental illness and psychological distress. Equally important, however, they were influential in calling attention to the importance of selection processes (both health and social) for understanding treatment patterns. In essence, they prompted scientific debate about whether one could understand causal processes in situations where the independent variables of interest were measured only for persons in treatment. Conclusions that the causes of mental illness could be determined by studying only treated samples were challenged and the utility of drawing these inferences seriously questioned (Dohrenwend, 1966; Mechanic, 1972). The questions of interest to researchers shifted from focusing solely on whether social conditions such as social class caused mental illness to whether social conditions also influenced entry into treatment. Research moved to samples in community settings to answer these questions.

Community Studies: The Treatment Gap

Studies using community samples addressed questions that were not answered with research using treated samples. These studies focused attention on why people with similar problems or similar levels of need for treatment varied in their utilization of mental health services. The community studies that were most influential for researchers in the United States are outlined in Table 15.1.

TABLE 15.1. Utilization of mental health services in community studies of mental illness.

Study	Year	Sample	Measure of mental health	Utilization of services
Midtown Manhattan Study (Srole & Fischer 1975)	1954	1,660 adults in midtown area of Manhattan	Ordinal scale of functioning from 'well to incapacitated' based on ratings by psychiatrists	*Total*: 13.9% saw specialist *Impaired group*: 27% saw specialist
Epidemiologic Catchment Area Program (Regier et al. 1993)	1980–1985	20,291 adults in five sites across the US	Specific disorders according to DSM-III criteria	*Total*: 10.9% in medical sector; 5.9% specialty care *With 12-month Disorder*: 21.9 in medical sector; 12.7% specialty care
National Comorbidity Survey (Kessler et al. 1994)	1990–1992	8,098 persons 15–55 years old in a national sample	Specific disorders consistent with DSM-III-R criteria	*Total*: not reported *With 12-month Disorder*: 20.9% in medical sector; 11.5% in specialty care
National Comorbidity Survey Replication (NCS-R) (Wang et al. 2005)	2001–2003	9,282 adults in a national sample	Specific disorders consistent with DSM-IV criteria	*Total*: 15% in medical sector; 9% in specialty care *With 12-month Disorder*: 36% in medical sector; 22% in specialty care

One of the most important early examples of community research on mental illness, the Midtown Manhattan Study, was conducted in 1954 (Srole & Fischer, 1975). Similar to research preceding it, the Midtown Manhattan Study included a complete census of psychiatric patients in mental hospitals, outpatient clinics, and private offices. Unlike previous studies, the research also included a home interview with approximately 1,900 adults. The interview asked about symptoms of mental illness, socio-demographics, attitudes, and use of services. Definitions of mental illness were made by psychiatrists based on information gathered about each respondent from the treatment census and the home interview. The measure of mental illness categorized respondents on a 7-point ordinal scale from "well" to "seriously incapacitated, unable to function." For much of the analyses, persons categorized as having "impaired" mental health (those with at least moderate symptoms and some impairment in functioning) were compared to the remainder of respondents.

The Midtown Manhattan Study found that approximately 14% of the sample had ever seen a mental health specialist (defined as nerve specialist or psychiatrist). Utilization of mental health specialists was positively associated with level of impairment. However, only about 27% of persons who met the criteria for being currently impaired by a mental health problem had ever been to a mental health specialist. Only 5% had visited a specialist in the month prior to the interview.

Srole (1975, p. 209) used the imagery of an iceberg to describe the treatment gap. Only a small proportion of those in the community who "need[ed]" mental health treatment were visible to service providers and thus they represented merely the tip of the iceberg. The majority of those with mental health problems did not receive care and were "submerged" and invisible to the treatment community.

Since the Midtown Manhattan Study, the iceberg metaphor has been supported by numerous community mental health surveys. The first study to provide national estimates of the "treatment gap" in the United States was conducted in five communities as part of the Epidemiologic Catchment Area (ECA) program (Robins & Regier, 1991). The ECA studies were the first to estimate the prevalence of specific types of mental disorders based on diagnostic criteria outlined in the American Psychiatric Association's Diagnostic and Statistic Manual of Mental Disorder (APA, 1980). The survey also asked about the use of health and other types of services. The ECA studies found that annually only about 1 in 5 adults who had a mental illness received treatment in the medical sector. Treatment by a mental health specialist was even less common; only about 13% of those with a disorder received specialty care. A decade later, the National Comorbidity Survey (NCS), a national sample of adults, found remarkably similar results: only 20% of persons with a mental illness received any treatment annually, and only 12% received treatment by a mental health specialist.

Rates of treatment for those with a mental health problem increased over the period between the NCS and the follow-up National Comorbidity Survey Replication (NCS-R) conducted between 2001 through 2003 (Kessler, Demler, Frank, Olfson, Pincus, Walters, Wang, Wells, & Zaslavsky, 2005). The NCS-R estimated that approximately 36% of the population with a mental disorder within the past

12 months received mental health care in the medical sector during the year prior to interview and 22% received specialty care (Wang, Lane, Olfson, Pincus, Wells, & Kessler, 2005).

While the estimates of treatment rates vary among surveys due to differences in the populations studied, time periods, and measurements of disorder and types of services used, all of these studies indicate that the majority of adults in the community with mental health problems do not receive treatment. One possible explanation of these findings is that definitions of need based simply on meeting diagnostic criteria are too broad and capture a large number of persons who do not need treatment (Mechanic, 2003). Of greatest concern are the low rates of treatment for persons with the most severe and disabling disorders. McAlpine and Mechanic (2000) estimated that approximately three-fifths of those in the community who meet the criteria for serious mental illness (e.g., schizophrenia or bipolar disorder) did not receive specialty mental health treatment in the year prior to interview. Even when need for treatment is more conservatively defined as disorders associated with the greatest impairment, a large treatment gap exists.

Community studies highlight the diversity of options for help with mental health problems and illnesses. Some individuals seek care in the non-medical sector including the "volunteer support network sector." Data from the ECA studies suggest that annually 37% of all visits among persons with a disorder were to self help groups and talking with family and friends about the problem (Narrow, Regier, Rae, Manderscheid, & Locke, 1993).

Research based on community samples suggests also that many individuals without a diagnosed mental illness receive services. Estimates from the NCS reveal that about 45% of persons not meeting criteria for a disorder used mental health services in the year prior to interview (Mechanic, 2003). These individuals may have a disorder not measured in the studies, or may not meet clinical criteria for a disorder, but define their feelings or symptoms as mental health problems likely helped with treatment.

These studies demonstrate that the presence of a mental illness is neither a necessary nor sufficient condition for entry into treatment nor the sole determinant for seeking help. Individuals with the greatest impairment are more likely to receive specialty mental health treatment, but recognizing and deciding to seek care is a complex social process. Attributing problems to a mental illness is another formidable barrier which may be complicated by stigma and fear. With such impressive evidence of variation in help-seeking, the search for explanations has logically extended to social conditions that select persons into care.

Social Characteristics Associated with Selection into Treatment

The long-standing interest in the impact of social class on treatment was generated by the research of Hollingshead and Redlich (1958) who produced the monograph, *Social Class and Mental Illness*. In addition to studying the correlation between social class and the prevalence of mental illness, the researchers examined patterns of treatment. Their work was influential for at least two reasons. First, it helped shape the conceptualization and measurement of social class in social science research. Second, it also suggested that social class was integral to understanding entry and selection into various treatment sites.

Operationalized as "shared patterns of consumption, taste, attitudes and other identifiable sociocultural characteristics" (Hollingshead & Redlich, 1958, p. 67), the Hollingshead Index of Social Position was one of the earliest measures of social class. The index used in the New Haven study combined information about an individual's area of residence, occupation and education. Five ordinal categories were created with Class V denoting the lowest class and Class I the highest. Hollingshead (1971) later refined this measure to be a two-factor index (education and occupation) that was then widely used by sociologists studying social class (Haug & Sussman, 1971).

In addition to this methodological contribution, the work by Hollingshead and Redlich (1958) informed the relationship between social class and patterns of treatment of mental health problems. One of the central hypotheses driving their work was that "the type of psychiatric treatment provided by psychiatrists is associated with a patient's position in the class structure" (Hollingshead & Redlich, 1958, p. 11). Treated cases of mental illness were much more likely to be from the lowest class than a comparison sample in the community. While 38% of treated cases were from the lowest social class (Class V), only 18% of the community sample was from Class V.

Social class also shaped the types of services that individuals received once in the treatment system. In their analysis of treatment for persons diagnosed with schizophrenia, Hollingshead and Redlich (1958) reported that persons in the lowest social class were more likely than those in the highest class to receive either organic treatment (e.g., psychotropic medications and surgery) or no treatment (simple custodial care) than persons in the upper class. The upper classes were more likely to be treated with individual psychotherapy.

The New Haven study also suggested a negative relationship between social class and hospitalization and quality of care. Other studies have focused on outpatient care and suggested a positive relationship between social class and treatment in these settings. Most community studies did not examine social class *per se*, but instead focused on socioeconomic status usually measured by some combination of occupation, income or education. Research from both the ECA and NCS showed that those with more education are significantly more likely to use outpatient mental health services than persons with less education (Howard, Cornille, Lyons, Vessey, Lueger, & Sanders, 1996).

The recent NCS-R reveals that the impact of income and education may depend on stage of treatment (Wang et al., 2005). These investigators reported that persons with lower income were less likely to have received treatment in the medical sector. However, among those in treatment, persons with less education were less likely to receive adequate treatment.

Differences between men and women in the utilization of mental health services have generated considerable research attention for decades. While some early research suggested that men and women did not differ in their use of services (Srole & Fischer, 1975), a much larger body of research has pointed to a gender difference. The ECA studies reported that among those with a current disorder, women were much more likely (23%) to have received recent treatment than were men (17%) (Robins & Regier, 1991). Using this finding with the same data Leaf and Bruce (1987) found that the higher use by women compared to men depended on the setting. Women were more likely than men to use mental health care in the general medical care sector, but no gender difference occurred in the use of specialty mental health care. However, much of the work documenting gender differences has focused primarily on outpatient care.

The Midtown Manhattan Study found that among persons with impaired mental health, older persons were much less likely to use services than younger persons (Srole & Fischer, 1975). This general pattern has been confirmed by numerous other community studies (Klap, Unroe, & Unutzer, 2003; Leaf, Bruce, Tischler, Freeman, Weissman, & Myers, 1988). In the NCS-R, older persons were significantly less likely than younger adults to receive any mental health treatment, and among those in treatment, older persons were less likely to access specialty mental health care.

Early studies of mental health services utilization often did not consider the role of race and ethnicity; generally those that did merely distinguished between white and African American patients. Hollingshead and Redlich (1958) found that Blacks were over-represented in mental hospitals compared to Whites. Studies using community samples reported that while African Americans and Whites had similar rates of disorder, African Americans were less likely to receive treatment (Cooper-Patrick, Gallo, Powe, Steinwachs, Eaton, & Ford, 1999). These differences did not appear to be explained by socio-economic differences between groups. The recent NCS-R also examined utilization of services for persons identified as Hispanic and those of other minority racial and ethnic groups (Wang et al., 2005). The NCS-R found that Blacks, Hispanics, and those of other race/ethnic groups were less likely than Whites to receive any treatment. However, noting some encouraging findings, access to specialty care and adequacy of treatment for those in treatment did not vary significantly by race or ethnicity.

Theories of Help-Seeking – Mental Health Service Utilization

We have argued that theories of help-seeking are essentially theories of selection. Social class, gender, age and race/ethnicity are among the social characteristics most frequently described as influencing selection into treatment. If these characteristics are associated with treatment simply because they reflect variation in levels of illness, severity of symptoms and functioning, then the study of treatment, help-seeking, and even involuntary use might be best described by health selection. Sociologists' roles might be then better exercised by turning attention to the social causes of health and illness. However, we have argued that "need" or illness characteristics do not fully explain variation in treatment, and that social factors matter.

Many studies that have documented social correlates of treatment simply include a number of variables in multivariate models that also include measures of illness characteristics. If the social factors emerge as significant correlates of treatment, they argue for the importance of considering the social context of people's lives for understanding help-seeking behavior. While informative, these studies lack a coherent conceptual framework from which we can examine *social* selection into care. With the following three bodies of work we provide this framework through the concepts of (1) societal reaction to mental disorder; (2) illness behavior, and (3) social networks.

Societal Reaction Theories

Much of the early interest in the treatment of mental illness was generated by observations of differences in rates of hospitalization by social characteristics. Some researchers located explanations for these differences in the societal reaction to persons defined as deviant (Scheff, 1999). According to Scheff, "mental illness" was essentially a label applied to persons exhibiting deviant feelings or behaviors. Much of the debate about the validity of labeling theory focused on claims that mental illness was but a label, and that the label could produce secondary deviance or further symptoms defined as mental illness (Scheff, 1999).

It is not our intent to revive this debate here (see Pescosolido & Martin, this volume); instead, we focus on the potential for societal reaction theorists to contribute to our understanding of variation in help-seeking. The central contribution of labeling theory to the field of mental health services was its emphasis on social control. While definitions vary, social control is a prominent concept in the language of sociologists (Janowitz, 1975; Meier, 1982). Classical theorists struggled with understanding the foundations of social order. Many argued that as societies became more heterogeneous and complex, the problem of social order was more imperative. Delineating and defining the mechanism of social control that produces social order occupied much attention. One argument was that formal institutions of control, such as the legal system, arose in modern societies to fulfill the roles once played by families and religion in exercising control over individuals' behaviors (Durkheim, 1947). Parsons (1951) saw the medical system as another institution of social control.

These functionalist accounts of social control saw institutions and agents exercising control for the benefit of the larger society. In contrast, conflict theorists' accounts of social control placed more emphasis on the power relationships that allowed some groups to define control over others (Meier, 1982). Within either perspective, most sociological accounts conceptualized society as requiring mechanisms through which to control individuals' behaviors.

Labeling theorists adopted the concept of social control to examine societal reactions to deviance for which mental illness was just one example. While much of the debate in the research focused on whether mental illness was best conceptualized from a psychiatric perspective or a labeling perspective (Townsend, 1980), the literature also suggested that social control was important for understanding differences in treatment. The application of a social control framework to understanding variations in rates of mental hospitalization suggested that it was the reaction of others to individuals, not the psychiatric distress or mental illness, that accounted for why some persons with a mental health problem were hospitalized and others were not. Hospitalization, particularly involuntary hospitalization, represented a method of social control over persons considered deviant.

The societal reaction framework generated an immense amount of literature in the 1960s through the 1980s that focused on understanding why social characteristics such as socioeconomic position were associated with selection into mental health treatment (Townsend, 1980). Under this framework, the selection of persons into treatment in a mental hospital can be understood as the result of differences in access to resources (Rushing, 1978). Statuses defined by lower socioeconomic position or minority group memberships are associated with less power, fewer opportunities, and reduced access to resources. Those in lower status positions are less able to resist social control and more likely to be involuntarily hospitalized. Rosenfield (1984) argued that status differences between the agents of social control (e.g., the psychiatrist, the hospital staff) and persons with mental health problems were most likely to generate a reaction leading to involuntary hospitalization. She found that taking into account illness characteristics and socioeconomic status, non-white men were more likely to be hospitalized than white men. Others argued that labeling accounted for the higher rates of treatment found among persons of lower social class or in immigrant groups (Gibbs, 1962; Rushing, 1978).

Given that gender generally affords more status to men than to women, societal reaction theories could not explain higher rates of involuntary hospitalization among men compared to women based on access to resources. Instead, they argued that sex-roles explained the different reaction (Rushing, 1979). Men exhibit more dangerous behaviors and thus the reaction is likely to be stronger than for women (and result in hospitalization). Moreover, because women are socialized to express distress and seek help voluntarily, coercive social control mechanisms are more likely to be used with men (Horwitz, 1977).

Walter Gove was the most vocal critic of labeling theories arguing that prior studies had not sufficiently accounted for need for treatment and misattributed selection into treatment as the result of social control, not of illness characteristics. Through a review of the literature and an examination of the social and illness characteristics of persons in a state mental hospital, Gove and Howell (1974) concluded that "when severity of disorder is controlled, married persons and persons from the upper classes are more likely to receive psychiatric treatment" (p. 98), a conclusion at odds with societal reaction theory.

As Scheff (1999) wrote in the update to his classic text, *Being Mentally Ill*, labeling theories of mental illness were generally abandoned in the 1980s largely a result of the criticism by Gove and colleagues. This was unfortunate because labeling processes provided important insights for understanding selection into treatment. As one example, Mechanic and colleagues (1991) used a labeling framework to explain differences in the selection into general medical and specialty mental health care. They argued that perceived risk explains why some patients are referred to specialty care while others are treated in the general medical sector.

More recent research showed that differential labeling based on social status did not account adequately for those with mental disorders recently hospitalized or pressured into treatment. Using data from the National Comorbidity Survey, Thoits (2005) tested both classical labeling theory and self labeling to compare hospitalization experiences with cases having no treatment history for persons with mental disorders and living in the community. Finding no support for classical labeling theory, those in lower status groups were not overrepresented among persons reporting that they had been pressured into treatment or hospitalized. However, those in lower status groups were the most underserved by the mental health system being less likely to be seen by a professional by their own choice.

The analysis of societal reactions to persons considered mentally ill was conducted within the broad tradition of the sociology of deviance. Initial theories of deviance focused attention on the etiology of deviant acts (Gibbs & Erickson, 1975). The study of mental illness as deviance highlighted that deviance is more broadly defined than the study of law breaking or criminology. More importantly, the literature on societal reactions to deviance drew attention to the reaction of others to the person considered deviant. It gave reason to question official statistics on treated prevalence. Moreover, it helped build a body of research focused more on the reaction to acts considered deviance than the etiology of deviance (Gibbs and Erickson, 1975). In doing so, it supported the development of literature focused on how societies react to deviance that was not based on assumptions about social definitions of deviance.

Studies of persons who were hospitalized for mental illness challenged the Parsonian conceptualization of institutions of social control acting benevolently to control deviance, in order to deter deviance and facilitating social order. The study of hospitalization for mental illness showed that control of persons considered mentally ill was selective; for example, involuntary hospitalization primarily affected those with less status or power. Thus, it emphasized a conceptualization of social control more in line with conflict rather than functionalist theories (Gibbs and Erickson, 1975).

The landscape of services has changed dramatically since Scheff's (1999) original application of labeling theory to mental illness. Whereas in 1969 there were approximately 487,000 admissions to state and county mental hospitals, admissions had declined to 218,000 by 2000. During this same period, admissions to private psychiatric hospitals substantially increased from about 92,000 admissions to 528,500 admissions in 2000 (Manderscheid, Atay, Male, Blacklow, Forest, Ingram, Maedke, Sussman, & Ndikumnwami, 2004). In recent decades, psychotherapy has become much less common and the use of psychotropic drugs has substantially increased. But while the nature of services has changed, there remain unanswered questions for which labeling theory may offer some direction.

Some of the most intriguing questions are derived from research about how treatment processes differ by race and ethnicity. A growing body of research has suggested that clinical decisions about diagnosis and treatment vary by the race or ethnicity of the patient independent of illness characteristics. Neighbors and colleagues (2003) reported that symptoms are identified based on patients' race or ethnicity. Black patients were more likely to receive a diagnosis of schizophrenia while white patients were more likely to be diagnosed with bipolar disorder. Treatment regimens also differ by race and ethnicity. Walkup and colleagues (2000) found that controlling for illness characteristics, African Americans with a diagnosis of schizophrenia were more likely than Whites to receive antipsychotic medication dosages higher than the recommended ranges. As yet, we cannot fully explain these and other similar findings, but social control theory offers some possible avenues for further research.

Illness Behavior

David Mechanic (1961, 1978) introduced the concept of illness behavior to explain variation in treatment for mental health problems. The study of illness behavior gives emphasis to the ways in which individuals or groups perceive "symptoms," define them as illness, and decide whether or not to seek help. Mechanic (1978) identified ten central dimensions of illness behavior that determine whether a "symptom" is interpreted as illness and whether it will initiate help-seeking behaviors: 1) visibility of symptoms; 2) perceived seriousness; 3) disruptions in functioning; 4) frequency and chronicity of symptoms; 5) tolerance; 6) knowledge and cultural assumptions; 7) need for denial; 8) competing needs; 9) alternative explanations; and 10) availability of treatment. At the most general level, symptoms that are defined as visible, frequent, serious or chronic, and those associated with greater impairment are more likely to be perceived as illness. The more tolerant persons are of symptoms, the more reasons they have to deny illness, and the greater the availability of alternative explanations for symptoms, the less likely they are to initiate help seeking. Individuals vary in their knowledge of specific illnesses and in their cultural assumptions about the causes and meanings of particular symptoms that will affect illness appraisal and subsequent help seeking. Finally, the availability of treatment will affect how persons interpret symptoms and whether they seek help.

Mechanic's (1978) conceptualization of illness behavior recognized explicitly the role of significant others in making judgments about whether an individual was considered ill, the nature of the illness, and whether help should be sought. Building on the work of Clausen and Yarrow (1955), Mechanic acknowledged that it was often the family who encouraged an individual into treatment as behaviors became sufficiently disturbing or disruptive. Although this conceptualization of illness behavior was not incompatible with societal reaction theories, it did show that labeling processes could not explain fully the variation in mental health services utilization.

The study of illness behaviors also focused on both the objective and subjective qualities of "illness." Individuals define a feeling or an emotion based not only on objective levels of distress or disturbance. While experiencing the same objective symptoms of depression—sadness, sleep problems, difficulties concentrating—individuals may differ substantially in whether they define their feelings as an illness, whether the feelings interfere with functioning, and whether (and to whom) to seek care. We know that many people experiencing similar distress will associate their symptoms with physical rather than mental causes (Schurman, Kramer, & Mitchell, 1985). It is not difficult to accept the proposition that individuals differ in how they appraise their own feelings and symptoms that then influences help-seeking.

The study of illness behaviors is essentially sociological in recognizing that how individuals and others in their social networks appraise symptoms is not the result of random processes, but instead is conditioned by social factors. Considerable work suggests that social positions affect illness appraisals. Gurin and colleagues' (1960) work in the late 1950s, *Americans View their Mental Health*, showed that women, younger persons, and those with more education were more likely to perceive a problem in terms of mental health than were men, older persons, and those with more education. Kessler and colleagues (1981) used data from four studies to explain gender differences in the use of mental health services. Women experienced higher levels of distress than men; this accounted for a large part of the difference in rates of treatment. At similar levels of distress women were more likely than men to perceive that they had a personal problem. Recognition of a problem translates into similar levels of help-seeking for men and women. They argued that the higher rates of women in treatment were due partially to their greater likelihood to define problems as a mental illness.

Others have shown that aspects of illness behavior may account for the race/ethnic differences in the utilization of mental health services. African Americans experiencing emotional problems have been less likely to believe that medical intervention was necessary and were more likely to be skeptical about the effectiveness of care (Schnittker, 2003; Schnittker, Freese, & Powell, 2000).

Perhaps the study of perceived need for mental health services best illustrates the potential contribution of the illness behavior perspective and highlights the complexity of help-seeking. Perceived need for care is a strong predictor of help-seeking (Katz, Kessler, Frank, Leaf, & Linn, 1997). But many persons in the community who meet clinical criteria for having a mental illness did not perceive a need for treatment. Using data from the NCS, Mojtabai and colleagues (2002) estimated that approximately 37% of persons with a mood, anxiety or substance use disorder did not perceive that they needed treatment. Decisions by individuals that they need care are complicated and are influenced by prior experiences with the mental health system, stigma, costs of care and many other social factors.

The conceptualization of illness behavior is ambitious in its scope; one can use this framework to integrate findings from a variety of studies that identify diverse social factors such as stigma, attitudes toward mental health services, insurance coverage and social support as correlates of help-seeking. This ambition is both a strength and a weakness of the framework. Despite substantial research that has investigated various aspects of illness behavior, we know little about the conditions under which specific dimensions are more important than others. Moreover, although Mechanic (1978) explicitly recognized the importance of power relationships for explaining variation in illness behavior, few studies have explored these processes for understanding the links between social position, illness appraisal and subsequent help-seeking behavior.

Social Network Perspectives

Mental health researchers who have contributed to our understanding of the importance of social networks do not deny that processes of social control and illness behavior shape selection into treatment. They differ from these perspectives in the emphasis placed on the involvement of individuals in socially structured relations. The focus on social networks is based on research that finds that help-seeking for psychiatric illnesses is not explained fully by various individual characteristics and predisposing, enabling and risk factors. Except in rare instances, seeking care and entering treatment result from social interaction rather than individual action (Pescosolido, 1992).

One of the major issues in mental health services utilization concerns the early and timely entry into treatment. Considerable effort is also directed to continuity of care and keeping individuals with severe mental illnesses in the treatment system to minimize their relapse and rehospitalization and to support recovery. Not only must mental health services be available and readily accessible, but treatment must be seen as necessary by those needing care and by those in close relationships to them. Social networks exert influence throughout the course of illness, its treatment and in long-term care and recovery.

Within the sequential process of help-seeking, several opportunities exist for social networks to intervene at various stages in recognizing and interpreting symptoms, weighing the risks and benefits of treatment, deciding to pursue formal or informal care and entering and continuing in treatment (Kadushin, 1969; Mechanic, 2002). Drawing from dual and social exchange theories (Ekeh, 1974; Homans, 1958; Uehara, 1990), the study of social networks in the utilization of mental health services targets the social structure, culture and interactions among inter-connected individuals at various points along the pathways to care.

A substantial literature exists on the structure, content and function of social networks (Freidson, 1970, Pescosolido & Levy, 2002), but a set of conclusions about their impact on mental health services utilization is not easily articulated. The field continues to grapple with complex methodological issues and the generalizability of findings beyond some fine ethnographic case studies (Uehara, 2001). There is an enormous richness to the data that have been amassed over recent years that detail the multiple and dynamic encounters of persons with mental health problems with family, friends, community members, the police and courts, non-medical professionals and clinicians. Other social entities within the social network include government agencies, mental health authorities, nonprofit organizations, and cities (Morrissey, Calloway, Bartko, Ridgely, Goldman & Paulson, 1994). Here the networks of community relationships can advance or deter mutual goals and clinical and policy initiatives.

Three major contributions to the larger sociological enterprise seem evident from research on social networks. First, the use of the social network perspective in mental health services research has reaffirmed and highlighted that multiple options and encounters exist along the pathway to care. No longer is the specification of services utilization solely in terms of the use or nonuse of services or deciding to seek or not seek treatment seen as especially informative in understanding how, why and where individuals get into treatment. Generally multiple sources of help, advice and care are sought in the pathway into professional treatment. While only 12% of a sample of individuals entering mental health care used complex patterns of lay and formal advisors in a study of access and entry into treatment among a sample in Puerto Rico, it was those with the most severe illnesses who involved multiple contacts (Pescosolido, Wright, Alegría, & Vera, 1998b).

Consumers themselves invest in self care that may or may not be consistent with ongoing treatment regimens, but open-mindedness by clinicians to these initiatives and the influential advisors and contacts along the pathway to care can help to bring client and network preferences in line with effective practices. Studies of nonadherence to antipsychotic medications have suggested that some client behaviors may be classified as "competent nonadherence." Certain adjustments and tailoring of timing and dosages allow enhanced well-being possibly without the danger of relapse. Through network contacts, individuals confront their psychiatric illness and can be helped to cope with symptoms and stigma. The roles played by consumers and their families, friends, neighbors and others in informal networks are critical to learning how to leverage their influence in facilitating appropriate care. In addition to encouragement or coercion by informal and formal networks (Pescosolido, Gardner & Lubell, 1998a) sophisticated interventions can facilitate movement along the pathway to treatment when it can be helpful and effective.

The second contribution from the social network perspective derives from two bodies of evidence about the impact of social networks on mental health services use. Social networks have been shown to facilitate as well as inhibit help-seeking and entry into care. In Kadushin's (1969) work, the "Friends and Supporters of Psychotherapy" provided referral advice and facilitated contact with the mental health system. Horwitz (1977) found also that "open networks," those with weak kin contacts, but with friends from diverse areas of social life, were more likely to prompt referrals for the least severe problems and result in contacts with treatment providers in the shortest periods of time. A contradictory finding occurred in the "closed networks" where delay in using professional help was identified (Horwitz, 1977, Pescosolido, Wright, Alegría, & Vera, 1998b). Here individuals were insulated by the strong instrumental and emotional support of kin until the family was unable to cope with the severe and disruptive behaviors of the illness. Clausen and Yarrow's (1955) research also revealed the "discontinuities and blocks to effective action" within families as well as the sometimes heroic efforts made in reaching psychiatric care once need for specialized treatment was recognized.

The framework of the Network Episode Model developed by Pescosolido (1991) allows for both positive and negative effects of social networks on service use. Operationalizing networks for their structure (size, density and dispersion) and describing their content (beliefs, values and attitudes) and function (sources of instrumental and emotional support, information and coercion) allow for diverse and contradictory efforts that can facilitate, delay, or hinder entry into psychiatric care and through one or more pathways. Identifying the content and function of social networks will enable well-designed, targeted interventions to facilitate timely entry into care.

The search for deeper knowledge of the resilience and stability of social networks as well as how they are disrupted needs to accompany future, ongoing work in mental health services utilization. The cognitive and behavioral disorganization that accompanies severe mental illnesses can have damaging effects on network ties. Both individuals and their families and friends struggle to cope with the illness and its effects on personal and social functioning (Clausen & Yarrow, 1955). Stigma and the burden of care add to the difficulties in support and management (Magliano, Fiorillo, De Rosa, Malangone, Maj & the National Mental Health Project Working Group, 2005; Mechanic, 1978; Smith, 2003). With the disruption and loss of former social ties, the formation and actions of newly established networks also require study for their development and persistence.

The third set of findings from research on social networks in mental health services utilization indicates that key socio-demographic characteristics might be of marginal importance relative to indicators of social network involvement. One of the most provocative aspects of studying entry into treatment among those with different social networks has been the finding of their being independent of the effects of many traditional covariates. Horwitz's (1977) study showed that social network categories predicted entering treatment more than social class. Kadushin (1969) noted that when membership in social groups was controlled, social class differences in entering care also disappeared. Members of social networks can be linked by similar values and beliefs that may be independent of different educational, racial and residential categories. Alternatively homogeneity in socio-economic status among some samples with little variation in their income and other social attributes results in only modest explanatory power in statistical models (Pescosolido et al., 1998b). Delving into the content of social networks, learning the directional tendencies about pursuing or delaying various treatment options can offer richer understanding and meaning than many of the socio-demographic characteristics. Pescosolido and colleagues (1998b) also suggest that socio-demographic categories have become less meaningful in contemporary societies and retain their influence more in traditional societies where closed systems of social networks exist (White, Boorman & Breiger, 1976).

The social network perspective offers the potential for explaining the specific mechanisms that operate when social selection occurs in mental health services utilization and in other sociological research on decision making and social action. How networks are mobilized, how they function in the unfolding of the complex social process of getting help and entering treatment and other roles, and how the temporal and causal sequences facilitate or hinder action hold much promise in sociological inquiries. We can learn about the preferences and values and contested decisions of the individuals and their networks, how their choices may be contradictory to evidenced-based treatment or other social, political and organizational outcomes and even be less than optimal for the efficiency of the mental health care system or other organizations. The social network perspective offers the opportunity for greater understanding of how different social class values and perspectives impact decisions made along a pathway to care or to entering other social roles. Living in poverty will impact decision-making, but learning about the structure and meanings within impoverished networks can be instructive for targeted interventions and policymaking. Understanding these dynamics can be helpful to fine tuning the process of receiving timely help or action and to intervening thoughtfully to achieve desired outcomes whether in health care, education, the work place or other social situations.

The networks that are studied in psychiatric help-seeking represent decision-making and social action in the face of psychological distress, a crisis, or traumatic experience. Studying this ongoing process during these periods provides a window into what transpires in the interaction with key contacts and the decisions made during crises. Not all networks will be activated to facilitate positive outcomes, and some networks will result in negative consequences. Using the social network perspective promises greater insight and understanding of the complex human responses in dealing with a range of transitions in the life course and so much of social life.

Conclusions

More than three decades ago, David Mechanic (1975; pp. 393–394) wrote that "The field is presently grasping for a theoretical framework that ties together disparate studies into a more coherent whole...What clearly seems necessary is not more studies in the same vein, but clarification of the theoretical problems, formulation of the issues that remain problematic, and review of the most adequate methodologies that facilitate their clarification." These statements were made in a paper that also used an overarching sociological framework of social selection.

In the years since this publication, there have been literally hundreds of studies that showed social variables are correlated with entry into treatment, quality of care, and recovery from mental illness. While informative, we echo Mechanic's concern that continuing to accumulate these types of studies has only limited value in improving our understanding of the variation in utilization of mental health services.

We have argued that three broad perspectives based on sociological traditions will help build the unifying framework that Mechanic called for: theories based on societal reaction to mental illness; illness behavior; and societal networks. These are not competing frameworks, but rather differ in their emphasis and scope. Moreover, they are not the only theories of help-seeking that are prevalent in the literature. We chose not to emphasize the perspectives of Andersen and Newman's Socio-Behavioral Model (Andersen & Newman, 1973) and Rosenstock's Health Belief Model (Rosenstock, 1966). These models are not targeted to understanding patterns of care for mental health problems and have been shown to have limited value in explaining variation in service use for psychiatric illnesses.

The theoretical perspectives that have been reviewed share two strengths. They are firmly rooted in sociological theories and thus offer the potential to unify findings from diverse studies of the correlates of mental health care utilization. They have also contributed to the accumulation of knowledge of selection processes as consequences of social contexts, structures and relationships. They challenge models of help-seeking that argue that people use care simply because they are sick or after weighing the costs and benefits of seeking help. Unfortunately, the potential of these theories has not been fully realized, perhaps because it is much simpler to continue to document social correlates of treatment.

Framing the study of variation in the use of mental health services with theories of social selection is not new; early studies in the area gave prominent attention to the concept (Fox, 1984; Greenley & Mechanic, 1976; Mechanic, 1978). More recently, however, health services researchers appear to have largely abandoned the language of social selection in studies of mental health services utilization. This is unfortunate, because in doing so we may have lost sight of the potential of studies in the area to contribute to the broader sociological concern with social selection.

Nowhere are theories of social selection more explicit than in the study of educational attainment (Kerckhoff, 1995). Students are continually sorted into groups throughout the education process from the schools they attend, the classrooms in which they learn, the teachers to whom they are exposed and the curriculum they study. Selection processes also operate sequentially and are cumulative; selection at one stage (e.g. ability groupings within schools) affects selection at later stages (e.g. college placements). However, studies of educational attainment have traditionally not looked to the field of research on mental health services utilization for explanation of the processes through which social selection occurs. But, the processes proposed are remarkably similar. It is not our intent to reproduce here the rich body of research that suggests that selection process matters for educational attainment. Suffice is to illustrate that the process of educational attainment in some way mirrors the study of selection into treatment.

Just as "need" does not fully explain selection into mental health treatment, so the literature on educational attainment suggests that ability does not fully explain selection into varying types of education. Moreover, the search for social factors that account for selection in both fields have tended to focus on social positions that are associated with access to resources, status and power. Sociologists have examined the roles of social class of origin and race or ethnicity as important to the selection of children and adolescents into education (Kerckhoff, 1995, Portes & Wilson, 1976).

While there remains significant debate about how selection processes operate to shape educational attainment, the mechanisms investigated mirror those identified in the three traditions of mental health services research reviewed here. Some researchers have emphasized the concept of labeling; research examining the concept of the self-fulfilling prophecy that was popular in the 1960s and 1970s (Wilkins, 1976), for example, argued that the labels applied to students shaped latter educational opportunities regardless of students' actual ability. Others have focused on social networks and social ties. There continues to be significant debate about whether closed or open social networks of parents and friends are associated with positive educational outcomes for students (Morgan & Sorensen, 1999). Still others have focused on aspirations of students for higher education (a concept analogous to that of perceived need in the mental health field), and suggest that aspirations are important for educational attainment independent of ability, especially for African American students (Portes & Wilson, 1976)

Similar strands of research are found in the literature on occupational attainment, (Kerckhoff, 1995; Lin, Vaughn, & Ensel, 1981). But with the exception of research in the sociology of deviance, it is rare for other sub-fields of sociology to turn to research about mental health services utilization for explanatory models of social selection. Herein lies the lost potential of the traditions of research reviewed in this chapter. The challenge remains to demonstrate the importance of these theories to selection process more generally.

The central tasks of this chapter did not include extensive consideration of the policy and practice implications of findings from these bodies of research. This is not to imply that they are unimportant. Typically, policy and practices interventions in the field of mental health are aimed at closing the treatment gap; the central assumption is that treatment in the medical sector is appropriate and helpful for persons experiencing psychological distress or disorder. And for some populations, most clearly individuals with the most severe and disabling conditions, this is a worthwhile pursuit. The body of research here has implications for targeted interventions for closing the treatment gap. Equally important, these theories draw attention to the possibility that there are many persons currently in treatment due to their social circumstances rather than their experience of illness. The potential of these theories to investigate and explain excess use of mental health services needs to be pursued in future work.

References

American Psychiatric Association (1980). *Diagnostic and statistical manual of mental disorders*. 3rd edition. Washington DC: American Psychiatric Association.

Andersen, R., & Newman, J. (1973). Societal and individual determinants of medical care utilization. *Milbank Memorial Fund Quarterly, 51*, 95–124.

Clausen, J. A., & Yarrow, M. R. (1955). Paths to the mental hospital. *The Journal of Social Issues, 11*, 25–32.

Cooper-Patrick, L., Gallo, J. J., Powe, N. R., Steinwachs, D. M., Eaton, W. W., & Ford, D. E. (1999). Mental health service utilization by African Americans and whites: The Baltimore Epidemiological Catchment Area follow-up. *Medical Care, 37*, 1034–1045.

Dohrenwend, B. P. (1966). Social status and psychological disorder: An issue of substance and an issue of method. *American Sociological Review, 31*, 14–34.

Durkheim, E. 1947. *The division of labor in society*. Glencoe, Ill: Free Press.

Ekeh, P. P. (1974). *Social exchange theory: The two traditions*. Cambridge, Mass: Harvard University Press.

Faris, R. E., & Dunham, W. H. (1960). *Mental disorders in urban areas; An ecological study of schizophrenia and other psychoses*. New York: Hafner Publishing.

Fox, J. W. (1984). Sex, marital status, and age as social selection factors in recent psychiatric treatment. *Journal of Health and Social Behavior, 25*, 394–405.

Freidson, E. (1970). *Profession of medicine*. New York: Dodd Mead.

Gibbs, J. P. (1962). Rates of mental hospitalization: A study of societal reaction to deviant behavior. *American Sociological Review, 27*, 782–792.

Gibbs, J. P., & Erickson, M. L. (1975). Major developments in the sociological study of deviance. *Annual Review of Sociology, 1*, 21–42.

Gove, W. R., & Howell, P. (1974). Individual resources and mental hospitalization: A comparison and evaluation of the societal reaction and psychiatric perspectives. *American Sociological Review, 39*, 86–100.

Greenley, J. R., & Mechanic, D. (1976). Social selection in seeking help for psychological problems. *Journal of Health and Social Behavior, 17*, 249–262.

Gurin, G., Veroff, J., & Feld. S. (1960). *Americans view their mental health*. New York: Basic Books.

Haug, M. R., & Sussman, M. B. (1971). The indiscriminate state of social class measurement. *Social Forces, 49*, 549–563.

Hollingshead, A. B. (1971). Commentary of "Indiscriminate State of Social Class Measurement." *Social Forces, 49*, 563–567.

Hollingshead, A. B., & Redlich, F. C. (1958). *Social class and mental illness: A community study*. New York: John Wiley & Sons, Inc.

Homans, G. C. (1958). Social behavior as exchange. *American Journal of Sociology, 63*, 597–606.

Horwitz, A. V. (1977). Social networks and pathways to psychiatric treatment. *Social Forces, 56*, 86–105.

Howard, K. I., Cornille, T. A., Lyons, J. S., Vessey, J. T., Lueger, R. J., & Saunders, S. M. (1996). Patterns of mental health service utilization. *Archives of General Psychiatry, 53*, 696–703.

Janowitz, M. (1975). Sociological theory and social control. *American Journal of Sociology, 81*, 82–108.

Kadushin, C. (1969). *Why people go to psychiatrists*. New York: Atherton Press.

Katz, S. J., Kessler, R. C., Frank, R. G., Leaf, P., & Linn, E. (1997). Mental health care use, morbidity and socioeconomic status in the United States and Ontario. *Inquiry, 34*, 38–49.

Kerckhoff, A. C. (1995). Institutional arrangements and stratification process in industrial societies. *Annual Review of Sociology, 21*, 323–347.

Kessler, R. C., Berglund, P. A., Bruce, M. L., Koch, J. R., Laska, E. M., Leaf, P. J., Manderscheid, R. W., Rosenheck, R. A., Walter, E. E., & Wang, P. S. (2001). The prevalence and correlates of untreated serious mental illness. *Health Services Research, 36*, 987–1007.

Kessler, R. C., Brown, R. L., & Broman, C. L. (1981). Sex differences in psychiatric help-seeking from four large-scale surveys. *Journal of Health and Social Behavior, 22*, 49–62.

Kessler, R. C., Demler, O., Frank, R. G., Olfson, M., Pincus, H. A., Walters, E. E., Wang, P., Wells, K. B., & Zaslavsky, A. M. (2005). Prevalence and treatment of mental disorders, 1990 to 2003. *New England Journal of Medicine, 352*, 2515–2523.

Klap, R., Unroe K. T., & Unutzer, J. (2003). Caring for mental illness in the United States: A focus on older adults. *American Journal of Geriatric Psychiatry, 11*, 517–524.

Leaf, P. J., & Bruce, M. L. (1987). Gender differences in the use of mental health-related services: A re-examination. *Journal of Health and Social Behavior, 28*, 171–183.

Leaf, P. J., Bruce, M. L., Tischler, G. L., Freeman, D. H., Weissman, M. M., & Myers, J. K. (1988). Factors affecting the utilization of specialty and general medical health services. *Medical Care, 26*, 9–26.

Lin, N., Vaughn, J. C., & Ensel, W. M. (1981). Social resources and occupational status attainment. *Social Forces, 59*, 1163–1181.

Magliano, L., Fiorillo, A., De Rosa, C., Malangone, C., Maj, M., & the National Mental Health Project Working Group. (2005). Family burden in long-term diseases: A comparative study in schizophrenia vs. physical disorders. *Social Science & Medicine, 61*, 313–322.

Manderscheid, R.W., Atay, J. E., Male, A., Blacklow, B., Forest, C., Ingram, L., Maedke, J., Sussman, J., & Ndikumwami, A. (2004). Highlights of organized mental health services in 2000 and major national and state trends. In R. W. Manderscheid & M. J. Henderson (Eds.), *Mental Health United States: 2002* (pp. 243–279). Rockville, Maryland: U.S. Department of Health and Human Services.

McAlpine, D. D., & Mechanic, D. (2000). Utilization of specialty mental health care among persons with severe mental illness: the roles of demographics, need, insurance, and risk. *Health Services Research, 35*, 277–292.

Mechanic, D. (1961). The concept of illness behavior. *Journal of Chronic Disease, 15*, 189–194.

Mechanic, D. (1962). Some factors in identifying behavior and defining mental illness. *Mental Hygiene, 46*, 66–74.

Mechanic, D. (1972). Social class and schizophrenia: Some requirements for a plausible theory of social influence. *Social Forces, 50*, 305–309.

Mechanic, D. (1975). Sociocultural and social-psychological factors affecting personal responses to psychological disorder. *Journal of Health and Social Behavior, 16*, 393–404.

Mechanic, D. (1978). *Medical sociology: A comprehensive text*. Second edition. New York: Free Press.

Mechanic, D. (1980). Introduction. In D. Mechanic (Ed.), *Readings in medical sociology* (pp. 1–13). New York: Free Press.

Mechanic, D. (2002). Removing barriers to care among persons with psychiatric symptoms. *Health Affairs, 21*, 137–147.

Mechanic, D. (2003). Is the prevalence of mental disorders a good measure of the need for services? *Health Affairs, 22*, 8–20.

Mechanic, D., Angel, R., & Davies, L. (1991). Risk and selection process between the general and the specialty mental health sectors. *Journal of Health and Social Behavior, 32*, 49–64.

Meier, R.F. (1982). Perspectives on the concept of social control. *Annual Review of Sociology, 8*, 35–55.

Minkin, E. B., Stoline, A., & Sharfstein, S. S. (1994). An analysis of the two-class system of care in public and private psychiatric hospitals. *Hospital & Community Psychiatry, 45*, 975–977.

Mojtabai, R., Olfson, M., & Mechanic, D. (2002). Perceived need and help-seeking in adults with mood, anxiety, or substance use disorders. *Archives of General Psychiatry, 59*, 77–84.

Morgan, S. L., & Sorensen, A. B. (1999). Parental networks, social closure, and mathematics learning: A test of Coleman's social capital explanation of school effects. *American Sociological Review, 64*, 661–681.

Morrissey, J. P., Calloway, M., Bartko, W. T., Ridgely, M. S., Goldman, H. H., & Paulson, R. I. (1994). Local mental health authorities and service system change: Evidence from the Robert Wood Johnson program on chronic mental illness. *Milbank Quarterly, 72*, 49–80.

Narrow, W. E., Regier, D. A., Rae, D. S., Manderscheid, R. W., & Locke, B. Z. (1993). Use of services by persons with mental and addictive disorders: Findings from the National Institute of Mental Health Epidemiologic Catchment Area Program. *Archives of General Psychiatry, 50*, 95–107.

Neighbors, H. W., Trierweiler, S. J., Ford, B. C., & Muroff, J. R. (2003). Racial differences in DSM diagnosis using a semi-structured instrument: The importance of clinical judgment in the diagnosis of African Americans. *Journal of Health and Social Behavior, 44*, 237–256.

Parsons, T. (1951). *The social system*. Glencoe, Ill: Free Press.

Pescosolido, B. A. (1991). Illness careers and network ties: A conceptual model of utilization and compliance. In G. Albrecht & J. Levy (Eds.), *Advances in medical sociology*, (pp.164–181). New York: JAI Press.

Pescosolido, B. A. (1992). Beyond rational choice: The social dynamics of how people seek help. *American Journal of Sociology, 97*, 1096–1138.

Pescosolido, B. A., Gardner, C. B., & Lubell, K. M. (1998a). How people get into mental health services: Stories of choice, coercion and "muddling through" from "first timers." *Social Science and Medicine, 46*, 275–286.

Pescosolido, B. A., & Levy, J. A. (2002). The role of social networks in health, illness disease and healing: the accepting present, the forgotten past, and the dangerous potential for a complacent future. In J.A. Levy & B.A. Pescosolido (Eds.), *Advances in medical sociology: Social networks and health* (pp. 3–25). New York: JAI Press.

Pescosolido, B. A., Wright, E. R., Alegría, M., & Vera, M. (1998b). Social networks and patterns of use among the poor with mental health problems in Puerto Rico. *Medical Care, 36*, 1057–1072.

Portes, A., & Wilson, K. L. (1976). Black-white differences in educational attainment. *American Sociological Review, 41*, 414–431.

Robins, L. N., & Regier, D. A. (1991). *Psychiatric disorders in America*. New York: Free Press.

Rosenfield, S. (1984). Race differences in involuntary hospitalization: Psychiatric vs. labeling perspectives. *Journal of Health and Social Behavior, 25*, 14–23.

Rosenstock, I. M. (1966). Why people use health services. *Milbank Memorial Fund Quarterly, 44*, 94–106.

Rushing, W. A. (1978). Status resources, societal reactions, and type of mental hospital admission. *American Sociological Review, 43*, 521–533.

Rushing, W. A. (1979). The functional importance of sex roles, and sex-related behavior in societal reactions to residual deviants. *Journal of Health and Social Behavior, 20*, 208–217.

Scheff, T. J. (1999). *Being mentally ill: A sociological theory.* Third Edition. Chicago: Aldine.

Schnittker, J. (2003). Misgivings of medicine? African American's skepticism of psychiatric medication. *Journal of Health and Social Behavior, 44,* 506–524.

Schnittker, J., Freese, J., & Powell, B. (2000). Nature, nurture, neither, nor: Black-white differences in beliefs about the cause and appropriate treatment of mental illness. *Social Forces, 78,* 1101–1130.

Schurman, R. A., Kramer, P. D., & Mitchell, J. B. (1985). The hidden mental health network: Treatment of mental illness by nonpsychiatric physicians. *Archives of General Psychiatry, 42,* 89–94.

Smith, G. C. (2003). Patterns and predictors of service use and unmet needs among aging families of adults with severe mental illness. *Psychiatric Services, 54,* 871–877.

Srole, L. (1975). Midtown and several other populations. In L. Srole & A. K. Fischer (Eds.), *Mental health in the metropolis: The Midtown Manhattan study* (pp.183–239). New York: McGraw-Hill.

Srole, L., & Fischer, A. K. (Editors). (1975). *Mental health in the metropolis: The Midtown Manhattan Study.* New York: McGraw-Hill.

Thoits, P. A. (2005). Differential labeling of mental illness by social status: A new look at an old problem. *Journal of Health and Social Behavior, 46,* 102–119.

Townsend, J. M. (1980). Psychiatry versus societal reaction: A critical analysis. *Journal of Health and Social Behavior, 21,* 268–278.

Uehara, E. S. (1990). Dual exchange theory, social networks, and informal social support. *American Journal of Sociology, 96,* 521–557.

Uehara, E.S. (2001). Understanding the dynamics of illness and help-seeking: Event-structure analysis and a Cambodian-American narrative of "Spirit Invasion." *Social Science and Medicine, 52,* 519–536.

Walkup, J. T., McAlpine, D. D., Olfson, M., Labay, L. E., Boyer, C.A., & Hansell, S. (2000). Patients with schizophrenia at risk for excessive antipsychotic dosing. *Journal of Clinical Psychiatry, 61,* 344–348.

Wang, P. S., Lane, M., Olfson, M., Pincus, H. A., Wells, K. B., & Kessler, R. C. (2005). Twelve-month use of mental health services in the United States. *Archives of General Psychiatry, 62,* 629–640.

Wheaton, B. (1978). The sociogenesis of psychological disorder: Reexamining the causal issues with longitudinal data. *American Sociological Review, 43,* 383–403.

White, H. C., Boorman, S. A., & Breiger, R. L. (1976). Social structure from multiple networks. I. Block models of roles and positions. *American Journal of Sociology, 81,* 730–780.

Wilkins, W. E. (1976). The concept of a self-fulfilling prophecy. *Sociology of Education, 49,* 175–183.

Winship, C., & Mare, R. D. (1992). Models for sample selection bias. *Annual Review of Sociology, 18,* 327–350.

16
An Organizational Analysis of Mental Health Care

Teresa L. Scheid and Greg Greenberg

Introduction

Mental health care organizations have been an important laboratory for sociological research. Classic studies on state mental hospitals focused on how the social structure of the hospital shaped therapeutic outcomes (Goffman, 1961; Strauss, Schatzman, Burcher, Ehrlich, & Sabshin, 1964). Organizational theorists (Etzioni, 1960; Perrow, 1965) found that state mental hospitals provided rich materials for understanding complex organizational structures and behavior, which led to significant advances in organizational theory. All of the aforementioned studies made significant contributions to sociological understanding of organizational control and power, and mental health care organizations continue to be excellent sites for understanding changing forms of organizational control as well as furthering understanding of conflict between professional and bureaucratic control. As organizational theory developed to include inter-organizational relations and networks of organizations, research on mental health care has contributed to knowledge about how organizations manage contradiction, conflict, and ambiguity (Meyer, 1986; Scott, 1983). Organizational theory also provides a powerful model for understanding changing systems of mental health care (Scheid, 2004; Schlesinger & Gray, 1999).

Because of changing societal preferences and demands, the type of care received by clients has undergone a series of historical shifts. There have been four major phases of mental health care which reflect different professional values, political preferences, and economic priorities (Scheid & Horwitz, 1999). First was the period of institutionalized care where the primary locus of care was the mental hospital. Next came deinstitutionalization, which emerged in the 1950s and began to recede in the mid 1980s, and was characterized by the movement of patients into the community. The third phase was the consolidation of community based care through the 1980s and 1990s where attention was placed on system coordination and integration. The fourth phase has been the movement to managed care, which has reshaped mental health care delivery systems and the organizations which deliver that care. During each phase of care, the types of organizations delivering care changed, as did entire mental health care system.

379

Our exploration of the theoretical and empirical exchange between organizational sociologists and mental health researchers is organized in terms of this historical progression from institutionalized care to the current era of managed care.

Our analysis is also organized by three levels of organizational analysis: the organization and its internal workings, the organizational field (i.e. networks of organizations) and changes to the population of organizations providing mental health care, and the influence of the institutional environment on organizational fields and individual organizations. In terms of the first level, mental health care is delivered by a diversity of complex organizations, most notably state mental institutions, community mental health care centers, and private mental health care organizations. State mental hospitals and community mental health centers have historically been part of the public mental health sector, which is funded by federal, state, and local monies. Clients are likely to be indigent, and to have severe, chronic mental illness. In contrast, mental health care in the private sector (private hospitals, group practices, and multi-disciplinary treatment centers) is more likely to be office based and provide therapy to clients with mental health care problems whose care is reimbursed by private insurance. Clients seen in private practice are also more likely to suffer from acute mental heath care problems.

The second level of organizational analysis focuses on the network of organizations sharing a common domain, referred to as the organization field. Organizational sociologists define the organizational field as those organizations which "constitute a recognized area of institutional life: key suppliers, resource and product consumers, regulatory agencies, and the other organizations that produce similar services or products" (DiMaggio & Powell, 1983, p. 143). Community mental health centers, state hospitals, the criminal justice system, and various types of social services all constitute the organizational field relevant to understanding the type of mental health care delivered to clients.

In turn, the organizational field is influenced by the external environment; forces existing outside the organization and the organization field that affect delivery systems. The relationship between the external environment and the organizational field (as well as individual organizations) constitutes the third level of organizational analysis. The environment consists of both technical forces (i.e. available treatment technologies) and institutional demands (i.e. social and normative forces) which influence definitions of appropriate care and treatment and consequently affects the way in which mental health care organizations are structured. The institutional environment is also the source of professional norms and practices which impinge upon the daily operations of organizations (DiMaggio & Powell, 1983). Mental health care organizations have been characterized as existing in primarily institutional environments (Hasenfeld, 1992; Scott, 1983; Scott & Meyer, 1991). Scott, Ruef, Mendel, and Caronna (2000) provide an exceptional organizational analysis of the health care sector and describe how health care changed due to differing institutional logics, moving from a professionally based system of care, to the era of federal involvement, to the current era of market driven care. While mental health care has evolved according to a somewhat different logic, it is now also driven by a market model of care (Brown and Cooksey, 1989).

We begin at the level of the organization and describe the ways in which mental health care organizations operate as complex organizations. We then move outside the organization to consider organizational fields and organizational environments. Population ecology and institutional theory work together to provide a powerful theoretical framework for understanding organizational change; they help us to understand how, and why, mental health care changed during the eras of institutionalization, deinstitutionalization, community based care, and finally managed care. Throughout each of these eras the study of mental health care organizations and systems of care has advanced sociological theorizing about various forms of organizational control and power. In the last sections of the paper we focus on our current system of care, and provide a discussion of managed care and how it may exacerbate traditional conflicts between bureaucratic and professional authority structures. Continued research at the organizational level has the potential to significantly contribute to both understandings of patient care as well as new forms of conflict between bureaucratic and professional systems of control.

Mental Health Care Organizations as Critical Laboratories for Research

In this section we describe how mental health care organizations operate as complex organizations. We introduce the reader to basic concepts in organization theory and also give the reader an understanding of the different types of organizations where mental health care is provided. We show how research on (and in) mental health organizations was critical to early understandings of professional authority and conflict with bureaucratic control. In addition, this section provides a preliminary discussion of professional and occupational identities. In short, this section attempts to elucidate why mental health organizations have been such fruitful laboratories for organizational research.

Individuals with mental health problems can receive care as either inpatients or as outpatients; the majority of this care is provided by multi-service mental health care organizations (referred to as MHO).[1] MHO provide a broad array of services to diverse client populations; individuals with severe persistent mental illnesses, individuals with developmental disabilities, and individuals with substance abuse problems. In addition to adults, MHO may also provide services to children, adolescents, and the elderly in specialized units or departments. What services are provided, and who is served, is a reflection of wider social values and priorities, which as discussed above, has undergone a number of historical

---

[1] Mental health care is increasingly referred to as behavioral health care, which includes both mental health and substance abuse services.

shifts. During the era of institutionalization, most clients received care as inpatients in public or private hospitals; today most clients receive care as outpatients and visit either a community mental health care center or a private practice.

Given the diversity in services and client populations, MHO are difficult to characterize. Researchers have described MHO as poor places to work, because of the difficulties faced by their clients, resource constraints, and because of the bureaucratic context. Clients with severe mental illness provide little positive feedback and have been labeled as "undesirable" (Atwood, 1982; Lang, 1981; Stern & Minkoff, 1979). In terms of resource constraints, MHO have generally operated in the public domain with funding by a diverse mix of federal, state and county funds with most clients receiving some form of Medicare, Social Security Income, or Social Security Disability Income. Historically the public mental health system has served as a safety net for those clients who are poorer, more disabled, and less desirable (Frank, Koyanagi, & McGuire, 1997; Institute of Medicine, 1997). Consequently resources in MHO are limited and providers are likely to be dissatisfied with opportunities for salary gains and promotion (Ben-Dror, 1994; Oberlander, 1990).

In part due to their historic reliance on governmental funds, MHO exemplify many of the characteristics of bureaucratic organizations. They are governed by a series of rules, specialization of functions, and hierarchical relationships. As first articulated by Weber (1946), bureaucracy is an important form of social control. However, the bureaucratic features of MHO may be undermined by the fact that they have been characterized as having contradictory and ambiguous objectives, loose-coupling of formal structure (work roles) and technical activities (the work performed) from client outcomes, and informal systems of organizational control and authority (Hasenfeld, 1992; Scheid-Cook,1990, 1991). In addition, MHO contain both professional and bureaucratic occupational groups, providing for the existence of conflict between expert (professional) and bureaucratic authority (Scott, 1985, 1992).

Researchers have generally found evidence of conflict between professional and bureaucratic authority in professional organizations (Hall, 1986). This is because bureaucratic decision making is hierarchical, rule governed, and based upon individual accountability while professional, or collegial, decision making is egalitarian, consensual, and based upon individual autonomy (Waters, 1989). However, the relationship between professional and bureaucratic authority is complex and conflict is not always evident, nor necessary. Scott (1992) distinguishes between heteronomous professional organizations, where professionals are subordinate to administrative authority, and autonomous professional organizations, where professionals have considerable power and authority. Conflict is less likely in autonomous professional organizations, where bureaucratic positions of organizational control are likely to be held by members of the profession. Furthermore, the non-routine nature of the work in professional organizations can mitigate centralized, bureaucratic control (Anderson, 1992).

Most MHO can be characterized as autonomous professional organizations; supervisors generally have a clinical background, consider themselves professionals, often have a caseload, and work on a fairly equal level with other providers. There are also relatively few layers of bureaucratic stratification and authority in outpatient MHO (although this is changing with managed care, as we will see). Despite the relatively few layers of management (low complexity) and professional orientation of mental health care administrators, there is still a bureaucratic ethos within most MHO. Drolen (1990) reported that MHO directors were more concerned with control and efficiency than creativity or innovation, despite the fact that Gowdy and Rapp (1989) found effective MHO were those with a "can-do" (i.e. innovative and creative) attitude. However, in a study of a counseling organization, Nijsmans (1991) found that professional imperatives were more powerful than organizational rules, which were often seen as incompatible with professional ideologies.

MHO also vary in the range of work roles and services provided, and, as has been found in other human service organizations (Glisson & Durick, 1988), there is likely to be variation in job characteristics even when similar tasks are performed. Another source of diversity is that mental health care is provided by a number of different types of professionals: psychiatrists, psychologists, social workers, and nurses (Scott & Lammers, 1985). Consequently there is much potential for inter-professional conflict. Because of this professional diversity and potential for conflict, MHO provide an excellent site for the study of different "segments," those occupational groups where members share common work activities, values, and identities (Halpern, 1992). Different segments may correspond to occupational or professional subcultures; differing occupations within an organization give rise to multiple organizational cultures (Gregory, 1993). One primary source of group identity is one's professional background; members of a profession share a common approach to their clients by virtue of their educational preparation and possession of a specialized body of knowledge. In addition to professional orientations, providers are also subject to the demands of their organizational work role. For example, case managers may be nurses, social workers, therapists, or rehabilitation counselors. A case manager with a RN license is a professional nurse, yet his/her occupation will be that of case manager. Likewise, a person with a M.S.W. is considered to be a professional social worker, yet if he/she is a case-manager, their occupation is that of case-manager. While professional orientations and training may vary, those performing "case management" are likely to face similar problems and have common experiences, leading to the formation of an occupational identity—which may then lead to the development of professional certification. Understanding the experiences of providers performing different work roles is critical because different segments will seek to protect their treatment domains with impending resource restrictions and rationing of services (Hafferty & Light, 1995).

Research on MHO has provided insight into the processes that influence occupational identities. Compared to other medical organizations, professionals in mental health organizations may have less authority within the organization than other groups of health care professionals (Scott, 1983; Scott & Lammers, 1985). This is due to the fact that treatment of the mentally ill is not as technically proficient or unambiguous as are many other medical practices. That is, there is a notable dearth of solutions or proven technologies to aid providers in their work (Mechanic, 1986, 1994; Rochefort, 1989).[2] This aspect of mental health work is part of the reason why MHO may have ambiguous and contradictory goals. In addition, many of the providers in mental health organizations are professions "in transition" seeking greater professional recognition; this is especially true of nurses and social workers (Guy, 1985) but other types of mental health workers (rehabilitation and substance abuse counselors) also would like greater professional recognition for their work. The conflict between bureaucratic and professional authority may be exacerbated in MHO because mental health professionals may have less professional authority than other groups of health care professionals.

In MHO inter-professional conflicts constitute another threat to professional status. Inter-professional conflict is often characterized by jurisdictional disputes (Abbott, 1988) that involve disagreements about treatment ideology, or which services to provide, or how best to achieve organizational objectives. Because MHO offer diverse services, they have a wide variety of professional and occupational (work-role) segments, and these groups are likely to disagree on treatment and service provision. For example, psychiatrists and nurses may emphasize the central role of medication, while social workers may stress rehabilitation and skills training. Shared organizational positions (i.e. shift or unit) can also lead to similar perceptions and treatment preferences (Doherty & Harry, 1976). The organization, and its structure of authority, is critical to resolution of these disputes. The organization may provide an arena in which disagreements can be resolved collegially, hence maintaining provider's sense of autonomy; or the organization may resolve disputes bureaucratically, hence limiting the provider's autonomy. Autonomy and a sense of control over one's work, as well as input into organizational decisions, contribute to a sense of self efficacy and self-esteem, and can have a critical impact on the provider's level of job satisfaction as well as the quality of care they provide.

Professional and occupational groups can also be viewed as an important aspect of the institutional environment of MHO. Beliefs about the etiology of mental illness and treatment technologies are produced and reproduced in the education and socialization of mental heath care providers, and these professional norms are an important form of institutional demand which shapes organizational structures and behavior. We move outside the organization where care is delivered to a consideration of the external forces which influence what type of care is provided. However, we first introduce the reader to those

---

[2] However, Cook and Wright (1995) argue that the lack of an unambiguous treatment technology actually gives mental health care professionals greater job latitude.

organizational theories which address the influence of the external environment on organizational behavior.

Understanding Changes in Mental Health Care Through the Lens of Organizational Theory

Institutional Theory and Population Ecology

In this section we provide a very brief discussion of those organization theories which address change – institutional theory and population ecology. Organizational theory emphasizes that organizations must be responsive to their external environments – they are open, rather than closed systems. Meyer and Scott (1983) expanded this insight into early formulations of institutional theory, which has had important implications for understanding mental health care services.[3] Meyer and Scott (1983) distinguish between the rational (or technical) model of organizational behavior where inputs, processes, and outcomes can be precisely measured and evaluated and the institutional model of organizational behavior where inputs, processes and outcomes are only loosely connected or coupled. Car manufactures are good examples of organizations which can be best understood under this technical model. Mental health organizations fit better into the institutional model of organizational behavior (Hasenfeld, 1992; Meyer 1986; Scott & Meyer, 1991).

Legitimacy is central to understanding the difference between technical and institutional environments. Legitimacy is necessary to resource acquisition and the institutional linkages that subsequently ensure organizational survival (Baum & Oliver, 1991; Tucker, Baum, & Singh 1992). Rather than attaining legitimacy primarily on the basis of demonstrated technical competence or successful client outcomes, mental health services are evaluated on the basis of their conformity to normative beliefs and societal preferences which exist in the institutional environment (Hasenfeld, 1992; Scheid-Cook, 1991; Scott & Meyer, 1991). That is, MHO must perform their role in the manner prescribed by the environment (for instance, providing community based care as opposed to institutionalized care). Consequently, legitimacy is based upon evaluations by various constituents that the organization is doing what it is believed it "ought to be doing."

Hasenfeld (1992, pp. 13–14) has argued that evaluations of organizational effectiveness involve "explicit or implicit moral choices that are embedded in the

---

[3] Organizational sociologists differentiate between institutional and neo-institutional theory. Neo-institutional theories place greater emphasis upon cognitive frameworks for action and institutional isomorphism (i.e. why are organizations within an organizational field so similar), while "old" institutional theory places greater emphasis upon competing values and conflict (i.e. how do organizations change with changes in their institutional environments?) Along with Rundall, Shortell, and Alexander (2004) we find "old" institutional theory to be more helpful in understanding changes in organizational structures and fields.

practices ideologies" of providers; practice ideologies refer to "beliefs about what is 'good' for the client." The effectiveness of service offerings is measured in light of these beliefs. That is, MHO will be viewed as effective if they are providing services mental health care providers consider necessary to mental health care. However, in mental health there is wide disagreement over the appropriateness of various treatment technologies and intervention strategies (Chandler, 1990; Rochefort, 1989). Furthermore, there is little consensus on what constitutes appropriate, adequate, or quality mental health care (Mechanic, 1994; Pollack, McFarland, George, & Angell, 1994; Rochefort, 1989). Mental health care providers also have very different views about the etiology of mental illness, and different approaches to treatment (Cook & Wright, 1995). As described above, mental health care is also provided by people with diverse professional, occupational, and educational backgrounds that contribute to a diversity of treatment ideologies. In addition to professional beliefs and values, governmental policies (and funding) are another important institutional force which affects the availability of services. Governmental regulators, funding agencies, and private insurers may also disagree about what constitutes appropriate mental health care (and consequently what they will fund). The need for MHO to meet demands from diverse institutional demands can result in ambiguity over goals as well as conflict over treatment or population priorities. In support of this argument, D'Aunno, Sutton, and Price (1991, p. 656) found that mental health organizations which also provided drug abuse services are characterized by "inconsistent treatment practices."

Additionally, MHO operate in turbulent institutional environments where there are multiple and often competing normative preferences for treatment and care. Consequently, they experience "cyclical legitimacy crises" (Hasenfeld, 1992, p. 1) as organizational form changes more slowly than do institutional demands. For example, community mental health centers were first critiqued for providing care to the "worried well" rather than to those with serious mental illnesses. To maintain their legitimacy (and funding), community mental health centers had to shift their organizational structures to provide care to those with chronic mental illnesses. Currently the worried well cannot get care from public sector mental health agencies, whose defined target population is now those with serious mental illness.

Ambiguity and inconsistency are obvious threats to legitimacy, which is critical to organizational survival. The importance of legitimacy for organizational survival links institutional theory to another organizational theory, population ecology. Population ecologists explore questions of organizational survival and decline. The ecological analysis of organizations focuses attention on an entire population, or community of organizations (Baum, 1996). The population could be state mental hospitals, comprehensive outpatient centers, providers in private practice, multi-disciplinary treatment teams or all of these organizational forms in a specified geographic area. Population ecologists study changes in organizational populations, examining sources of variation, selection, retention, and competition (Baum, 1996). The central concern is with understanding why new organizational forms emerge (foundings), why (and especially how) some organizational forms survive, and what factors account for organizational failure (decline or death).

Population ecology is linked to institutional theory in that for some populations of organizations survival (as well as processes of selection and variation) is dependent on responding to wider institutional demands (Alexander & Amburgey, 1987; Alexander & D'Aunno, 1990). A population ecology perspective is certainly useful for understanding recent changes to mental health care organizations because managed care incorporates principles of competition among providers and organizations. A series of articles published in *Medical Care* applied population ecology perspectives to health care organizations (Alexander & Amburgey, 1987; Aldrich, 1987; Hurley & Kaluzny, 1987).

In the following sections, we apply institutional theory and population ecology to the four major phases of mental health care identified in the introduction: institutionalized care, deinstitutionalization, community based care, and managed care. During each historical phase we examine how research in MHO has been used to advance sociological understanding of complex organizational processes, and how organizational research has contributed to understanding of mental health care.

Institutionalized Care and Social Control

The first phase of mental health care, institutionalization, is also a time when organizational sociologists focused primarily upon single organizations and how formal structures operate. Mental hospitals were fruitful research sites in that research on these organizations led to a better understanding of social control in organizations. Researchers were interested in how the social structure of mental institutions shaped therapeutic outcomes. Erving Goffman (1961, p. 4) described the state mental hospital as a "total" institution where all of an individual's needs are met and life is highly regimented and controlled. Mental hospitals were designed to care for those who are "felt to be incapable of looking after themselves and a threat to the community." Goffman analyzed the two sub-cultures of the mental hospital: staff and patient, and showed how patients have to conform to institutional expectations which ultimately undermine their sense of self. While we tend to remember Goffman for his insights into patient life and the reality of the stigma of mental illness, he also provided insight into how mental health care organizations work and how mental health care providers think about their patients and their problems. While diagnosis of mental illness was based on some form of medical criteria, treatment was largely custodial. Furthermore, because of the involuntary nature of most commitments to a mental hospital, as well as the small numbers of mental health professionals to deal with increasingly large patient populations, custodial care became a matter of social control.

Anselm Strauss also studied mental health care and the treatment ideologies of mental health professionals. Strauss, Schatzman, Burcher, Ehrlich, and Sabshin (1964, p. 8) defined a psychiatric ideology as "shared or collective sets of psychiatric ideas" about the causes and treatment of mental illness. In their study of two psychiatric hospitals, Strauss et al. (1964) identified three philosophies of care: somatotherapeutic (or organic), psychotherapeutic, and milieu or sociotherapeutic (environmental). In today's terminology, these ideologies correspond to the biomedical, psychosocial, and social models of treatment. Strauss et al. (1964) described the conflict between ideologies that emphasized treatment and those that emphasized custodial care, and how these ideologies are shaped by organizational and professional factors. Custodial care is dehumanized care, and was the result of strict professionalism, reliance on technologies and medications, and the large size of health care organizations (Strauss, 1975). Strauss has also focused on how the widespread prevalence of chronic illness necessitates a different treatment philosophy, and will require organizational restructuring in order to meet therapeutic and moral goals for treatment (Strauss, Fagerhaugh, Suczek, & Wiener, 1985).

Mental hospitals were also rich sources of theoretical innovation for organizational sociologists. Amitai Etzioni (1960) advanced organizational theory by providing a critique of human relations approaches to human behavior within organizations. He found that in state mental hospitals communication and participation were not just ways of sharing power (as argued by human relations theorists), but rather could be used as techniques of manipulation. By over-emphasizing the importance of communication and the benefits of participation, organizational researchers had neglected to examine important structural and external forces which influence organizational activities.

Another leading organizational theorist, Charles Perrow, also conducted research in mental hospitals. Perrow's research (1965) contributed to the understanding of the source of the conflict between therapeutic goals (care and treatment) and custodial goals (maintenance and control of patients). Perrow (1965) argued that organizations are influenced by a cultural system which sets legitimate goals (i.e., therapy), a technology which determines the means available to the attainment of these goals (i.e., psychiatrists or counselors), and a social structure (the mental hospital) in which these technologies are embedded. State mental hospitals were at that time described as resource deprived institutions, with little means or technology available to meet therapeutic goals. Consequently, treatment goals were only symbolic, and the real function of the state mental hospital was custodial. In other words, the authoritarian structure of state mental hospitals observed by Etzioni was consistent with available technologies. While the advent of psychotropic drugs certainly provided state mental hospitals with a viable treatment technology, it still is not clear whether medication serves therapeutic or custodial goals.

Following the theoretical insights of Etzioni and Perrow, there has been a large body of research which points to the importance of organizational factors in understanding the treatment careers of individuals with mental illnesses (Brissendum & Lennard, 1971; Mechanic, 1968; Morrissey, Goldman, & Klerman, 1980; Tessler & Goodman, 1982). For example, Holland, Konick, Buffum, Smith, & Petcher (1981) studied the influences of alternative organizational structures in state mental hospitals on the care of patients and patient level outcomes and found that organizational structure influences the behavior of staff and hence patient level outcomes. O'Driscoll and Evans (1988) found that perceptions of the atmosphere in three psychiatric wards (reflecting organizational climate) affected the treatment programs offered on those wards. That is, the care delivered to clients is a product of organizational processes. While we know that the care provided to clients is influenced by the treatment ideologies of providers (Strauss et al., 1964), we are less likely to remember that Strauss et al. (1964) also argued that treatment ideologies are shaped by organizations within which providers work. While treatment ideologies are learned in formal educational settings, they are shaped and modified by concrete organizational experiences (for a discussion of how organizational context influences the treatment practices of psychiatrists, see Luhrmann, 2000). At the same time, professional preferences for care can also shape organizational structures providing care, as was seen in the transition from institutional to community based care.

Deinstitutionalization and the Transitions to Community Based Care

When mental health care began to move into the community, organizational researchers were also extending their gaze to the organizational field. Organizational theories moved from an emphasis on closed systems (with a focus on internal organizational structures) to open system models, which emphasize the relations organizations have with each other and the external environment. Baker (1969) applied the open system model of organizational behavior to a mental hospital as it changed to a community mental health care system. The community mental health ideology changed the goals and structure of the hospital. More recently, Gudeman (1988) has described how state mental hospitals have diversified and now provide a broad range of outpatient and rehabilitation services to different patient populations, although Dowdall (1996) argues that state hospitals still provide custodial care to those who cannot survive in the community.

State mental hospitals were slated for extinction with the advent of community based care. Deinstitutionalization began in the 1950s and reflects a change in the wider social environment—both technical and institutional. Psychotropic drugs developed in the 1950s provided health care workers with the technology to treat patients in the community and to control the bizarre behavior associated with psychosis. At the same time, the more liberal attitudes of the 1960s resulted in a series of court rulings that mandated care in the least restrictive environment. There were also important economic reforms which led to new forms of public funding for community based health in the 1960s. The political mechanism for deinstitutionalization was President Kennedy's Community Mental Health Centers Act of 1963 which provided funding for community mental health centers (CMHC) to serve clients in a catchment area of 75,000 to 200,000 people. The legislation was designed so that the National Institute of Mental Health (NIMH) dealt directly with communities and CMHC while state governments had authority over state mental hospitals, which resulted in conflict between state and local authorities and states continued to direct the majority of their funding to state mental hospitals. The problem would be exacerbated with Reagan's 1980 Omnibus Reconciliation Act which block-granted federal monies for mental health to states, by-passing communities. We will talk more about CMHC in the next section; here we focus on what happened to state mental hospitals.

Dowdall (1996, p. 23) describes state mental hospitals as "maximalist" organizations; they live very long lives and are unusually resistant to change. One might describe them more unkindly as "permanently failing" organizations (Meyer & Zucker, 1988). State mental hospitals exhibited remarkable stability from the mid 1960s to the 1980s. This is partly because states had legal monopoly over involuntary admissions, which were the "natural, or taken-for-granted institutional response to mental illness" (Dowdall, 1996, p. 31). Most of the several hundred state mental hospitals created since 1773 remain in existence, although patient censuses dropped drastically with deinstitutionalization. While some state mental hospitals have closed, in the past two decades most changed their organizational form to meet new institutional demands. Dowdall (1996) describes the new functions taken on by the Buffalo State Hospital, which now provides rehabilitation, day treatment, case management, sheltered workshops, and family care. In 1992, the NIMH reported that the average state spends 57 percent of their state mental health care dollars on hospitals, despite the fact that most people need outpatient care in their communities. This is because state mental hospitals are deeply intertwined into the local economies within which they reside (many state mental hospitals are major employers in their largely rural communities), or else they continue to serve vital functions by caring for those individuals that do need inpatient care. Consequently, CMHC have had to struggle for resources and have also had to work to define their relevant domain (Wagenfeld & Robin, 1976). David Mechanic (1974) argued that CMHC operated under conditions of uncertainty, had diffuse goals, and lacked clear performance standards.

Community Based Care and System Integration

In theory, CMHC were to provide individualized competency based programs, to coordinate those agencies that provided services to clients with mental illnesses, and to promote social support networks for these individuals (Adler, 1982). These functions specify a social model of care, rather than a medical one, and the locus of care moved from the confines of a single organization to the organizational field.

As mental health care moved into the community there was a need to understand how services which had once been delivered within one institution could be delivered by a number of organizations within the community. At the same time, organizational researchers were also focusing their attention on the organizational field (i.e. the system of organizations around a given organizational entity such as the CMHC) and utilizing network theory and population ecology to understand dynamic relations among organizations. Consequently, there was a concern with coordination and integration of services and mental health researchers began to draw upon organizational theories in order to understand relations between organizations (i.e. inter-organizational relations). Network theories were used to understand not only the social support networks of clients (Perrucci & Targ, 1982), but to understand whether the various organizations providing services were integrated whether services were coordinated (Morrissey & Lindsey, 1987).

Outpatient community mental health care organizations have clearly suffered from the "liability of newness." As described by organizational ecologists, newer organizations have higher failure rates (Baum, 1996). Small organizations are also more likely to fail, in part because larger organizations (such as state mental hospitals) are less likely to fail due to their greater inertia (i.e. their resistance to change). Small organizations are also more likely to fail because they have lower visibility and recognition, and a lower degree of embeddedness in their communities. Outpatient community mental health care organizations are fairly invisible and often do not have strong ties to other organizations in the mental health field. In contrast, state mental hospitals have established high levels of normative legitimacy and also meet standards for external accountability. Additionally, they are deeply rooted in their communities and in the mental health field; hence they have been able to maintain resource flows. As predicted by organizational ecology, outpatient mental health care organizations have had problems gaining and maintaining resources, both in terms of funding and qualified staff. Organizations attempting reorganization are also more unstable, and may ultimately fail in their reorganization attempts. In part because of their large size, state mental hospitals have been able to take on new roles or tasks, often performing the same functions traditionally associated with outpatient care. Consequently, most state mental hospitals have survived structural reorganization while many outpatient mental health care organizations have been less successful.

While organizational structure was still an important influence on the quality of care received by patients (Greenley, 1973; Mechanic, 1968; Schulbegt & Bromet, 1981), researchers pointed to the need for increased coordination of community services, and organizational studies of mental health care emphasized inter-organizational relations and organizational boundaries (Morrissey, 1982; Morrissey, Tausig, & Lindsay, 1984). A persistent theme has been that mental health services are fragmented and inaccessible to clients (Gruenberg & Huxley, 1970; Mechanic & Rochefort, 1990; Shadish, Lurigio, & Lewis, 1989). Several researchers (Goldman, Morrissey, Rosenheck, Cocozza, Blasinsky, & Randolph, 2002; Morrissey, Calloway, Bartko, Ridgeley, Goldman, & Paulson, 1994; Rosenheck, Lam, Morrissey, Calloway, Stolar, & Randolph, 2002) have evaluated the effect of system integration on patient level outcomes, significantly advancing mental health services research with their creative use of organizational sociology. At the same time, Provan and Milward (1995) used their study of four community mental health systems to advance organizational theory on network effectiveness. Issues of system integration and coordination are still critical to understanding mental health care systems, and mental health services researchers must also address ways in which different systems of care (i.e. substance abuse, physical health care, and vocational rehabilitation) can be integrated in order to provide needed social supports for clients. Research in this area will most certainly benefit from the inclusion of organizational researchers, and will no doubt lead to further advances in our understanding of inter-system as well as inter-organizational linkages.

Population ecology is also important to understanding relations between organizations within an organizational field. An important distinction made by population ecologists is between specialist and generalist organizations. Specialist organizations operate in one domain, or provide one service, while generalist organizations operate in multiple domains or provide multiple services (Singh, Tucker, & Meinhard, 1991). While all mental health care organizations perform multiple services, they can be characterized as specialist or generalist by examining the range of services they provide, and how many populations they provide services to. Specialist mental health care organizations provide highly specialized services to a single, or narrowly, delineated client population. Generalist organizations provide a broader range of services to more diverse client populations. Scheid and Greenley (1997) utilized this distinction between generalist and specialist organizations in an examination of 29 outpatient mental health programs in Wisconsin (these programs were purposefully selected on the basis of having good reputations and organizational stability). Specialist programs provided tailored services to those with chronic mental illnesses, while generalist organizations provided comprehensive services to a wide array of clients with mental health problems. The two types of mental health organizations had different organizational structures, faced different environmental demands, and had very different work climates. Specialist mental health organizations had more positive work environments, more coherent, clearly articulated program philosophies, and lower levels of goal incongruence (disagreements about organizational priorities). Consequently, participants in specialist mental health organizations evaluated their organization as being more significantly more effective than participants in generalist organizations (Scheid & Greenley, 1997). One explanation for the effectiveness (and survival) of specialist organizations is that they are able to exploit resources by not competing with generalist organizations (Baum, 1996).

The development of community based mental health was associated with new funding which focused on individuals with chronic mental illnesses, who had been neglected in the generalist, comprehensive mental health centers. While mental health care is important, clients with chronic illnesses must access diverse systems of care and social support (Schlesinger & Mechanic 1993). Medical services, housing, rehabilitation services, and social supports must be integrated to meet the diverse service needs of clients with mental health problems. When service agencies focus on only one type of problem or client population (as specialist organizations do), or when there are categorical funding streams that pay for one type of service, but not another (i.e. substance abuse or mental health care), then service system fragmentation will occur (Provan & Sebastian 1998). Managed care has the potential to increase system coordination and efficiency by combining funding streams and reorganizing systems of care (Feder, Komisar, & Niefeld, 2000), although there is obvious concern that such integration will favor acute medical services over the long term supportive services needed by chronic care patients (Cohen, 1998).

Managed Care and the Logic of Cost Containment

We are currently in the era of managed care, or market driven health care (Scott et al., 2000). Managed care refers to processes or techniques used by, or on behalf of, purchasers of health care which seek to control or influence the quality, accessibility, utilization, and costs of health care. Managed care began to have an effect on mental health organizations in the early 1990s, appearing first in the private sector as private insurance companies imposed managed care mechanisms to control costs. Public mental health care systems soon followed suit (Essok & Goldman, 1995; Mechanic, 1999). Managed care practices have even spread to integrated public health systems such as the Veterans Administration, which in 1995 introduced prospective payment and implemented performance monitoring systems tied to administrators' compensation (Greenberg & Rosenheck, 2003).

Utilization review has been the most common form of public sector managed care, though some states are turning to capitation to control costs. Three types of utilization review can occur: prospective, concurrent, and retrospective. Prospective review refers to denying or modifying the availability of services before they are provided (pre-authorization or pre-certification and gatekeeping). Concurrent review refers to ongoing review of treatment at regular intervals (either during inpatient stay or during outpatient visits) to determine whether treatment is still necessary. Retrospective review is the evaluation of services that have already been provided and can involve the use of aggregate data to evaluate levels and types of services provided by individuals or groups (often called provider profiling), or to identify under and over utilization of services for a specific population.

Managed care emphasizes a treatment modality in keeping with a medical model of illness; decisions to reimburse care are based upon determinations of "medical necessity." If a mental health problem meets established diagnostic criteria, results in impaired social functioning, and can be treated efficaciously, then conditions of "medical necessity" are met (Birne-Stone, Cypres, & Winderbaum, 1997; Mechanic, 1999). Treatment goals are set in terms of short term improvements in functional ability rather than longer term goals of community stability and integration, producing what Hoge, Davidson, Griffith, Sledge, and Howenstine (1998) refer to as the crisis of care.

In order to determine if treatment is indeed cost effective, managed care organizations must also emphasize measurable outcomes (i.e. evidence based medicine). As noted above, an important obstacle to evaluating managed mental health care is the difficulty in assessing treatment effectiveness. There is little consensus about the etiology of mental illness, appropriate treatments, or the effectiveness of various treatments (Cook & Wright, 1995; Mechanic, 1999). In terms of chronic and severe mental illness, there may not be noticeable signs of improvement, even within excellent programs (Mechanic, Schlesinger, & McAlpine, 1995). However, managed care organizations do rely upon the assessment of client outcomes and have propelled the development of a bureaucratic system of treatment and practice guidelines (i.e. cookbook medicine). Thus, there is now a good bit of literature on outcome assessment in mental health (Essock & Goldman, 1997; MacFarland, 2001; Salzer, 1999) and a focus on the development of measures of quality care (Hermann, Left, Palmer, Yang, Teller, Provost, Jakubiak, & Chan, 2000) as well as procedures for ensuring quality improvement. It is clear that managed care represents an extension of bureaucratic control, although the driving force is not increased effectiveness or efficiency, but cost containment (Scheid, 2003).

What have been the consequences of managed care? Managed care has resulted in fewer inpatient care episodes and reduced hospital stays (Durham, 1995; Manderscheid, Henderson, Witkin, & Atay, 2000), but this has been at the expense of restricted access to care (Weisman, Pettigrew, Stosky, & Regier, 2000). Managed care plans generally do not cover chronic mental illness in their standard benefit packages, and the amount of money allocated for mental health care is not sufficient for adequate treatment (Inglehart, 1996; Manderscheid et al., 2000). Fried, Topping, Morrissey, Ellis, Stroup, & Blank (2000) found that providers in managed care felt their clients had less access to long term services, and that they had less confidence in external review. Kirschner and Lachiocotte (2001) found that providers felt threatened by managed care. Ware, Lachiocotte, Kirschner, Cortes, and Good (2001) reported that these same providers feared that the quality of care would deteriorate. Scheid (2004) provides an extensive analysis of how the work of mental health care providers (both in the public and the private sector) has changed with managed care, and finds that organizational environments are less supportive of provider's work and that providers have lower levels of autonomy than before managed care. Consequently, providers report less satisfaction with work and higher levels of burnout. Not only are providers highly critical of managed care, they felt it undermined the quality of care delivered to clients. Empirical analysis of changes in service system offerings confirm provider's beliefs that under managed care utilization review has limited the types and availability of services, and that there is less emphasis on the provision of services and supports necessary for community stability.

Another consequence of managed care has been the breakdown of the historic divide between public and private sector health care. Most public sector mental health care is paid for by Medicaid dollars, and states have been moving their Medicaid enrollees to managed care plans in order to save money, effectively privatizing public sector mental health. There is a great deal of state to state variability in the degree of managed care penetration, as well as in how managed care services are reimbursed. Some states use integrated programs where the state Medicaid agency contracts with managed care organizations to provide both physical and mental health, while others "carve-out" mental health services. Researchers (Hodgkin, Horgan, & Garnick, 1997; Vogelsang, 1999) have begun to examine the efficiency of separating primary from mental health in this manner from an institutional economics approach known as Transaction Costs theory. Although research is preliminary, carve outs may allow managed care organizations to avoid the inefficiencies that are associated with providing too many diverse services. At the same time, Transaction Costs theory would also allow for the possibility that carve outs may increase inefficiencies due to opportunism or a lack of competition.

Traditional providers of mental health services will be able to survive in the managed care environment to the degree that they develop organizational structures that conform to the institutional demands of managed care. This means developing new departments to manage care, provide utilization and concurrent review, and to provide outcome assessment. However, there is concern that managed care cannot meet the long term care needs of individuals with chronic illnesses because of its inherent focus on short term outcomes (Schlesinger &

Mechanic, 1993). The Bazelon Center (2000, 2001) found that in many states privatized managed care resulted in fewer services to those with serious mental illness and neglect of rehabilitation care. We have come full circle to concerns raised in the 1960s and 1970s about therapeutic treatment versus custodial care, and conflict between professional authority and bureaucratic control.

The Exacerbation of Conflict Between Professional Authority and Bureaucratic Control

As we noted in the introduction, one of the central contributions of research on MHO has been to sociological understanding of conflicting forms of authority and control in organizations. In particular, MHO have been excellent sources for advancing our understanding of the relationship between bureaucratic control and professional status. As we discussed earlier, central to professional status is autonomy and control over one's work. Summarizing the various definitions of professional Hafferty and Wolinsky (1991) identify three characteristics of professionalism: monopolization of knowledge (i.e. expert identification), autonomy in work performance, and authority over clients. Central to legitimacy as a professional is licensure and the authority and control over one's work (Freidson, 1984).

Managed care represents a direct challenge to the autonomy and control mental health professionals have over the care they provide; "by design, managed care is intended to alter clinical practices" (Schlesinger & Gray, 1999, p. 441). Managed care sets limits to the types of care authorized, limits treatment sessions, subjects clinical decisions and client records to third party review, and imposes bureaucratic controls over therapeutic relationships (Scheid, 2004). Rather than advocating for their clients, providers must meet the standards of care determined by the managed care entity. There is a great deal of literature on the ethical dilemmas experienced by mental health care providers (Backlar, 1996; Fletcher, 1998; Furman, 2003; Galambos, 1999; Kirschner & Lachicotte 2001; Moffic, 1997; Phillips, 1997; Ware et al., 2000). However, there has been little research on how mental health care organizations have changed with institutional demands for managed care (for an exception, see Scheid 2004). This is partly due to the fact that there is tremendous diversity at both the state and local levels in mental health care organizations, and in approaches to managed care (Hanson & Huskamp, 2001).

Within MHO psychiatrists and psychologists are the ultimate "legitimate" professionals, welding considerable power and authority (Luhrmann, 2000). Yet the majority of care is increasingly provided by nurses and social workers; both "professional" groups have traditionally sought greater professional recognition, power and autonomy. With greater professional status, providers are in a better position to challenge organizational (or bureaucratic) forms of control. The central issue is whether work is guided by standardized rules and formal procedures, or whether the provider has a wide degree of skill discretion, decision latitude, and autonomy. With greater standardization, or rationalization, the work of professionals is subject to deprofessionalization, or the loss of autonomy and control over one's work (Hafferty & Wolinsky, 1991).

Anderson (1992) refers to the replacement of internalized professional norms and standards with organizational arrangements which monitor practice as corporate rationalization (Anderson, 1992), which does have the effect of de-legitimating the decision making power of the individual (Scott, 1985). As described by Starr (1982), organizational control over the pace and routines of work as well as the close scrutiny of mistakes, has contributed to the loss of professional autonomy of individual doctors. However, since doctors themselves have served as agents of formal control, the profession itself does not become deprofessionalized (Friedson, 1984; Scott, 1985; Starr, 1982). Managed care represents an obvious extension of the logic of corporate rationality, and may also involve some degree of deprofessionalization, depending on the specific mechanisms whereby care is managed and how much input providers have into the management of care.

While the work of physicians is indeed subject to greater bureaucratic oversight in managed care organizations, physicians have been able to maintain control over their work by virtue of claims to professional expertise (Griffiths & Hughs, 1999; Hoff & McCaffrey, 1996; Lupton 1997; Weiss & Fitzpatrick, 1997). This is because decisions about clinical care rely upon medical expertise. For example, Weiss and Fitzpatrick (1997) found that while physicians in Great Britain were conforming to principles of cost containment, clinical autonomy was maintained. Professional logics of care had changed to incorporate bureaucratic and corporate principles. However, healthcare providers with less legitimate claim to expert knowledge (such as mental health care providers) may have more difficulty maintaining clinical autonomy. In 1990, Dumont wrote in an editorial that managed mental health care represented the "final subordination of professionalism to the market" (p. 166) and the loss of the ideals of community based mental health care. Another consequence of managed care relevant to deprofessionalization is the use of lower level professional to provide care. The mental health workforce is increasingly made up of fewer psychiatrists and Ph.D. psychologists and more clinical social workers and advanced practice nurses (Scheffer, Ivey, & Garrett, 1998; Scheffer & Kirby, 2003). However, there has been little research on the effects of changing patterns of provider mix on either the quality or the effectiveness of mental health care. It is likely that where treatment technologies are ambiguous or contradictory (as in mental health) there is an increased likelihood that bureaucratic standards of care will prevail.

Current Controversies and Research Possibilities

Mental health organizations have been excellent sources of information for organizational sociologists studying the consequences of bureaucracy, conflict between bureaucratic and professional authority, and the degree of control and autonomy individuals have in bureaucratic settings. In addition, mental health care researchers have drawn upon organizational theory to understand the factors which affect the delivery of mental health care and the quality of care received. We have shown how the study of the mental health care sector has led to advances in organizational sociology, and how organizational sociology has enabled mental health researchers to make sense of the effects of these changes in the mental health sector. With the realization that the organization of care matters, mental health services research has maintained close ties to organizational theory, while mental health organizations have remained fertile grounds for organizational researchers. In 1974, David Mechanic argued that mental health services are characterized by unclear objectives and outcomes, conflict between different groups of providers or units over responsibilities for patient care, and diverse external pressures from the community and other agencies. This is still an apt description for today's mental health care organizations, and consequently they remain an excellent laboratory for studying how organizations manage contradiction, conflict, and ambiguity.

We are in the early stages of a new era of mental health care. Managed care constitutes a fundamental change and represents the rationalization of care-giving with emphasis placed upon efficiency and cost containment. Managed care imposes a rational business ethic and corresponding systems of bureaucratic control on organizations which had previously operated on the basis of a professionally based moral foundation (Scheid, 2003). The conflict between these two logics is reflected in the often used phrase, "managing costs versus managing care." Managed care also reinforces a medical model of care and has led to a greater reliance upon pharmacological approaches to treatment (Luhrmann, 2000; Scheid, 2004). Consequently, managed care presents a threat to the professional autonomy and decision making power of providers and may also result in lower quality care.

Managed care is providing new opportunities for sociologists to study how institutional demands can change the structure, organization, and delivery of mental health care. As we have elucidated above, managed care represents a fundamental change and may intensify conflict between bureaucratic (or entrepreneurial) and professional logics of care. Scheid (2003) found that professional based standards for effective, quality care were being displaced in a public sector mental health organization which sought to implement managed care. However, this research needs to be supplemented by more case studies as well as more extensive research on various forms of managed care, as well as the effect of managed care practices on diverse professional and occupational groups. We feel continued study of MHO will lead to further advances in organizational theorizing about the resolution of conflict between different principles of organizational control, and in lieu of a conclusion, we offer some promising directions for future research.

Neo-institutional theorists have emphasized institutional isomorphism where organizations in a shared organizational field exhibit similarity and homogeneity in response to institutional demands (Baxter, 1983; DiMaggio & Powell, 1983; Edelman, 1990). However, organizations also provide the context within which institutional demands are interpreted and worked out. When institutional demands are ambiguous and contradictory, organizational activities may be less easily understood in terms of isomorphism or homogeneity. Instead, the processes by which organizations confront their environment must also be understood in terms of enactment (Scheid-Cook, 1992). Enactment refers to the reality that the external environment exists within the constructions of organizational members (Weick, 1977). Enactment processes create the very information organizations are usually portrayed as responding to, and focuses attention on the ways in which organizational members select, manipulate, and/or ignore information (Pfeffer & Salanick, 1978). One reason for the diversity of response to managed care is that enactment processes logically result in variability (rather than homogeneity) of organizational response, especially for those organizations residing in turbulent institutional environments (such as mental health care organizations). Consequently, the diversity of forms of organizational response to managed care provides a new laboratory for sociological investigation, and may well lead to important advances in sociological theory. In the remaining paragraphs, we point to some important avenues researchers should draw upon in order to advance understanding of the social organization of mental health care.

In 1995 *The Journal of Health and Social Behavior* published an extra issue to assess the state of medical sociology and provide directions for future research. Flood and Fennel (1995) wrote a chapter on the role of organizational sociology in understanding the health care system. They provide a thorough (and still relevant) discussion of how the professional model of organizations and work, institutional theory, ecological theory, exchange theory, and various economic models can be used to guide research as well as understanding the shifting dynamics of health care policy and reform. We encourage the readers of this chapter interested in the organizational analysis of mental health care to study Flood and Fennel's article carefully.

In 2004 *The Journal of Health and Social Behavior* published an extra issue on the social organization of health care. Michael Hughes was editor of the Journal of Health and Social Behavior at that time, and asked for the special issue because so few articles in the journal have addressed the social organization of health care (Hughes, 2004). One article in that issue is highly relevant to understanding the diversity in the mental health care sector. Rundall, Shortell, and Alexander (2004) draw from institutional and market theories to develop a series of hypothesis to guide research on changing organizational forms of physician-hospital integration. One larger theoretical issue they address is the relationship between institutional and market logics of care. In this chapter, we have viewed market logics as one form of institutional demand, which is in line with the more common view that markets operate within institutional environments (Baum, 1996). It is certainly plausible that market forces can promote changes in the institutional environment, and this thinking is in line with Meyer's (1990) commodity model (for a full description of this model and its relevance to mental health care, see Scheid, 2003). Not surprisingly, the commodity model arises from the work of economists and views organizational structures as being guided by financial controls and the desire to accumulate wealth (or to save public monies). Along with Scott et al., (2000) we have taken the view that professional logics and market logics (which both exist in the institutional environment) are in conflict. As we have argued, the outcome of this conflict is not clear.

However, Rundall et al. (2004) provide a very good framework for investigating this conflict. They use the concept of domain separation to conceptualize the degree to which organizations and professional groups in a given geographic area operate in institutional and market environments that are relatively separate (high domain separation) or relatively integrated (low domain separation). The degree of domain separation will affect how competing institutional logics are enacted, the conflict between competing logics, and the degree to which market or professionally based logics will prevail. Researchers studying the evolving system of mental health care should draw upon the concepts introduced by Rundall et al. (2004, p. 114) to make predictions about the different types of organizational structures likely to prevail in different types of domains.

A second article in the special issue argues that economic transactions are embedded in networks of social relationships (Wholey, Christianson, Draper, Lesser, & Burns, 2004). Understanding of social and economic embeddedness is one way to approach the degree of domain separation, and is also important in understanding variability in community and organizational responses to competing institutional and market demands. Consequently, as they respond to institutional demands for managed care, states and communities are creating new opportunities for sociological investigation of changing organizational forms as well as exploration of the dynamics of community networks. The diversity of responses to managed care should be considered as an opportunity rather than an obstacle to research, and we hope we are entering a new era of research which links organizational and mental health researchers.

References

Abbott, A. (1988). *The system of professions*. Chicago: The University of Chicago Press.

Adler, P. T. (1982). An analysis of the concept of competence in individuals and social systems. *Community Mental Health Journal, 18*, 34–45.

Alexander, J. A., & Amburgey, T. L. (1987). The dynamics of change in the American hospital industry: Transformation or selection." *Medical Care Review, 44*, 279–321.

Alexander, J. A., & D'Aunno, T. A. (1990). Transformation of institutional environments: Perspectives on the corporatization of U.S. health care. In S. S. Mick (Ed.), *Innovations in health care delivery* (pp. 53–85). San Francisco: Jossey-Bass Publishers.

Aldrich, H. (1987). New paradigms for old: The population perspectives contribution to health services research." *Medical Care, 44*, 257–277.

Anderson, J. G. (1992). The deprofessionalization of American medicine. *Current Research in Occupations and Professions, 7*, 241–256.

Atwood, N. (1982). Professional prejudice and the psychotic client. *Social Work, 27*, 172–177.

Backlar, P. (1996). Managed mental health care: Conflicts of interest in the provider/client relationship. *Community Mental Health Journal, 32*, 101–106.

Baker, F. (1969). An open systems approach to the study of mental hospitals in transition. *Community Mental Health Journal, 5*, 403–412.

Baum, J. (1996). Organizational ecology. In S. R. Clegg, C. Hardy, & W. R. Nord (Eds.), *Handbook of organization studies*. (pp. 76–114). London: Sage Publications.

Baum, J., & Oliver, C. (1991). Institutional linkages and organizational mortality. *Administrative Science Quarterly, 36*, 187–218.

Baxter, V. (1989). The process of change in public service organizations. *Sociological Quarterly, 30*, 283–304.

Bazelon Center for Mental Health Law. (2000). Effective public management of mental health care: Views from states on Medicaid reforms that enhance service system integration and accountability. Washington, DC. See *http://www.bazelon.org*.

Bazelon Center for Mental Health Law (2001). Disintegrating systems: The state of State's public mental health systems. Washington, DC. See *http://www.bazelon.org*.

Ben-Dror, R. (1994). Employee turnover in community mental health organizations: A developmental stages model. *Community Mental Health Journal, 30*, 243–257.

Birne-Stone, S., Cypres, A., & Winderbaum, S. (1997). Case-management and review strategies. In R. N. Alperin & D. C.Phillips (Eds.), *The impact of managed care on the practice of psychotherapy* (pp. 51–56). New York: Brunner/Mazel Publishers.

Brissendum, R., & Leonard, H. (1971). Organization of mental health services and Its effect on the treatment career of the patient. *Mental Hygiene, 54*, 416–420.

Brown, P., & Cooksey, E. (1989). Mental health monopoly: Corporate trends in mental health services. *Social Science and Medicine*, 28, 1129–1139.

Chandler, S. (1990). *Competing realities: The contested terrain of mental health advocacy*. New York: Praeger.

Cohen, M. A. (1998). Emerging trends in the finance and delivery of long-term care: Public and private opportunities and challenges. *The Gerontologist, 38*, 80–89.

Cook, J., & Wright, E. (1995). Medical sociology and the study of severe mental illnesses: Reflections on past accomplishments and directions for future research. *Journal of Health and Social Behavior, (Special Issue)*, 95–114.

D'Aunno, T., Sutton, R., & Price, R. (1991). Isomorphism and external support in conflicting institutional environments: A study of drug abuse treatment units. *Academy of Management Review, 34*, 636–661.

DiMaggio, P., & Powell, W. W. (1983). The iron cage revisited: Institutional isomorphism and collective rationality in organization fields. *American Journal of Sociology, 48*, 147–60.

Doherty, E. G., & Harry, J. 1976. Structural dissensus in a therapeutic community. *Journal of Health and Social Behavior, 17*, 272–279.

Dowdall, G. (1996). *The eclipse of the state hospital: Policy, stigma and organization*. NY: State University of New York Press.

Drolen, C. S. (1990). Current community mental health center operations: Entrepreneurship or business as usual? *Community Mental Health Journal, 26*, 547–558.

Dumont, M. P. (1990). Managed care, managed people, and community mental health. *American Journal of Orthopsychiatry, 60*, 166–67.

Durham, M. L. (1995). Can HMOs manage the mental health benefit? *Health Affairs, 14*, 116–122.

Edelman, L. B. (1990). Legal environments and organizational governance: The expansion of due process in the American work-place. *American Journal of Sociology, 95*, 1401–1440.

Essock, S. M., & Goldman, H. H.. (1995). States' embrace of managed mental health care. *Health Affairs, 14*, 34–44.

Etzioni, A. (1960). Interpersonal and structural factors in the study of mental hospitals. *Psychiatry, 23*, 13–22.

Feder, J., Komisar, H. L., & Niefeld, M. (2000). Long term care in the United States: An overview. *Health Affairs, 19*, 40–55.

Fletcher, J. J. (1998). Mental health nurses: Guardians of ethics in managed care. *Journal of Psychosocial Nursing and Mental Health Services, 36*, 34–7.

Flood, A. B., & Fennell, M. L. (1995). Through the lens of organizational sociology: The role of organizational theory and research in conceptualizing and examining our health care system. *Journal of Health and Social Behavior, (Special Issue)*, 154–169.

Frank, R. G., Koyanagi, C., & McGuire, T. G. (1997). The politics and economics of mental health "parity" laws. *Health Affairs, 16*, 108–120.

Freidson, E (1984). The changing nature of professional control. *Annual Review of Sociology, 10*, 1–20.

Fried, B. J., Topping, S., Morrissey, J. P., Ellis, A. R., Stroup, S., & Blank, M. (2000). Comparing provider perceptions of access and utilization management in full risk and no risk Medicaid programs for adults with serious mental illness. *Journal of Behavioral Health Services and Research, 18*, 73–91.

Furman, R. (2003). Frameworks for understanding value discrepancies and ethical dilemmas in managed mental health for social work in the U.S. *International Social Work, 46*, 37–52.

Galambos, C. (1999). Resolving ethical conflicts in a managed health care environment. *Health and Social Work, 24*, 191–198.

Glisson, C., & Durick, M. (1988). Predictors of job satisfaction and organizational commitment in human service organizations. *Administrative Science Quarterly, 33*, 1–81.

Goffman, E. (1961). *Asylums*. New York: Anchor Books.

Goldman, H. H., Morrissey, J. P., Rosenheck, R. A., Cocozza, J., Blasinsky, M., & Randolph, F. (2002). Lessons from the evaluation of the ACCESS program: Access to community care and effective services. *Psychiatric Services, 53*, 967–9.

Gowdy, E., & Rapp, C. A. (1989). Managerial behavior: The common denominators of effective community based programs. *Psychosocial Rehabilitation Journal, 13*, 31–51.

Greenberg, G., & Rosenheck, R. (2003). Change in mental health service delivery among Blacks, Whites and Hispanics in the Department of Veterans Affairs. *Administration and Policy in Mental Health, 31*, 31–43.

Greenley, J. R. (1973). Organizational characteristics of agencies and the distribution of services to applicants. *Journal of Health and Social Behavior, 14*, 70–79.

Gregory, K. (1983). Native-view paradigms: Multiple cultures and culture conflicts in organizations. *Administrative Science Quarterly, 28*, 359–376.

Griffiths, L., Hughes, D. (1999). Talking contracts and taking care: Managers and professionals in the British National Health Service internal market. *Social Science and Medicine, 44*, 1–13.

Gruenberg, E., & Huxley, J. (1970). Mental health services can be organized to prevent chronic disability. *Community Mental Health Journal, 6*, 431–436.

Gudeman, J. E. (1988). The evolution of a public psychiatric hospital and its system of care. In M. F. Shore & J. E. Gudeman (Eds.), *Serving the chronically mentally ill in an urban setting: New directions for mental health services*, No. 39, (pp. 25–32). San Francisco: Jossey-Bass Publishers.

Guy, M. E. (1985). *Professionals in organizations: Debunking a myth*. New York: Praeger.

Hafferty, F. W., & Light, D. W. (1995). Professional dynamics and the changing nature of medical work. *Journal of Health and Social Behavior (Special Issue)*, 154–167.

Hafferty, F. W., & Wolinsky, F. D. (1991). Conflicting characterizations of professional dominance. *Current Research in Occupations and Professions, 6*, 225–249.

Hall, P. (1986). *Dimensions of work*. Beverly Hills: Sage Publications.

Halpern, S. A. (1992). Dynamics of professional control: Internal coalitions and crossprofessional boundaries. *American Journal of Sociology, 97*, 994–1021.

Hanson, K. W., & Huskamp, H. A. (2001). State health care reform: Behavioral health services under Medicaid managed care. *Psychiatric Services, 52*, 447–50.

Hasenfeld, Y. (1992). *Human services as complex organizations*. Newbury Park: Sage Publications.

Hermann, R. C, Left, S. H., Palmer, H. R., Yang, D., Teller, T., Provost, S., Jakubiak, C., & Chan, J. (2000). Quality measures for mental health care: Results from a national inventory. *Medical Care Research and Review, 57*, 136–55.

Hodgkin, D., Horgan, C. M., & Garnick, D. W. (1997). Make or buy: MHOs contracting arrangements for mental health care. *Administration and Policy in Mental Health, 24*, 359–76.

Hoff, T., & McCaffrey, D. P. (1996). Adapting, resisting, and negotiating: How physicians cope with organizational and economic change. *Work and Occupations, 23*, 165–89.

Hoge, M. A., Davidson, L., Griffith, E., Sledge, W. H., & Howenstine, R. A. (1994). Defining managed care in public-sector psychiatry. *Hospital and Community Psychiatry, 45*, 1085–1089.

Holland, T. P., Konick, A., Buffum, W., Smith, M., & Petcher, M. (1981). Institutional structure and patient outcomes. *Journal of Health and Social Behavior, 22*, 433–44.

Hughes, M. (2004). Editor's introduction. *Journal of Health and Social Behavior, 45 (Extra Issue)*, iv.

Hurley, R. E., Kaluzny, A. D. (1987). Organizational ecology and health services research: New answers for old and new Questions. *Medical Care, 44*, 235–55.

Igelhart, J. (1996). Managed care and mental health. *The New England Journal of Medicine, 334*, 131–135.

Institute of Medicine. (1997). *Managing managed care: Quality improvement in behavioral health*. Washington, DC: National Academy Press.

Karasek, R., & Theorell, T. (1990). *Healthy work: Stress, productivity, and the reconstruction of working life*. New York: Basic Books.

Kirschner, S. R., & Lachiotte, W. S. (2001). Managing managed care: Habitus, hysteresis and the end(s) of psychotherapy. *Culture and Medicine in Psychiatry, 25*, 441–456.

Lang, C. L. (1981). Good cases – bad cases: Client selection and professional prerogative in a community mental health center. *Urban Life, 10*, 289–309.

Lupton, D. (1997). Doctors on the medical profession. *Sociology of Health and Illness, 19*, 480–97.

Luhrmann, T. M. (2000). *Of two minds: The growing disorder in American psychiatry*. New York: Alfred Knoff.

McFarland, B. (2001). Assessments, interventions, and outcomes: Who cares? *Community Mental Health Journal, 37*, 93–5.

Manderscheid, R. W., Henderson, M. J., Witkin, M. J., & Atay, J. E. (2000). The U.S. mental health system of the 1990s: The challenges of managed care. *International Journal of Law and Psychiatry, 23*, 245–59.

Mechanic, D. (1968). *Medical sociology: A selective view*. New York: The Free Press.

Mechanic, D. (1974). *Politics, medicine, and social science*. New York: John Wiley & Sons.

Mechanic, D. (1986). The challenge of chronic mental illness: A retrospective and prospective view. *Hospital and Community Psychiatry, 37*, 891–896.

Mechanic, D. (1994). Establishing mental health priorities. *Milbank Quarterly*, 72, 501–514.

Mechanic, D. (1999). *Mental health and social policy: The emergence of managed care.* Boston: Allyn and Bacon.

Mechanic, D., & Rochefort, D. (1990). Deinstitutionalization: An appraisal of reform. *Annual Review of Sociology, 16*, 301–327.

Mechanic, D., Schlesinger, M., & McAlpine, D. D. (1995). Management of mental health and substance abuse services: State of the art and early results. *Milbank Quarterly, 73,* 19–55.

Meyer, J. W. (1986). Institutional and organizational rationalization in the mental health system. In W. R. Scott & B. L. Black (Eds.), *The organization of mental health services: Societal and community systems* (pp. 15–19). Beverly Hills, CA: Sage Publications.

Meyer, J. W., & Scott, W. R. (1983). *Organizational Environments: Ritual and rationality.* Beverly Hills: Sage.

Meyer, M. M. (1990). The Weberian tradition in organizational research. In C. Calhoun, M. W. Meyer, & W. R. Scott (Eds.), *Structures of power and constraint* (pp. 191–215). Cambridge: Cambridge University Press.

Meyer, M. M., & Zucker, L. G. (1988). *Permanently failing organizations.* Huntington Park: Sage Publications.

Moffic, H. S. (1997). *The ethical way: Challenges and solutions for managed behavioral health care.* San Francisco: Jossey-Bass Publications.

Morrissey, J. P. Assessing interorganizational linkages: Toward a system analysis of community support programs at the local level. In R. Tessler & H. Goldman (Eds.), *The chronically mentally ill: Assessing community support programs* (pp. 159–191). Cambridge, MA: Ballinger.

Morrissey, J. P., Calloway, M. O., Bartko, W. T., Ridgeley, M. S., Goldman, H. H., & Paulson, R. J. (1994). Local mental health authorities and service system change: Evidence from the Robert Wood Johnson Program on Chronic Mental Illness. *Milbank Quarterly, 72*, 49–80.

Morrissey, J. P., Goldman, H. H., & Klerman, L. V. (1980). *The enduring asylum.* New York: Grune and Stratton.

Morrissey, J. P., & Lindsey, M. (1987). *Organizational structure and continuity of care: A study of community mental health centers.* Albany: New York State Office of Mental Health.

Morrissey, J. P., Tausig, M., & Lindsay, M. L. (1984). *Interorganizational networks in mental health services. Assessing community programs for the chronically mentally ill.* Presented at the Workshop for Organizations and Mental Health. National Institute of Mental Health. September 17–18.

Nijsmans, M. (1991). Professional cultures and organizational morality: An ethnographic account of a therapeutic organization. *British Journal of Sociology, 42*, 1–19.

Oberlander, L. B. (1990). Work satisfaction among community-based mental health service providers: The association between work environment and work satisfaction. *Community Mental Health Journal, 26*, 517–532.

O'Driscoll, M. P., & Evans, R. (1988). Organizational factors and perceptions of climate in three psychiatric units. *Human Relations, 41*, 371–388.

Perrow, C. (1965). Hospitals, technology, structure, and goals. In J. March (Ed.), *Handbook of organizations* (pp. 910–971). Chicago: Rand McNally.

Perrucci, R., & Targ, D. (1982). *Mental patients and social networks.* Boston, MA: Auburn House Publishing Co.

Pfeffer, J., & Salanick, G. (1978). *The external control of organizations: A resource dependency perspective.* New York: Harper and Row.

Phillips, D. G. (1997). Legal and ethical issues in the era of managed care. In R. M. Alperin & D. G. Phillips (Eds.), *The impact of managed care on the practice of psychotherapy*, (pp. 171–184). New York: Brunner/Mazel Publishers.

Pollack, D., McFarland, B. H, George, R. A., & Angell, R. H. (1994). Prioritization of mental health services in Oregon. *Milbank Quarterly, 72*, 515–550.

Provan, K., & Milward, H. B. (1995). A preliminary theory of interorganizational network effectiveness: A comparative study of four community health systems. *Administrative Science Quarterly, 40*, 1–33.

Provan, K. G., & Sebastian, J. G. (1998). Networks within networks: Service link overlap, organizational cliques, and network effectiveness. *The Academy of Management Journal, 41*, 453–483.

Rochefort, D. (1989). *Handbook on mental health policy in the U.S.* New York: Greenwood Press.

Rosenheck, R. A., Lam, J., Morrissey, J. P., Calloway, M., Stolar, M., & Randolph, F. (2002). Service systems integration and outcomes for mentally ill homeless persons in the ACCESS program: Access to community care and effective services and supports. *Psychiatric Services, 53*, 958–66.

Rundall, T. G., Shortell, S. M., & Alexander, J. (2004). A theory of physician-hospital integration: Contending institutional and market logics in the health care field. *Journal of Health and Social Behavior (Extra Issue)*, 102–17.

Salzer, M. (1999). The outcomes measurement movement and mental health services research. *Mental Health Services Research, 1*, 59–63.

Scheffer, R. M., & Kirby, P. B. (2003). The occupational transformation of the mental health system. *Health Affairs, 22*, 177–88.

Scheffer, R. M., Ivey, S. L., & Garrett, A. B. (1998). Changing supply and earning patterns of the mental health workforce. *Administration and Policy in Mental Health, 26*, 85–99.

Scheid, T. L. (2003). Managed care and the rationalization of mental health services. *Journal of Health and Social Behavior, 44*, 142–61.

Scheid, T. L. (2004). *Tie a knot and hang on: Providing mental health care in a turbulent environment*. New York: Aldine de Gruyter.

Scheid, T. L., & Greenley, J. R. (1997). Evaluations of organizational effectiveness in mental health care programs. *Journal of Health and Social Behavior, 38*, 403–26.

Scheid, T. L., & Horwitz, A. V. (1999). Mental health systems and policy. In. A. V. Horwitz & T. L. Scheid (Eds.), *A handbook for the study of mental health*. Cambridge, UK: Cambridge University Press.

Scheid-Cook, T. L. (1990). Ritual conformity and organizational control: Loose-coupling or professionalization? *The Journal of Applied Behavioral Science, 26*, 183–99.

Scheid-Cook, T. L. (1991). Outpatient commitment as both social control and least restrictive alternative. *Sociological Quarterly, 32*, 433–60.

Scheid-Cook, T. L. (1992). Organizational enactments and conformity to environmental prescriptions. *Human Relations, 6*, 537–554.

Schlesinger, M. J., & Gray, B. H. (1999). Institutional change and its consequences for the delivery of mental health services. In A. V. Horwitz & T. L. Scheid (Eds.), *A handbook for the study of mental health* (pp. 427–448). Cambridge: Cambridge University Press.

Schlesinger, M. J., & Mechanic, D. (1993). Challenges for managed competition from chronic illness. *Health Affairs, 12*, 123–137.

Schulberg, H. C., & Bromet, E. (1981). Strategies for evaluating the outcome of community services for the chronically mentally ill. *American Journal of Psychiatry, 138*, 7, 930–5.

Scott, R. W. (1983). Health care organizations in the 1980's: The convergence of public and professional control systems. In J. W. Meyer & R. W. Scott (Eds.), *Organizational Environments* (pp. 99–114). Beverley Hills: Sage.

Scott, W. R. (1985). Conflicting levels of rationality: Regulators, managers, and professionals in the medical care sector. *The Journal of Health Administration Education, 3*, 113–131.

Scott, W. R. (1992). *Organizations: Rational, natural, and open systems*. 3rd Edition. Englewood Cliffs, N.J.: Prentice-Hall.

Scott, W. R., & Lammers, J. C. (1985). Trends in occupations in the medical care and mental health sectors. *Medical Care Review, 42*, 37–76.

Scott, W. R., & Meyer, J. W. (1991). The organization of societal sectors: Propositions and early evidence. In W. W. Powell & W. W. DiMaggio (Eds.), *The new institutionalism in organizational analysis* (pp. 108–140). Chicago: University of Chicago Press.

Scott, W. R., Ruef, M., Mendel, P., & Caronna, C. A. (2000). *Institutional change and organizational transformation of the health care field*. Chicago: University of Chicago Press.

Shadish, W. R., Lurigio A. J., & Lewis, D. A. (1989). After deinstitutionalism: The present and future of mental health long-term policy. *Journal of Social Issues, 45*, 1–15.

Singh, J. V., Tucker, D. J., & Meinhard, A. G. (1991). Institutional change and ecological dynamics. In W. W. Powell and D. P. DiMaggio (Eds.), *The new institutionalism in organizational analysis* (pp. 390–433). Chicago, IL: University of Chicago Press.

Soderfeldt, B., Soderfeldt, M. Muntaner, C., O'Campo, P., Warj, L., & Ohlsom, C. (1996). Psychosocial work environment in human service organizations: A conceptual analysis and development of the demand-control model. *Social Science and Medicine, 42*, 1217–1226.

Starr, P. (1982). *The social transformation of American medicine*. New York: Basic Books.

Stern, R., & Minkoff, K. (1979). Paradoxes in programming for chronic patients in a community clinic. *Hospital and Community Psychiatry, 30*, 613–617.

Strauss, A. (1975). A sociologist's perspective. In J. Howard & A. Strauss (Eds.), *Humanizing health care* (pp. 277–284). New York: John Wiley & Sons.

Strauss, A., Fagerhaugh, S., Suczek, B., & Wiener, C. (1985). *Social organization of medical work*. Chicago: University of Chicago Press.

Strauss, A., Schatzman, L., Burcher, R., Ehrlich, D., & Sabshin, M. (1964). *Psychiatric ideologies and institutions*. London: The Free Press.

Tessler, R., & Goldman, H.. (1982). *The chronically mentally ill: Assessing community support programs*. Cambridge, MA: Ballinger.

Trice, H. M. 1993. *Occupational subcultures in the workplace*. Ithaca, NY: ILR Press.

Tucker, D. J., Baum, J., & Singh, J. V. (1992). The institutional ecology of human service organizations. In Y. Hasenfeld (Ed.), *Human services as complex organizations* (pp. 47–72). Newbury Park: Sage Publications.

Vogelsang, I. (1999). Economic aspects of mental health carve outs. *The Journal of Mental Health Policy and Economics, 2*, 29–41.

Wagenfeld, M., & Robin, S. S. (1976). Boundary busting in the community mental health center. *Journal of Health and Social Behavior, 17*, 112–122.

Ware N. C., Lachiocotte, W. S., Kirschner, S. R., Cortes, D. E., & Good, B. J. (2000). Clinician experiences of managed mental health: A rereading of the threat. *Medical Anthropology Quarterly, 14*, 3–27.

Waters. M. (1989). Collegiality, bureaucratization, and professionalization: A Weberian analysis. *American Journal of Sociology, 94*, 945–72.

Weber, M. (1946). *From Max Weber: Essays in sociology*, edited and translated by H. H. Gerth & C. W. Mills. Oxford University Press.

Weick, K. E. (1977). Enactment processes in organizations. In B. M. Shaw & G. Salanick (Eds.), *New directions in organizational behavior* (pp. 267–300). Chicago: St. Clair Press.

Weiss, M., & Fitzpatrick, R. (1997). Challenges to medicine: The case of prescribing. *Sociology of Health and Illness, 19*, 297–327.

Weissman, E., Pettigrew, K., Stosky, S., & Regier, D. A. (2000). The cost of access to mental health services in managed care. *Psychiatric Services, 51*, 664–6.

Wholey, D. R., Christianson, J. B., Draper, D. A., Lesser, C. S., & Burns, L. R. 2004. Community response to national health care firms. *Journal of Health and Social Behavior, (Extra Issue)*, 118–135.

17
Recognizing a Role for Structure and Agency: Integrating Sociological Perspectives into the Study of Recovery from Severe Mental Illness

Philip T. Yanos, Edward L. Knight, and David Roe

Introduction

Background: A Gap in Emphasis

Mental health practitioners have traditionally regarded the long-term prognosis for severe mental illness[1] to be poor, with a steady deterioration of functioning over the lifespan (Harding, Zubin, & Strauss, 1987). Influenced by findings from long-term outcome studies that called this view into question (for a review, see Calabrese & Corrigan, 2005), prominent researchers of the 1980's (e.g., Cohen & Cohen, 1984; Harding et al., 1987) called for the field to adopt a more optimistic outlook with regard to potential outcome for severe mental illness. In an influential paper, Anthony (1993) discussed the concept of "recovery" from severe mental illness as an idea with important implications for mental health services and policy. Drawing heavily from descriptions of recovery in the personal accounts of mental health consumers (e.g., Deegan, 1988; Lovejoy, 1984), he stressed that achieving or being in recovery does not require that one be completely free of symptoms, but rather that one has found "a way of living a satisfying, hopeful, and contributing life even with the limitations caused by illness."[2]

---

[1] Severe mental illness is a category which is generally agreed to include individuals diagnosed with major psychiatric disorders such as schizophrenia, bipolar disorder, and major depression.

[2] Recently, there has been debate over how exactly recovery should be defined and operationalized (Corrigan & Ralph, 2005). Ralph (2005) emphasized the subjective aspects, defining recovery as a form of personal growth, including elements such as finding hope, a positive sense of self, and a sense of well-being. Liberman and Koplewicz (2005), however, maintained that a definition of recovery related to clearly delineated functional criteria is necessary; their definition requires that one demonstrate independence, involvement in work or school, and involvement in social and recreational activities to be considered "recovered." Our view is that recovery is a

A principal focus of this chapter is to use sociological conceptions of structure and agency to inform our understanding of the recovery process. Despite a long history of emphasis on biological determinism, there is growing research evidence that both social factors and individual agency can play an important role in shaping individual outcomes and recovery for people with severe mental illness. Nevertheless, biomedical conceptualizations of severe mental illness continue to pay relatively little attention to both social structure and agency in influencing recovery, emphasizing genetic and biological explanations for outcome variation in this population. For example, the most recent edition of the Diagnostic and Statistical Manual-IV-TR (APA, 2000) states that "worse outcome" for schizophrenia is most likely explained by "poorer premorbid adjustment, lower educational achievement . . . structural brain abnormalities, more prominent negative signs and symptoms, more evidence of cognitive impairment." The most socially oriented of these variables—educational achievement—is typically viewed as a result of poorer premorbid adjustment, which is considered to be genetically determined. This emphasis on factors of presumed biological origin leaves little room for either social structure or individual agency, and in fact often explicitly excludes them. This perspective was exemplified by a response to an article discussing the impact of poverty on conditions such as homelessness in this population, where the author stated that it is misguided to emphasize economic disadvantage since it is the "clinical consequences" of mental illness that lead to any associated social disability. In a lament over the psychiatric establishment's inability to take the impact of social factors seriously, Cohen (2000) charged that the field suffers from "social amnesia."

From another vantage, psychological researchers have increasingly found evidence supporting the role of personal agency, usually in the form of "coping," on outcomes for people severe mental illness (e.g., Andres, Pfammatter, Fries, & Brenner, 2003; Boschi, Adams, Bromet, Lavelle, Everett, & Galambos, 2000; Roe & Chopra, 2003; Yanos, Primavera, & Knight, 2001; Yanos, Knight, & Bremer, 2003). This research has begun to demonstrate that the types of coping strategies chosen can in fact impact important functional outcomes for people with severe mental illness. Others have demonstrated that active involvement in the process of goal-setting and the pursuit of personal goals can influence outcomes for this population (Anthony, 1978). However, what is lacking within these studies is a consideration of how and the extent to which coping, goal striving and other expressions of personal

---

multi-dimensional construct and that a diverse array of experiences may reflect recovery. For example, some individuals with severe mental illness may achieve independence and employment,and may find a sense of fulfillment in these roles, but may lack involvement in their communities. Others may not be employed but may lead rich social lives and may make contributions to their communities. Still others may achieve personal well-being through the pursuit of relatively solitary, but enriching activities (e.g., creating art). In the present chapter, we will conceptualize recovery broadly to consider these types of experiences.

agency are constrained by and respond to social structural factors to influence outcomes.

Though a relatively muted voice in mental illness research, medical sociologists have long carried the torch for the impact of social factors in this area, typically focusing either on the role of social factors as antecedents to the onset of mental illness, or on the social consequences of mental illness (Aneshensel & Phelan, 1999). Beyond a concern with labeling processes, however, an important omission in most sociological analyses has been the way in which social factors can impact on outcomes (including recovery) after mental illness has developed (Markowitz, 2005).

Structure and Agency

The tension between structure and agency in determining human action has been a longstanding concern of sociology and the social sciences more generally (Sewell, 1992). This debate concerns how and how much social structures and practices constrain individuals' choices of action (Fine, 1992); in essence, the degree to which people are "free" to determine their own destinies. Although we have not previously seen the issue of structure versus agency explicitly addressed in the context of the recovery of people with severe mental illness, we believe that a careful treatment of it is essential and long overdue in this area. We begin with a discussion of both constructs.

While clarifications of both structure and agency seldom appear and conceptualizations vary, there have been recent attempts to formally define them. Sewell (1992) defined structure as including both "mutually sustaining schemas" (i.e., social rules and procedures) "and resources" (including naturally-occurring and manufactured resources) "that empower or constrain human action." This definition therefore includes both codified and non-codified social rules and procedures, as well as social resources such as wealth and goods that can facilitate social power. In the present analysis, our consideration of structure will incorporate these aspects, as well other aspects of structure such as socially influenced rituals and roles described by Fine (1992). Fine (1992) attempted to form a "synthesis" between structural sociology and symbolic interactionism in an effort to clarify the structure-agency dichotomy. He highlighted several aspects of the social structure that can have a meaningful impact on individual choice of action, including: "obdurateness" (relating to material social resources and codified rules), "ritualization" (referring to cultural traditions and practices, including culturally-influenced "lifestyles"), "symbolization" (referring to the socially-influenced process of assigning identities to other people and things), and "identification" (referring to the socially-influenced process of identity formation).

Emirbayer and Mische (1998) recently defined agency as "the temporally constructed engagement of actors of different structural environments—the temporal-relational contexts of action—which, through the interplay of habit, imagination, and judgment, both reproduces and transforms those structures in interactive response to the problems posed by changing historical situations." As we interpret this definition, it characterizes agency as the process by which individuals consider past, present and future to make choices of action that can influence their environments. Considering the interplay between structure and agency therefore concerns the manner in which people make choices of action within the constraints imposed by social rules and social resources, and how these constraints limit the types of choices individuals can make. This conceptualization informs our analysis of agency in recovery, as we examine how individuals with severe mental illness use judgment (problem-solving in the present), and imagination (considering future choices) to respond to structural constraints such as institutionalized poverty. Following Fine (1992) and others, our conceptualization of agency includes both individual and collective forms of action.

Framework for the Current Analysis

The primary aim of this chapter is to respond to the assessed gap in emphasis by providing the field with a discussion of the impact of social structure and individual agency on recovery that is well-grounded in theory and an understanding of the issues relevant to the lives of people with severe mental illness. Although our analysis draws upon a wealth of sociological theory from both the macro (Giddens, 1984) and micro (i.e., symbolic interactionist) frameworks (Blumer, 1969; Stryker, 2002), its principal theoretical foundation is Fine's (1992) "synthetic interactionism," discussed above. Using Fine's analysis as a springboard, and his consideration of the processes of "obdurateness," "ritualization," "symbolization" and "identification," we have developed a framework for conceptualizing the relationship between social structure, agency, and recovery-related outcomes among persons with severe mental illness. A visual representation of this framework is represented in Figure 17.1. Our analysis considers important "obdurate" factors such as laws and codified social processes that constrain the lives of people with severe mental illness, ritualized forms of stigma and discrimination, as well as the ways in which internalized identity processes come to impact the lives of persons in this population. Through a review of research and other evidence, our analysis considers the manifestations of these structural characteristics that impact the lives of people with severe mental illness. Simultaneously, we examine how people with severe mental illness work within constraints to make choices of action that can help them work toward recovery and gain greater control over their lives. Specifically, we consider individual and collective forms of agency whenever appropriate. Finally, we examine both subjective (e.g., improved self-esteem) and objective (e.g., increased financial independence) outcomes related to recovery that can result from these choices of action.

A secondary aim of our analysis is to inform sociology's understanding of structure and agency in human action by way of an examination of how they

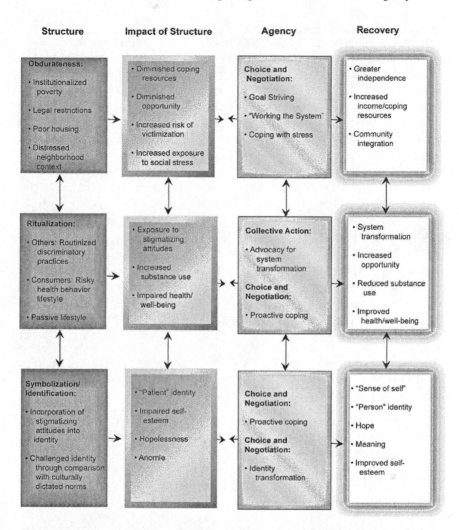

FIGURE 17.1. Graphical Representation of Model for Impact of Structure and Agency on Recovery from Severe Mental Illness.

operate in recovery from severe mental illness. This aim will be addressed by providing "real-world" examples, informed by our clinical and personal experience, throughout our analysis, that can provide substance to this essential but sometimes obscure social science concern. These illustrations will demonstrate that the process of recovery offers a unique lens into the way both structure and agency impact the human condition. People with severe mental illness are a heavily marginalized and stigmatized social group, and the manner in which many of these persons are able to negotiate and overcome constraints to achieve recovery can be highly illustrative of the deeply human struggle embedded in abstract conceptualizations of "structure vs. agency."

It should be noted that our analysis generally does not attempt an examination of the sources of variation for the choices that individuals with severe mental illness make in response to structural constraints (i.e., why one person may make a particular choice in responses to a structural constraint that can facilitate recovery, while another will not). An examination of this difficult issue would largely delve into issues regarding variables such as personality and symptom severity that were regarded to be beyond the scope of this chapter. For the reader who is interested in such issues, we recommend the first author's recent review (Yanos & Moos, In Press) and Avison and Speechley's (1987) earlier review.

Obdurateness

As it is used by Fine (1992), the term "obdurateness" refers to the "consequential reality of objects, behaviors, and reactions" (the term appears to have been originated by Blumer, [1969]). Thus, obdurateness refers to both physical limits and the very real consequences that can be imposed by the social structure that can constrain action. Legally-codified aspects of the power structure, which can marshal constraining forces such as the police and criminal justice system, are implicitly included in this category.

Obdurate Structural Constraints Affecting People with Severe Mental Illness

People with severe mental illness are forced to contend with many obdurate aspects of the social structure. The obdurateness of the physical constraints contained in involuntary hospitalization and imprisonment, which still confront substantial numbers of persons with severe mental illness, are certainly undeniable. Historically, long-term involuntary hospitalization was a major constraint placed upon people with mental illness, by design making it nearly impossible to live functional lives in the community (Grob, 1994). However, even in the current era of short-term hospitalization, no less tangible are the impact of laws and codified aspects of the disability and housing system which some have characterized as an insidious "network of control" (Chamberlain, 1978). These laws and systems can greatly limit the rights and opportunities of people with severe mental illness living in the community. Below, we discuss existing research on this issue in greater detail.

Legal Restrictions. Legal restrictions on the rights of people with mental illness are not often acknowledged. Nevertheless, a legal analysis confirmed that as of 2000, every state in the U.S. had a law which explicitly restricted the rights of persons with "mental illness" to either vote, sit on a jury, hold political office, remain married, or parent; 5 states had laws which restricted all of these rights (Hemmens, Miller, Burton, & Milner, 2002). Legal restrictions in other areas, such as in obtaining drivers' licenses, have not been discussed in the literature, but also exist.

No analysis has yet been conducted on the extent to which such laws are enforced and exert a practical influence on the lives of people with mental illness. However, our experience working within mental health service systems suggests that the impact of some of these restrictions can be quite real. For example, in New Jersey (and most likely many other states) individuals are required to report if they suffer from a "nervous or psychiatric disorder, e.g., severe depression" if they are applying for a driver's license. If a person with a mental illness responds honestly to this question, he or she must provide an affidavit from a psychiatrist attesting to his or her competency in order to receive a license. As a result of this process, individuals with mental illness may not be able to receive permission to drive, or may become discouraged enough to choose not to obtain the right to drive even if they can afford to buy a car; lacking a driver's license can severely limit social and employment opportunities in areas without comprehensive public transportation systems (i.e., most of the United States) (Duany, Plater-Zybeck, & Speck, 2001).

Institutionalized Poverty. Even more palpable than laws in the lives of people with severe mental illness are the codified restrictions imposed by the disability, health insurance and housing systems. In the United States, the decision to accept entrance into the disability system and apply for the federal entitlement programs Supplemental Security Income (SSI) or Social Security-Disability Insurance (SSDI) is one that many people with severe mental illness make with reluctance (Estroff, Patrick, Zimmer, & Lachicotte, 1997). The motivation is typically perceived necessity to insure survival following a period of acute symptomatology that may have led to the loss of a previous income source. In other instances, application for SSI or SSDI may be required to enable one to continue residing in a homeless shelter after state public assistance has expired. However, although the immediate goal of application for disability may be to provide short-term security, the implications of this process are enduring. Individuals obtaining SSI payments receive monthly incomes of between $579 and $812 per month, depending on state of residence *(http://www.ssa.gov/notices/supplemental-security-income)* (this income may be supplemented by only a $10 monthly Food Stamp voucher). These monthly stipends dictate annual incomes that are in almost all cases well below the 2005 Federal Poverty Line of $9,570 *(http://aspe.hhs.gov/poverty/05poverty.shtml)*. This places people with mental illness who have accepted entrance into the disability system in a category of poverty that is shared with many working Americans. Individuals living in poverty have been found to be at increased risk of exposure to both chronic and acute social stressors, and to have diminished financial coping resources to deal with these stressors (see McLeod & Nonnemaker, 1999, for a review); there is no reason to expect that people with mental illness will be any less impacted by poverty than others. In fact, there is considerable evidence that people with mental illness are at increased risk of exposure to criminal victimization and other forms of traumatic stress relative to the general population (Teplin, McLelland, Abram, & Weiner, 2005; Hiday, Swartz, Sawanson, Borum, & Wagner, 1999).

As significant as living in poverty is, for the subset of individuals with severe mental illness who are compelled to reside in "board-and-care" and similar custodial facilities due to the limitations of the low-income housing market (discussed further below), the reality of poverty is considerably more drastic. Although it is not known exactly how many people with mental illness reside in these types of facilities, in some states it may be as high as 30%, depending on the availability of other types of affordable housing (Mares, Young, McGuire, & Rosenheck, 2002). These facilities typically require that residents contract with the housing operator to become their "representative payee," in return for the provision of room and board (but not clothing or personal hygiene supplies); residents are then allowed to keep a monthly "personal needs allowance" (PNA) of no less than $30 (up to $85 in some states) *(http://www.ssa.gov/payee/faqrep.htm)*.

The incredible constraints that a monthly PNA of $30–85 can place on coping resources have been little appreciated in the mental health literature. Only recently did a discussion of the experience of living on such severely limited means among Canadians with severe mental illness appear (Wilton, 2004). Individuals participating in this study stated that they typically run out of money from their PNA 2–3 weeks into the month after buying essential clothes (e.g., underwear) and personal care items (e.g., soap), and have no money left over for such minor luxuries as eating at a fast food restaurant once per month. If a person with serious mental illness has a smoking habit, then there is almost a guarantee that he or she will be in debt to others by the end of the month.

Our experience working with people with severe mental illness supports the conclusion that residence in a board-and-care and related facilities, and resultant dependence on very restricted PNA's, can have a drastic effect on individuals' ability to cope with symptoms and other life stressors. Well-established treatment approaches which emphasize building up routines of meaningful activity to combat symptoms of depression, anxiety and social withdrawal (for example, the Wellness Recovery Action Plan [Copeland, 1997], and Illness Management and Recovery [Mueser, Corrigan, & Hilton, 2002]) typically emphasize activities that may necessitate the spending of at least some money (e.g., going to movies, eating out; even attending religious services, which carries the expectation of contributing to the collection basket). These are resources that board-and-care residents most often do not have the ability to participate in.

Conversely, experimental research has found that simply providing people with mental illness who live in poverty with extra monthly income can lead to significant improvements in social functioning and quality of life (Lafave, de Souza, Prince, & Atchison, 1995; Davidson, Shahar, Stayner, Chinman, Rakfeldt, & Tebes, 2004). Davidson et al. (2004) found such effects for a study of supported socialization that provided participants in the "control" condition with a $28 per month stipend; these participants ended up showing as much improvement in psychiatric symptoms and global functioning as participants in the experimental condition, which involved pairing individuals with community partners for socialization. These findings support the view that extreme poverty creates substantial constraints on functioning and that easing poverty can have a measurable impact on these outcomes.

Housing Type, Quality and Location. One's living circumstances can be one of the most important "obdurate" structural aspects of one's life. Several aspects of housing can impact people's lives: the size and condition of the housing, degree of privacy and sense of safety that is available, and the conditions of the neighborhood surrounding the housing. A continuum of compromised housing possibilities exists for people with severe mental illness, ranging from homelessness, to residence in custodial and quasi-institutional settings, to residence in independent apartments in neighborhoods with concentrated poverty. These types of housing outcomes have typically been seen as the result of mental illness symptoms, which function as a "risk factor," for example, for homelessness (e.g., Weitzman, Knickman, & Shinn, 1992). However, as many have argued, this perspective ignores the essential way in which housing choice is dictated by structural factors such as the availability of affordable or subsidized housing for low-income persons (Hopper, 1988; Schwartz, 1994).

Limitations of the housing market dictate that many people with mental illness do not have much opportunity to reside in independent, as opposed to group-based, housing. Existing research has only skimmed the surface of how housing status and location can impact the range of choices that people with mental illness have to achieve recovery. For example, most research on the impact of housing type among people with mental illness has emphasized the association between independence and housing satisfaction (Newman, 2001); however, our research suggests that housing independence may also be strongly associated with meaningful recovery-related outcomes such as sense of self-worth, independence in self-care, and involvement in leisure activities (Yanos, Barrow, & Tsemberis, 2004; Yanos, Felton, Tsemberis, & Frye, in press). This can occur for reasons that are relatively straightforward when one considers the conditions of most group-based housing: residents typically lack private rooms, almost always have to share bathrooms and kitchen facilities with others, and have to obey rules such as curfews that can restrict personal freedom. One can certainly imagine how lack of privacy and personal space can compromise one's ability to pursue productive leisure activities such as painting or playing a musical instrument, or to maintain intimate relationships with others.

Another potentially important aspect of housing is its location. Despite a large sociological literature on the impact of "neighborhood context" on social outcomes such as crime and health status (Browning & Cagney, 2002; Sampson & Raudenbush, 1999), only a small number of studies have addressed the impact of neighborhood location on outcomes among people with mental illness. The research that has been conducted to date, however, suggests that controlling for structural characteristics of neighborhoods (e.g., neighborhood social disadvantage) can statistically account for behavior that is typically seen as resulting directly from the symptoms of mental illness (e.g., violent behavior [Silver, 2000]). Similarly, neighborhood socioeconomic and political environment have been found to account for a significant proportion of the variance in degree of community integration for people with severe mental illness (Segal, Baumohl, & Moyles, 1980). These findings have important implications for how many of the behaviors of people with severe mental illness that are often seen as "symptomatic" are viewed; they suggest that looking at the larger picture of social disadvantage that many people with severe mental illness, as frequent members of an "underclass" residing in neighborhoods with concentrated poverty, are exposed to, is necessary (Draine, Salzer, Culhane, & Hadley, 2002). For example, violent behavior may partly result from criminal victimization, which people with severe mental illness have been found to be at a high risk of experiencing, especially when homeless or living in poor urban areas (Hiday et al., 1999).

Personal Agency and Obdurateness

Obdurateness is an aspect of the social structure that is particularly resistant to the impact of personal agency (Fine, 1992). Nevertheless, despite often devastating symptoms and their personal and social consequences, there is increasing evidence that people with severe mental illness use a range of strategies to negotiate the legal, financial and housing constraints discussed above. These strategies have not always been discussed in the research literature, so our discussion relies in some cases on our experiences as mental health practitioners and service recipients.

Choice and Negotiation. A strategy that many individuals with severe mental illness choose to take to cope with the institutionalized poverty created by the disability system is to work to supplement income. Work situations chosen can range from casual work for extra spending money (e.g., performing odd jobs such as mowing lawns, shoveling snow and running errands for others), to part-time transitional employment obtained through mental health programs, to "off-the-books" competitive employment, to declared part-time or full-time competitive employment. Earning income that is not tied to the disability system then gives people the flexibility to pursue additional community activities that they may not otherwise be able to afford.

Although estimates vary, it is clear that a minority of individuals with severe mental illness who live in the United States work (this is similar to other industrialized countries but stands in strong contrast with data from developing countries [Marawah & Johnson, 2004]). Why is this the case? Beyond the impact of psychiatric symptoms and the difficulties of finding work due to job discrimination, our experience and ethnographic research confirms that the act of enrolling in the disability system discourages many from working (Estroff, 1981). A study of the effect of disability receipt on participation and outcomes in vocational rehabilitation programs supported this conclusion (Drew, Drebing, Van Ormer, Losardo, Krebs, Penk, & Rosenheck, 2001), finding that individuals with severe mental illness who were receiving disability benefits worked fewer hours, had poorer job success, and had a higher dropout rate from the program than comparable individuals who were not receiving disability. The reason why enrollment in disability confers such a disadvantage is not yet known, but it appears to be the case both because of the impact of the process of applying for disability, which forces one to declare and document "permanent" inability to work, as well as what many perceive to be a penalty for reporting legal income ($1 is deducted from SSI for every $2 earned in employment).

Although little research has explored factors influencing the likelihood that a person with severe mental illness will be employed, the research that has been conducted suggests that a strong sense of self-efficacy and positive attitudes toward work make it more likely for one to select obtaining work as a goal and to take the action necessary to contend with the numerous barriers to finding employment (Mowbray & Bybee, 1995). Why and how do some individuals develop a positive attitude toward work despite mental illness and enrollment in the disability system? While the traditional psychological and psychiatric orientation would seek "premorbid" or "personality" characteristics associated with having such attitudes, an alternate perspective, consistent with symbolic interactionist and social cognitive positions, is that people exercise choice in how to define and "negotiate" the constraints that they are confronted by (Fine, 1992). In lay terms, some people see constraints imposed by the system as challenges and take efforts to "work the system." Those choosing to "work the system," however, may exercise a more flexible approach, and may see disability as more of a "safety net" that provides some degree of security, while work may be interpreted as both a means to the end of having more income, and as an opportunity for engaging in productive activity that may have its own positive effects. Individuals who do not take this position interpret the state of unemployment following enrollment in the disability system as a symbolic surrender and are not able to reconcile returning to work while remaining on disability simultaneously. They may view employment or disability as categorical states and may find it difficult to reconcile the idea that both may coexist. Of course, the degree to which people possess such attitudes and make such interpretations are likely to be influenced by structural factors associated with identity that will be discussed in more detail below.

Exercising choice in defining and negotiating situations can also apply to how persons with mental illness address housing constraints. For example, many mental health consumers who reside in board-and-care housing may qualify for independent housing but may not receive it because they have not benefited from sufficient advocacy from a professional or family member who is willing to help them negotiate the complex process of applying for subsidized independent housing. However, in our experience, there are many mental health consumers who, despite lacking a strong advocate, take on this role themselves and "beat on the doors" of the system until they are able to receive what they feel they rightly deserve (usually a decent, independent apartment in an acceptable neighborhood). Some may in fact choose the option of becoming homeless rather than accepting the rules, lack of privacy, and financial compromise associated with board-and-care living arrangements (Howie the Harp, 1990). Ironically, in many locations, the decision to become homeless may in fact speed up the process of receiving independent housing since many locations have developed streams of funding that are specifically targeted (and only available) to individuals who have been homeless. For example, in New York City, since 1990 the

"New York/New York" agreement has funded and set aside 3,000 housing units for formerly homeless persons with severe mental illness – persons with mental illness who have remained stably housed but who require better housing are not eligible for these housing units *(http://www.cucs.org/ny-nyagr.htm)*. Persons with mental illness who have become savvy to these rules may choose to "work the system" by arranging for an eviction from a group-based setting in order to spend enough time in a homeless shelter to qualify for subsidized independent housing.

Collective Agency. Another important way in which consumers are able to exercise agency in response to obdurate structural constraints is by organizing with each other for collective action. Bandura (2002) has described how perceptions of "collective efficacy," which are acquired through organized action, can be an important force for societal change. In fact, sociological theorists have emphasized that, through time and concerted effort, collective action can be a force by which larger social structures are ultimately reconfigured (Sewell, 1992; Snow, 2001).

In the last 40 years, people diagnosed with mental illness have organized throughout the United States, Canada, the United Kingdom and elsewhere in what has variously been termed the "mental health consumer movement" (Van Tosh, Ralph, & Campbell, 2000), the "ex-patients movement" (Chamberlain, 1978) and the "psychiatric survivors' movement" (Everett, 2000) (the term consumer movement will be used from this point on). This movement has consisted of a variety of efforts, including political organization and advocacy (participating in protests, public testimony, letter writing, etc.) for system change and funding initiatives, the development of mutual-aid groups for social support, the development of non-treatment oriented "consumer-run" businesses which can provide job opportunities, and the development of funded "consumer-run" treatment organizations which provide a variety of services. Since it began, the consumer movement has impacted the opportunities available to people with mental illness and the mental health service system in a variety of direct and indirect ways.

Many effects that this collective action has had on other aspects of society and the service system will be discussed in greater detail below; however, one way in which the consumer movement has clearly impacted upon the obdurate constraints discussed in the present section is by creating a greater variety of work opportunities for people with mental illness. Specifically, "consumer-run" service organizations have created opportunities for people with mental illness to obtain competitive employment as service providers or administrators in organizations in which personal quirks and temporary work disruptions that may be related to mental illness are not only tolerated but seen as potential assets. Similarly, treatment experience within the mental health system and "street smarts," which in other cases are viewed as liabilities, are in these settings often seen as an essential asset. In other ways, people with mental illness have been able to apply job skills from prior employment experience (e.g., in accounting, grantwriting, or law) within supportive work environments to facilitate the organizational survival of consumer-run services.

Ritualization

Structural Constraints Imposed by Ritualization

According to Fine (1992), ritualization refers to cultural traditions and practices that have accumulated over time and that have become "routinized." Ritualization is an important sociological notion that began with Durkheim (Collins & Makowsky, 1989) and that can be seen as related to Bourdieu's (1990) more contemporary notions of "practice" and "habitus." As discussed by Frohlich, Corin, & Potvin (2001), a useful way to make sense of these somewhat abstract concepts in the arena of health behavior is by considering the notion of "collective lifestyle." For example, in order to understand why there might be particularly high rates of smoking or drug use in a given neighborhood, it is important to understand the collective lifestyle practices that have become ingrained within the routines of that particular location, such as "hanging out" in front of liquor or corner stores, socializing and drinking alcohol from paper bags.

In applying the concept of ritualization to factors that impact the lives of people with mental illness, it may be helpful to think about both the routinized practices of individuals with mental illness themselves as well as the routinized practices of individuals who can influence the lives of people with mental illness. Both types of ritualized practice will be discussed in this chapter.

Ritualized Practices of Mental Health Consumers. It is important to consider the routinized practices of individuals with mental illness themselves and the impact that these practices can have on recovery. A body of research has documented that "unhealthy lifestyles," including lack of exercise, smoking, and high-fat dietary intake predominate among people with schizophrenia; these unhealthy practices exceed those of the general population, even when controlling for socioeconomic status, (e.g., Brown, Birtwistle, Roe, & Thompson, 1999). Time-use studies have also documented how greater reliance on passive leisure activities (such as watching television) characterizes the daily routines of people with schizophrenia (Hayes & Halford, 1996), even when compared with unemployed individuals from the general population. Other studies have documented some of the "risky" lifestyle practices associated with people with severe mental illness who abuse substances, such as panhandling and prostitution (Cohen & Henkin, 1995). Collectively, these types of practices can have considerable impact on the health and well-being of persons with mental illness, leading to high rates of health conditions such as diabetes, hypertension, heart disease, HIV/AIDS, and hepatitis (see Bartels, 2004, for a review). These health complications can, in turn, have a negative impact on the recovery process by leading to diminished well-being and ability to function independently as a result of health complications (e.g., as a result of foot swelling related to diabetes).

While some assume these behaviors to be somehow endemically linked to the symptoms of mental illness (for example, as a manifestation of negative symptoms), an alternate interpretation is that they are practices that have become a ritualized part of the "culture" of the settings that many individuals with mental illness are compelled to frequent. Ethnographic studies have documented how activities such as smoking, substance use, prostitution and pahhandling may be associated with aspects of "lifestyle" that are present in settings such as neighborhood streets, homeless shelters, hospitals, and day treatment programs where mental health consumers tend to spend time (Estroff, 1981; Weinberg & Koegel, 1995; Cohen & Henkin, 1995; Cohen, 2001). From this perspective, many risky behaviors seen among individuals living on the street or in other marginalized settings are "survival strategies" that are learned and maintained within these types of environmental contexts. Herman (1994) similarly characterized groups of mental health consumers she studied ethnographically in Canada and Michigan as "subcultures." In addition to providing support to each other, members of these subcultures instructed each other in survival strategies such as prostitution, petty theft and panhandling.

In interview-based qualitative research, behaviors such as smoking (Lawn, Pols, & Barber, 2002), and inactivity (Shaw, 1991) have also been found to be socially conditioned ways of coping with profound boredom, lack of control and need for meaning in life among people with mental illness. For example, in Shaw's study within a board and care setting, a new resident described a subgroup of other residents he called "rocks," who sat without moving for long stretches of time. While the resident was critical of the "rocks," he found himself becoming one of them over the course of the study as he was subjected to numbing routine and lack of autonomy within the boarding home: "I can feel myself getting passive. And I'm told exactly what to do ... I was hoping to find some work, but these sheltered workshops are only for the very worst. So [these people] spend time vegetating ... I find myself doing that now" (Shaw, 1991, p. 300).

Ritualized Practices of Others: Media and Employers. With regard to the ritualized practices of others, discriminatory practices which are the expression of widely-held stigmatizing views are particularly salient. For example, stigmatizing and discriminatory practices have become a strongly routinized part of the ethos of the United States media (Corrigan, Markowitz, & Watson, 2004), where the view that stories emphasizing the dangerousness of people with mental illness are newsworthy and profitable appears to have become deeply ingrained. In the U.S., stories are routinely published and broadcast which wildly exaggerate the dangerousness of people with mental illness (a 2000 *New York Daily News* front page headline titled "Get the Violent Crazies of the Street" stands out powerfully in our memory). A recent analysis of all U.S. newspaper media stories referring to mental illness during a 6 week period in 2002 (Corrigan, Watson, Gracia, Slopen, Rasinski, & Hall, 2005) found that the largest proportion of stories emphasized dangerousness and violence, while only a small minority emphasized recovery. Stories emphasizing dangerousness were also most prominently featured and were typically found on the front pages of newspapers.

The negative effect that the routinized practices of the media can have on the intensity of stigmatizing attitudes in the general public has been supported by experimental research, which found that exposure to an article emphasizing violence was related to harsher subsequent attitudes toward people with mental illness (Thornton & Wahl, 1996). We expect that the exposure to newspaper and other media portrayals emphasizing dangerousness among people with mental illness can negatively bias the attitudes of both people who can influence the opportunities of people with mental illness (e.g., landlords, family members, police officers), as well as people with mental illness themselves (this will be discussed further under identification, below).

In addition to the practices of the media, there are other areas where routinized practices can have a powerful impact on the lives of people with mental illness. For example, a dated but nevertheless impressive body of research found that landlords and employers systematically discriminate against potential applicants with mental illness (see Farina [1998] for a review). These discriminatory practices can reinforce many of the "obdurate" barriers in the areas of housing and poverty discussed previously.

Ritualized Practices of Mental Health Professionals. Less frequently studied but likely no less important are the practices of people who work within the mental health system. Many mental health consumers contend that the practices of professionals working in mental health system are dehumanizing; that mental health practitioners often insult the dignity of people with mental illness by making statements and taking actions that reduce people to diagnoses, ignoring their strengths, and discounting or minimizing their successes (Deegan [2000] has called this "spirit breaking"; many of these views are also described in Everett [2000]).

A small body of relatively dated ethnographic research has provided evidence supporting the existence of dehumanizing practices among mental health professionals. Rosenhan's (1972) classic study involving "pseudopatients" who gained entry into a psychiatric hospital after complaining of auditory hallucinations, found that the "pseudopatients," who no longer feigned any signs of symptoms of mental illness after they were admitted, were treated as non-entities by the hospital staff. In an inpatient ethnographic study, Goldin (1990), found that "institutional control" practices tended to overwhelm efforts to facilitate personal choice by way of rehabilitation interventions. In ethnographic work conducted in the 1980's with treatment providers in a community mental health system, Scheid (1992; Scheid-Cook, 1990) discussed the process by which treatment providers demonstrate "ritual conformity" to biomedical concepts such as "compliance" and the need for social control, in both their behavior and espoused ideologies. While a more recent study conducted in the early 1990's (Scheid, 1994) found that some providers adhered to an "empowerment" ideology, suggesting that professional views may be changing, many professions continued to adhere to a care-taking ideology.

Other, more recent, research supports both that stigmatizing views persist among professionals, and that the types of attitudes professionals hold can impact mental health consumer outcomes. For example, Van Dorn, Swanson, Elbogen, & Swartz (2005) found that mental health professionals in a U.S. state did not differ from the general public in their desire for social distance from people with mental illness (36% indicated they were somewhat or very likely to maintain social distance), and that 30% of professionals endorsed views that people with mental illness are somewhat or very likely to be violent. Killian, Lindenbach, Lobig, Uhle, Petsheleit, & Angermeyer's (2003) qualitative research with German mental health consumers offers some insight into the relationship between types of professional practices and consumers' sense of empowerment. This research found that the majority of mental health consumers described treatment that did not meet criteria for "empowering" practice (i.e., practices that actively involved the consumer in decision-making). Participants who described experiencing less empowering practices also tended to have a more passive attitude and a greater sense of helplessness in their lives. Though causal inferences are difficult to draw from this type of study, it provides some support for the view that treatment practices can influence consumers' own attitudes.

Agency and Ritualization

Choice and Negotiation. Personal agency can be exercised by people with mental illness to change individual ritual behaviors and practices that have been acquired over time and replace them with new practices of their own choice. From our perspective, this process can be linked to research on the importance of coping, and especially what has been recently called "proactive coping" (Yanos, 2001). Proactive coping consists of coping efforts that are undertaken as part of a regular routine in order to prevent problems or symptoms from arising. For example, a person who has previously engaged in the routine of watching television for several hours per day may choose to take on a routine of physical exercise and volunteer work. Qualitative researchers have described how people with mental illness who show significant improvement in functioning over time acquire new sets of activities that provide a sense of meaning and "sense of self" and replace previous activities and routines which did not support this process (Davidson, Sells, Sangster, & O'Connell, 2005; Davidson & Strauss, 1992).

While the impact that individual agency can have on ritualized practices may seem somewhat straightforward, these forces may act to constrain behavior insidiously, as their impact on behavior may lie outside of conscious awareness (Bourdieu, 1979). How do people with mental illness come to become aware of their routinized behavior and transform their practices and routines? Little systematic research has examined this issue; however, models of the recovery process based on personal accounts of mental health consumers identify the importance of an internal "awakening" or realization that change is possible (Ralph, 2005). This "turning point" (Strauss, Hafez, Lieberman, & Harding, 1985) is a moment or period of time when a chance event or a remark from another person can lead to a change in perspective. After this moment, an individual begins to redefine his or her interpretation of what it means to have a mental illness and begins to seek out ways to change. As a result, the person becomes determined to develop an action plan to construct alternate ways of living that can advance recovery.

Collective Agency. Collective action through the activity of the consumer movement is an important vehicle by which many people with severe mental illness work to change important practices of others that have a direct impact upon their lives (Roe & Davidson, 2005). In part, this is done by creating new practices. Notably, mental health consumers have combated the practices of mental health professionals which they consider to be degrading and dehumanizing by "speaking out" about such activities in public forums and taking other forms of organized action. Herman and Musolf (1998) found that acts of speaking out could be characterized as "rituals of resistance," learned by mental health consumers as ways to express anger and combat stigma experienced in the mental health system. Crossley and Crossley (2001) have described how the practice "speaking out" in the British mental health consumer movement represents the construction of an alternative "habitus" to the predominant practice of the mental health system. As a result, over the past 20 years the mental health system has begun to undergo a gradual transformation that explicitly has adopted some of the recommendations of the consumer movement (Jacobson, 2004). Although change continues to be slow, it is hard for whoever has worked within the mental health system over this period to deny that the spirit of the treatment system is beginning to take on greater respect for personal choice and consumer inclusion in decision-making.

Organized protest, especially when conducted through strategic alliances with mental health professionals and family groups, can also lead to changes in the practices of the media. For example, organized protests (including picketing and letter-writing campaigns) have been conducted against films and television shows that depict people with mental illness in a stigmatizing light. While these protest efforts do not necessarily lead to immediate changes in practice, they may over time lead to adjustments in practices. There is evidence, for example, that news media depictions of people with mental illness became on balance more benign between 1989 and 1999 (Wahl, 2003).

Symbolization and Identification

Structural Constraints Imposed by Symbolization and Identification

Related to ritualization are the processes of symbolization and identification. As used by Fine (1992), symbolization refers to the collective process by which meanings are attached to objects; similarly, identification refers to the collective process by which meanings are attached to people and groups of people. Thus, for example, groups of people may come to identify psychiatric medication as a "crutch" for people lacking self-reliance and willpower, and may identify persons who have been treated in psychiatric hospitals as "mental patients" who are incapable of establishing normal social roles. These processes can be partially determined by one's position in the social hierarchy (as Stryker [2002] explains- "if the social person is shaped by interaction, it is social structure that shapes the possibilities for interaction" [p. 66]); in turn, tendencies to attach certain types of meaning to people and objects become attached to social position over time through the process of "sedimentation" (Berger & Luckman, 1966).

An important way in which symbolization and identification can impact people with severe mental illness is through their impact on individual identity formation. Identity can relate to both the social categories that individuals use to describe themselves and the social categories that others use to describe them (Thoits, 1999). These categories need not be the same (for example, a person may see himself as a competent and committed professional, while others may see him as a buffoon), but there is little question that identity is impacted by others' perceptions of one's identity when one is made aware of these views. In the case of people with mental illness, strongly-held stigmatizing attitudes held by others in society can impinge upon self-concept and make it more difficult to establish distinct identities than many others in society. This is partially determined by long-standing attitudes that have been passed on through time, and the low-status position that many people with mental illness occupy in the social hierarchy,

Role Engulfment. The process by which many people with mental illness may come to lose previously held identities (e.g., as students, workers, parents, etc.) and internalize some of the negative views held by others has been characterized by some in the mental health consumer movement as "learned hopelessness" (Deegan, 1992). It has been stated that learned hopelessness is transmitted by the messages of professionals and leads to passivity and a sense of powerlessness among many people with mental illness. Thus, if one hears that he or she will never amount to anything enough times, this view may become internalized.

A variant of the process of identity loss that has been discussed by mental health researchers is "role-engulfment." The term role-engulfment was used by Lally (1989) to describe the process of "acceptance of the patient role as the primary definition of self." Lally (1989) identified three stages of the engulfment process. In the early stage, individuals deny and minimize their psychiatric problems, compare themselves with less fortunate individuals, and thus view themselves as better off than others. Important transitional events linking the early stage to the middle phase include the onset of major symptoms and repeated hospitalizations. In the middle stage persons accept that they have psychiatric problems, but minimize their potentially devastating implications and meaning by focusing primarily on normality and the commonality of mental illness. Transitional events leading to the final stage include hearing a diagnosis, applying for disability and resigning oneself to the permanence of the illness. In the final stage ("true" engulfment) an all-encompassing definition of self as "mentally ill" is established. Loss of hope, acceptance of a life with illness, and a deep sadness for the loss of a previous and future life without illness characterize this stage. As a person becomes increasingly engulfed with his or her illness, "patient"-related activities may gradually expand to a point where they have, in effect, taken over his or her life and become the main, or even only, surviving context for self evaluation (Skaff & Pearlin, 1992).

Engulfment is conceptualized as a passive, powerless, identity. Although one cross-sectional study found that greater engulfment was strongly associated with better insight (Williams & Collins, 2002), another found that it was associated with poorer social functioning (McCay & Seeman, 1998). Thus, adopting a patient identity may lead to greater acceptance of the mental illness label, but may restrict one's ability to improve social functioning. There is some support for this conclusion from a prospective study of "internalized stigma" (Ritsher & Phelan, 2004), that assessed the degree to which individuals felt alienated from others due to having mental illness. This study found that greater alienation and stereotype endorsement at baseline were significantly related to greater depressed mood at follow-up.

Link and colleagues' research on a "modified labeling perspective," though not explicitly addressing identity, has also provided support for the impact that internalizing the label of "mentally ill" can have on a person's self-concept. Link's theory posits that generally-held stereotypical attitudes about people with mental illness take on personal relevance when a person is diagnosed with mental illness; people incorporate these attitudes and direct them inward, which then impacts upon self-image in a variety of ways (Link, Cullen, Struening, Shrout, & Dohrenwend, 1989). There is some prospective evidence that the degree to which a person with mental illness agrees that "most people" have devaluing and discriminating attitudes toward the mentally ill is related to impaired self-esteem (Link, Streuning, Neese-Todd, Asmussen, & Phelan, 2001), sense of mastery (Wright, Gronfein, & Owens, 2000), and life satisfaction (Markowitz, 1998).

Role Expectations. Although the incorporation of stigmatizing views into one's identity is an obvious way in which identification can impact people with mental illness, there is another manner in which identification can adversely impact outcomes. This roughly corresponds to what Merton (1938) described as the "anomie" (or demoralization) that results when one is unable to live up to culturally-dictated norms for what one "should" be doing. So, for example, a man with mental illness who is unable to achieve expected social roles of becoming a husband, breadwinner and father, may experience a strong sense of demoralization. This sense of demoralization may be independent of or may compound any self-denigration that accompanies taking on the identity of having a mental illness. Quantitative support for the importance of this process was recently found by a study which observed that higher socioeconomic status of origin and resultantly higher job expectations were related to greater hopelessness among people with schizophrenia (Lewine, 2005). Shaw's (1991) study also provided a poignant qualitative illustration of this process, as she described the increasing hopelessness of a boarding home resident with "middle class" aspirations who was constantly confronted with what he perceived as his "failure" in his institutional surroundings. As a sad footnote to her report, Shaw indicated that the participant committed suicide some time after her research ended. According to Merton, in addition to demoralization, anomie is a major explanation for "deviant" behavior among individuals from socially disadvantaged groups, and thus may partially explain behaviors such as substance use that are frequently observed among people with severe mental illness.

Agency, Symbolization, and Identification

Choice and Negotiation. An important assertion of symbolic interactionism is that individuals can exercise choice in selecting and constructing their identities (Snow, 2001). Thus, individuals with mental illness may actively negotiate the personal and social meaning of their illness, often as part of the process of constructing alternate identities that can replace previously held "patient" identities (Roe & Ben-Yishai, 1999). There is empirical support that people with mental illness make deliberate efforts to choose and construct alternate identities, and that this process has important implications for recovery. As we discussed above, qualitative research has described how the process of constructing a new "sense of self" has been found to be an important part of the process of recovery from mental illness (Davidson & Strauss, 1992; Davidson et al., 2005). These studies describe how persons with severe mental illness who displayed significant improvement in global functioning expressed themes of the discovery of ways of recapturing a sense of purpose through daily activities.

A related longitudinal qualitative study assessing the process of recovery from schizophrenia has supported this conclusion, finding that individuals who improved in functioning over a 1 year period showed a progression from the identity of "patient" to "person" in their narratives (Roe, 2001). This study observed that finding ways to engage in regular and meaningful activities may help persons to construct an identity that is independent of being a "patient." The transition from "patienthood" to "personhood" was found to not occur in a vacuum but rather through ongoing interactions between the person and others (Roe, 2001).

Collective Agency. While the process of identity transformation described above may occur independently of involvement in the consumer movement, the process by which involvement in this movement allows individuals to transform their identities has been the specific subject of some research. Anspach (1979) discussed how the early mental health consumer movement engaged in "identity politics" by trying to redefine the social meanings attached to the status of having a psychiatric label. According to Anspach, the early consumer movement attempted to change these social meanings by highlighting the abuses of the mental health system and redefining their experiences as enlightening and potentially positive.

While less radical versions of the consumer movement have predominated since Anspach's discussion, more recent analyses suggest that their role in identity transformation persists. In a study combining ethnographic and historical document analysis methods, McCoy and Aronoff (1994) described how the growth and development of a self-help program in Michigan became a vehicle for both social activism and identity transformation for those involved in it. The organization, through rituals of self-disclosure and advocacy, encouraged members to transform identities of "mental patient" to "consumer advocate." This transformation enabled consumers to reframe the experience of mental illness so that it no longer carried a negative connotation but instead was seen as something that is "okay," or even a mark of social advantage. Experience with mental illness and mental health treatment was used by some self-help members as form of "expertise" that could then be used to advise mental health professionals and policy-makers in how to best design mental health services. In a similar interview-based qualitative study, Onken and Slaten (2000) described how people with mental illness who were involved in self-help programs described a process of "coming out of shame" and achieving "positive disability identities" as a result of their participation in consumer-run programs.

Conclusions

We have attempted to establish a connection between the concepts of structure and agency as they are discussed in the sociological literature, and the everyday reality of people diagnosed with severe mental illness. We have demonstrated that both structure and agency are indeed important factors in influencing the recovery of people with severe mental illness. Our analysis has taken an implicit symbolic interactionist position in that we have rejected determinism by assuming that individual choice does exist, and that collective agency can play a role in reconfiguring social structures. We have found that obdurateness, ritualization, identification and symbolization are important aspects of the social structure that place constraints on individual agency, but that coping, goal setting and collective action can have an important impact on people's ability to negotiate these structural constraints, and increase the likelihood of recovery.

It was also our goal to inform sociology's understanding of structure and agency in human action by way of an analysis of how these processes impact recovery from severe mental illness. As we have discussed, individuals with severe mental illness are a heavily marginalized and stigmatized social group, and the manner in which these persons are able to negotiate and overcome constraints to achieve recovery illustrates the deeply human struggle embedded in the abstract notions of "structure" and "agency." We have demonstrated that despite the highly marginalized position that individuals with severe mental illness occupy, there is clear evidence that such individuals are able to alter their own personal destinies to negotiate and influence their environments as part of the recovery process. This provides a real-world illustration of the manner in which socially marginalized persons are able to manipulate their destinies. Furthermore, we have learned that individuals with severe mental illness, through the process of collective action, have succeeded in many ways in transforming the nature of the mental health system and altering some of the structures within which they are able to operate. This, we believe, is highly illustrative of the process by which agency and structure are intertwined, as Giddens (1984) has discussed.

Notably, we have ignored an examination of how factors of presumed biological or genetic origin influence recovery, as these factors have received ample discussion elsewhere (e.g., Liberman & Kopelowicz, 2005). However, by doing so, we do not mean to minimize the impact that these factors have on the lives of people with severe mental illness, as their influence is undoubtedly considerable — we have simply tried to "balance the scales" by emphasizing the other variables that influence the possibility of recovery.

Acknowledgment. Preparation of this manuscript was supported in part by a grant from the National Institute of Mental Health (5K23MH066973–02) to Philip T. Yanos.

References

Amercian Psychiatric Association. (2000). DSM-IV-TR. Washington, DC: Author.

Andres, K., Pfammatter, M., Fries, A., & Brenner, H. D. (2003). The significance of coping as a therapeutic variable for the outcome of psychological therapy in schizophrenia. *European Psychiatry, 18*, 149–154.

Aneshensel, C. S., & Phelan, J. C. (1999). The sociology of mental health: Surveying the field. In C. S. Aneschensel & J. C. Phelan (Eds.). *Handbook of the sociology of mental health* (pp. 3–17). New York: Kluwer.

Anspach, R. (1979). From stigma to identity politics: Political activism among the physically disabled and former mental patients. *Social Science and Medicine, 13*, 765–773.

Anthony, W. A. (1978). *The principles of psychiatric rehabilitation (2nd Ed.).* Amherst, MA: Human Resource Development Press.

Anthony, W. A. (1993). Recovery from mental illness: The guiding vision of the mental health service system in the 1990's. *Psychosocial Rehabilitation Journal, 16*, 11–23.

Avison, W. R., & Speechley, K. N. (1987). The discharged psychiatric patient: A review of social, social-psychological, and psychiatric correlates of outcome. *American Journal of Psychiatry, 144*, 10–18.

Bandura, A. (2002). Social cognitive theory in a cultural context. *Applied Psychology: An International Review, 51*, 269–290.

Bartels, S. J. (2004). Caring for the whole person: Integrated health care for older adults with severe mental illness and medical comorbidity. *Journal of the American Geriatric Society, 52*, 249–257.

Berger, P. L., & Luckman, T. (1966). *The social construction of reality: A treatise in the sociology of knowledge.* New York: Doubleday.

Blumer, H. (1969). *Symbolic interactionism: Perspective and method.* Englewood Cliffs, NJ: Prentice Hall.

Boschi, S., Adams, R. E., Bromet, E. J., Lavelle, J. E., Everett, E., & Galambos, N. (2000). Coping with psychotic symptoms in the early phases of schizophrenia. *American Journal of Orthopsychiatry, 70*, 242–252.

Bourdieu, P. (1990). *The logic of practice.* Stanford, CA: Stanford University Press.

Brown, S., Birtwistle, J., Roe, L., & Thompson, C. (1999). The unhealthy lifestyle of people with schizophrenia. *Psychological Medicine, 29*, 697–701.

Browning, C. R., & Cagney, K. A. (2002). Neighborhood structural disadvantage, collective efficacy, and self-rated physical health in an urban setting. *Journal of Health and Social Behavior, 43*, 383–399.

Calabrese, J. D., & Corrigan, P. W. (2005). Beyond dementia praecox: Findings from long-term follow-up studies of schizophrenia. In R. O. Ralp & P. W. Corrigan (Eds.), *Recovery in mental illness: Broadening our understanding of wellness* (pp. 63–84).Washington, DC: American Psychological Association.

Chamberlain, J. (1978). *On our own: Patient-controlled alternatives to the mental health system*. New York: Hawthorn Books.

Cohen, A. (2001). The search for meaning: Eventfulness in the lives of homeless mentally ill persons in the Skid Row district of Los Angeles. *Culture, Medicine and Psychiatry, 25*, 277–296.

Cohen, C. I. (2000). Overcoming social amnesia: The role for a social perspective in psychiatric research and practice. *Psychiatric Services, 51*, 72–78.

Cohen, E., & Henkin, I.. (1995). Substance abuse and lifestyle among an urban schizophrenic population: Some observations. *Psychiatry, 58*, 113–120.

Cohen, P., & Cohen, J. (1984). The clinician's illusion. *Archives of General Psychiatry, 41*, 1178–1182.

Collins, R., & Makowsky, M. (1989). *The discovery of society (4th Ed.)*. New York: Random House.

Copeland, M. E. (1997). *Wellness recovery action plan*. Brattleboro, VT: Peach Press.

Corrigan, P. W., Markowitz, F. E., & Watson, A. C. (2004). Structural levels of mental illness stigma and discrimination. *Schizophrenia Bulletin, 30*, 481–491.

Corrigan, P. W., & Ralph, R. O. (2005). Introduction: Recovery as consumer vision and research paradigm. In R. O. Ralph & P. W. Corrigan (Eds.), *Recovery in mental illness: Broadening our understanding of wellness* (pp.3–17).Washington, DC: American Psychological Association.

Corrigan, P. W., Watson, A. C., Gracia, G., Slopen, N., Rasinski, K., & Hall, L. L. (2005). Newspaper stories as measures of structural stigma. *Psychiatric Services, 56*, 551–556.

Crossley, M. L., & Crossley, N. (2001). "Patient" voices, social movements and the habitus; how psychiatric survivors "speak out." *Social Science and Medicine, 52*, 1477–1489.

Davidson, L., Sells, D., Sangster, S., & O'Connell, M. (2005). Qualitative studies of recovery: What can we learn from the person? In R. O. Ralph & P. W. Corrigan (Eds.), *Recovery in mental illness: Broadening our understanding of wellness* (pp.147–170).Washington, DC: American Psychological Association.

Davidson, L., Shahar, G., Stayner, D. A., Chinman, M. J., Rakfeldt, J., & Tebes, J. K. (2004). Supported socialization for people with psychiatric disabilities: Lessons from a randomized controlled trial. *Journal of Community Psychology, 32*, 453–477.

Davidson L., & Strauss J. S. (1992). Sense of self in recovery from severe mental illness. *British Journal of Medical Psychology, 65*, 131–145.

Deegan, P. E. (1988). Recovery: The lived experience of rehabilitation. *Psychosocial Rehabilitation Journal, 11*, 11–19.

Deegan, P. E. (1992). The Independent Living Movement and people with psychiatric disabilities: Taking back control over our own lives. *Psychosocial Rehabilitation Journal, 15*, 3–19.

Deegan, P. E. (2000). Spirit breaking: When the helping professions hurt. *Humanistic Psychologist, 28*, 194–209.

Draine, J., Salzer, M. S., Culhane, D. P., & Hadley, T. R. (2002). Role of social disadvantage in crime, joblessness, and homelessness among persons with serious mental illness. *Psychiatric Services, 53,* 565–573.

Drew, D., Drebing, C. E., Van Ormer, A., Losardo, M., Krebs, C., Penk, W., & Rosenheck, R. A. (2001). Effects of disability compensation on participation in outcomes of vocational rehabilitation. *Psychiatric Services, 52,* 1479–1484.

Duany, A., Plater-Zyberk, E., & Speck, J. (2001). *Suburban nation: The rise of sprawl and the decline of the American dream.* New York: North Point Press.

Emirbayer, M., & Mische, A. (1998). What is agency? *American Journal of Sociology, 103,* 962–1023.

Estroff, S. E. (1981). *Making it crazy: An ethnography of psychiatric clients in an American community.* Berkeley: University of California Press.

Estroff, S. E., Patrick, D. L., Zimmer, C. R., & Lachicotte, W. S. (1997). Pathways to disability income among persons with severe, persistent psychiatric disorders. *Milbank Quarterly, 75,* 495–532.

Everett, B. (2000). *A fragile revolution: Consumers and psychiatric survivors confront the power of the mental health system.* Waterloo, Ontario, Canada: Wilfrid Laurier University Press.

Farina, A. (1998). Stigma. In K. T. Mueser & N. Tarrier (Eds.). *Handbook of social functioning in schizophrenia* (pp. 247–279). Needham Heights, MA: Allyn & Bacon.

Fine, G. A. (1992). Agency, structure, and comparative contexts: Toward a synthetic interactionism. *Symbolic Interaction, 15,* 87–107.

Frohlich, K. L., Corin, E., & Potvin, L. (2001). A theoretical proposal for the relationship between context and disease. *Sociology of Health and Illness, 23,* 776–797.

Giddens, A. (1984). *Constitution of society.* Oxford, UK: Polity Press.

Goldin, C. S. (1990). Stigma, biomedical efficacy, and institutional control. *Social Science and Medicine, 30,* 895–900.

Grob, G. N. (1994). *The mad among us: A history of the care of America's mentally ill.* New York: Free Press.

Harding, C. M., Zubin, J., & Strauss, J. S. (1987). Chronicity in schizophrenia: Fact, partial fact, or artifact? *Hospital and Community Psychiatry, 38,* 477–485.

Hayes, R. L., & Halford, W. K. (1996). Time use of unemployed and employed single male schizophrenia subjects. *Schizophrenia Bulletin, 22,* 659–669.

Hemmens, C., Miller, M., Burton, V. S., & Milner, S. (2002). The consequences of official labels: An examination of the rights lost by the mentally ill and mentally incompetent ten years later. *Community Mental Health Journal, 38,* 129–140.

Herman, N. J. (1994). "Mixed nutters," "looney tuners," and "daffy ducks:" A research update. In E. Rubington & M. Weinberg (Eds.), *Deviance: The interactionist perspective* (pp. 254–265). New York: McMillan.

Herman, N. J., & Musolf, G. R. (1998). Resistance among ex-psychiatric patients: Expressive and instrumental rituals. *Journal of Contemporary Ethnography, 26,* 426–449.

Hiday, V. A., Swartz, M. S., Swanson, J. W., Borum, R., & Wagner, H. R. (1999). Criminal victimization of persons with severe mental illness. *Psychiatric Services, 50,* 62–68.

Hopper, K. (1988). More than passing strange: Homelessness and mental illness in New York City. *American Ethnologist, 15,* 155–167.

Howie the Harp. (1990). Independent living with support services: The goal and future for mental health consumers. *Psychosocial Rehabilitation Journal, 13,* 85–89.

Jacobson, N. (2004). *In recovery: The making of mental health policy.* Amsterdam, Netherlands: VU University Press.

Killian, R., Lindenbach, I., Lobig, U., Uhle, M., Petsheleit, A., & Angemeyer, M. C. (2003). Indicators of empowerment and disempowerment in the subjective evaluation of the psychiatric treatment process by persons with severe and persistent mental illness: A qualitative and quantitative analysis. *Social Science and Medicine, 57*, 1127–1142.

Lafave, H. G., de Souza, H. R., Prince, P. N., Atchison, K. et al (1995). Partnerships for people with serious mental illness who live below the poverty line. *Psychiatric Services, 46*, 1071–1073.

Lally, S. J. (1989). "Does being in here mean there is something wrong with me?" *Schizophrenia Bulletin, 15*, 253–265.

Lawn, S. J., Pols, R. G., & Barber, J. G. (2002). Smoking and quitting: A qualitative study with community-living psychiatric clients. *Social Science & Medicine, 54*, 93–104.

Lewine, R. R. J. (2005). Social class of origin, lost potential, and hopelessness in schizophrenia. *Schizophrenia Research, 76*, 329–335.

Liberman, R. P., & Kopelowicz, A. (2005). Recovery from schizophrenia: A criterion-based definition. In R. O. Ralph & P. W. Corrigan (JEds.), *Recovery in mental illness: Broadening our understanding of wellness* (pp. 101–129).Washington, DC: American Psychological Association.

Link, B. G., Cullen, F., Struening, E. L., Shrout, P. E., & Dohrenwend, B. P. (1989). A modified labeling theory approach to mental disorders: An empirical assessment. *American Sociological Review, 54*, 400–423.

Link, B. G., Struening, E. L., Neese-Todd, S., Asmussen, S., & Phelan, J. C. (2001). The consequences of stigma for the self-esteem of people with mental illness. *Psychiatric Services, 52*, 1621–1626.

Lovejoy, M. (1984). Recovery from schizophrenia: A personal odyssey. *Hospital and Community Psychiatry, 35*, 809–812.

Marawah, S., & Johnson, S. (2004). Schizophrenia and employment: A review. *Social Psychiatry and Psychiatric Epidemiology, 39*, 337–349.

Mares, A. S., Young, A. S., McGuire, J. F., & Rosenheck, R. A. (2002). Residential environment and quality of life among seriously mentally ill residents of board and care homes. *Community Mental Health Journal, 38*, 447–458.

Markowitz, F. E. (1998). The effects of stigma on the psychological well-being andlife satisfaction of persons with mental illness. *Journal of Health and Social Behavior, 39*, 335–347.

Markowitz, F. (2005). Sociological models of recovery. In R. O. Ralph & P. W. Corrigan (Eds.), *Recovery in mental illness: Broadening our understanding of wellness* (pp. 85–99).Washington, DC: American Psychological Association.

McCay, E. A., & Seeman, M. V. (1998). A scale to measure the impact of a schizophrenic illness on an individual's self-concept. *Archives of Psychiatric Nursing, 12*, 41–49.

McCoy, M. L., & Aronoff, M. (1994). Against all odds: Revitalization of local self-help alternatives by longterm mental health consumers. *Qualitative Sociology, 17*, 365–381.

McLeod, J. D., & Nonnemaker, J. N. (1999). Social stratification and inequality. In C. S. Aneshensel & J. C. Phelan (Eds). *Handbook of sociology of mental health* (pp. 321–344).New York: Kluwer.

Merton, R. K. (1938). Social structure and anomie. *American Journal of Sociology*, 672–682.

Mowbray, C. T., & Bybee, D. (1995). Predictors of work status and future work orientation in people with a psychiatric disability. *Psychiatric Rehabilitation Journal, 19*, 17–28.

Mueser, K. T., Corrigan, P. W., Hilton, D. (2002) Illness management and recovery for severe mental illness: A review of the research. *Psychiatric Services, 53*, 1272–1284.

Newman, S. J. (2001). Housing attributes and serious mental illness: Implications for research and practice. *Psychiatric Services, 52*, 1309–1317.

Onken, S. J., & Slaten, E. (2000). Disability identity formation and affirmation: The experiences of persons with severe mental illness. *Sociological Practice: A Journal of Clinical and Applied Sociology, 2*, 99–111.

Ralph, R. O. (2005). Verbal definitions and visual models of recovery: Focus on the recovery model. In R. O. Ralph & P. W. Corrigan (Eds.), *Recovery in mental illness: Broadening our understanding of wellness* (pp. 131–145).Washington, DC: American Psychological Association.

Ritsher, J. B., & Phelan, J. C. (2004). Internalized stigma predicts erosion of morale among psychiatric outpatients. *Psychiatry Research, 129*, 257–265.

Roe, D. (2001). Progressing from patienthood to personhood across the multidimensional outcomes in schizophrenia and related disorders. *Journal of Nervous and Mental Disease, 189*, 691–699.

Roe, D., & Ben-Yishai, A. (1999). Exploring the relationship between the person and the disorder among individuals hospitalized for psychosis. *Psychiatry, 62*, 370–380.

Roe, D., & Chopra, M. (2003). Beyond coping with mental Illness: Towards personal growth. *American Journal of Orthopsychiatry, 73*, 334–344.

Roe, D., & Davidson, L. (2005). Self and narrative in schizophrenia: Time to author a new story. *Journal of Medical Humanities, 31*, 89–94.

Rosenhan, D. L. (1973). On being sane in insane places. *Science, 179*, 250–258.

Sampson, R. J., & Raudenbush, S. W. (1999). Systematic social observation of public spaces: A new look at disorder in urban neighborhoods. *American Journal of Sociology, 105*, 603–651.

Scheid, T. L. (1994). An explication of treatment ideology among mental health providers. *Sociology of Health and Illness, 16*, 668–693.

Scheid-Cook, T. L. (1990). Ritual conformity and organizational control: Loose coupling or professionalization? *Journal of Applied Behavioral Science, 26*, 183–199.

Scheid-Cook, T. L. (1992). Organizational enactments and conformity to environmental prescriptions. *Human Relations, 45*, 537–554.

Schwartz, S. (1994). The fallacy of the ecological fallacy: the potential misuse of a concept and the consequences. *American Journal of Public Health, 84*, 819–24.

Segal, S. P., Baumohl, J., & Moyles, E. W. (1980). Neighborhood types and community reaction to the mentally ill: A paradox of intensity. *Journal of Health and Social Behavior, 21*, 345–359.

Sewell, W. H. (1992). A theory of structure: Duality, agency, and transformation. *American Journal of Sociology, 98*, 1–29.

Shaw, L. L. (1991). Stigma and the moral careers of ex-mental patients living in board and care. *Journal of Contemporary Ethnography, 20*, 285–305.

Silver, E. (2000). Race, neighborhood disadvantage, and violence among persons with mental disorders: The importance of contextual measurement. *Law and Human Behavior, 24*, 449–456.

Skaff, M. M., & Pearlin, L. I. (1992). Caregiving: Role engulfment and the loss of self. *Gerontologist, 32*, 656–664.

Snow, D. A. (2001). Extending and broadening Blumer's conceptualization of symbolic interactionism. *Symbolic Interaction, 24*, 367–377.

Strauss J. S., Hafez H., Lieberman P., & Harding C. M. (1985). The course of psychiatric disorders III: Longitudinal principles. *British Journal of Psychiatry, 155*, 128–132.

Stryker, S. (2002). *Symbolic interactionism: A social structural version.* Caldwell, NJ: Blackburn Press.

Teplin, L. A., McClelland, G., Abram, K. M., & Weiner, D. A. (2005). Crime victimization in adults with severe mental illness: Comparison with the National Crime Victimization Survey. *Archives of General Psychiatry, 62,* 911–921.

Thoits, P. A. (1999). Self, identity, stress, and mental health. In C. S. Aneshensel & J. C. Phelan (Eds.), *Handbook of sociology of mental health* (pp. 321–344).New York: Kluwer.

Thornton, J. A., & Wahl, O. F. (1996). Impact of a newspaper article on attitudes toward mental illness. *Journal of Community Psychology, 24,* 17–25.

Van Dorn, R. A., Swanson, J. W., Elbogen, E. B., & Swartz, M. S. (2005). A comparison of stigmatizing attitudes toward persons with schizophrenia in four stakeholder groups: Perceived likelihood of violence and desire for social distance. *Psychiatry, 68,* 152–163.

Van Tosh, L., Ralph, R. O., & Campbell, J. (2000). The rise of consumerism. *Psychiatric Rehabilitation Skills, 4,* 383–409.

Wahl, O. F. (2003). News media portrayal of mental illness: Implications for public policy. *American Behavioral Scientist, 46,* 1594–1600.

Weinberg, D., & Koegel, P. (1995). Impediments to recovery in treatment programs for dually diagnosed homeless adults: An ethnographic analysis. *Contemporary Drug Problems, 22,* 193–236.

Weitzman, B. C., Knickman, J. R., & Shinn, M. (1992). Predictors of shelter use among low-income families: Psychiatric history, substance abuse, and victimization. *American Journal of Public Health, 82,* 1547–1550.

Williams, C. C., & Collins, A. (2002). Factors associated with insight among outpatients with serious mental illness. *Psychiatric Services, 53,* 96–98.

Wilton, R. (2004). Putting policy into practice? Poverty and people with serious mental illness. *Social Science and Medicine, 58,* 25–39.

Wright, E. R., Gronfein, W. P., & Owens, T. J. (2000). Deinstitutionalization, social rejection, and the self-esteem of former mental patients. *Journal of Health and Social Behavior, 41,* 68–90.

Yanos, P. T. (2001). Proactive coping among persons diagnosed with severe mental illness: An exploratory study. *The Journal of Nervous and Mental Disease, 189,* 121–123.

Yanos, P. T., Barrow, S., & Tsemberis, S. (2004). Community integration in the early phase of housing among homeless persons diagnosed with severe mental illness: Successes and challenges. *Community Mental Health Journal, 40,* 133–150.

Yanos, P. T., Felton, B., Tsemberis, S., & Frye, V. A. (In press). Exploring the role of housing type, neighborhood characteristics, and lifestyle factors in the community integration of formerly homeless persons diagnosed with mental illness. *Journal of Mental Health.*

Yanos, P. T., Knight, E., L., & Bremer, L. (2003). A new measure of coping with symptoms for use with persons diagnosed with severe mental illness. *Psychiatric Rehabilitation Journal, 27,* 168–176.

Yanos, P. T., & Moos, R. H. (In Press). Determinants of functioning and well-being among individuals with schizophrenia: An integrated model. *Clinical Psychology Review.*

Yanos, P. T., Primavera, L.H., & Knight, E. L. (2001). Consumer-run service participation, recovery in social functioning, and the mediating role of psychological factors. *Psychiatric Services, 52,* 493–500.

Part V
Mental Health, Social Mirror:
Looking Forward, Reflecting Back

18
Mainstream Sociology and Sociological Specialties: Toward Understanding the Gap and Its Consequences

Sheldon Stryker

Noting that mental health held an important place in the writings of classical sociologists but that contemporary sociologists often fail to see mental health research as more than marginal with respect to the "real" work of the discipline, the editors of this volume hope to bridge the gap (or breach), in part current and in part potential, between mainstream sociology and the specialty area of the sociology of mental health. That is, the editors, through the volume's contents, seek to convince sociologists in general that mental health research has contributed and can continue to contribute to the resolution of theoretical debates in mainstream sociology. At least implicitly, the editors also seek to encourage mental health researchers to continue to draw on mainstream theories and concepts in their work, if they already do so, or to begin drawing on such theories and concepts if they are not already doing so. Too, and again at least implicitly, the argument the editors present is that unless the gap between the mainstream and the specialty is bridged in important degree, the marginalization and devaluation of mental health research by the mainstream will continue and the specialty will produce work that does not contribute as much as it can to the further development of general sociological theory. In short, the argument is that the consequences for both mainstream and specialty will be beneficial to neither mainstream nor specialty.

I fully agree with that argument. The particular consequences motivating this volume are, of course and quite properly, the impoverishment of the sociology of mental health through failure to take advantage of the theoretical leverage available in sociological theory in advancing knowledge in the specialized field, and the impoverishment of mainstream sociology through a reciprocal failure to see the larger theoretical relevance of knowledge gained through the work of specialists in the sociology of mental health.

These consequences are of primary import, and the work reported in the volume itself makes the editors' case, to which I do not have any thing in particular to add. However, there are other consequences worthy of note and concern, consequences that do not speak directly to the quality of the intellectual product of mainstream sociology and the specialty area of mental health, but nevertheless are important to consider because they have longer-term and indirect implications for and impact on the sociological enterprise. What I think these consequences are and why I think they are important is the burden of the discussion that follows.

In part, my views on such matters stem from being a participant in an early attempt to deal with a gap—I am not at all certain that the word "breach" fits the earlier case at the time of my participation although it does apply in more recent times—of mainstream sociology and another specialty area, namely, the sociology and social psychology of the family. I will focus my attention on this case, since through it I became an interested and concerned witness to what I saw as the unhealthy consequences of this particular separation; and I have given it most thought. In part, however, it also stems from the fact that, having been a participant in the earlier case, I perceived still other gaps (or, and in at least some of the cases, breaches) between mainstream sociology and specialty areas, specifically criminology and applied sociology, and I will give some attention to each of these as well.

In brief, then, the problematic relations of mainstream sociology and the sociology of mental health to which this volume is addressed have been and are found in the relations of mainstream sociology and other sociological specializations. My hope is that what little insight I may offer into what is at stake for both the mainstream and specialty areas in such gaps or breaches will reinforce the editors' aims with respect to bridging the gap between mainstream sociology and the sociology of mental health. I also hope that what is said will have some impact on thinking about similar breaches that exist elsewhere in the discipline.

The Starting Point: An Interlude in the History of the Sociology and the Social Psychology of the Family, Circa 1960s

As indicated, my interest in the problems generating this volume began not with a concern with the sociology of mental health but rather with the sociology and social psychology of the family. As a student and later colleague of Clifford Kirkpatrick (see Kirkpatrick, 1947; 1955), a leading presence in the sociology of the family from the 1930's through the 1960's, my earliest work (see, e.g., Stryker, 1956; 1959) identified me as a family sociologist, and I pursued that earliest work drawing on assumptions and conceptions stemming from George Herbert Mead (1934) and symbolic interactionist thought more generally.

A major concern of family sociologists (not all, but some of the most active) at the time—post-World War II and through the next decade into the 1960's—was that their specialty field was not being given the respect it warranted because it was seen by many sociologists as a-theoretical, despite contrary evidence in the work of sociologists like Willard Waller (1938), William Goode (1956, 1963) and Reuben

Hill (1949), and as more devoted to describing rather than explaining these behaviors by reference to the theoretical ideas of classical sociology.[1] It was also seen as more motivated by doing good rather than doing good science,[2] and as more attuned to the "trivialities" of interpersonal interaction and relationships—dating and "courtship" processes, spousal relations, and parent-child interaction—as, for example, in Locke (1951), Burgess and Cottrell (1939) and Burgess and Wallin (1953), rather than the "obviously" more socially significant central issues of classical sociology.

Led by Hill, family sociologists who believed that at least some of these perceptions had some validity and that family research could benefit from being grounded in general sociological theory sought to stimulate awareness among family sociologists of the relevance of extant general sociological theory for their specialized interests. Clearly, too, these sociologists saw their effort as potentially serving to counter the devaluation and marginalization of their specialized field by sociologists outside the family area. That effort led in the mid-1960's to the organization of a 1966 plenary session of the ASA Section on the Family that invited participants to develop papers arguing the potential contributions to research on the family of the theoretical frames underlying their own work. I presented a paper that concerned itself with the usefulness of a symbolic interactionist frame for family research in which I initially outlined what came to be known as Identity Theory (Stryker, 1968, 1980). Although I had already given up thinking of myself as a family sociologist, preferring an identity as a social psychologist (Stryker, 2002), I nevertheless remained sensitive to developments in family sociology, especially some I believed to be either products or by-products of the gap with which Reuben Hill and other family sociologists had been concerned earlier.

What developments did I observe (or more interpretatively, did I believe I was observing)? Most important from the standpoint of the health of the family subfield of sociology, I witnessed an erosion of the field's long-standing concerns with family interactive processes and relationships: such concerns appeared to me to have either dissipated or at least to an important degree gone underground.[3] One bit of evidence in this regard: in my earlier years in sociology, articles by sociologists about family interpersonal processes and relations often appeared in the general sociological journals. More recently, such articles are rare if not non-existent. I am certain that sociological writings about family matters are considerable, perhaps larger than they have ever been. But much of these writings have been devoted to the social history of the family, to the comparative description and institutional analysis of family forms across extant societies and within American society (a turn evidenced by the plethora of family texts with these

---

[1] I tended to share these views, I am somewhat chagrined to say (see Stryker, 2001).
[2] I choose not to "name names" here. However, I am struck by how many of the sociologists characterized as having followed pioneering paths in their work on families in Steinmetz and Peterson (2002) develop their self-portraits in ways that fit this charge, a fact that cannot surprise given the important role of clergy in early American sociology.
[3] This discussion incorporates ideas and language appearing in Stryker (2001).

emphases in recent decades), and to demographic inquiry.[4] Further, much of the work by contemporary sociologists involving family interaction and relationships data of one sort or another is subsidiary to other concerns, undertaken largely if not entirely because the data are germane to a diverse set of other interests—for example, in feminist theory, gender relations, equity issues more generally, delinquency, sexuality—rather than in family interaction and relationships *per se*.

Accompanying this shift away from interest in and work on family interaction and relationships, it seems to me that there has been a gradual but steady decline in the course offerings that focus on the family in departments of sociology. Certainly, departments continue to offer an undergraduate family course, but graduate programs emphasizing that specialization (e.g., like that led by Reuben Hill at the University of Minnesota, involving a specialized family research training program, from the late 1950's into the 1980's, now absorbed into a Life Course program) have essentially disappeared.[5]

Relatedly, and unsurprisingly, as sociology has retreated from an interest in such topics as processes of entering and leaving marital or marriage-like relationships as well as other interactional processes related to the family, a variety of disciplines ranging across a wide spectrum but including psychology, family studies, communication, home economics, human development, health and recreation, what used to be called home economics, and social work have been absorbing these interests. Thus, for example, "love" as well as other intimate relationships (e.g. Harvey & Weber, 2002; Honeycutt & Cantril, 2001) have become important topics among psychologists as have marital conflict and conflict resolution processes (e.g. Gottman, Katz, & Hooven, 2002; Hetherington & Kelley, 2003).[6] Noting this migration of family interactional and relationship topics to non-sociology departments should not be read as saying or even implying that the intellectual work on these topics by non-sociologists is necessarily inferior to that done by sociologists. Nevertheless, that work typically will be different: it will be even less guided by and relevant to classical sociological theory than there-to-fore. For me, and I presume for most other sociologists, this counts as an important loss for the discipline. However, and whatever may be the case on the quality score or for that matter on the degree to which a sociological sensibility is present in work on intimate

---

[4] A quick check of the 2005 Guide to Graduate Departments of Sociology published by the ASA indicates that in seventeen departments commonly cited as top-ranked, five have no full-time faculty who list family as a major scholarly interest. Of the 30 faculty who do cite family as a major interest, 22 are clearly demographers, and none is unambiguously focused on family relationships and interaction processes.

[5] As far as I know, Hill's program was unique in continuity of federal training grant support and broad focus on family interaction and relationships, although Murray Strauss headed a NIMH-supported program on family violence at the University of New Hampshire. Other graduate programs focusing on family existed at Case Western University, the University of Florida, Brigham Young University, and I presume other universities as well without looking systematically for them. Only four of the 17 departments of footnote 4 include family in their listings of special programs in the family; of these departments, one has no full-time faculty who include family as being within their scholarly interests.

[6] Intimate relations, of course, have long been a central concern of clinical psychology.

relationships and interactions, it is still other implications of this shift that will be drawn shortly that makes its discussion here pertinent.

Beyond Family Sociology, but More of the Same

As I watched the sociology of the family turn away in important degree from what had been earlier focal concerns in family interactions and relationships, I came to think that I was at the same time witnessing comparable developments in other sociological specialty areas. The cases of criminology and delinquency seem to repeat a particularly important feature of the case of family sociology: fewer departments of sociology are teaching courses in criminology and delinquency, even at the undergraduate level, and fewer have graduate programs featuring these topics. Rather, these topics and both undergraduate and graduate curricula dealing with them have transferred to schools or departments of criminal justice or their equivalents. To be sure, in some degree these topics are incorporated into the newer specialty area of the sociology of law, but the very emergence of that specialty makes a relevant point: my sense is that the willingness of departments of sociology to accept without strong demurrer the transfer of crime and delinquency to criminal justice reflects the attitudes of mainstream sociology with respect to these topics, which attitudes are not unlike those relating the mainstream to work on family interactional processes and relationships. Again, this is a matter to which the discussion will return shortly.

Mainstream responses to the emergence of yet another sociological specialty, namely, sociological practice, seem to me to have much in common with those relating mainstream to family interaction and to crime and delinquency work. Sometime in the early 1970's, I participated in a conference devoted to (whatever its formal title may have been) the deprecation of the social policy and practice efforts of some sociologists and what might be done to overcome that response from mainstream sociology (see Demerath, Larsen, & Schuessler, 1975, reporting papers and discussion from that conference). Despite the American Sociological Association's strong efforts to find a meaningful place for sociological policy and practice activities and research over recent years, it is my sense that little real change has taken place in mainstream attitudes in the thirty-some years since that conference.[7] Recalling that a major (if sometimes only implicit) theme of the conference was the negative impact on the status of those working on public policy

---

[7] Social psychology is yet another sociological specialty seen by many sociologists as being outside the mainstream, "nicely" (if that word is appropriate here) illustrated by Alvin Gouldner's (1970) vitriolic attack on Erving Goffman, whose work Gouldner believed focused on the trivial in contrast to work in the tradition of Marx and Weber. That mainstream response to social psychology, although importantly mitigated, still exists today and may well enter into contemporary mainstream attitudes toward the sociology of mental health, given that mental health issues are often approached from a social psychological perspective. However, this case is different in many ways from the other sociological specialties discussed above and will not be pursued further here.

and in sociological practice of attitudes held by a self-appointed sociological elite, I would guess that something of the same sort operates today, old attitudes dying hard, in particular with respect to sociological practice. (It is, after all, sociological practice, rather than the "high level" public policy issues that draw the attention of the government commissions and the more "intellectual" media, that come closest to work on everyday issues of family interaction and relationships, crime and delinquency, and sociological practice.)

What is it about the specialty areas of the work on family interaction and relationships, criminology and delinquency, and sociological practice that makes them germane to this volume's concern with the breach that separates mainstream sociology from the sociology of mental health? Posing this question immediately provides the answers to it: each finds much of its motivation not in sociological theory per se but in everyday problems of human beings and the attempts of these human beings to resolve those everyday problems. And each finds some part of its motivation in social policy issues that emerge around alternative ways of meeting these problems through collective (essentially governmental) action. Clearly, neither problem-focused interests nor sociological practice represents "pure" sociology, either in the sense propounded by Donald Black (1995) or by mainstream theorists in general. It reveals no secret of sociology as a discipline—nor does it take any deep sociological inquiry—to note that American sociology for almost a century has taken pains to dissociate itself from ameliorative interests of social work and from the religious personnel who constituted a major segment of its 19th and early 20th century professorial cadre. In that process, mainstream sociology found its major motivation largely in the logic and societal level concerns of its European forebears. While there can be no quarrel with such logic and concerns as at the very core of the sociological enterprise (and I certainly have no quarrel with these), a number of unfortunate consequences have followed for both mainstream and specialties, albeit not necessarily.

The first of these consequences is the devaluation and marginalization of sociological specialties that have their substantive focus on problems of everyday life of ordinary people, that is, on the topic on which this volume focuses attention, mental health, as well as on the other sociological topics that have been noted above.[8] A set of auxiliary consequences follow such devaluation and marginalization. One is the pattern of present and probably future migration of substantive fields—the present day exemplar is the movement of criminology and

---

[8] There is one area of sociology that has largely if not entirely escaped the attitudes toward work dealing with everyday problems of human beings I have attributed to mainsteam sociology, and that is the area of race, especially racial segregation. Why that may be so is an interesting question. Likely strongly implicated in the answer is the fact that race and ethnicity are closely related to issues of social class and social power, and class and power analyses are the heart of the foundational contributions of Marx and Weber to the discipline. An important element in this part of the answer lies in that which is noted in the text, above, as well as in the just prior sentence: sociological theory itself provides more than sufficient motivation for work in race relations. Sociology's historic affinity for the underdog may enter the answer as well. Some might include an element of political correctness in the answer; I do not believe that is the case.

delinquency to criminal justice programs—from sociology to other disciplines. Another is that major talent among recruits to sociology becomes diverted from the devalued and marginalized fields as the recognition of such denigration sinks in and as they receive career advice from mainstream representatives. Still further, a perhaps inevitable accompaniment of devaluation and marginalization of specialty fields is some degree of alienation of those who remain within sociology itself, a phenomenon that seems to have occurred among those with interests in family interaction and relationships and in criminology who seek to pursue those interests in the context of non-sociological organizations.

But it is perhaps a longer term consequence of the gap between mainstream sociology and specializations like mental health, crime and delinquency, and sociological practice that may be even more fateful for sociology as a discipline and a profession. It is this possibility that initially caught my own attention as I witnessed the noted changes in work on the family among sociologists. In the main, students entering sociology as undergraduate majors (and it is such students who ultimately enter graduate programs of sociology and eventually are employed as sociologists) do so because some everyday social problem has attracted them to the field: interactional problems centering around their own social relationships; difficulties in family relationships that eventuate in parental divorce or in their own "divorce" from parents or siblings; mental health problems of friends or family members, their own delinquent behavior or such behavior that has in one way or another impacted them; the aspiration to do something to mitigate such problems. As far as I can see, we recruit few persons directly through interest in abstract theoretical issues; and they become interested in theoretical problems only as they begin to see the relevance of these for illuminating their own initiating concerns. If this is so, to denigrate those initiating concerns, directly or by implication, may rob sociology of a significant portion of its potential recruits.

That is my fear, and it is a fear that generalizes beyond work on the family and other "marginal" specialties within sociology to work on mental health: denial of the relevance and potential import for sociological theory of any of its specialty areas by mainstream sociology closes off important processes by which students become interested in sociology and truncates the potential contributions to sociological theory of those who maintain their interests in one or another non-mainstream sociological specialty. Doing whatever can be done to make more visible the reciprocal links between mainstream and specialty areas serves the interests of both specialty and mainstream, and benefits sociology as a whole.

Can anything be done? In my more optimistic moments, I think some possibilities exist to stem the tide. Volumes such as the present one can certainly help, though its impact is likely to be more limited to one side of its intended audience than one might hope. But suppose the underlying rationale and principle involved in the volume—increasing the specialty's awareness of the utility of sociological theory to enrich its research and increasing sociological theorists' awareness of the potential of specialty contributions to "growing" sociological theory—were extended to sessions at ASA meetings as well as regional association meetings jointly sponsored and organized by theory and specialty sections. Suppose, too, that editors of specialty journals (including theory) could be persuaded to sponsor special issues of their journals pursuing the same tack? Might we reasonably expect such communication across the specialty-mainstream gap (as well as other efforts generated by more imaginative minds than mine) to contribute strongly to making each side of that gap aware of the intellectual and professional costs of their separation?

I hope so.

References

Burgess, E. W., & Cottrell, L. S. (1939). *Predicting success or failure in marriage.* New York: Prentice-Hall.

Burgess, E. W., & Wallin, P (1953). *Engagement and marriage.* Philadelphia: J. B. Lippincott.

Demerath, N. J., Larsen, O., & Schuessler, K. (Eds.) (1975). *Social policy and sociology.* NY: Academic Press.

Goode, W. J. (1963). *World revolution and family patterns.* New York: Free Press of Glencoe.

Goode, W. J. (1956). *After divorce.* Glencoe IL. Free Press.

Gottman, J. (1994). *Why marriages succeed or fail.* New York: Simon & Schuster.

Gottman, J. M., Katz, L. F., & Hooven, C. (1997). *Meta emotion: How families communicate emotionally.* Mahwah, NJ: L. Erlbaum Associates.

Gouldner, A. W. (1970). *The coming crisis of western sociology.* New York: Basic Books.

Harvey, J., & Weber, A. L. (2002). *Odyssey of the heart: Close relationships in the 21st century.* Mahwah, NJ.: L. Erlbaum Associates.

Hetherington, E. M., & Kelly, J. (2002). *For better or worse: Divorce reconsidered.* New York: Norton.

Honeycutt, J. M., & Cantril, J. G (2001). *Cognition, communicatiaon, and romantic relationships.* Mahwah, NJ: L. Erlbaum Associates.

Hill, R. (1947). Families under stress: *Adjustments to the crises of war separation and return.* Westport, CT: Greenwich Press.

Kirkpatrick, C. (1955*). The family as process and institution.* New York: The Ronald Press.

Kirkpatrick, C. (1947). *What science says about happiness in marriage.* Minneapolis, MN: Burgess Publishing Company.

Locke, H. J. (1951). *Predicting adjustment in marriage.* New York: Henry Holt.

Mead, G. H. (1934). *Mind, self, and society.* Chicago: University of Chicago Press.

Steinmetz, S. K., & Peterson, G. W. (Eds.) 2002. *Pioneering paths in the study of families: The lives and careers of family scholars.* New York: Haworth Press.

Stryker, S. (2002) Soft ideas and hard methods: Family sociologist or social psychologist? In S. Steinmetz & G. W. Peterson (Eds.), *Pioneering paths in the study of families: The lives and careers of family scholars* (pp. 623–633). New York: Haworth Press.

Stryker, S. (1980). *Symbolic interaction: A social structural version.* Menlo Park, CA: Benjamin/Cummings Publishing Company.

Stryker, S. (1968). Identity salience and role performance. *Journal of Marriage and the Family, 30,* 558–564.

Stryker, S. (1959). Symbolic interaction as an approach to family research. *Marriage and Family Living, 31,* 111–119.

Stryker, S. (1956). Relationships of married offspring and their parents: A test of Mead's theory. *American Journal of Sociology, 62,* 308–319.

Waller, W. (1938). *The family.* New York: Dryden.

Index

Page number with 'f' and 't' denotes footnotes and tables

Printed in the USA